PEDIATRIC EMERGENCY MEDICINE

MEDICINE

SECRETS

PEDIATRIC EMERGENCY MEDICINE

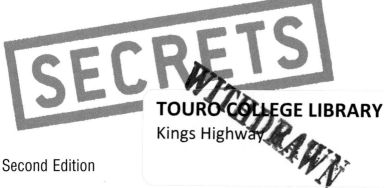

Second Edition

Steven M. Selbst, MD, FAAP, FACEP
Professor of Pediatrics
Vice Chair for Education
Director of Pediatric Residency Program
Jefferson Medical College
Thomas Jefferson University
Philadelphia, Pennsylvania
Attending Physician
Division of Emergency Medicine
A.I. duPont Hospital for Children
Wilmington, Delaware

Kate M. Cronan, MD, FAAP
Associate Professor of Pediatrics
Jefferson Medical College
Thomas Jefferson University
Philadelphia, Pennsylvania
Chief, Division of Emergency Medicine
A.I. duPont Hospital for Children
Wilmington, Delaware

MOSBY

ELSEVIER

MOSBY
ELSEVIER

1600 John F. Kennedy Blvd.
Ste 1800
Philadelphia, PA 19103-2899

PEDIATRIC EMERGENCY MEDICINE SECRETS,   ISBN: 978-1-4160-2990-8
SECOND EDITION

Copyright © 2008, 2001 by Mosby, Inc., an affiliate of Elsevier Inc.

NOTICE

Knowledge and best practice in this field are constantly changing. As new research and experience broaden our knowledge, changes in practice, treatment and drug therapy may become necessary or appropriate. Readers are advised to check the most current information provided (i) on procedures featured or (ii) by the manufacturer of each product to be administered, to verify the recommended dose or formula, the method and duration of administration, and contraindications. It is the responsibility of the practitioner, relying on their own experience and knowledge of the patient, to make diagnoses, to determine dosages and the best treatment for each individual patient, and to take all appropriate safety precautions. To the fullest extent of the law, neither the Publisher nor the Authors assume any liability for any injury and/or damage to persons or property arising out of or related to any use of the material contained in this book.

The Publisher

Library of Congress Cataloging-in-Publication Data
Pediatric emergency medicine secrets / [edited by] Steven M. Selbst,
Kate Cronan.—2nd ed.
    p. ; cm.
Includes bibliographical references and index.
ISBN 978-1-4160-2990-8
1. Pediatric emergencies—Examinations, questions, etc. 2. Pediatric intensive care—Examinations, questions, etc. I. Selbst, Steven M. II. Cronan, Kate, 1953-
[DNLM: 1. Emergencies—Examination Questions. 2. Child.
3. Emergency Medicine—Examination Questions. 4. Infant. WS 18.2 P36995 2008]

RJ370.P4533 2008
618.92'0025076—dc22

                    2007044368

Acquisitions Editor: James Merritt
Developmental Editors: Stan Ward and Nicole DiCicco
Senior Project Manager: Mary Stermel

Working together to grow
libraries in developing countries

www.elsevier.com | www.bookaid.org | www.sabre.org

ELSEVIER   BOOK AID International   Sabre Foundation

Printed in China

Last digit is the print number: 9 8 7 6 5 4 3 2 1

4/30/09

DEDICATION

To my wife, Andrea
To my children, Lonn and Eric
To my parents, Sidney and Sophie Selbst
And (yes) to my in-laws, Marvin and Dolores Kushner

S. Selbst

To my husband, Steve
To my children, Olivia, Colin, and Natalie
To my parents, Charles and Joan Cronan
To my siblings, Bob, Beth, Jamie, Brian, and Maggie

K. Cronan

CONTENTS

III. MEDICAL EMERGENCIES

IV. SURGICAL EMERGENCIES

V. TRAUMA

VI. ENVIRONMENTAL EMERGENCIES

VII. SPECIAL TOPICS

CONTRIBUTORS

Sarah W. Alander, MD
Clinical Assistant Professor, University of Missouri, Columbia, Missouri; Attending Physician, Emergency Department, St. John's Mercy Medical Center, St. Louis, Missouri

Evaline A. Alessandrini, MD, MSCE
Associate Professor of Pediatrics and Emergency Medicine, University of Pennsylvania School of Medicine; Attending Physician, Division of Emergency Medicine, The Children's Hospital of Philadelphia, Philadelphia, Pennsylvania

Elizabeth R. Alpern, MD, MSCE
Assistant Professor, Department of Pediatrics, University of Pennsylvania; Attending Physician, Division of Emergency Medicine, The Children's Hospital of Philadelphia, Philadelphia, Pennsylvania

Linda D. Arnold, MD
Assistant Professor of Pediatrics, Yale University School of Medicine; Attending Physician, Section of Emergency Medicine, Yale-New Haven Children's Hospital, New Haven, Connecticut

Magdy W. Attia, MD
Professor of Pediatrics, Jefferson Medical College, Thomas Jefferson University, Philadelphia, Pennsylvania; Fellowship Director, Attending Physician, Division of Emergency Medicine, A.I. duPont Hospital for Children, Wilmington, Delaware

Jeffrey R. Avner, MD
Professor of Clinical Pediatrics, Albert Einstein College of Medicine; Director, Children's Emergency Service, Children's Hospital at Montefiore, Bronx, New York

M. Douglas Baker, MD
Professor of Pediatrics, Sarah M. and Charles E. Seay Chair in Pediatrics, University of Texas Southwestern Medical Center; Director of Medical Services, Director of Pediatric Emergency Medicine, Children's Medical Center of Dallas, Dallas, Texas

Robert G. Bolte, MD
Professor, Department of Pediatrics, University of Utah School of Medicine; Attending Physician, Division of Pediatric Emergency Medicine, Primary Children's Medical Center, Salt Lake City, Utah

Linda L. Brown, MD
Assistant Professor of Pediatrics, Yale University School of Medicine; Attending Physician, Section of Emergency Medicine, Yale-New Haven Children's Hospital, New Haven, Connecticut

James M. Callahan, MD, FAAP, FACEP
Associate Professor of Clinical Pediatrics, Department of Pediatrics, University of Pennsylvania School of Medicine; Attending Physician, Director of Medical Education, Division of Emergency Medicine, The Children's Hospital of Philadelphia, Philadelphia, Pennsylvania

Brian Coleman, MD, MS
Assistant Professor, Department of Pediatrics; Attending Physician, Division of Pediatric Emergency Medicine, University of Washington, Children's Hospital & Regional Medical Center, Seattle, Washington

Howard M. Corneli, MD
Professor of Pediatrics, University of Utah College of Medicine; Attending Physician, Emergency Department, Primary Children's Medical Center, Salt Lake City, Utah

Julie-Ann Crewalk, MD
Pediatric Infectious Disease Fellow, Children's National Medical Center, George Washington University, Washington, District of Columbia; Formerly a Pediatric Resident at A.I. duPont Hospital for Children, Thomas Jefferson University, Wilmington, Delaware

Kate M. Cronan, MD, FAAP
Associate Professor of Pediatrics, Jefferson Medical College, Thomas Jefferson University, Philadelphia, Pennsylvania; Chief, Division of Emergency Medicine, A.I. duPont Hospital for Children, Wilmington, Delaware

Lauren P. Daly, MD
Associate Professor of Pediatrics, Jefferson Medical College, Thomas Jefferson University, Philadelphia, Pennsylvania; Attending Physician, Division of Emergency Medicine, A.I. duPont Hospital for Children, Wilmington, Delaware

Reza J. Daugherty, MD
Assistant Professor of Pediatrics, Jefferson Medical College, Thomas Jefferson University, Philadelphia, Pennsylvania; Attending Physician, Emergency Department, Division of Emergency Medicine, A.I. duPont Hospital for Children, Wilmington, Deleware

Andrew D. DePiero, MD
Assistant Professor of Pediatrics, Jefferson Medical College, Thomas Jefferson University, Philadelphia, Pennsylvania; Attending Physician, Division of Emergency Medicine, A.I. duPont Hospital for Children, Wilmington, Delaware

Maria Carmen G. Diaz, MD
Assistant Professor of Pediatrics, Jefferson Medical College, Thomas Jefferson University, Philadelphia, Pennsylvania; Attending Physician, Division of Emergency Medicine, A.I. duPont Hospital for Children, Wilmington, Delaware

Nanette C. Dudley, MD
Associate Professor of Pediatrics, University of Utah School of Medicine; Attending Physician, Primary Children's Medical Center, Salt Lake City, Utah

Susan Duffy, MD
Associate Professor, Departments of Emergency Medicine and Pediatrics, Brown Medical School; Attending Physician, Emergency Department, Hasbro Children's Hospital, Providence, Rhode Island

Yamini Durani, MD
Attending Physician, Department of Pediatrics, Division of Emergency Medicine, A.I. duPont Hospital for Children, Jefferson Medical College, Wilmington, Delaware

Stephen C. Eppes, MD
Associate Professor of Pediatrics, Department of Pediatrics, Jefferson Medical College, Thomas Jefferson University, Philadelphia, Pennsylvania; Division of Pediatric Infectious Diseases, A.I. duPont Hospital for Children, Wilmington, Delaware

Deirdre Fearon, MD, MA
Assistant Professor, Departments of Emergency Medicine and Pediatrics, Brown Medical School; Attending Physician, Emergency Department, Hasbro Children's Hospital, Providence, Rhode Island

Joel A. Fein, MD, MPH
Associate Professor of Pediatrics and Emergency Medicine, University of Pennsylvania School of Medicine; Attending Physician, Division of Emergency Medicine, The Children's Hospital of Philadelphia, Philadelphia, Pennsylvania

Fred A. Fow, MD
Attending Physician, Division of General Pediatrics, A.I. duPont Hospital for Children, Wilmington, Delaware

Marla J. Friedman, DO
Attending Physician, Division of Emergency Medicine, Miami Children's Hospital, Miami, Florida

Susan Fuchs, MD
Professor of Pediatrics, Feinberg School of Medicine, Northwestern University; Attending Physician, Division of Pediatric Emergency Medicine, Children's Memorial Hospital, Chicago, Illinois

Ronald A. Furnival, MD
Department of Pediatric Emergency Medicine, Banner Desert Children's Hospital, Mesa, Arizona

Javier A. Gonzalez del Rey, MD, MEd
Professor of Pediatrics, Director, Pediatric Residency Programs, Associate Director, Division of Emergency Medicine, Cincinnati Children's Hospital Medical Center, Cincinnati, Ohio

Marc H. Gorelick, MD, MSCE
Professor of Pediatrics, Medical College of Wisconsin; Chief, Pediatric Emergency Medicine, Children's Hospital of Wisconsin, Milwaukee, Wisconsin

Hazel Guinto-Ocampo, MD
Assistant Professor of Pediatrics, Jefferson Medical College, Thomas Jefferson University, Philadelphia, Pennsylvania; Attending Physician, Division of Emergency Medicine, A.I. duPont Hospital for Children, Wilmington, Delaware

Fred M. Henretig, MD
Professor of Pediatrics and Emergency Medicine, University of Pennsylvania School of Medicine; Senior Toxicologist, Associate Medical Director, Poison Control Center; Director, Section of Clinical Toxicology, Attending Physician, Division of Emergency Medicine, The Children's Hospital of Philadelphia, Philadelphia, Pennsylvania

Dee Hodge III, MD
Associate Professor of Pediatrics, Washington University School of Medicine; Associate Director, Clinical Affairs Emergency Services, St. Louis Children's Hospital, St. Louis, Missouri

Allen L. Hsiao, MD
Assistant Professor, Department of Pediatrics, Section of Pediatric Emergency Medicine, Yale University School of Medicine; Chief Medical Information Officer, Yale-New Haven Hospital, New Haven, Connecticut

James Edward Hulse III, MD
Associate Professor, Department of Pediatrics, University of Missouri School of Medicine; Director, Electrophysiology Cardiology Services, Children's Mercy Hospital, Kansas City, Missouri

Paul Ishimine, MD
Assistant Clinical Professor of Medicine and Pediatrics, University of California at San Diego School of Medicine; Director, Pediatric Emergency Medicine, Children's Hospital and Health Center, San Diego, California

Mark D. Joffe, MD
Associate Professor of Pediatrics, University of Pennsylvania School of Medicine; Director, Community Pediatric Medicine, Department of Pediatrics; Attending Physician, Division of Emergency Medicine, The Children's Hospital of Philadelphia, Philadelphia, Pennsylvania

Laurie H. Johnson, MD
Assistant Professor of Clinical Pediatrics, University of Cincinnati College of Medicine; Attending Physician, Division of Emergency Medicine, Cincinnati Children's Hospital Medical Center, Cincinnati, Ohio

Howard Kadish, MD
Associate Professor of Pediatrics, University of Utah School of Medicine; Attending Physician, Emergency Department, Primary Children's Medical Center, Salt Lake City, Utah

Jenny Kim, MD
Attending Physician, Division of Hematology/Oncology, Children's Specialists of San Diego; Co-Director, Comprehensive Sickle Cell Center, Children's Hospital and Health Center, San Diego, California

Brent R. King, MD, FACEP, FAAEM, FAAP
Professor of Emergency Medicine and Pediatrics, Chairman, Department of Emergency Medicine, The University of Texas Medical School at Houston; Chief, Emergency Medicine, Memorial Hermann Hospital, Houston, Texas

Christopher King, MD, FACEP
Associate Professor of Emergency Medicine and Pediatrics, University of Pittsburgh School of Medicine; Attending Physician, Emergency Medicine, UPMC-Presbyterian Hospital, Children's Hospital of Pittsburgh, Pittsburgh, Pennsylvania

Joel D. Klein, MD, FAAP
Professor of Pediatrics, Jefferson Medical College, Thomas Jefferson University, Philadelphia, Pennsylvania; Chief, Division of Pediatric Infectious Diseases, A.I. duPont Hospital for Children, Wilmington, Delaware

Jane F. Knapp, MD
Vice Chair of Pediatrics, Director of Graduate Medical Education, University of Missouri-Kansas City School of Medicine; Attending Physician, Division of Emergency Medicine, Children's Mercy Hospital, Kansas City, Missouri

Susanne Kost, MD
Clinical Assistant Professor, Department of Pediatrics, Jefferson Medical College, Thomas Jefferson University, Philadelphia, Pennsylvania; Attending Physician, Division of Emergency Medicine, A.I. duPont Hospital for Children, Wilmington, Delaware

Jane M. Lavelle, MD
Associate Professor, Department of Pediatrics, University of Pennsylvania; Associate Director, Pediatric Emergency Medicine, The Children's Hospital of Philadelphia, Philadelphia, Pennsylvania

John M. Loiselle, MD
Associate Professor of Pediatrics, Jefferson Medical College, Thomas Jefferson University, Philadelphia, Pennsylvania; Assistant Director, Emergency Services, A.I. duPont Hospital for Children, Wilmington, Delaware

Stephen Ludwig, MD
Professor and Associate Chair, Department of Pediatrics, University of Pennsylvania School of Medicine; Associate Physician-in-Chief for Education, Attending Physician, Division of Emergency Medicine, The Children's Hospital of Philadelphia, Philadelphia, Pennsylvania

Constance M. McAneney, MD, MS
Associate Professor of Pediatrics, University of Cincinnati College of Medicine; Associate Director, Division of Emergency Medicine, Cincinnati Children's Hospital Medical Center, Cincinnati, Ohio

Douglas M. Nadel, MD
Private Practice, Otorhinolaryngology, Doylestown, Pennsylvania

Frances M. Nadel, MD, MSCE
Assistant Professor, Department of Pediatrics, University of Pennsylvania School of Medicine; Attending Physician, Division of Emergency Medicine, The Children's Hospital of Philadelphia, Philadelphia, Pennsylvania

Douglas S. Nelson, MD, FAAP, FACEP
Professor of Pediatrics, University of Utah School of Medicine; Medical Director, Emergency Department, Primary Children's Medical Center, Salt Lake City, Utah

Robert P. Olympia, MD
Assistant Professor, Department of Emergency Medicine and Pediatrics, Penn State College of Medicine; Attending Physician, Emergency Department, Penn State Milton S. Hershey Medical Center, Hershey, Pennsylvania

Kevin C. Osterhoudt, MD, MSCE
Associate Professor of Pediatrics, University of Pennsylvania School of Medicine; Attending Physician, Division of Emergency Medicine, The Children's Hospital of Philadelphia; Medical Director, Poison Control Center, Philadelphia, Pennsylvania

Kathy Palmer, MD
Clinical Instructor of Pediatrics, Jefferson Medical College, Thomas Jefferson University, Philadelphia, Pennsylvania; Attending Physician, Urgent Care Center, Division of Emergency Medicine, A.I. duPont Hospital for Children, Wilmington, Delaware

Ronald I. Paul, MD
Professor of Pediatrics, University of Louisville; Chief, Pediatric Emergency Medicine, Kosair Children's Hospital, Louisville, Kentucky

Melanie Pitone, MD, FAAP
Clinical Instructor, Jefferson Medical College, Thomas Jefferson University, Philadelphia, Pennsylvania; Attending Physician, Division of Emergency Medicine, A.I. duPont Hospital for Children, Wilmington, Delaware

Jill C. Posner, MD
Assistant Professor of Pediatrics, University of Pennsylvania School of Medicine; Attending Physician, Division of Emergency Medicine, The Children's Hospital of Philadelphia, Philadelphia, Pennsylvania

Amanda Pratt, MD
Clinical Assistant Professor, Department of Pediatrics, UMDNJ, Robert Wood Johnson Medical School; Attending Physician, Emergency Department, Robert Wood Johnson University Hospital, New Brunswick, New Jersey

Linda Quan, MD
Professor, Department of Pediatrics, University of Washington School of Medicine; Attending Physician, Division of Emergency Medicine, Children's Hospital & Regional Medical Center, Seattle, Washington

Eileen C. Quintana, MD, MPH
Assistant Professor of Pediatrics and Emergency Medicine, Drexel University College of Medicine; Attending Physician, Emergency Department, St. Christopher's Hospital for Children, Philadelphia, Pennsylvania

Richard M. Ruddy, MD
Professor of Clinical Pediatrics, University of Cincinnati College of Medicine; Director, Division of Emergency Medicine, Cincinnati Children's Hospital Medical Center, Cincinnati, Ohio

Robert E. Sapien, MD, FAAP
Associate Professor of Emergency Medicine and Pediatrics, University of New Mexico Health Sciences Center; Chief, Division of Pediatric Emergency Medicine, Albuquerque, New Mexicio

Richard J. Scarfone, MD, FAAP
Associate Professor of Pediatrics, University of Pennsylvania School of Medicine; Attending Physician, Division of Emergency Medicine, The Children's Hospital of Philadelphia, Philadelphia, Pennsylvania

Robert D. Schremmer, MD
Associate Professor, Department of Pediatrics, University of Missouri-Kansas City School of Medicine; Attending Physician, Division of Emergency Medical Services, Children's Mercy Hospitals and Clinics, Kansas City, Missouri

Jeff E. Schunk, MD
Professor, Department of Pediatrics, University of Utah School of Medicine; Chief, Division of Pediatric Emergency Medicine, Primary Children's Medical Center, Salt Lake City, Utah

Sara A. Schutzman, MD
Assistant Professor, Department of Pediatrics, Harvard Medical School; Assistant in Medicine, Division of Emergency Medicine, Children's Hospital, Boston, Massachusetts

Sandra H. Schwab, MD
Pediatric Emergency Medicine Fellow, Division of Emergency Medicine, The Children's Hospital of Philadelphia, Philadelphia, Pennsylvania

Philip V. Scribano, DO, MSCE
Associate Professor, Clinical Pediatrics, The Ohio State University College of Medicine; Medical Director, Center for Child and Family Advocacy, Columbus, Ohio

Steven M. Selbst, MD, FAAP, FACEP
Professor of Pediatrics, Vice Chair for Education, Director of Pediatric Residency Program, Jefferson Medical College, Thomas Jefferson University, Philadelphia, Pennsylvania; Attending Physician, Division of Emergency Medicine, A.I. duPont Hospital for Children, Wilmington, Delaware

Kathy N. Shaw, MD, MSCE
Professor of Pediatrics, The Nicholas Crognale Endowed Chair in Pediatric Emergency Medicine, University of Pennsylvania School of Medicine; Chief, Division of Emergency Medicine, The Children's Hospital of Philadelphia, Philadelphia, Pennsylvania

Joan E. Shook, MD, MBA
Professor of Pediatrics, Baylor College of Medicine; Head, Section of Emergency Medicine, Texas Children's Hospital, Houston, Texas

Sabina B. Singh, MD, FAAP
Assistant Professor of Pediatrics and Emergency Medicine, Drexel University School of Medicine; Attending Physician, Division of Pediatric Emergency Medicine, St. Christopher's Hospital for Children, Philadelphia, Pennsylvania

Martha W. Stevens, MD, MSCE
Assistant Professor, Department of Pediatrics, Medical College of Wisconsin; Attending Physician, Emergency Department and Trauma Center, Children's Hospital of Wisconsin, Milwaukee, Wisconsin

Bambi Taylor, MD
Attending Physician, Department of Pediatrics, Division of Emergency Medicine, A.I. duPont Hospital for Children, Wilmington, Delaware

Nicholas Tsarouhas, MD
Associate Professor of Clinical Pediatrics, University of Pennsylvania School of Medicine; Medical Director, Emergency Transport Services, Attending Physician, Division of Emergency Medicine, The Children's Hospital of Philadelphia, Philadelphia, Pennsylvania

James F. Wiley II, MD, MPH
Professor of Pediatrics and Emergency Medicine/Traumatology, University of Connecticut School of Medicine; Medical Toxicology Consultant, Connecticut Regional Poison Control Center; Attending Physician, Emergency Department, Connecticut Children's Medical Center, Hartford, Connecticut

Kristine G. Williams, MD, MPH
Instructor in Pediatrics, Washington University School of Medicine; Pediatric Emergency Medicine Physician, St. Louis Children's Hospital, St. Louis, Missouri

George A. Woodward, MD, MBA
Professor of Pediatrics, Adjunct Professor of Medicine, University of Washington School of Medicine; Chief, Division of Emergency Medicine, Children's Hospital & Regional Medical Center, Seattle, Washington

Martha S. Wright, MD
Associate Professor of Pediatrics, Case Western Reserve University School of Medicine; Director, Pediatric Residency Education, Attending Physician, Pediatric Emergency Medicine, Rainbow Babies and Children's Hospital, Cleveland, Ohio

Theoklis Zaoutis, MD, MSCE
Assistant Professor of Pediatrics and Epidemiology, University of Pennsylvania School of Medicine; Director, Antimicrobial Stewardship Program, Division of Infectious Diseases, The Children's Hospital of Philadelphia, Philadelphia, Pennsylvania

ACKNOWLEDGMENTS

We are very much indebted to our spouses and our children for their patience and understanding as we worked on our second edition. We especially thank Elaine Fusco for her dedication to keeping track of our manuscripts and our contributors during the evolving process. We also acknowledge Debbie Campbell, Joan Culver, and Cindy Chuidian for their invaluable assistance. We very much appreciate the help of Linda Belfus, James Merritt, Stan Ward, Nicole DiCiccio, and Richard Hund at Elsevier. In addition, we thank our colleagues and friends who authored excellent chapters and contributed very important questions while caring for children in emergency departments all over the country.

We acknowledge the very talented members of our Division of Emergency Medicine at the A.I. duPont Hospital for Children (Magdy Attia, MD; Jonathan Bennett, MD; Lauren Daly, MD; Reza Daugherty, MD; Andrew DiPiero, MD; Maricar Diaz, MD; Fred Fow, MD; Hazel Guinto-Ocampo, MD; Sue Kost, MD; John Loiselle, MD; Kathy Palmer, MD; Parul Patel, MD; Melanie Pitone, MD; Alexandra Taylor, MD; and Bambi Taylor, MD) for their continuous support and encouragement. We also recognize the enthusiastic support of Jay Greenspan, MD, Chairman of the Department of Pediatrics at Jefferson Medical College, and B.J. Clark, MD, Executive Vice President at Nemours, as well as J. Carlton Gartner, MD, Pediatrician-in-Chief of the A.I. duPont Hospital for Children. Furthermore, we are grateful to the dedicated nurses and clerical staff of our emergency department. We sincerely thank our residents who continuously motivate us with their passion for learning and their quest for evidence-based medicine. Finally, we thank our patients and their families who unknowingly provided us with many of the "secrets" for our book.

Steven M. Selbst, MD, FAAP, FACEP
Kate M. Cronan, MD, FAAP

PREFACE

Those who care for children in the emergency department (ED) know they will be challenged on every shift. Anticipating which challenge will come in next engenders a certain thrill and perhaps some apprehension as well. Clinical questions arise with each patient. Likewise, astute young trainees often challenge senior physicians with relevant queries in bedside discussion of pediatric patients. Physicians rarely have time to sort through lengthy texts or volumes of information to get their answers. This book tackles the difficult questions that are often generated by pediatric patients and trainees in the ED. It offers succinct, up-to-date answers.

This second edition of *Pediatric Emergency Medicine Secrets* is divided into seven sections. The first section addresses life-threatening conditions and immediate stabilization of children. The second section features common chief complaints that are often managed in the ED. Later sections focus on important medical emergencies, surgical emergencies, major and minor trauma, and environmental emergencies. Finally, questions relating to special topics in pediatric emergency medicine (procedural sedation, bioterrorism, risk management, and the transport of children to specialized centers) are included.

Several new chapters are featured in this second edition, including Acute Care of Technology-Assisted Children, Sports Injuries, Emergency Medical Services and Prehospital Care, and Patient Safety in the Emergency Department. All other chapters have been revised and revamped with new questions and current references. References and relevant websites are frequently listed with their related questions to allow for further study. Many chapters have classic photographs and radiographs to enhance learning. Each chapter now features Key Points that highlight essential tips and pearls. The Top 100 Secrets have been collated for rapid review and summary. The new style of this edition makes the book very user friendly.

This book is unique in its question and answer format. We hope it will prove useful to those caring for ill and injured children and those preparing for examinations or board certification. Some questions focus on "fun trivia." Most provide valuable insight into common and unusual pediatric conditions seen in the ED. All the questions should inform, challenge, amuse, and motivate the reader, as do our patients and our trainees.

Steven M. Selbst, MD, FAAP, FACEP
Kate M. Cronan, MD, FAAP

TOP 100 SECRETS

These secrets are 100 of the top board alerts. They summarize the basic concepts, principles, and most salient details of pediatric emergency medicine.

1. Children most commonly develop respiratory failure prior to cardiac arrest. Early intervention, before cardiac arrest, offers the best chance for successful outcome.

2. The poor prognosis for children in cardiopulmonary arrest probably reflects the terminal nature of asystole, the most common rhythm. Long-standing tissue hypoxemia and acidosis from antecedent prolonged respiratory insufficiency add to the poor prognosis.

3. The two-thumb method of chest compressions is preferred for newborns, with the depth of compression being one-third of the anterior–posterior diameter of the chest rather than a fixed depth. Compression should be deep enough to generate a pulse.

4. Newborn infants do not tolerate cold, and hypothermia can prolong acidosis. Prevent heat loss as much as possible.

5. Because hypoxemia may be clinically inapparent, pulse oximetry is important; some call it the "fifth vital sign."

6. Respiratory failure may be present without respiratory distress. Work of breathing may appear normal in children with reduced level of consciousness (ingestion, metabolic derangements, head trauma), neuromuscular dysfunction (muscle disease), or fatigue, despite the presence of significant hypoventilation.

7. Shock is not defined by the blood pressure (BP) or any other vital sign. Shock exists when the patient's metabolic demand exceeds the body's ability to deliver oxygen and nutrients.

8. The greatest error that you can make in the treatment of shock is to use pressor agents to treat hypovolemia. Even in cases of distributive shock, fluids should be used for initial treatment.

9. Analgesia should not be withheld from a child with abdominal pain of unknown etiology simply for fear of delaying diagnosis or causing misdiagnosis.

10. Parents of children with abnormal mental status may try to minimize the extent of their child's illness by saying that the patient missed his nap that day or is always difficult to wake up. Don't send the child home without seeing him or her awake and alert.

11. An infant can have a normal physical examination even though the baby "looked dead" at the time of the apneic episode. If you are convinced by the history that a significant episode of apnea has occurred, admit the child for observation and further diagnostic evaluation even if no specific cause is identified in the emergency department (ED).

12. Chest pain in children is rarely related to previously undiagnosed cardiac disease, but children with this symptom deserve careful evaluation. Pediatric chest pain is concerning when it is

induced by exercise, associated with fever, or accompanied by an abnormal physical examination.

13. A young child who has persistent coughing following a severe choking episode has a foreign body in one of the mainstem bronchi until proven otherwise.

14. There is no reliable evidence that any pediatric cough suppressant medications are more effective than placebo.

15. Crying and irritability in an infant may indicate only colic or a life-threatening condition. A careful history and physical examination may detect treatable causes for crying in infancy.

16. A clear liquid diet is not necessary for most children with acute gastroenteritis. Full-strength milk or formula and an age-appropriate diet offer superior nutrition and are well tolerated by most children with diarrhea.

17. Oral rehydration therapy, when properly administered, is as effective as intravenous rehydration in the majority of children with mild-to-moderate dehydration due to gastroenteritis.

18. Relieve pain from a live insect in the ear by promptly immobilizing the insect with mineral oil or viscous lidocaine.

19. There is no single value for normal body temperature because there is individual variation; a variety of factors affect temperature, including time of day and age of the child.

20. The height of the fever by itself is a poor predictor of serious bacterial illness. Temperatures $< 42°C$ have not, by themselves, been associated with any serious sequelae.

21. When a child presents with new respiratory symptoms, inquire about the possibility of a choking episode, especially while eating nuts, popcorn, raw apples, or carrots.

22. Migraine and tension-type headaches are common in children and adolescents. Many children also suffer from headaches that include both migraine and tension-type characteristics.

23. A multitude of factors may cause headaches, but most are benign. Emergent neuroimaging is rarely indicated. A well-balanced diet, adequate hydration, regular sleep, and exercise can help prevent many headaches in children.

24. Urinary tract infections are the most common cause of hematuria in children. Any child presenting with gross hematuria or hematuria with associated symptoms, such as headache, edema, or hypertension requires emergent evaluation.

25. Confirm elevated BP readings with an appropriate-size cuff, when the child is calm and not in pain.

26. In addition to a thorough history and physical examination, perform screening laboratory testing on children with BPs greater than the 95th percentile. If the child's BP is greater than the 99th percentile or if there is evidence of end-organ damage, lower the BP as slowly as is safely possible, and admit the child to the hospital.

27. All neonates with conjugated hyperbilirubinemia have a pathologic process that requires further diagnostic studies, admission, and appropriate supportive and definitive care. Jaundice in children older than 3 months is almost always due to a pathologic process.

28. Normal radiographs do not equate with no pathology. Fractures, infections, and early destructive processes may not be apparent on x-ray.

29. Transient synovitis can mimic septic arthritis. However, patients with transient synovitis usually have little or no fever, appear well, and have less pain and limitation of motion than those with septic arthritis.

30. Neoplastic neck masses are generally painless, firm, fixed cervical masses. Neck masses that are tender, warm, and erythematous are more likely to be infectious (cervical adenitis).

31. Stevens-Johnson syndrome and toxic epidermal necrolysis represent a spectrum of the same disease; erythema multiforme is a separate process.

32. A computed tomographic (CT) scan may help distinguish orbital cellulitis from preseptal cellulitis when the child has severe edema and eye examination is difficult. Orbital cellulitis is often associated with a sinus infection.

33. Always examine the genitalia of a boy reporting abdominal pain. A history of trauma does not preclude the diagnosis of testicular torsion.

34. Children with group A β-hemolytic streptococcus (GABHS) pharyngitis usually do not have cough or coryza, but submandibular lymphadenopathy is usually present with GABHS pharyngitis.

35. Perform a lumbar puncture to rule out meningitis for any child with stiff neck, fever, and ill appearance.

36. Children who present with a stiff neck after trauma should be immediately immobilized in a cervical collar and have a complete radiographic evaluation.

37. Laryngomalacia is the most common cause of stridor in infants. It is generally benign and resolves spontaneously as the child grows.

38. Stridor may be caused by a number of pathologic processes that are not directly related to airway anatomy, such as cardiac, gastrointestinal, or neurologic.

39. Syncope in children is usually benign and neurocardiogenic in origin, but other, potentially serious causes must be eliminated through a thorough history and physical and review of an electrocardiogram (ECG) in all patients. The initial history, physical examination, and ECG guide further investigations, but further testing usually is of high cost and low yield.

40. Syncope that recurs, occurs during infancy, occurs when the patient is in a supine position, is associated with an injury related to the patient's fall, occurs with exertion, or is associated with chest pain, is very likely to be due to a cardiac abnormality and requires further testing, referral to a cardiologist, and possible admission to the hospital.

41. Consider hospitalization of a patient with pelvic inflammatory disease in the following instances: pregnancy, unclear diagnosis, vomiting, peritoneal signs, a young teenager (age < 15 years), tubo-ovarian abscess present or suspected, failed outpatient treatment, or patient's inability to follow the outpatient regimen.

42. Vomiting that persists for more than 24 hours without the development of diarrhea is unlikely to be caused by gastroenteritis. Vomiting can be caused by abnormalities in almost any organ

system. Always consider nongastrointestinal causes when evaluating a pediatric patient with vomiting.

43. Delays in administration of epinephrine during anaphylaxis are common and associated with a higher frequency of biphasic reactions and increased fatality rates. Oral diphenhydramine, the medication most commonly prescribed for allergic reactions, may have a limited role in the acute treatment of moderate or severe anaphylaxis.

44. During respiratory syncytial virus season, always check for hepatomegaly in infants with bronchiolitis. It may help you clinically distinguish the rare child with heart failure from the many others with tachypnea, tachycardia, and pulmonary rales caused by bronchiolitis.

45. To treat a child with hemodynamically compromising bradycardia, first assess the airway. Remove any foreign body from the airway, if present, and reposition the patient (jaw-thrust maneuver). Next, assist respiration with 100% oxygen and perform chest compressions if the heart rate is <80 beats per minute in newborns and <60 beats per minute in infants and children. If the child is not improved, give epinephrine (1:10,000; 0.01 mg/kg IV) or atropine (0.02 mg/kg IV, with 0.1 mg as a minimum dose and 0.5 mg as the maximum dose).

46. Imaging of a well-appearing child after a nontraumatic seizure can be delayed, thereby avoiding radiation exposure with urgent CT.

47. A child with severe headache and a suspicion or diagnosis of sphenoid sinusitis warrants a careful evaluation for an intracranial complication.

48. Remember to administer stress doses of intravenous hydrocortisone for acute adrenal insufficiency.

49. In diabetic ketoacidosis, high initial blood urea nitrogen, low arterial carbon dioxide, inadequate increase in serum sodium concentration, and bicarbonate administration are associated with the development of cerebral edema.

50. In many cases of gastroenteritis, it is beneficial to begin oral rehydration in the waiting area. Offer oral electrolyte solution: 1 mL/kg for mild dehydration and 2 mL/kg for moderate dehydration, every 5 minutes.

51. A quick estimate of degree of dehydration can be obtained by checking for four examination findings: capillary refill at the fingertip > 2 seconds, ill general appearance, dry mucous membranes, and absence of tears. If two or more are found, the child is likely dehydrated.

52. A currant-jelly stool is a late finding in intussusception. Not all red or black stools are due to blood.

53. Symptoms of pregnancy in teens can be vague, and the diagnosis can be missed if testing is done only in the scenario of a missed period.

54. A history of recent vigorous activity may provide a clue to the diagnosis of ovarian torsion in a female with symptoms of stabbing abdominal pain.

55. Patients with sickle cell disease and fever are at high risk for bacterial infection and should usually receive broad-spectrum antibiotic coverage even if no source is identified.

56. Anticipate tumor lysis syndrome in patients with newly diagnosed leukemia or lymphoma. Patients should receive aggressive hydration with intravenous fluids that contain sodium bicarbonate and do not contain potassium.

57. Vincent's angina is a necrotizing ulcerative gingivitis known as "trench mouth" during World War II. It occurs on the gingivae between the teeth and has a clinical triad of pain, bleeding, and ulceration between the teeth. It is associated with poor dental hygiene and is caused by fusobacteria and spirochetes.

58. Ludwig's angina is an indurated cellulitis of the submandibular or sublingual spaces. It usually results from trauma to the floor of the mouth or dental infection.

59. Characterizations of a poisoned patient's mentation, vital signs, pupil size and reactivity, bowel sounds, and skin appearance are usually more useful to the clinician than urine drug screening.

60. Careful support to a poisoned patient's airway and breathing, circulation, and neurologic function will help more patients than antidotal therapies.

61. The most significant risk factors for adolescent suicide include male sex, age > 16 years, previous suicide attempt, mood disorder, substance abuse, poor social support, and access to firearms or other lethal means.

62. If a child requires restraint, the least restrictive efforts should be attempted (verbal de-escalation) prior to physical restraint or use of medications for restraint. When necessary, benzodiazepines, neuroleptics, and antihistamines are the most common drugs of choice to use for restraint.

63. All that wheezes is not asthma or bronchiolitis, though the vast majority is. Consider other causes in atypical cases (e.g., poor response to treatment, more severe course).

64. Warm water is more effective than vinegar or soda to unclog a gastrostomy tube.

65. Dental caries are contagious.

66. Dental abscess is a common cause of facial swelling in young children.

67. Bilious emesis in infants is often related to a surgically correctable abdominal process that can progress quickly to severe morbidity or death. Infants with bilious emesis should have a prompt physical examination, and radiologic evaluation is mandatory.

68. Normal laboratory values may not exclude a surgical abdomen. A thorough examination, detailed history, and experience are the best tools to diagnose most abdominal surgical emergencies.

69. Seventy to eighty percent of shunt infections occur within 2 months of shunt placement; 80–90% occur within 4 months.

70. Ventriculitis may occur in the absence of cerebrospinal fluid abnormalities if the ventricles are not communicating with the lumbar spinal fluid.

71. A Marcus Gunn pupil represents an afferent papillary defect and may detect optic nerve or retinal disease. It is demonstrated with a swinging flashlight test. Swinging the light to the

normal eye causes both pupils to constrict normally. Swinging the light to the affected eye causes both pupils to redilate, reflecting defective conduction.

72. Flashers, floaters, and visual defects are hallmarks of partial retinal tear, which may lead to retinal detachment.

73. Magnetic resonance imaging is the best imaging test for the diagnosis of osteomyelitis.

74. Knee pain is a common presenting symptom of slipped capital femoral epiphysis. A thorough hip evaluation is mandatory in the evaluation of an adolescent with knee pain. Avoid movement of the hip when obtaining plain radiographs in cases of suspected slipped capital femoral epiphysis; it may cause further slippage.

75. If a young child presents with a foul odor from his or her mouth and green nasal drainage after treatment for sinusitis, think of nasal foreign body, which is often misdiagnosed as sinusitis or an upper respiratory tract infection.

76. Ureteropelvic junction obstruction presents more commonly on the left side.

77. Serial examinations of the abdomen are crucial to detect abdominal injuries in children. Clinical instability is the most important indication for an emergent laparotomy in the child with an abdominal injury.

78. Prevention is more effective than medical intervention in decreasing morbidity and mortality from burn and smoke inhalation injury. Most children involved in fires die from the effects of smoke inhalation as opposed to burn injuries.

79. Most sexually abused children have a normal physical examination.

80. Rib fractures, metaphyseal chip fractures, spine and scapula fractures, and complex skull fractures have a high probability of being caused by child abuse.

81. Avulsed permanent teeth should be immediately reimplanted to preserve tooth viability. If immediate reimplantation is not possible, temporarily store the tooth in cool milk, saliva, or saline.

82. The physis is the weakest link in the pediatric musculoskeletal system and will fracture before the ligament fails.

83. Chemical burns and suspicion of globe perforation are true ophthalmologic emergencies and require immediate recognition and initiation of treatment and stabilization. Both warrant emergent (same-day) ophthalmologic consultation or referral.

84. Eye irrigation should begin as soon as possible after potential chemical burn to the eye is recognized. If possible, it is begun with any bland fluid at the scene of the injury and continued at the medical facility, immediately on arrival, with normal saline or lactated Ringer's solution.

85. A young infant with a nonfrontal, large scalp hematoma often has a skull fracture and may have an intracranial injury.

86. Managing hypoxia, hypoperfusion, and metabolic derangements after head trauma may prevent secondary brain injury.

87. Consult with a surgical or orthopedic specialist for wounds associated with a fracture; violation of a joint cavity; injury to a tendon, nerve, or vessel; those wounds that seem difficult to repair; or those located in areas of high cosmetic concern.

88. Puncture wounds have a greater incidence of infectious complications, such as cellulitis, soft tissue abscess, pyarthrosis, osteomyelitis, and foreign-body granuloma.

89. The smaller the individual, the larger the body surface-to-volume ratio. This places pediatric trauma patients at risk for hypothermia, both at the scene of injury and during the ED resuscitation.

90. In the trauma patient, the ABCs (airway, breathing, circulation) must be frequently reassessed. Deteriorating vital signs despite "appropriate" resuscitation efforts demand operative intervention.

91. Use of steroids for children with spinal injury is controversial.

92. A hard cervical collar does not provide complete neck immobilization.

93. Hematuria, a hallmark for genitourinary trauma, is absent with some pedicle and penetrating injuries. CT scan is the diagnostic test of choice for *stable* patients with suspected renal injury.

94. Avulsion fractures of the ischial tuberosity or iliac spine may occur from sudden muscle contraction during vigorous running or jumping.

95. A child struck in the chest by a pitched baseball may develop commotio cordis and sudden cardiac arrest.

96. Tension pneumothorax is diagnosed clinically, without taking time for radiographs, in a child with respiratory distress or cardiovascular compromise.

97. Pulmonary contusion often occurs without obvious chest wall injury or fracture of the thorax.

98. DEET (N, N diethyl-m-toluamide) is a broad-spectrum repellant effective against mosquitoes (including those carrying West Nile virus), chiggers, ticks and fleas, and gnats.

99. Treatment for a brown recluse spider bite is supportive and not specific: local wound care, analgesics, and tetanus immunization are mainstays of therapy. Extensive dermal injury may require skin grafting.

100. Drowning is a hypoxic injury; addressing the basic ABCs and correcting hypothermia to 32°C are the cornerstones of resuscitation, postresuscitation, and cerebral resuscitation management. Because of the lack of 100% reliable outcome predictors, resuscitation should be attempted for all patients arriving in the ED.

I. ADVANCED LIFE SUPPORT

CHAPTER 1

CHILDHOOD RESUSCITATION

Allen L. Hsiao, MD, and M. Douglas Baker, MD

1. What is the incidence of pediatric cardiopulmonary arrests?

The estimates of incidence of pediatric cardiopulmonary arrests vary by location. In suburban King County, Washington, Eisenberg et al reported an annual pediatric cardiopulmonary arrest rate of 12.7 per 100,000 of the population younger than age 18 years. From rural community emergency departments, Thompson et al reported a range of 1.3 to 5.3 cardiopulmonary arrests per 10,000 of the population younger than age 5 years. Ronco et al estimated 63 cardiopulmonary arrests per 150,000 of the population younger than age 15 years in Birmingham, Alabama. Schoenfeld and Baker noted that 0.25% of patient visits to the emergency department of Children's Hospital of Philadelphia involved management in the resuscitation room. A prospective study by Ong et al found an overall annual incidence of cardiopulmonary arrests of 59.7 per million children, with the highest incidence, 175 per million children, noted in the youngest age group (under 4 years).

Eisenberg M, Bergner L, Hallstrom A: Epidemiology of cardiac arrest and resuscitation in children. Ann Emerg Med 12:672–674, 1983.

Ong ME, Stiell I, Osmond MH, et al: Etiology of pediatric out-of-hospital cardiac arrest by coroner's diagnosis. Resuscitation 68:335–342, 2006.

Ronco R, King W, Donley DK, et al: Outcome and cost at a children's hospital following resuscitation for out-of-hospital cardiopulmonary arrest. Arch Pediatr Adolesc Med 149:210–214, 1995.

Schoenfeld PS, Baker MD: Management of cardiopulmonary and trauma resuscitation in the pediatric emergency department. Pediatrics 91:726–729, 1993.

Thompson JE, Bonner B, Lower GM Jr: Pediatric cardiopulmonary arrests in rural populations. Pediatrics 86:302–306, 1990.

2. Is the pathophysiology of cardiopulmonary arrest in children similar to that in adults?

No. cardiopulmonary arrests in children most commonly involve primary respiratory failure with subsequent cardiac arrest. Furthermore, cardiopulmonary arrests in children generally follow progressive deterioration and usually do not occur as sudden events. Exceptions to this statement include cases of sudden infant death syndrome (SIDS), major trauma, or certain primary cardiac events.

3. What are the common causes of cardiopulmonary arrest in children?

Common causes of cardiopulmonary arrest in children are numerous, but most fit into the classifications of respiratory, infectious, cardiovascular, traumatic, or central nervous system (CNS) diseases (Table 1-1). Respiratory diseases and SIDS together consistently account for one-third to two-thirds of all pediatric cardiopulmonary arrests in published series.

4. What is the typical age distribution of pediatric cardiopulmonary arrests?

Almost regardless of the underlying disease, the age distribution of cardiopulmonary arrest in children is skewed toward infancy. In published series of childhood cardiopulmonary arrests, 56% (range, 43–70%) of patients are younger than 1 year, 26% (range, 21–30%) are between 1 and 4 years of age, and 18% (range, 6–28%) are older than 4 years. For general emergency medicine practice settings, this finding is particularly important. Equipment and skills preparedness for this young age range are crucial to achieve best outcomes.

TABLE 1-1. COMMON CAUSES OF CARDIOPULMONARY ARREST IN CHILDREN	
Respiratory	**Central Nervous System**
Pneumonia	Seizures, or complications thereof
Near drowning	Hydrocephalus, or shunt malfunction
Smoke inhalation	Tumor
Aspiration and obstruction	Meningitis
Apnea	Hemorrhage
Suffocation	**Other**
Bronchiolitis	Trauma
Cardiovascular	Sudden infant death syndrome
Congenital heart disease	Anaphylaxis
Congestive heart failure	Gastrointestinal hemorrhage
Pericarditis	Poisoning
Myocarditis	
Arrhythmia	
Septic shock	

5. **What are the outcomes of pediatric cardiopulmonary arrests?**
    In four reviews published since 1983, the survival rates for children experiencing isolated respiratory arrests ranged from 75% to 97%, while survival rates for children experiencing full cardiopulmonary arrests ranged from 4% to 16%. One recent comprehensive review of 41 articles on pediatric arrest found that of 5363 out-of-hospital pediatric arrests, only 12.1% of patients survived until discharge and only 4% were neurologically intact. Another study prospectively followed 474 patients having out-of-hospital pediatric cardiac arrest and found that only 1.9% survived to discharge. The poor prognosis of full cardiopulmonary arrests probably reflects the terminal nature of asystole, which is often preceded by prolonged respiratory insufficiency and its resultant long-standing tissue hypoxemia and acidosis. This is one reason why initial management is directed toward improvement of oxygenation and ventilation.

    Donoghue AJ, Nadkarni V, Berg RA, et al: Out-of-hospital pediatric cardiac arrest: An epidemiologic review and assessment of current knowledge. Ann Emerg Med 46:512–522, 2005.

    Kuisma M, Suominen P, Korpela R: Pediatric out-of-hospital cardiac arrests: Epidemiology and outcome. Resuscitation 30:141–150, 1995.

    Lopez-Herce J, Garcia C, Dominguez P, et al: Outcome of out-of-hospital cardiorespiratory arrest in children. Pediatr Emerg Care 21:807–815, 2005.

    Nadkarni VM, Larkin GL, Peberdy MA, et al: First documented rhythm and clinical outcome from in-hospital cardiac arrest among children and adults. JAMA 295:50–57, 2006.

    Schindler MB, Bohn D, Cox PN, et al: Outcome of out-of-hospital cardiac or respiratory arrest in children. N Engl J Med 335:1473–1479, 1996.

6. **What are some prognostic factors for pediatric cardiopulmonary arrests?**
    For out-of-hospital arrests, bystander or paramedic initiation resuscitation of witnessed arrest has repeatedly been found to improve survival by as much as fourfold compared to initial resuscitation by physicians after patient arrival at the hospital. Similarly, in eight reviews

published since 1983, 96 of 542 (17.7%) children experiencing out-of-hospital cardiopulmonary arrest survived versus 137 of 342 (40%) experiencing in-hospital cardiopulmonary arrest.

Survival of patients presenting in ventricular fibrillation is much higher than among those in asystole, severe bradycardia, or pulseless electrical activity (PEA). Prolonged resuscitation over 20 minutes is often thought to be the strongest indicator of mortality. Trauma- and submersion injury–associated arrests are associated with better survival rates compared with isolated cardiac-origin arrests (21.9% and 22.7% versus 1.1%, respectively).

Scribano PV, Baker MD, Ludwig S: Factors influencing termination of resuscitative efforts in children: A comparison of pediatric emergency medicine and adult emergency medicine physicians. Pediatr Emerg Care 13:320–324, 1997.

7. **Does the initial approach to childhood resuscitation differ from that for adults?**
    The initial approach to pediatric resuscitation is similar to that for adults: **A** (airway), **B** (breathing), **C** (circulation), **D** (drugs), **E** (exposure). Attention to proper positioning, oxygenation, and ventilation comes first, and drug therapy comes "last." It is always advisable to preassign resuscitation duties to available staff. This eliminates confusion during the heat of the action. Care should always be taken to protect the cervical spine (and spinal cord) during resuscitation, especially during manipulation of the neck and jaw.

8. **After establishing a clear chain of command and assigning specific duties to all members of the resuscitation team, what should the order of priorities be?**
    The order of priorities is:
    1. Identify the patient's level of responsiveness.
    2. Properly position the patient on a firm surface, considering the potential for head or cervical spine injury.
    3. Establish a patent airway.
    4. Assure proper oxygenation and ventilation.
    5. Attend to circulation.
    6. Consider drug therapy.

9. **What is the recommended way to establish a patent airway?**
    - The first attempt to establish airway patency should be through **proper airway positioning**. Often, this alone will be effective. Since most airway obstruction is due to the effect of gravity on the mandibular block of soft tissues, it can be relieved by either a head tilt–chin lift or jaw-thrust maneuver.
    - Vomitus or other foreign material can also obstruct airways. Inspect the airway for these materials, and **suction early and frequently**.
    - In selected patients with altered levels of consciousness, **nasopharyngeal or oropharyngeal airway stents** are useful. Semiconscious children generally tolerate the softer nasopharyngeal airways better than the harder, less comfortable oropharyngeal airways. Children, such as those in postictal states, who have sustained spontaneous respiratory effort but have upper airway obstruction due to poor muscle tone often benefit from the use of these devices.
    - The **laryngeal mask airway** is a relatively new supraglottic advanced airway device that may be a very useful tool to the experienced user in certain situations. However, at this time, the American Heart Association states that there is insufficient evidence to recommend for or against the routine use of this device during arrests.

10. **What is the recommended way to deliver supplemental oxygen to a child?**
    Supplemental oxygen can be delivered to a child by a variety of different means. For the sickest patient, oxygen should be delivered in the highest concentration and by the most direct method possible. Children who demonstrate spontaneous breathing might require less invasive means

of administration of supplemental oxygen. Table 1-2 lists some different methods of oxygen delivery with their associated delivery capabilities.

Children without adequate spontaneous breathing effort require mechanical support. Different bag-valve mask devices have different oxygen delivery capabilities. Self-inflating bag-valve devices are capable of delivering 60–90% oxygen, while non–self-inflating devices (anesthesia ventilation systems) deliver 100% oxygen to the patient. Endotracheal intubation offers the most secure and direct means of delivery of 100% oxygen to the patient.

Mondolfi AA, Greiner BM, Thompson JE, et al: Comparison of self-inflating bags with anesthesia bags for bag-mask ventilation in the pediatric emergency department. Pediatr Emerg Care 13:312–316, 1997.

TABLE 1-2. METHODS OF OXYGEN DELIVERY AND THEIR DELIVERY CAPABILITIES

Nasal cannula: 30–40% oxygen

Simple masks: 30–60% oxygen

Partial rebreather masks: 50–60% oxygen

Oxygen tents: 30–50% oxygen

Oxygen hoods: 80–90% oxygen

Nonrebreather masks: ~100% oxygen

---

11. **Which children require intubation?**

While the most obvious indication for endotracheal intubation is sustained apnea, a number of other indications exist. These include:
- Inadequate central nervous system control of ventilation
- Functional or anatomic airway obstruction
- Strong potential for developing airway obstruction (e.g., inhalation airway burns, expanding airway hematoma)
- Loss of protective airway reflexes
- Excessive work of breathing, which might lead to fatigue and respiratory insufficiency
- Need for high airway pressures to maintain effective alveolar gas exchange
- Need for mechanical ventilatory support
- Potential occurrence of any of the above during patient transport

In many instances, bag-mask ventilation and bag–endotracheal tube ventilation are equally effective for the patient. In such circumstances, it is logical to employ the method that the rescuer is best able to deliver. A recent prospective study randomized the use of bag-mask ventilation and endotracheal intubation by paramedics in 830 out-of-hospital pediatric arrests. There was no difference in survival (30% versus 26%, respectively) or good neurologic outcome (23% versus 20%) between the two groups of children.

Gausche M, Lewis RJ, Stratton SJ, et al: Effect of out-of-hospital pediatric endotracheal intubation on survival and neurological outcome: A controlled clinical trial. JAMA 283:783–790, 2000.

12. **When selecting an endotracheal tube, what sizing guidelines are suggested?**

There are a number of ways to ensure selection of properly sized endotracheal tubes (ETTs) for children. The most often cited is the following age-based formula:

$$\text{ETT internal diameter (mm)} = (16 + \text{years of age})/4$$

Another "rule of thumb" is really a "rule of finger." Research has demonstrated that the width of the child's fifth fingernail is approximately equal to the outer width of the appropriately sized ETT. Most emergency physicians use uncuffed tubes for children younger than 10 years because in these patients, the anatomic narrowing at the level of the cricoid cartilage provides a natural "cuff." However, in the in-hospital setting, a cuffed tube has been shown to be as safe as an uncuffed tube for infants beyond the newborn period. In some circumstances (e.g., poor lung compliance, high airway resistance, or a large glottic leak), a cuffed tube may be preferable.

American Heart Association: 2005 Guidelines for Cardiopulmonary Resuscitation and Emergency Cardiovascular Care. Part 12: Pediatric Advanced Life Support. Circulation 112:167–187, 2005.

KEY POINTS: HOW TO DETERMINE THE PROPER PLACEMENT OF THE ETT ✔

1. Check to see that the tube is inserted at a depth that is three times the internal diameter of the ETT (from the point of the patient's central incisors).

2. Observe for symmetric chest expansion.

3. Auscultate for symmetric breath sounds.

4. Look for distention of the abdomen, indicating misplacement of the tube.

5. Measure end-tidal carbon dioxide using a colorimetric detector. In infants and children with a perfusing rhythm, a purple color on the device indicates a problem, whereas a yellow color implies that the tube is in the trachea.

6. Confirm tube placement with a chest radiograph.

13. **How can I determine if ETT placement is appropriate?**
Proper depth for ETT insertion from the point of the patient's central incisors can be estimated to be three times the internal diameter of the ETT. Measurement of end-tidal carbon dioxide using a colorimetric detector, observation for symmetric chest expansion, and auscultation for symmetric breath sounds can help to ensure proper placement. Confirmation of placement is probably best determined with a chest radiograph. Prior to an x-ray, the colorimetric detector offers a rapid bedside determination to detect CO_2 to confirm endotracheal tube placement (Fig. 1-1).

14. **What are the best methods to assess a child's circulatory status?**
Assessment of a child's circulatory status should always include appraisal of:
- Skin and mucous membrane color
- Presence and quality of pulses
- Capillary refill
- Heart rate and blood pressure

Always keep in mind that in the instance of acute blood loss, the protective mechanisms of increased heart rate and increased vascular resistance maintain a child's blood pressure within a normal range in spite of losses as high as 25% of total body blood volume.

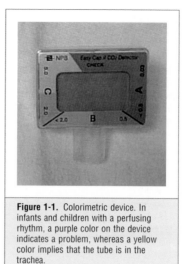

Figure 1-1. Colorimetric device. In infants and children with a perfusing rhythm, a purple color on the device indicates a problem, whereas a yellow color implies that the tube is in the trachea.

15. **To whom and how should external cardiac compression be delivered?**
Apply external cardiac compression to any child with ineffectual pulses. The optimal compression–ventilation ratio for two-rescuer cardiopulmonary resuscitation (CPR) is 15 to 2. It takes a number of compressions to raise coronary perfusion pressure, which drops with each pulse. Interruptions in chest compressions are associated with decreased rate of return of spontaneous circulation. It is currently recommended that in infants, compressions be applied evenly over the lower half of the sternum. The two thumb-encircling hands technique is preferred for two-rescuer CPR because it produces higher coronary perfusion pressure and more consistently results in appropriate depth of compression. For children and adolescents, compress the lower half of the sternum with the heel of one hand or with two hands, but do not press over the xiphoid process or ribs.

American Heart Association: 2005 Guidelines for Cardiopulmonary Resuscitation and Emergency Cardiovascular Care. Part 11, Pediatric Basic Life Support. Circulation 112:1567–1166, 2005.

Plaisance P, Adnet F, Vicaut E, et al: Benefit of active compression-decompression cardiopulmonary resuscitation as a prehospital advanced cardiac life support: A randomized multicenter study. Circulation 95:955–961, 1997.

16. **What are the golden rules of vascular access?**
1. Attempt first the technique that has yielded best personal success.
2. One small-sized line beats none at all.
The messages are obvious. During resuscitation, procedures should be done by those most talented, and they should do what they do best. While it is better to have large-gauge vascular access for resuscitation, small-gauge vascular access is adequate to deliver medications and slower infusions of fluids.

17. **What are the options for vascular access in children?**
There are many options for vascular access in children. Depending on the situation at hand, some might not be as available or achievable as others. Conditions permitting, **peripheral venous access** is generally preferred over other means. Antecubital, hand, wrist, foot, and ankle veins are the most popular access sites. Saphenous veins in the ankle are deep but often accessible. External jugular veins are also reliably accessible but require difficult positioning of the child to be successful. Scalp veins are potential sites of access in infants but are located on a portion of the body that might be difficult to access while managing the patient's airway.

Central access sites include bone marrow, femoral veins, and subclavian veins. Subclavian access should be attempted only by those skilled in the procedure. Intraosseous access should be considered early, especially in the case of apnea and pulselessness in an infant.

18. **Why does intraosseous infusion work?**

    The bone marrow serves as a "stiff" vascular bed. It is composed of interconnected sinusoids that are fed and drained by veins that traverse the cortex of the bone and connect with the central circulation. Fluids infused anywhere into the marrow cavity enter these vascular channels and find their way to the central venous system. In animal models, transit times from the tibia to the heart are short (less than 60 seconds). Numerous medications and fluids have been shown to be effective when administered via this route.

19. **What are the dos and don'ts surrounding intraosseous infusion?**

    Although there is no age limit for use of intraosseous infusion, it is easiest to accomplish in younger patients, whose bones are less calcified. Remember that intraosseous infusion was developed in the 1930s as a technique of vascular access in adults. Numerous studies using adult patients have demonstrated a cumulative 98% success rate. Preferred sites of intraosseous needle placement are the proximal tibia in children younger than 2 years and the distal tibia in those age 2 or older. The distal femur may also be used. Any IV fluid or medication can be safely and effectively administered via the intraosseous route. Rates of infusion are limited by needle gauge and length. When infusion is delivered with pressure, flow rates of saline through 20-G needles have been measured as high as 25 mL per minute.

    Intraosseous needle placement is painful, and time-limited in its effectiveness. It should be reserved for emergency vascular access needs. Complications encountered most often include needle damage (bending or breaking), fluid extravasation at the needle entry site, and puncture through both sides of the bone. Intraosseous infusion will not succeed with bones that have breaks or holes in them because fluid will extravasate through these openings.

20. **What role does drug therapy play in pediatric resuscitation?**

    Drug therapy during resuscitation is reserved for patients who do not respond adequately to the ABCs. Other than oxygen, most pediatric resuscitations require few drugs. Other useful chemical agents include:

    - Epinephrine (to increase heart rate, myocardial contractility, and systemic vascular resistance)
    - Atropine (to increase heart rate in nonneonates)
    - Dextrose (to increase glucose)
    - Sodium bicarbonate (to increase pH)
    - Amiodarone or procainamide (to reverse ventricular arrhythmias)
    - Naloxone (to reverse the effects of narcotics)
    - Adenosine (to reverse supraventricular tachycardia)
    - Dopamine (to increase vasoconstriction and blood pressure)
    - Dobutamine (to increase myocardial contractility)
    - Benzodiazepines (to achieve sedation and control seizures)

    Keep in mind that administration of any of these drugs should never be considered as a first line of management for any disorder. During resuscitation, drug therapy should always be preceded by another intervention. *Oxygenation and ventilation are always the first priorities for any seriously ill child.* Other appropriate supportive measures (e.g., chest compressions for pulselessness or fluid infusion for shock) should also precede administration of drugs during resuscitation.

21. **What are the new recommendations regarding epinephrine administration during pediatric resuscitation?**

    Epinephrine dosing recommendations have undergone much debate recently. Reports have cited observations of "increased effectiveness" of high doses of epinephrine on cerebral resuscitation of children who sustained witnessed cardiopulmonary arrest. Other reports have demonstrated no increased effectiveness of higher doses. Pending the results of properly conducted prospective investigations of the issue, the American Heart Association and American Academy of Pediatrics, through their pediatric advanced life support (PALS) program, have issued recommendations for administration of epinephrine during management of asystole. Generally, with management of asystole in children, epinephrine should be used differently than if it were being administered to reverse bradycardia. However, in both situations, a dose-response method of epinephrine should be employed.

PALS recommendations for pulseless arrest (PES, asystole)
- If the first asystole-countering dose is intravascularly (IV or IO route) administered: give as a standard dose (0.01 mg/kg). This can be delivered as 0.1 mL/kg of a 1:10,000 solution of epinephrine. Vasopressin is used in place of epinephrine for the first or second dose in adult resuscitations but is considered *Class Indeterminate* (not enough evidence to recommend for or against) in pediatric arrests.
- If the first asystole-countering dose is endotracheally administered: give as a higher dose (0.1 mg/kg). This can be delivered as 0.1 mL/kg of a 1:1000 solution of epinephrine. An IV or IO route of administration is preferred, however, if at all possible.
- Higher-dose epinephrine (0.1 mg/kg; 0.1 mL/kg of a 1:1000 solution) is no longer routinely recommended for subsequent doses of epinephrine given through an IV or IO route.

PALS recommendations for bradycardia
- Any intravascularly (IV or IO route) administered doses should be given as standard doses (0.01 mg/kg). This is generally delivered as 0.1 mL/kg of a 1:10,000 solution of epinephrine.
- Any endotracheally administered doses should be given as higher doses (0.1 mg/kg). This can be delivered as 0.1 mL/kg of a 1:1000 solution of epinephrine.

American Heart Association: 2005 Guidelines for Cardiopulmonary Resuscitation and Emergency Cardiovascular Care. Part 12: Pediatric Advanced Life Support. Circulation 112:167–187, 2005.

Carpenter TC, Stenmark KR: High-dose epinephrine is not superior to standard-dose epinephrine in pediatric in-hospital cardiopulmonary arrest. Pediatrics 99:403–408, 1997.

22. **Which resuscitation drugs are effective when given via an endotracheal tube?**
There are four "traditional" resuscitation drugs that are effective when administered through the ETT. Those four are **l**idocaine, **a**tropine, **n**aloxone, and **e**pinephrine. The acronym **LANE** is an easy way to remember them. **V**ersed (midazolam) also is useful and is effective when administered endotracheally. Adding this drug to the list yields a different acronym: **NAVEL**. With the exception of epinephrine, endotracheal doses are the same as intravascular doses. All endotracheal doses of epinephrine should be a higher dose (0.1 mg/kg).

KEY POINTS: DRUGS THAT CAN BE GIVEN VIA THE ENDOTRACHEAL ROUTE ✔

1. Lidocaine
2. Atropine
3. Naloxone
4. Epinephrine

23. **Are there minimum dosing requirements for any resuscitation drugs?**
    - **Atropine** (usual dose, 0.02 mg/kg) has a minimum dosing requirement for effective reversal of bradycardia. It appears that at doses lower than 0.1 mg, atropine exerts an effect that might actually worsen bradycardia. Thus, if its use is considered for reversal of bradycardia in a child who weighs less than 5 kg, a minimum of 0.1 mg should be administered.
    - **Dopamine** also has different effects when administered at different doses. At lower doses (1–5 μg/kg/min), dopaminergic effects are seen. When administered at these lower doses, dopamine tends to augment renal blood flow and enhance urinary output. During resuscitation, dopamine typically is used to bolster blood pressure through increased vasoconstriction. For that α-adrenergic effect, higher doses (10–20 μg/kg/min) are required.

24. **What are the recommendations for use of adenosine?**
    Adenosine is the drug of choice in the acute management of supraventricular tachycardia. It is a short-acting agent (half-life of approximately 10 seconds) that slows atrioventricular node conduction. The initial dose is 0.1 mg/kg, given as a rapid intravascular push with an immediate saline flush. If the drug is not given rapidly, its effectiveness is diminished. If the first dose is properly administered but ineffective, give a larger second dose of 0.2 mg/kg. Usual adult doses are 6 mg (first dose), followed by 12 mg (second dose). Expect that the first dose might be completely ineffective or only transiently effective. Administration of subsequent higher doses generally yields success.

    Ros SP, Fisher EA, Bell TJ: Adenosine in the emergency management of supraventricular tachycardia. Pediatr Emerg Care 197:222–223, 1991.

25. **Does calcium have any usefulness in pediatric resuscitations?**
    The American Heart Association does not recommend the routine use of calcium in pediatric cardiac arrest. While the use of calcium during resuscitation has declined considerably, there remain specific instances when it has significant value. Use calcium to remedy the following disorders:
    - Documented hypocalcemia
    - Documented hyperkalemia
    - Documented hypermagnesemia
    - Calcium-channel blocker excess

    When administered, calcium should be infused slowly. Rapid infusion results in severe bradycardia. Take care to avoid back-to-back infusion of calcium- and sodium bicarbonate–containing solutions. If mixed, these agents form calcium carbonate (chalk) in the IV tubing.

    American Heart Association: 2005 Guidelines for Cardiopulmonary Resuscitation and Emergency Cardiovascular Care. Part 12: Pediatric Advanced Life Support. Circulation 112:167–187, 2005.

26. **Does sodium bicarbonate still have a role in pediatric resuscitations?**
    Sodium bicarbonate is not recommended for routine use in pediatric resuscitations. Although it is a useful agent for the reversal of documented metabolic acidosis, it is effective only in the presence of adequate ventilation. When bicarbonate combines with hydrogen, it forms a complex molecule that splits into carbon dioxide and water. The carbon dioxide has only one route of exit, the respiratory tract. Without effective ventilation, this by-product is not removed, and the buffering capacity of the bicarbonate is eliminated. A randomized, controlled trial found no benefit from sodium bicarbonate use in neonatal resuscitation. After provision of effective ventilation and chest compressions and administration of epinephrine, consider sodium bicarbonate for prolonged cardiac arrest.

    American Heart Association: 2005 Guidelines for Cardiopulmonary Resuscitation and Emergency Cardiovascular Care. Part 12: Pediatric Advanced Life Support. Circulation 112:167–187, 2005.

Lokesh L, Kumar P, Murki S, Narang A: A randomized controlled trial of sodium bicarbonate in neonatal resuscitation—effect on immediate outcome. Resuscitation 60:219–223, 2004.

27. **Is there an easy method to calculate mixtures of constant infusions of drugs?**
Several methods are used. Here is one easy method:
- For constant infusion of drugs (epinephrine, isoproterenol) beginning at **0.1 µg/kg/min:** 0.6 times the weight in kg equals the number of milligrams of drug to add to enough water to make a total of 100 mL of solution. The resultant solution is then infused at a rate of 1 mL per hour, delivering 0.1 µg/kg/min.
- For constant infusion of drugs (dopamine, dobutamine) beginning at **1 µg/kg/min:** 6 times the weight in kg equals the number of milligrams of drug to add to enough water to make a total of 100 mL of solution. The resultant solution is then infused at a rate of 1 mL per hour, delivering 1 µg/kg/min.

28. **What role does defibrillation play in pediatric resuscitation?**
Historically, pediatric resuscitation has focused on pulmonary etiologies; defibrillation is a relatively uncommon intervention in pediatric resuscitation. While asystole remains the most commonly observed arrhythmia during pediatric cardiac arrests, recent research indicates that ventricular fibrillation may occur much more frequently than originally thought. The National Registry of Cardiopulmonary Resuscitation, the largest inpatient pediatric cohort reported to date, found ventricular fibrillation occurred in 14% of pediatric arrests. In that study, pediatric patients with ventricular fibrillation had a higher survival rate (29%) than those with asystole (24%) or PEA (11%). A recent study of out-of-hospital pediatric arrests found ventricular fibrillation as the presenting rhythm in 17.6% of cases, with children older than 7 years of age having the highest incidence (38/141, 27.0%). Survival of patients with ventricular fibrillation was threefold greater (31.3% versus 10.7%) than in those without a shockable rhythm.

Smith BT, Rea TD, Eisenberg MS: Ventricular fibrillation in pediatric cardiac arrest. Acad Emerg Med 13:525–529, 2006.

29. **How is defibrillation best accomplished?**
As with any resuscitation, rhythm should be carefully checked after airway and breathing are established. Ventricular fibrillation should be carefully confirmed before defibrillation is attempted. Unmonitored defibrillation of a child is not recommended.

Defibrillation works by producing a mass polarization of myocardial cells with the intent of stimulating the return of a spontaneous sinus rhythm. Once ventricular fibrillation is diagnosed, prepare the patient for defibrillation and correct acidosis and hypoxemia. High-amplitude (coarse) fibrillation is more easily reversed than low-amplitude (fine) fibrillation. Administration of epinephrine can help coarsen fibrillation.

Defibrillation is most effective with use of the largest paddle that makes complete contact with the chest wall. Using the larger (8-cm diameter) paddle lowers the intrathoracic impedance and increases the effectiveness of the defibrillation current.

Take care to use an appropriate interface between the paddles and the chest wall. Electrode cream, paste, gel pads, or self-adhesive monitoring–defibrillation pads are preferred. Do not use saline-soaked gauze pads, ultrasound gel, alcohol pads, or bare paddles. Placement of the paste or pads must be meticulous, since electrical bridging across the surface of the chest results in ineffective defibrillation and, possibly, skin burns. When attempting defibrillation, guideline updates (2005) from the American Heart Association now state that immediate CPR should follow the delivery of one shock, rather than delivery of up to three shocks before CPR. These recommendations are based on the fact that the first shock eliminates ventricular fibrillation 85% of the time and studies have shown long delays typically occur between shocks when automated external defibrillators (AEDs) are used.

30. **Are AEDs useful for children with sudden collapse?**
    PALS guidelines as of 2005 now recommend use of AEDs for children 1 year of age and older. Newer models of AEDs have been shown to be able to reliably recognize shockable rhythms in children. There is not enough evidence to recommend use of AEDs for children under 1 year of age (*Class Indeterminate*).

    American Heart Association: 2005 Guidelines for Cardiopulmonary Resuscitation and Emergency Cardiovascular Care. Part 12: Pediatric Advanced Life Support. Circulation 112:167–187, 2005.

CHAPTER 2

NEONATAL RESUSCITATION

Constance M. McAneney, MD, MS

1. **What physiologic changes take place during the transition from intrauterine to extrauterine life?**
   The cardiopulmonary systems undergo a rapid change from fetal to extrauterine life. At birth the umbilical cord is clamped, and systemic vascular resistance rises. With the newborn's first breaths (increasing the neonate's PaO_2 and pH), pulmonary vascular resistance decreases, thereby causing an increase in pulmonary blood flow. Blood flow through the foramen ovale and the ductus arteriosus reverses direction, and then these structures eventually close. The ductus arteriosus is usually closed functionally by 15 hours of age.
   If the pulmonary vascular resistance does not fall adequately, a persistent right-to-left shunt will occur (persistent pulmonary hypertension). Inability to expand alveolar spaces can cause intrapulmonary shunting of blood (hypoxia). Disruption of fetal maternal circulation (placenta previa, abruption placentae) can result in acute blood loss and hypovolemia in the newly born infant.

2. **What preparation is necessary for the unexpected emergency department (ED) delivery?**
   Preparation is key, as most ED deliveries are "unexpected." A prearranged plan should be set in motion as soon as birth is imminent. That plan should include the assembly of personnel who are best able to take care of the newly born infant. A brief history should be obtained if possible because it may affect the resuscitation. Equipment and medications specifically for a neonatal resuscitation should be kept in a designated tray so they are quickly available (Table 2-1). Periodic inspection of this equipment for proper functioning and expiration dates of medication should become part of the routine upkeep of the neonatal resuscitation tray.

3. **What problems should be anticipated for a preterm delivery ($<$ 37 weeks' gestation)?**
   Preterm babies have immature lungs that may be more difficult to ventilate and more prone to injury by positive-pressure ventilation. Premature infants are also more prone to intracranial hemorrhage because they have immature blood vessels in the brain. In addition, these infants are at risk for rapid heat loss because of their thin skin and large surface area. Finally, premature infants are at increased risk for infection and hypovolemic shock caused by small blood volume.

   American Heart Association: Part 13: Neonatal Resuscitation Guidelines. Circulation 112:IV-188–195, 2005.

4. **What are the critical facts in the history that should be elicited, if possible, prior to delivery?**
   The **standard maternal history** is important but may need to wait until after delivery because of the imminent birth of the infant. Critical information may need to be narrowed to facts that may affect the immediate preparation (equipment and personnel) for the delivery:

TABLE 2-1. EQUIPMENT AND DRUGS FOR THE NEONATAL RESUSCITATION

Equipment

- Gowns, gloves, and masks
- Warm towels and blankets
- Bulb syringe
- Meconium aspirator
- Suction catheters (sizes 5–10 Fr)
- Face masks (sizes premature, newborn, and infant)
- Oral airways (sizes 000, 00, 0)
- Anesthesia bag with manometer (preferably 500 mL, no larger than 750 mL)
- Laryngoscope with straight blades (sizes 0 and 1)
- Spare bulbs and batteries
- Stethoscope
- Endotracheal tubes (sizes 2.5, 3.0, 3.5, 4.0) and stylet
- Tape
- Umbilical catheters (3.5 and 5 Fr)
- Oxygen source with flow meter
- Umbilical catheter tray
- Three-way stopcocks
- Nasogastric feeding tubes (8 and 10 Fr)
- Needles and syringes
- Chest tubes (8 and 10 Fr)
- Magill forceps
- Radiant warmer
- Cardiorespiratory monitor with electrocardiography leads
- Pulse oximeter with neonatal probes
- Suction equipment and tubing
- Pulse oximeter with newborn probe
- End-tidal CO_2 detector
- Laryngeal mask airway (optional)

Drugs

- Epinephrine 1:10,000
- Naloxone
- Sodium bicarbonate
- Dextrose in water 10%
- Normal saline, lactated Ringer's
- Resuscitation drug chart

- It is important to know if the expectant mother knows **if she is having twins.** Additional resuscitation equipment as well as personnel should be quickly gathered. Ideally there should be a resuscitation area, equipment, and personnel for each expected newly born infant.

- The **expected due date** is crucial to determine if the newly born infant will be premature and, if so, approximately how premature. Infants born at less than 36 weeks' gestation are more likely to be born "unexpectedly" and will have an increased risk of needing resuscitation. Smaller-caliber equipment will be needed.

- The **color of the amniotic fluid** is important. If the fluid is meconium stained (greenish), then one should anticipate a distressed newly born infant with or without airway obstruction from the meconium. The infant may require intubation with suctioning. Equipment should be available and personnel should be aware of this clinical situation.

Hazinski MF (ed): Textbook of Pediatric Advanced Life Support. Dallas, American Heart Association, 2002.

5. **What steps should be taken initially to care for the newly born infant?**
Since newly born infants do not tolerate cold, and hypothermia can prolong acidosis, prevent heat loss as much as possible. Dry the infant of the amniotic fluid and place the newborn in slight Trendelenburg position, on his or her back with the neck slightly extended, under a prewarmed radiant warmer. Suction the mouth and then nose with the bulb syringe or catheter. Duration of the suctioning should not exceed 5 seconds, and the tip should not be passed farther than 5 cm. Vigorous suctioning will cause bradycardia. Usually by drying and suctioning the infant, he or she is adequately stimulated to begin effective respirations. Gently flicking the heels and rubbing the back are additional stimulation methods. Avoid vigorous stimulation. Wrapping the newly born infant in warmed blankets will reduce heat loss.

6. **How can a very–low-birthweight premature newborn infant (< 1500 gm) be kept warm in the ED?**
Drying and swaddling, warming pads, increased environmental temperature, covering with a blanket, and placing the baby skin-to-skin with the mother have all been used to keep newborns warm. These techniques have not been evaluated in controlled trials and may not be enough to warm very small newborns. Very–low-birthweight infants may need additional warming techniques, such as covering the infant in plastic wrapping (food-grade, heat-resistant plastic) and placing him or her under radiant heat.

Costeloe K, Hennessy E, Gibson AT, et al: The EPICure study: Outcomes to discharge from hospital for infants born at the threshold of viability. Pediatrics 106:659–671, 2000.

7. **How do you assess the condition of a newly born infant?**
The basic principles for the newly born infant are the same as for any patient. However, there are particular problems of the neonate that bear special attention. After placing the neonate under the prewarmed radiant warmer on his or her back, dry and suction the baby (see Question 5). Carefully observe the respiratory effort and rate. If cyanosis or other signs of distress are noticed, administer oxygen. If the respiratory response is inadequate, stimulate the infant again and reposition. Adequacy of respirations is based on the rate (usually 35–60 breaths per minute), the effort (lack of retractions and grunting), and breath sounds. If the respiratory effort continues to be suboptimal (absent, slow, shallow), begin positive-pressure ventilation. If the respiratory effort is adequate, then evaluate the heart rate.

The **heart rate** is a critical measurement in determining the condition of the infant. Determine the heart rate by listening to the apical area with a stethoscope or palpating the pulse at the base of the umbilical cord. The normal heart rate of the newly born infant is above 100 beats per minute and is generally 120–150 beats per minute. If the heart rate is less than 100 beats per minute, begin positive-pressure ventilation. If the heart rate is greater than 100 beats per minute with spontaneous respirations, continue the assessment.

Assess the **newborn's color** for the presence of pallor and cyanosis. Pallor could indicate hypovolemia, anemia, hypoglycemia, decreased cardiac output, or acidosis. Cyanosis of the distal extremities or acrocyanosis is common and not a sign of hypoxia. Central cyanosis requires oxygen administration. If the neonate is still cyanotic despite oxygen therapy and positive-pressure ventilation, begin an organized workup for life-threatening illnesses, such as heart disease, sepsis, congenital anomalies, and diaphragmatic hernia.

Finally, assign an **Apgar score** at 1 minute and at 5 minutes of life (Table 2-2). The Apgar score assesses heart rate, respirations, muscle tone, reflex irritability, and color. It indicates how the infant is doing or the responsiveness to the resuscitation. If the Apgar score is less than 7 at 5 minutes, continue scoring every 5 minutes. *Do not delay resuscitative efforts to obtain an Apgar score.*

Owen CJ, Wyllie JP: Determination of heart rate in the baby at birth. Resuscitation 60(2):213–217, 2004.

8. **When does the newly born infant need assistance with ventilation?**
    Approximately 10% of newly born infants require some assistance to begin breathing at birth, and 1% require extensive resuscitation measures. After the infant has been quickly assessed and found to have apnea or gasping respirations, initiate positive-pressure ventilation with oxygen. Also, initiate positive-pressure ventilation if the heart rate is less than 100 beats per minute because bradycardia in a newborn is usually due to hypoxia. Persistent central cyanosis despite 100% oxygen is another indication to begin positive-pressure ventilation.

    American Heart Association: Part 13: Neonatal Resuscitation Guidelines. Circulation 112:IV-188–195, 2005.

9. **What is the proper technique to assist ventilations in the newly born infant?**
    The mask should fit around the nose and mouth but not cover the eyes or go below the chin. Assisted ventilations should be at a rate of 40–60 breaths per minute (30 breaths per minute when chest compressions are being performed), but controversy exists over the rate. The initial breaths may require higher inflation pressures and longer inflation times. The effectiveness of the assisted ventilations is judged by the movement of the chest, adequacy of breath sounds, and the heart rate. If the condition of the neonate does not improve, then reposition the head, check for patency of the airway, improve the seal of the mask on the face, and increase the inflating pressure of the bag.

TABLE 2-2. APGAR SCORE

Sign	Score		
	0	1	2
Heart rate	Absent	Slow (<100/min)	>100/min
Respirations	Absent	Slow, irregular	Good, crying
Muscle tone	Limp	Some flexion	Active motion
Reflex irritability (catheter in nares)	No response	Grimace	Cough Sneezes
Color	Blue or pale	Pink body with blue extremities	Completely pink

10. **What are the indications for tracheal intubation of the newly born infant?**
    Indications for intubation vary but are based on the degree of respiratory depression, the success of ventilation efforts, the presence of meconium, the degree of prematurity, and the skill of the health care provider. There is controversy at every turn. For instance, some neonatal experts feel that early intubation in infants younger than 28 weeks is indicated, while others suggest that these infants can be handled with mask or nasal prong continuous positive airway pressure.
    Endotracheal intubation is indicated if a neonate:
    ■ Has not responded to assisted ventilations with a bag-mask
    ■ Is extremely low birthweight (< 1000 gm)
    ■ Requires chest compressions
    ■ Needs tracheal administration of medications
    ■ Has signs of respiratory depression with meconium
    ■ Has special circumstances (diaphragmatic hernia)
    Laryngeal masks may be used as an alternative airway method by trained providers when bag-mask ventilation is ineffective or attempts at endotracheal intubation have been unsuccessful.

    American Heart Association: Part 13: Neonatal Resuscitation Guidelines. Circulation 112:IV-188–195, 2005.

11. **How should endotracheal intubation of the newborn be performed?**
    Perform the tracheal intubation by the oral route, using an uncuffed endotracheal tube and a laryngoscope with a straight blade (size 0 for premature baby, size 1 for term baby). If a stylet is used, it should not protrude beyond the end of the tube. Cricoid pressure may be needed. After the endotracheal tube is passed through the vocal cords, check the position by observing symmetrical chest wall movement, listening for breath sounds at the axillae, and noting the absence of breath sounds over the stomach. Confirm the absence of gastric inflation; watch for condensation in the endotracheal tube during exhalation; and note the improvement in heart rate, color, and activity of the newborn. A prompt increase in heart rate is the best indicator that the tube is in the tracheobronchial tree and providing effective ventilation. Confirm tube placement with a CO_2 monitor. Exhaled CO_2 detection is effective for confirmation of endotracheal tube placement in infants, including very–low-birthweight infants. Confirmation of tube placement by radiograph is also recommended. The guide for the proper size of the endotracheal tube size is:

    Endotracheal tube size = gestational age in weeks/10

    The proper depth of insertion can be estimated by:

    Insertion depth at lip in centimeters = weight in kilograms + 6 cm

    American Heart Association: Part 13: Neonatal Resuscitation Guidelines. Circulation 112:IV-188–195, 2005.
    Aziz HF, Martin JB, Moore JJ: The pediatric disposable end-tidal carbon dioxide detector role in endotracheal intubation in newborns. J Perinatol 19:110–113, 1999.

12. **When are chest compressions indicated in the resuscitation of the newly born infant?**
    Effective ventilation usually restores vital signs to normal in a newborn, and chest compressions are generally not needed. Because chest compressions make effective ventilations more difficult and the heart rate usually responds to assisted ventilation, chest compressions are not initiated until assisted ventilation has been started. The indications for the initiation of chest compressions during the resuscitation of the newly born infant are absent heart rate, or heart rate less than 60 beats per minute despite adequate assisted ventilation for 30 seconds.

13. **What is the proper technique for chest compressions in the newborn?**
The two acceptable techniques for performing chest compressions are applying two thumbs superimposed or next to each other on the sternum with the fingers surrounding the chest, or two fingers placed on the sternum at a right angle to the chest with the other hand supporting the back. Data suggest that the two-thumb method may have the advantage of generating peak systolic and coronary perfusion, and it is preferred by providers. Placement on the chest is at the lower third of the sternum. The rate should be approximately 90 times per minute at a 3:1 ratio with assisted ventilations. Take care not to simultaneously provide a breath while compressing the chest. Compress the chest to one-third of the anterior–posterior diameter of the chest. Compressions must be adequate to generate a pulse. Reassess the heart rate every 30 seconds during this time and continue compressions until there is a spontaneous heart rate over 60 beats per minute.

American Heart Association: Part 13: Neonatal Resuscitation Guidelines. Circulation 112:IV-188–195, 2005.
David R: Closed chest cardiac massage in the newborn infant. Pediatrics 81:552–554, 1988.

14. **How does the resuscitation of the newly born infant differ if meconium is present in the amniotic fluid?**
Current recommendations no longer advise routine intrapartum oropharyngeal and nasopharyngeal suctioning for infants born to mothers with meconium staining of amniotic fluid. If the newborn has meconium-stained fluid and is not vigorous (decreased tone, absent or depressed respirations, or a heart rate less than 100 beats per minute), intubate the trachea immediately to suction out meconium. This is accomplished by suctioning while withdrawing the endotracheal tube from the airway. Repeat intubation with suctioning until no more meconium is suctioned. If the heart rate falls below 60 beats per minute, keep the endotracheal tube in place and initiate positive-pressure ventilation. Newer research indicates this technique is of no value if the infant is vigorous. Delay gastric suctioning until the initial resuscitation is complete. Meconium-stained newborns who develop respiratory depression should receive tracheal suctioning prior to positive-pressure ventilation.

American Heart Association: Part 13: Neonatal Resuscitation Guidelines. Circulation 112:IV-188–195, 2005.
Wiswell TE, Gannon CM, Jacob J, et al: Delivery room management of the apparently vigorous meconium stained neonate: Results of the multicenter, international collaborative trial. Pediatrics 105:1–7, 2000.

15. **What are the most common drugs used in a neonatal resuscitation, and when are they indicated?**
Drugs are rarely used in neonatal resuscitation as most problems are improved by addressing airway, breathing, and circulation. Bradycardia in the newborn infant is usually due to inadequate lung inflation and hypoxemia, so adequate ventilation is most important.
- **Epinephrine** is recommended when the heart rate remains below 60 beats per minute despite adequate ventilation with 100% oxygen and chest compressions for 30 seconds. Evidence from neonatal models shows increased diastolic and mean arterial pressures in response to epinephrine. The current recommended dose for epinephrine during the neonatal resuscitation is 0.01 to 0.03 mg/kg of 1:10,000 concentration (0.1–0.3 mL/kg). High-dose epinephrine is not recommended for neonates because of the rare incidence of ventricular fibrillation and the theoretical risk of a hypertensive response, which could result in intraventricular hemorrhage.
- **Atropine** is a parasympathetic drug that decreases vagal tone and **is not** recommended in neonatal resuscitation. Bradycardia in the neonate is usually caused by hypoxia, and therefore atropine is unlikely to be beneficial.
- **Naloxone** is a narcotic antagonist that is indicated in the newborn with respiratory depression thought to be secondary to drugs given to the mother during delivery. The dose of naloxone is 0.1 mg/kg, delivered through the IV or IM route. Because of the short half-life relative to most narcotics, repeat doses may be required, and careful observation of the neonate after

administration is necessary. Do not give naloxone to infants of mothers who have recently abused narcotics because it will precipitate an acute withdrawal syndrome in the newborn. Endotracheal administration of naloxone to newborns is not recommended because of lack of clinical data.

- **Sodium bicarbonate** helps to reverse systemic acidosis and is indicated in neonatal resuscitation after adequate ventilation is established and metabolic acidosis is suspected. If adequate ventilation is not established, the metabolic acidosis will be replaced by respiratory acidosis. Other complications from bicarbonate include hypernatremia and intraventricular hemorrhage. The recommended dose of sodium bicarbonate is 1 to 2 mEq/kg in a dilute solution of 0.5 mEq/mL given slowly at 1 mEq/kg/min.
- Volume expanders such as **crystalloids** (normal saline or lactated Ringer's) and **colloids** (blood) are indicated for signs of hypovolemia. Signs of hypovolemia in the neonate include pallor, weak pulses, or poor response to resuscitative efforts. The dose for volume expanders is 10 mL/kg, with reassessment after each dose. Isotonic crystalloids are the first choice in volume expanders. Red blood cells (O negative) are indicated in situations of large blood loss. Albumin is less frequently used because of limited availability, risk of infection, and an association with increased mortality.

Gibbs J, Newson T, Williams J, et al: Naloxone hazard in infants of opioid abusers. Lancet 2:159–160, 1989.

Lokesh L, Kumar P, Murki S, Narang A: A randomized controlled trail of sodium bicarbonate in neonatal resuscitation—effect on immediate outcome. Resuscitation 60:219–223, 2004.

Oca MJ, Nelson M, Donn SM: Randomized trial of normal saline versus 5% albumin for the treatment of neonatal hypotension. J Perinatol 23:473–476, 2003.

Perondi MB, Reis AG, Paiva EF, et al: A comparison of high-dose and standard-dose epinephrine in children with cardiac arrest. N Engl J Med 350:1722–1730, 2004.

16. **Where is the best place to obtain IV access?**
    The easiest and most direct access is the umbilical cord. Any medication, as well as volume expanders, can be given through the umbilical vein. Note that it is not recommended to administer resuscitative drugs via the umbilical artery. Peripheral veins in the extremities and the scalp can also be used but generally require more skill to access. Intraosseous lines can be used when no other access can be obtained. Drugs (e.g., epinephrine) can also be given via the endotracheal tube.

KEY POINTS: MAJOR GUIDELINE CHANGES AND RECOMMENDATIONS OF THE PEDIATRIC WORKING GROUP OF THE INTERNATIONAL LIAISON COMMITTEE ON RESUSCITATION ✓

1. Prevent hypothermia. Although some studies have suggested that cerebral hypothermia of the asphyxiated infant may protect against brain injury, it is not routinely recommended pending controlled human studies.

2. Prevent hyperthermia because it has been associated with perinatal respiratory depression.

3. Use 100% oxygen with positive-pressure ventilation. Although some studies have shown that lower inspired oxygen is useful in some settings, this is not recommended because of insufficient data.

4. A laryngeal mask may be used as an alternative airway method by trained providers when bag-mask ventilation is ineffective or attempts at endotracheal intubation have been unsuccessful.

5. Confirm endotracheal intubation with CO_2 detectors.

6. The two-thumb method of chest compressions is preferred for newborns, with the depth of compression being one-third of the anterior–posterior diameter of the chest rather than a fixed depth. Compression should be deep enough to generate a pulse.

7. Administer epinephrine if the heart rate remains 60 beats per minute after 30 seconds of adequate ventilation and chest compressions.

8. Albumin-containing solutions are no longer the fluid of choice for initial volume expansion. Isotonic crystalloids are the first choice.

9. Intraosseous access can be used if the umbilical vein is not readily available.

17. **Are there circumstances when resuscitation of the newly born infant may not be the appropriate action?**

Since all ED deliveries are considered "unexpected" and the ED physician rarely has a previous relationship with the delivering mother, conversations about withholding resuscitation are difficult at best. Antenatal information can be incomplete or inaccurate. In the ED, it may not be possible to gather this information quickly with precision and reliability. Guidelines should be developed after discussion with local resources and review of the most recent literature. Review the guidelines regularly and modify them on the basis of changes in resuscitation and neonatal intensive care practices.

If gestational age, birthweight, or congenital anomalies are associated with almost certain early death or high morbidity, resuscitation is not indicated. Examples include extreme prematurity (gestational age < 23 weeks, birthweight < 400 gm), anencephaly, and chromosomal abnormalities incompatible with life (trisomy 13).

American Heart Association: Part 13: Neonatal Resuscitation Guidelines. Circulation 112:IV-188–195, 2005.

RESPIRATORY FAILURE

Mark D. Joffe, MD

1. **Why is it so important to know about respiratory failure in children?**
   Children are at greater risk of respiratory failure than adults. Respiratory symptoms are one of the most common reasons children are taken to emergency departments (EDs) and the most frequent cause of cardiopulmonary arrest. The potential for progression of respiratory distress to respiratory failure necessitates prompt evaluation of children with respiratory symptoms. Much of the morbidity and mortality from respiratory disease in children can be prevented by competent pediatric emergency care.

2. **Why are children at greater risk for respiratory failure?**
   Children have greater metabolic requirements and greater need for oxygen on a per-kilogram basis when compared to adults. **Anatomic factors** put infants, in particular, at high risk for respiratory failure. Infants breathe almost exclusively through their noses because the nasopharynx is in close proximity to the more cephalad glottis and the infant tongue fills most of the oropharynx. Nasal obstruction, therefore, can cause significant respiratory signs and symptoms in infants. The caliber of infant airways is small, so respiratory resistance is much higher in infants, especially when they have inflammation of the respiratory tree. Alveoli have less collateral ventilation in infants. Thus, obstruction of small, peripheral airways is more likely to lead to atelectasis and hypoxemia. A compliant chest wall facilitates passage through the birth canal but leads to respiratory problems when airway resistance is increased. The diaphragm of infants is weaker and more easily fatigued compared with the diaphragm of older children and adults. Also, the inability of younger children to verbalize their symptoms may cause delayed presentations of respiratory problems.

3. **What are the clinical features of respiratory failure?**
   - Poor color (ashen or central cyanosis)
   - Obtunded mental status
   - Decreased chest wall movement, with or without signs of respiratory distress
   - Bradypnea or marked tachypnea

   American Heart Association, Subcommittee on Pediatric Resuscitation: Recognition of respiratory failure and shock. In Zritsky AL (ed): Pediatric Advanced Life Support Provider Manual, Dallas, American Heart Association, 2002, p 81.

4. **Why does respiratory resistance increase so significantly with inflammation of the respiratory tree?**
   The resistance to laminar air flow through a tube is inversely related to the radius to the fourth power (Poiseuille's law). Modest decreases in the radius of the lumen of the airway can lead to dramatic increases in respiratory resistance when airway caliber is small (Fig. 3-1).

5. **Why do children get respiratory infections so frequently?**
   The immature immune system puts infants at risk for respiratory infections. Children have less immunologic memory, so exposure to a particular respiratory pathogen is more likely to be a child's first. Young children playing together in a group tend to exchange contaminated

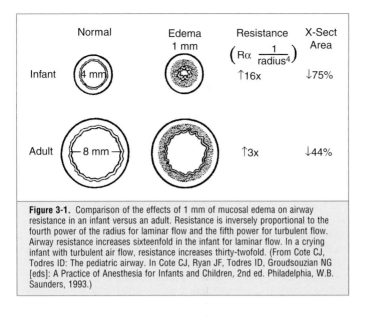

Figure 3-1. Comparison of the effects of 1 mm of mucosal edema on airway resistance in an infant versus an adult. Resistance is inversely proportional to the fourth power of the radius for laminar flow and the fifth power for turbulent flow. Airway resistance increases sixteenfold in the infant for laminar flow. In a crying infant with turbulent air flow, resistance increases thirty-twofold. (From Cote CJ, Todres ID: The pediatric airway. In Cote CJ, Ryan JF, Todres ID, Groudsouzian NG [eds]: A Practice of Anesthesia for Infants and Children, 2nd ed. Philadelphia, W.B. Saunders, 1993.)

respiratory secretions with particular aplomb. They do not know that frequent handwashing can dramatically reduce the spread of respiratory infections. Many adult caregivers do not recognize this as well.

6. **Are there different types of respiratory failure?**
   Some clinicians divide respiratory failure into two categories. The first type is generally caused by mismatch of ventilation and perfusion resulting from problems in the lung. This type of respiratory failure is characterized by hypoxemia with normal or low PCO_2. Other patients with respiratory failure have an overall decrease in alveolar ventilation that is usually the result of upper airway obstruction, neuromuscular disease, thoracic trauma, or muscle fatigue. These patients have relatively proportional decreases in PO_2 and increases in PCO_2. The physiology in most children with respiratory failure is a combination of these two types because one type often leads to the other. For instance, an infant with bronchiolitis initially may have hypoxemia from atelectasis and ventilation–perfusion mismatch, but may progress to inadequate alveolar ventilation when airway resistance is high and respiratory muscle fatigue supervenes.

7. **How do I know which of the numerous children with respiratory symptoms will progress to respiratory failure?**
   Predicting the future is difficult, but many clinical skills can be employed. A detailed history can give information about the vulnerability of the child to respiratory decompensation. Children who are very young, were born prematurely, have chronic pulmonary or cardiac diseases, or have immunodeficiencies are at particular risk. Recent medical advances, including the development of home nursing capabilities, have resulted in many "graduates" of intensive care nurseries living in our communities. EDs are confronted with these medically fragile children more than ever before.

   Diseases have a natural history that must be considered. If a child is evaluated early in the course of respiratory infection, you can anticipate that the child is likely to worsen before improvement will be noted. Intervention may vary depending upon the stage in the natural history of the disease a child is in at the time of the visit. Children with significant respiratory distress may worsen as their disease process progresses or as they become fatigued.

Young children are more difficult to assess for respiratory problems. Histories are obtained secondhand, as the parent interprets behaviors and relays observations that have been made. Young children with significant respiratory distress may remain happy and playful until fatigue suddenly sets in. A careful clinical assessment of the current degree of respiratory distress is necessary to identify those sicker patients who are more likely to develop respiratory failure.

8. **How do I assess respiration in a baby who screams every time I approach him?**
"Stranger anxiety" normally develops in the second half of the first year of life. The child's alertness to your presence is certainly a positive sign. Observing the child from across the room provides valuable information. General appearance, state of hydration, respiratory rate, nasal flaring, retractions, paradoxical respirations, and grunting can be appreciated without close proximity to the child. In many cases, the child is more cooperative if your approach is delayed, slow, and accompanied by soothing speech.

9. **What are paradoxical respirations? Why do they occur?**
Infants who have increased airway resistance need to generate high negative intrathoracic pressures to inflate their lungs. As the diaphragm moves downward and intrathoracic pressure becomes negative, the cartilaginous bones and weak intercostal musculature cannot maintain the thoracic circumference. As the abdomen moves outward, the chest collapses inward (rather than the normal expansion) on inspiration; hence the terms *paradoxical respirations*, *thoracoabdominal asynchrony*, or *see-saw breathing*. Paradoxical respirations are often a sign of impending respiratory failure.

10. **How can one tell if the respiratory failure is caused by an upper airway disease or by lower airway disease?**
Distinguishing upper from lower respiratory disease is a difficult but important part of clinical evaluation. Many children have disease processes that involve the upper and lower respiratory tracts simultaneously, for example, bronchiolitis caused by respiratory syncytial virus. In general, respiratory sounds reflecting upper airway inflammation are most prominent during inspiration, when negative intraluminal pressure causes upper airway narrowing. Conversely, intrathoracic (lower airway) processes produce wheezing and other sounds of airway obstruction primarily during expiration, when positive intrapleural pressure compresses intrathoracic airways. If breath sounds are more obstructed on inspiration, the upper airway is probably involved. Wheezing or other sounds more prominent during expiration suggests lower respiratory tract disease.

11. **Is wheezing a reliable sign of severe lower airway disease?**
No. Prominent wheezing requires significant airflow through narrowed small airways. Children with severe obstruction of small airways may have such great reduction of airflow that audible wheezing is not present. These children usually have decreased inspiratory breath sounds and increased work of breathing. Administration of bronchodilators to these patients will often increase wheezing because more air flows through the narrowed airways.

12. **What is the value of a chest radiograph in evaluation of a child with suspected respiratory failure?**
In previously normal children, respiratory failure is generally preceded by clinically identifiable respiratory distress. Young children with fever and tachypnea may benefit from a chest radiograph because bacterial pneumonia can be difficult to diagnose by history and physical examination alone. Foreign-body aspiration, pneumothorax/pneumomediastinum, and cardiac disease are a few of the diagnoses that can also be suspected on the basis of a chest radiograph. Children with minor respiratory illnesses generally do not need chest radiographs, even if they seek care in an ED. If there is concern about impending or existing respiratory failure, a chest radiograph can be very useful.

13. **Why do some people call pulse oximetry the fifth vital sign?**
    Hypoxemia is not always obvious from the physical examination. "The fifth vital sign" is a phrase used by those who feel pulse oximetry should become routine in the assessment of pediatric patients. Most children who are hypoxemic from a respiratory illness have signs of respiratory distress, but in some cases hypoxemia may be clinically inapparent. Hypoxemia is a less potent stimulator of the respiratory center than is hypercarbia. Thus, the increase in minute ventilation that occurs with mild hypoxemia is modest, and may be difficult to detect by physical examination. Cyanosis requires 3–5 gm of unsaturated hemoglobin per deciliter to be visible. If a child has a total hemoglobin of 12 gm/dL, cyanosis is not apparent until the oxygen saturation drops below 75%. Most clinicians believe it is useful to be aware of hypoxemia before it is severe enough to cause visible cyanosis.

14. **What's the big deal if the oxygen saturation is 2–3% below normal?**
    The relationship between PO_2 and saturation is not linear but sigmoidal. While there is little difference in PO_2 between saturations of 99% and 96%, there is a much greater difference between 93% and 90%. In children with bronchiolitis, oxygen saturation below 95% during feeding was the most useful factor in identifying infants who would have a more severe course of illness. Sleeping children with respiratory illnesses often have transient periods of desaturation that require no intervention. Oxygen therapy and closer monitoring should be considered if the desaturation is persistent (Fig. 3-2).

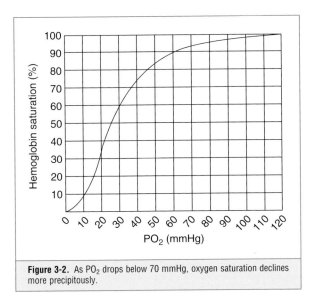

Figure 3-2. As PO_2 drops below 70 mmHg, oxygen saturation declines more precipitously.

15. **What causes pulse oximeter readings to be inaccurate?**
    The most common problem is the oximeter probe not consistently registering the pulsatile arterial flow through the skin. This is often caused by movement, poor perfusion of the skin, or bright ambient light. Careful attention to the graphical display of pulsatile flow on the pulse oximeter can almost always distinguish a falsely low saturation due to poor signal capture from true hypoxemia. Occasionally, hemoglobin is abnormal. Carboxyhemoglobinemia will cause a

falsely elevated measurement of oxygen saturation by pulse oximetry; methemoglobinemia in significant concentrations will cause a modest lowering.

Lee WW, Mayberry K, Crapo R, et al: The accuracy of pulse oximetry in the emergency department. Am J Emerg Med 18:427, 2000.

16. **Why are some children with severe respiratory distress well saturated, while others who look comfortable are hypoxemic?**

In most cases, hypoxemia is due to a mismatch of ventilation and perfusion, not to alveolar hypoventilation. As long as unventilated areas of the lung are not perfused because of hypoxic pulmonary vasoconstriction, systemic oxygen saturation may remain normal. Many children with respiratory distress have hypoxemia and hypocarbia, suggesting ventilation–perfusion mismatch despite alveolar hyperventilation. The absence of hypoxemia is not, by itself, reassurance that the child's respirations are adequate.

17. **Why do some patients with wheezing have a reduction in their oxygen saturation after bronchodilator treatment when they otherwise appear to be improving?**

Albuterol and other bronchodilators are β-adrenergic agents that are somewhat β2 selective. β2 receptor stimulation causes vasodilation as well as bronchodilation. One explanation for decreases in oxygen saturation noted after treatment with bronchodilators is that the agents cause some pulmonary vasodilation, resulting in increased perfusion of poorly ventilated areas of the lung and thereby worsening ventilation–perfusion matching. This is seen in a minority of patients; is usually a transient phenomenon; and is not a contraindication to continued, aggressive bronchodilator therapy in children with severe lower airway disease.

18. **Can respiratory failure be present without respiratory distress?**

Absolutely. Children may hypoventilate because of reduced level of consciousness (ingestion, metabolic derangements, head trauma) or neuromuscular dysfunction. After prolonged respiratory distress, children may become fatigued, and their work of breathing may appear normal in the presence of significant hypoventilation. Elevation of the PCO_2 may signal the presence of fatigue and hypoventilation.

19. **What is ARDS in children? Doesn't the "A" stand for *ADULT*?**

Acute respiratory distress syndrome (ARDS) occurs in children, so the "A" was changed from *adult* to *acute*. It is a common cause of respiratory failure at all ages. ARDS is a diffuse pulmonary process that develops after another condition injures the lung. Some causes of ARDS that are treated in EDs include sepsis, hypotension, pneumonia, aspiration of gastric contents, smoke or other inhalation injury, near drowning, and chest trauma with pulmonary contusion. Chest radiographs show diffuse, bilateral infiltrates that resemble left-sided congestive heart failure, but left atrial pressures must be normal for the diagnosis of ARDS. The diagnostic criteria for ARDS are as follows:

- Acute onset
- Severe hypoxemia ($PO_2 < 200$ mmHg regardless of fraction of inspired oxygen and positive end-expiratory pressure)
- Diffuse bilateral infiltrates on chest radiography
- Normal left atrial pressure

Bernard GR: Acute respiratory distress syndrome: A historical perspective. Am J Respir Crit Care Med 172:798, 2005.

20. **How is respiratory failure defined? When does respiratory *distress* become respiratory *failure*?**

A general definition of respiratory failure is inadequate oxygenation to meet metabolic needs and/or inadequate excretion of CO_2. Many specific definitions have been proposed, but the best clinicians individualize their decisions about therapy according to the particulars of the case. One definition is PO_2 <60 mmHg or O_2 saturation <93% on >60% oxygen, PCO_2 >60 mmHg and rising, or clinical apnea.

21. **Why are some patients who meet the definition for respiratory failure not intubated and mechanically ventilated to normalize their blood gases?**
Children tolerate hypercarbia better than adults do. If oxygenation is adequate, and hypercarbia is likely to be reversed in the near future, some intensivists permit the hypercarbia to persist for a period of time. So-called **permissive hypercarbia** reduces barotrauma to the lungs that results from mechanical ventilation. In patients with reactive airway disease or asthma, positive-pressure ventilation is fraught with risk of pneumomediastinum and pneumothorax. Since there are effective medications to reverse airway obstruction in a relatively short period of time, some patients can be closely monitored without endotracheal intubation and mechanical ventilation, despite levels of CO_2 that define respiratory failure.

22. **Is endotracheal intubation the only way to manage an airway in respiratory distress?**
No. In fact, bag-valve-mask ventilation is adequate for many children with transient, reversible airway problems. Positioning the child with some extension of the neck and moving the mandible forward by lifting the angles of the jaw pulls the tongue off the posterior pharynx, often relieving airway obstruction. Oral or nasal airways can be used to maintain the patency of the upper airway in selected patients. All children should receive effective bag-valve-mask ventilation with 100% oxygen prior to intubation.

American Heart Association: 2005 Guidelines for Cardiopulmonary Resuscitation and Emergency Cardiovascular Care. Part 11: Pediatric Basic Life Support. Circulation 112:156–166, 2005.

KEY POINTS: INDICATIONS FOR ENDOTRACHEAL INTUBATION ✓

1. Progressive respiratory exhaustion—unlikely to reverse quickly

2. Apnea, hypoventilation that requires mechanical ventilation

3. Need for airway protection (upper airway obstruction, loss of protective airway reflexes)

4. Shock

5. Need to improve pulmonary toilet

23. **What are the indications to intubate the trachea of a child?**
    - Respiratory failure that is unlikely to be reversed quickly, especially if hypoxemia is present despite >60% oxygen administration
    - Apnea, hypoventilation, or progressive respiratory exhaustion that requires ongoing mechanical ventilation
    - Need for airway protection for children who have upper airway obstruction or an inability to protect their airway from aspiration
    - Desire to decrease the work of breathing for patients in shock (under normal circumstances, work of breathing requires less than 5% of the total energy expenditure, but with respiratory

distress it can demand up to 50%; in a shock state, energy can be better utilized for other essential body functions)

- Therapeutic interventions, such as tracheal administration of medications and suctioning for pulmonary toilet (mechanical ventilation is also required)

KEY POINTS: STEPS TO PERFORM ENDOTRACHEAL INTUBATION ✓

1. Preoxygenate with 100% oxygen by bag-valve-mask device.

2. Prepare equipment (e.g., suction, endotracheal tubes, laryngoscopes).

3. Confirm functioning IV line.

4. Apply cricoid pressure (Sellick maneuver).

5. Administer medications (atropine, sedative, paralytic agent).

6. Intubate the trachea, observing the tube pass through the vocal cords.

7. Verify proper placement—auscultate the chest, check for CO_2 by capnometry, chest radiograph.

8. Secure the endotracheal tube.

24. **What are the steps for emergency endotracheal intubation of a child?**
Bag-valve-mask ventilation with 100% oxygen should begin as soon as the need for positive-pressure ventilation is identified. Emergency endotracheal intubations are generally treated as "full-stomach" intubations. The steps for a rapid sequence intubation are:
    1. Preoxygenate with bag-valve-mask ventilation with 100% oxygen.
    2. Prepare all equipment, including suction, endotracheal tubes, and laryngoscopes.
    3. Make certain an IV catheter is functioning well.
    4. Apply cricoid pressure (Sellick maneuver) to prevent passive regurgitation and aspiration. (Keep applying pressure until endotracheal tube is known to be in the trachea.)
    5. Administer atropine (for younger children), followed by a sedative agent and then a paralytic agent.
    6. Perform laryngoscopy once paralysis is complete, and watch the endotracheal tube go through the vocal cords into the trachea.
    7. Auscultate for equal breath sounds, and check for gurgling over the stomach, which suggests esophageal intubation. Observe symmetric chest expansion, misting in the tube with exhalation, improvement in oxygen saturation by pulse oximetry, and presence of CO_2 by capnometry.
    8. Release cricoid pressure.
    9. Secure the tube with tape.
    10. Obtain chest radiograph to check position of the tube and adjust accordingly.

American Heart Association: 2005 Guidelines for Cardiopulmonary Resuscitation and Emergency Cardiovascular Care. Part 12: Pediatric Advanced Life Support. Circulation 112:167–187, 2005.

King C, Stayer SA: Emergent endotracheal intubation. In Henretig FM, King C (eds): Textbook of Pediatric Emergency Procedures. Baltimore, Williams & Wilkins, 1997.

25. **Can a difficult endotracheal intubation be predicted?**

Not always, so it is important to have people experienced with airway management available, especially when a difficult intubation is anticipated. The following conditions often result in difficult intubations:

Congenital	Acquired
Micrognathia	Hoarseness/stridor/drooling
Macroglossia	Facial burns/singed facial hairs
Cleft or high-arched palate	Facial fractures/oral trauma
Protruding upper incisors	Foreign body
Small mouth	
Limited mobility of temporomandibular joint	

26. **What should you consider if a patient deteriorates after endotracheal intubation?**

If an intubated patient's condition deteriorates after endotracheal intubation, consider **DOPE**:

- **D**isplacement of the endotracheal tube—no longer in the trachea
- **O**bstruction of the tube—perhaps by mucus
- **P**neumothorax
- **E**quipment failure—perhaps the ventilator is malfunctioning or perhaps you are not actually delivering 100% oxygen as you thought

American Heart Association: 2005 Guidelines for Cardiopulmonary Resuscitation and Emergency Cardiovascular Care. Part 12: Pediatric Advanced Life Support. Circulation 112:167–187, 2005.

SHOCK

Brent R. King, MD, FACEP, FAAEM, FAAP

1. **What blood pressure defines shock in the pediatric patient?**

   Shock is not defined by the blood pressure or by any other vital sign. Shock exists when the patient's metabolic demand exceeds the body's ability to deliver oxygen and nutrients. This occurs most commonly when metabolic demand is normal or slightly elevated but delivery of oxygen and nutrients is dramatically reduced. Examples include excessive blood loss (hemorrhage) or excessive fluid loss (diarrhea). The shock state can and often does exist in the presence of a "normal" blood pressure.

   Bell LM: Shock. In Fleisher GM, Ludwig S, Henretig FM (eds): Textbook of Pediatric Emergency Medicine, 5th ed. Philadelphia, Lippincott Williams & Wilkins, 2006, pp 51–62.

KEY POINTS: DEFINITION OF SHOCK ✓

1. Shock is a condition in which the patient's metabolic requirements are unmet.

2. The shock state is a complex interplay between the physiologic insult and the host's response to that insult; both play a role.

3. In its earliest phase, shock might be recognized only by abnormal results of laboratory tests that measure tissue acid–base status (e.g., serum lactate). Overt clinical signs are seen as the shock state progresses.

2. **How can shock be recognized?**

   To recognize shock, consider both the consequences of inadequate perfusion and the patient's compensatory mechanisms. The clinical manifestations of shock are those of **inadequate perfusion** and **compensation**. Inadequate perfusion of the brain results in an alteration in the child's level of consciousness. Inadequate perfusion of the kidneys results in decreased urine output.

   As perfusion decreases, compensatory changes occur. These changes improve delivery of oxygen and nutrients and direct blood flow to the vital organs. The first compensatory mechanism is usually an **increased heart rate**. Since cardiac output is equal to the rate multiplied by the stroke volume, an increased heart rate can maintain cardiac output in the face of decreased stroke volume. Additionally, peripheral vasoconstriction helps to maintain blood flow to the central organs and to the brain. The patient therefore has pale, cool extremities and a delayed capillary refilling time. This increased vascular tone also affects the measured blood pressure. The diastolic pressure is slightly elevated, so the difference between the systolic and diastolic pressures—the pulse pressure—is smaller. This is referred to as a "narrowed" pulse pressure.

   To compensate for both the decreased oxygen delivery and the acidosis created by underperfusion of peripheral tissues, the respiratory rate increases. The blood pressure eventually falls, but this is a late finding and may signal that the shock state is irreversible.

3. **What are the stages of shock?**
   Shock is a spectrum of illness, so any division into discrete segments is somewhat artificial. However, shock is usually divided into two stages: *compensated shock* and *uncompensated shock*.

4. **What is compensated shock?**
   In early shock, various physiologic changes allow continued delivery of oxygen and nutrients to the heart, kidneys, brain, and other vital organs. Tachycardia is usually the first compensatory mechanism. The increased heart rate helps to maintain cardiac output in the face of low blood volume, excessive vasodilation, or pump failure. Increased vasomotor tone shunts blood away from the skin and the extremities to more vital organs. In compensated shock, the patient is able to continue to meet his or her metabolic demand, even if only marginally.

5. **Are there exceptions to the compensatory mechanisms described above?**
   Yes. In **septic shock** the patient sometimes develops so-called warm shock or warm distributive shock. In this state the patient has flushed skin and bounding pulses associated with a hyperdynamic precordium. This state can be explained by the cascade of inflammatory mediators that is responsible for the condition called septic shock. Likewise, in **neurogenic shock**, loss of sympathetic tone can result in bradycardia in the face of profound hypotension.

6. **What is uncompensated shock?**
   If the shock state progresses without interruption, the patient's compensatory mechanisms eventually fail. Hypoperfusion of organ systems causes acidosis and further release of inflammatory mediators. As blood flow to the brain decreases, the patient can become irritable or stuporous and eventually slips into coma. Likewise, decreased renal blood flow causes decreased urine output and finally results in anuria. The gastrointestinal tract is similarly affected, so the patient often has decreased bowel motility followed by distention and edema of the bowel wall. As tissue ischemia and acidosis progress, the inflammatory mediators cause diffuse vascular injury and capillary leakage. The pulmonary bed is especially sensitive to this type of injury. Damage to the pulmonary tissues exacerbates tissue hypoxemia. The ultimate result of progressive shock is multiorgan system failure and acute respiratory distress syndrome. At some point during this process the patient's blood pressure falls.

7. **What are the types (or mechanisms) of shock?**
   There are multiple mechanisms for shock. These include:
   - **Hypovolemic shock:** Hypovolemia, such as might occur with blood loss, vomiting, and/or diarrhea, decreases perfusion to the tissues and leads to shock.
   - **Distributive or vasodilatory shock:** This type of shock is the final common pathway of a variety of conditions that result in vasodilation. Neurogenic distributive shock is caused by a spinal cord injury that eliminates sympathetic innervation to the blood vessels, causing profound vasodilation and bradycardia. Accidental ingestion of vasodilating medications can also result in distributive shock. Anaphylaxis results in vasodilation, and, although anaphylaxis has many other components, shock is a part of the clinical picture. Septic shock is largely distributive in nature but is a complex process (see below).
   - **Cardiogenic shock:** Pump failure is the primary mechanism for cardiogenic shock. Decreased myocardial contractility makes adequate delivery of oxygen and nutrients impossible. Since children are very dependent on a normal heart rate to produce an adequate cardiac output, drugs and other conditions that cause bradycardia can lead to shock. The patient will have evidence of congestive heart failure, such as rales on pulmonary auscultation and peripheral edema. Viral myocarditis, hypertrophic cardiomyopathy, and certain myocardial depressant drugs can cause cardiogenic shock.
   - **Septic shock:** Many consider septic shock to be another form of distributive shock. In septic shock, a stimulus causes the formation of inflammatory mediators that result in profound

vasodilation and shock. However, some of these mediators also directly depress myocardial activity; thus, septic shock can have features of both distributive and cardiogenic shock.

Jones AE, Craddock PA, Tayal VS, Kline JA: Diagnostic accuracy of left ventricular function for identifying sepsis among emergency department patients with nontraumatic, symptomatic, undifferentiated hypotension. Shock 24:513–517, 2005.

8. **Is the pathophysiology of shock really that simple?**
No, it is exceedingly complex. What we refer to as "shock" is the final common pathway for a variety of physiologic insults. Whether the process starts with acute blood loss or with an overwhelming infection, eventually the host mounts a response to the insult, and this response—at least in some cases—seems to contribute to the shock state.

9. **What usually initiates septic shock?**
The most common and potent initiator of the inflammatory cascade called septic shock is exposure to **endotoxin**. Endotoxin is the lipopolysaccharide (LPS) coat of gram-negative bacteria. Other bacterial and viral agents can also start this process. Examples include certain viral proteins and teichoic acid.

10. **Is septic shock caused by gram-positive organisms different from septic shock caused by gram-negative organisms?**
Yes, gram-negative septic shock is more severe. The expected mortality from gram-negative septic shock is 20–50%, while that from gram-positive septic shock is 10–20%.

11. **How do proteins such as endotoxin cause septic shock?**
This is a trick question. Endotoxin and the other bacterial and viral proteins do not actually cause septic shock. Instead, their presence in the body leads to a response from the host. This response involves a **cascade of inflammatory mediators** that are responsible for most of the symptoms of shock.

12. **What are these inflammatory mediators called?**
They are called cytokines.

13. **Which of the cytokines is the most important?**
Tumor necrosis factor appears to be the most important of the cytokines. Its formation seems to initiate and propagate the remainder of the inflammatory cascade.

Glauser MP: The inflammatory cytokines: New developments in the pathophysiology and treatment of septic shock. Drugs 52(2 Suppl):9–17, 1996.

14. **Describe how the cascade of septic shock begins.**
Most commonly, endotoxin (LPS) is bound by a plasma protein called LPS-binding protein (LBP). The LPS–LBP complex then binds to the CD14 receptor on the surfaces of macrophages. This process stimulates the formation of both tumor necrosis factor and interleukin. These two cytokines begin the cascade that leads to septic shock.

15. **What is the role of activated protein C in the treatment of pediatric septic shock?**
Sadly, this agent does not have a role in the treatment of pediatric septic shock. While studies of adults showed that activated protein C conferred a modest survival advantage, a large phase IIIb pediatric trial was terminated following a recommendation by the Data Monitoring Committee based on "futility due to an unfavorable benefit/risk profile."

16. **Which is more important in the management of the child with septic shock: aggressive resuscitation at the referring hospital or excellent care at the tertiary care center?**
While both are important, a recent study demonstrated that children in shock from sepsis who are aggressively resuscitated at the referring hospital have better outcomes than those who

do not receive such care. Theses results support the notion that management of shock must begin as soon as it is recognized.

Han YY, Carcillo JA, Dragotta MA, et al: Early reversal of pediatric-neonatal septic shock by community physicians is associated with improved outcome. Pediatrics 112:793–799, 2003.

17. **What is the most common cause of shock in children?**
Hypovolemia is the most common cause of shock in children.

18. **What is the usual cause of hypovolemia?**
Throughout most of the world, hypovolemia is caused by diarrheal illness. Millions of children die of hypovolemia caused by diarrhea each year.

19. **What are some ways in which trauma can cause shock?**
Posttraumatic hemorrhage is the most common way that trauma causes shock. Because young children have abdominal wall muscles that are poorly developed, they are at risk for liver and spleen injury after blunt abdominal trauma.
   In addition to hemorrhagic shock, blunt chest trauma can result in a tension pneumothorax. Tension pneumothorax causes increased intrathoracic pressure, which in turn reduces venous return to the heart and causes shock. Similarly, blunt chest trauma can result in pericardial tamponade (essentially a form of restrictive cardiomyopathy).
   Finally, cervical spine injury can result in neurogenic shock.

20. **How does isolated head trauma cause shock?**
It doesn't. If a patient has shock after what appears to be isolated head trauma, there must be another explanation for the shock.

KEY POINTS: ETIOLOGY OF SHOCK IN CHILDREN ✓

1. Hypovolemia (not enough circulating volume to deliver oxygen and nutrients)
2. Impaired cardiac function (ineffective pumping of the circulating volume)
3. Inappropriate vasodilation (the circulating volume exists primarily in the venous capacitance system and is unavailable to deliver oxygen and nutrients)

21. **How is hemorrhage classified?**
Hemorrhage is divided into four classes based on the amount of blood loss. Class I hemorrhage produces the least amount of blood loss, and class IV, the greatest.

22. **How do the classes of hemorrhage relate to shock?**
There is no direct relationship. In fact, a patient can experience class I hemorrhage without demonstrating signs of shock. However, as patients experience greater degrees of hemorrhage, they are more likely to have symptoms of shock.

23. **What are the classes of hemorrhage?**
   ■ **Class I hemorrhage:** The patient has lost up to 15% of his or her blood volume. Otherwise healthy patients are likely to have minimal tachycardia and no other symptoms. Unless there is ongoing hemorrhage, the patient should require no treatment.
   ■ **Class II hemorrhage:** The patient has lost 15–30% of his or her blood volume. Loss of this amount of blood stimulates the compensatory mechanisms usually associated with early,

compensated shock. Tachycardia, increased respiratory rate, and narrowed pulse pressure are seen. Urine output is usually maintained, but the patient may have signs of early central nervous system impairment. Such signs may include fright or anxiety.

- **Class III hemorrhage:** The patient has lost 30–40% of his or her blood volume. This amount of blood loss is clearly associated with signs of compensated shock but may also be associated with uncompensated shock. Even healthy individuals may have a drop in systolic blood pressure with this degree of blood loss. Urine output is likely to be decreased, and the patient may be very anxious or confused.
- **Class IV hemorrhage:** This represents loss of more than 40% of the circulating blood volume. This degree of hemorrhage is uniformly fatal if untreated. The shock state may, in some cases, be irreversible. The patient has a markedly decreased blood pressure. He or she can be expected to have complete peripheral vasoconstriction, extreme tachycardia, and little or no urinary output. Mental status is very depressed, and the patient may be unconscious.

24. **How can emergency physicians make a presumptive diagnosis of cardiogenic shock?**

Recent studies have demonstrated that emergency physicians using bedside ultrasonography can correctly identify cardiac wall motion abnormalities. This technology makes it easy for the emergency physician to identify patients with abnormal cardiac function.

Dey I, Sprivulis P: Emergency physicians can reliably assess emergency department patient cardiac output using the USCOM continuous wave Doppler cardiac output monitor. Emerg Med Austr 17:193–199, 2005.
Hollenberg SM, Kavinsky CJ, Parrillo JE: Cardiogenic shock. Ann Intern Med 131:47–59, 1999.

25. **How can neurogenic shock be distinguished from hemorrhagic shock?**

The patient with hemorrhagic shock has a rapid and possibly irregular pulse, while the patient with neurogenic shock has a slow and regular pulse.

26. **In general, what is the initial treatment for shock?**

There is no single treatment for shock: Therapy is aimed at the cause. That being said, most types of shock respond well to fluid therapy, so if the cause cannot be identified, a single bolus of 20 mL/kg of either normal saline or lactated Ringer's may be helpful and, at worst, is unlikely to cause serious harm. Additionally, the patient should receive supplemental oxygen and may require assisted ventilation to ensure that oxygen delivery is maximized.

27. **Which treatments should be avoided?**

The greatest error that you can make in the treatment of shock is to use pressor agents to treat hypovolemia. Even in cases of distributive shock, fluids should be used for initial treatment. Note that excessive fluid administration can be harmful in cardiogenic shock.

28. **How should hypovolemic shock be treated?**

Treat hypovolemia with volume. Initial therapy is usually crystalloids. Acceptable crystalloids are lactated Ringer's and normal saline. Give boluses of 20 mL of fluid per kilogram of body weight. Up to 60 mL/kg can be given before considering other therapy. Patients with severe (class III and IV) hemorrhage usually require blood replacement therapy.

29. **What is the treatment for neurogenic shock?**

In neurogenic shock, injury to the spinal cord results in decreased sympathetic input to the vascular system. Most of the patient's blood supply is left in the venous or capacitance system. **Fluid therapy** is an appropriate initial treatment, but pressor agents may also be needed. **Norepinephrine** is a powerful α-agonist and is often recommended for neurogenic shock. **Metaraminol** is an excellent alternative to norepinephrine. If the patient has profound bradycardia, **atropine** may be used to increase the heart rate and, therefore, the cardiac output.

In field situations or as a temporizing measure in the emergency department, a military antishock garment (MAST) can be applied to patients with neurogenic shock. The garment increases peripheral vascular resistance and thus compensates for some of the loss of sympathetic innervation.

Chiles BW III, Cooper PR: Current concepts: Acute spinal injury. N Engl J Med 334:514–520, 1996.

30. **Is the MAST garment useful in other kinds of shock?**
    The MAST garment has been the subject of intense research since it was introduced during the Vietnam War. The available literature suggests that the MAST garment has a very limited role in the management of shock. It may help to stabilize pelvic fractures and may be of some use in patients who require prolonged transport to a definitive care center. As discussed, it may also be useful in the management of certain patients in neurogenic shock.

31. **When should the MAST garment be avoided?**
    There is only one absolute contraindication to the use of the MAST garment. The garment increases peripheral vascular resistance (afterload) and therefore is contraindicated in patients with cardiogenic shock or potential cardiogenic shock (pulmonary edema). In general, it should be avoided in patients with impaled objects in the chest or abdomen, evisceration of the abdominal contents, and pregnancy. There is strong evidence against the use of MAST garments in patients with penetrating injuries to the chest, particularly in cases of penetrating cardiac injury.

32. **How should the patient with septic shock be treated?**
    Treatment of septic shock is difficult and complex. Fluid therapy is usually employed first, but pressor agents are often required. Treatment with antibodies directed against the inflammatory mediators has not proven to be effective, but as our understanding of this complex process evolves, effective immunomodulator therapy may be developed. Interestingly, although antibiotics are needed to limit the infectious process, they alone are not sufficient treatment for septic shock. In certain cases, they may actually increase the antigen load in the system by destroying gram-negative organisms, which results in more LPS in the circulatory system. However, patients who do not receive adequate antibiotic therapy have a higher mortality than those receiving such therapy.

Carcillio JA, Fields AI, Task Force Committee Members: Clinical practice parameters for hemodynamic support of pediatric and neonatal patients in septic shock. Crit Care Med 30:1365–1378, 2002.

33. **How should I choose an appropriate antibiotic for the patient in septic shock?**
    Septic shock is a severe and life-threatening condition and should be treated promptly. It may, however, be impossible to identify the causative organism in a timely fashion. Therefore, empirically administer antibiotic therapy. In most cases, it is prudent to choose broad-spectrum agents that are effective against a wide range of likely pathogens.

Schexnayder SM: Pediatric septic shock. Pediatr Rev 20:303–308, 1999.

34. **Under what circumstances might the drug phenylephrine be useful in the management of shock?**
    Phenylephrine causes vasoconstriction without causing excessive tachycardia. In the patient whose shock state is caused primarily by vasodilation, phenylephrine might be indicated.

35. **What is early, goal-directed therapy?**
    Early, goal-directed therapy is a management scheme that has been shown to be effective in the treatment of adult patients with sepsis and septic shock. There are four basic components of early, goal-directed therapy: (1) early recognition of the patient who is at risk for physiologic compromise using metabolic markers such as serum lactate; (2) correction of hypovolemia

and cardiovascular function using predetermined goals or endpoints (e.g., fluid resuscitation until the central venous pressure has reached 8–12 mmHg); (3) prevention of sudden cardiopulmonary dysfunction; and (4) interruption of the inflammatory cascade created by cellular hypoxemia.

Rivers E, Nguyen B, Havstad S, et al: Early goal-directed therapy in the treatment of severe sepsis and septic shock. N Engl J Med 345:1368–1377, 2001.

36. How should anaphylactic shock be treated?
Most manifestations of anaphylaxis, including hypotension, respond well to intramuscular epinephrine. Epinephrine has both α- and β-receptor agonist effects, so it can effectively treat bronchospasm and hypotension.

American Heart Association: 2005 Guidelines for Cardiopulmonary Resuscitation and Emergency Cardiovascular Care. Part 10.6: Anaphylaxis. Circulation 112:143–145, 2005.

37. What is toxic shock syndrome (TSS)?
TSS is an illness characterized by fever, erythroderma, hypotension, and involvement of several other organ systems. It is caused by strains of *Staphylococcus aureus* that produce an exotoxin (TSST-1, enterotoxin B, enterotoxin C). It is most often associated with prolonged use of tampons, but young children (boys and girls) with open skin wounds or minor abrasions can also develop toxic shock syndrome.

38. How do the exotoxins cause shock?
TSST-1 and the other exotoxins are profound vasodilators, and their effect causes distributive shock. Additionally, vasodilation seems to cause rapid movement of fluids and serum proteins to the extravascular space, leading to intravascular volume depletion. Exotoxins also have a direct effect upon the heart that results in decreased myocardial function. Finally, many patients with TSS experience vomiting or diarrhea, which leads to further volume depletion.

39. Are there other forms of TSS?
Yes, a clinical syndrome very similar to TSS has developed in association with group A streptococcal infections (*Streptococcus pyogenes*). Group A streptococci produce exotoxins very similar to those produced by staphylococci. These toxins are called streptococcal pyogenic exotoxins (SPEs). There are three of these: SPEs A, B, and, C. SPE A has long been associated with the clinical features of scarlet fever. Exactly why these toxins have recently become more virulent is unknown.

ABDOMINAL PAIN

Reza J. Daugherty, MD, and Jill C. Posner, MD

1. **Why is the evaluation of abdominal pain especially challenging in the pediatric patient?**

   Infants with abdominal pain may present with nonspecific signs, such as irritability, poor feeding, and lethargy. Toddlers and preschool children may report pain but are unable to provide further details, such as the quality or location of the pain. The physical examination of a child requires time and patience on the part of the examiner. The history and a physical examination of the abdomen may be more difficult to obtain with children. In addition to the more common causes, the differential diagnosis of abdominal pain in children includes a host of disorders unique to the pediatric patient, such as congenital anatomic abnormalities, Henoch-Schönlein purpura, abdominal migraines, or metabolic disorders.

   McCollough M, Sharieff GO: Abdominal surgical emergencies in infants and young children. Emerg Med Clin North Am 21:909–935, 2003.

   Pollack ES: Pediatric abdominal surgical emergencies. Pediatr Ann 25:448–457, 1996.

2. **How can I organize my approach to the patient?**

   In the unstable patient, the initial approach should begin with an assessment of the patient's airway, breathing, and circulation. Following stabilization, obtain a complete history and perform a physical examination. The history and physical examination are the essential components of the evaluation. Elicit the nature of the pain, such as its onset, quality, location, and duration, as well as the presence of any associated symptoms. The differential diagnosis of abdominal pain in children is extensive (Table 5-1). The age of the patient and the most likely diagnoses in that age group can be used in concert with the history and physical examination to narrow the differential and guide further diagnostic testing.

3. **What are the life-threatening causes of abdominal pain?**
   - Appendicitis
   - Intussusception
   - Incarcerated hernia
   - Trauma (accidental or inflicted injury)
   - Tumors
   - Sepsis
   - Volvulus
   - Ectopic pregnancy
   - Diabetic ketoacidosis
   - Intra-abdominal abscess (pelvic inflammatory disease, inflammatory bowel disease)
   - Aortic aneurysm
   - Toxic ingestion (iron, lead, aspirin)

4. **What are some extraintestinal causes of abdominal pain?**

   Pain originating at sites distant from the abdomen can be manifest by abdominal pain. In processes such as lower lobe pneumonia, afferent nerves from the parietal pleura share central pathways with those that originate from the abdominal wall. Similarly, scrotal pain may be

TABLE 5-1. CAUSES OF ACUTE ABDOMINAL PAIN

Infancy (<2 y)	Preschool Age (2–5 y)	School Age (>5 y)	Adolescent
Common			
Colic (age <3 mo)	Acute gastroenteritis	Acute gastroenteritis	Acute gastroenteritis
Acute gastroenteritis	Urinary tract infection	Trauma	Gastritis (primary or alcohol-induced)
"Viral syndromes"	Trauma	Appendicitis	Colitis (food intolerance)
	Appendicitis	Urinary tract infection	Trauma
	Pneumonia, asthma	Functional abdominal pain	Constipation
	Sickling syndromes	Sickling syndromes	Appendicitis
	"Viral syndromes"	Constipation	Pelvic inflammatory disease
	Constipation	"Viral syndromes"	Urinary tract infection
		Strep pharyngitis	Pneumonia, bronchitis, asthma
			"Viral syndromes"
			Dysmenorrhea
			Epididymitis
			Lactose intolerance
			Sickling syndromes
			Mittelschmerz
			Ovarian cyst

Relatively Uncommon

Trauma (possible child abuse)	Meckel's diverticulum	Pneumonia, asthma, cystic fibrosis	Ectopic pregnancy
Intussusception	Henoch-Schönlein purpura (anaphylactoid purpura)	Inflammatory bowel disease	Testicular torsion
Intestinal anomalies	Toxin	Peptic ulcer disease	Ovarian torsion
Incarcerated hernia	Cystic fibrosis	Cholecystitis, pancreatic disease	Renal calculi
Sickling syndromes	Intussusception	Diabetes mellitus	Peptic ulcer disease
	Nephrotic syndrome	Collagen vascular disease	Cholecystitis or pancreatic disease
		Testicular torsion	Meconium-ileus equivalent (cystic fibrosis)
			Collagen vascular disease
			Inflammatory bowel disease
			Toxin

Rare

Appendicitis	Incarcerated hernia	Rheumatic fever	Rheumatic fever
Volvulus	Neoplasm	Toxin	Tumor
Milk allergy	Hemolytic uremic syndrome	Renal calculi	Abdominal abscess
Tumors (e.g., Wilms' tumor)	Rheumatic fever, myocarditis, pericarditis	Tumor	
Toxin (heavy metal)	Hepatitis	Ovarian torsion	
Disaccharidase deficiency	Inflammatory bowel disease	Meconium-ileus equivalent (cystic fibrosis)	
Malabsorptive syndromes	Choledochal cyst	Intussusception	
	Hemolytic anemia	Pyomyositis of abdomen	
	Diabetes mellitus		
	Porphyria		

Reproduced from Ruddy RM: Pain—abdomen. In Fleisher GR, Ludwig S, Henretig FM (eds): Textbook of Pediatric Emergency Medicine, 5th ed. Philadelphia, Lippincott Williams & Wilkins, 2006, p 470, with permission.

referred to the abdomen. Other illnesses that are associated with abdominal pain include streptococcal pharyngitis, renal calculi, urinary tract infections, diabetes mellitus, ovarian disease (cyst, torsion, pelvic inflammatory disease), testicular disease, cholecystitis, pancreatitis, sickle cell vaso-occlusive crisis, lead toxicity, and porphyria.

5. **How can I maximize the physical examination of the pediatric patient with abdominal pain?**
The physical examination of a child requires patience on the part of the examiner, who must take time to establish rapport. Begin with observation, often best accomplished while unseen by the child. Notice the general appearance of the child. Is he lying still on the stretcher, suggesting peritonitis, or writhing with colicky pain? Is she able to climb off or onto the stretcher? Commence further inspection, auscultation, and palpation by examining the least threatening areas first and saving particularly invasive aspects of the examination for last (e.g., otoscopy). Lying the child with his or her knees flexed may facilitate relaxation of the rectus muscles. The child's "help" can be elicited during the abdominal examination by allowing him to place his hands on top of the examiner's during palpation. Apply gentle pressure beginning in a location away from the area identified by the child as the most painful. If a surgical consultation is anticipated, the physicians should agree on who will perform the digital rectal examination, thus minimizing the number of examinations.

McCollough M, Sharieff GO: Abdominal surgical emergencies in infants and young children. Emerg Med Clin North Am 21:909–935, 2003.

KEY POINTS: ABDOMINAL EMERGENCIES ✓

1. Analgesia should not be withheld from a child with abdominal pain of unknown etiology simply for fear of delaying diagnosis or causing misdiagnosis.

2. Children are at particularly high risk of ruptured appendicitis, with the youngest children possessing the highest risk.

6. **Does the use of IV analgesia affect the diagnostic accuracy of the physical examination in children with significant abdominal pain of unknown etiology?**
It is imperative that health care practitioners caring for children make every effort to safely and effectively treat pain whenever possible. Multiple studies with adults and one with children have shown that giving IV narcotics at adequate doses to decrease pain does not adversely affect the physical examination or diagnostic accuracy in patients with abdominal pain of unknown etiology. In fact, pain control might facilitate localization of the origin of the pain, thereby improving the diagnostic accuracy of the physical examination. Therefore, avoid delaying administration of proper analgesia simply because the diagnosis is unknown or the child is awaiting examination by a consultant.

Kim MK, Strait RT, Sato TT, et al: A randomized clinical trial of analgesia in children with acute abdominal pain. Acad Emerg Med 9:281–287, 2002.

Thomas SH, Silen W, Cheema F, et al: Effects of morphine analgesia on diagnostic accuracy in emergency department patients with abdominal pain: A prospective, randomized trial. J Am Coll Surg 196:18–31, 2003.

7. **Which blood tests may be useful in the evaluation of abdominal pain?**
Patients who have experienced unremitting vomiting and appear dehydrated may have electrolyte abnormalities. In young infants, patients who will undergo surgery, or patients who are more severely ill, it may be more important to obtain blood studies to evaluate abdominal pain. The benefit of the complete blood count (CBC) remains controversial. While

an elevated white blood cell count is common in appendicitis, this finding is neither sensitive (many patients with appendicitis will have a normal white blood cell count) nor specific (many patients without appendicitis will have an elevated count). Measurement of liver aminotransferase values is useful in patients with scleral icterus or right-upper-quadrant tenderness. An elevation of one or both of serum amylase and lipase in the appropriate clinical context supports the diagnosis of pancreatitis.

8. **What other laboratory testing may be helpful in certain patients?**
A urinalysis is relatively inexpensive and easy to obtain. It can be helpful in diagnosing urinary tract infections and renal calculi but can be misleading if pyuria is due to cervicitis or bladder/ureteral irritation from an adjacent inflamed appendix. A urine pregnancy test is indicated in most postpubertal females. Additionally, diagnostic testing for gonorrhea and chlamydia should be included when indicated.

9. **What are the two most common causes of acute abdominal emergencies in children?**
Appendicitis is the most common cause in the United States, followed by intussusception.

Pollack ES: Pediatric abdominal surgical emergencies. Pediatr Ann 25:448–457, 1996.

10. **What is the typical presentation of appendicitis in children?**
There is no typical presentation of appendicitis; thus, the diagnosis can be difficult to make and easy to miss. Classically, periumbilical abdominal pain precedes the onset of vomiting and is associated with low-grade fever and anorexia. As the inflammation of the appendix advances and touches the adjacent peritoneum, the pain localizes to the right lower quadrant at McBurney's point. Since the clinical course often does not follow the "textbook" description, the physician must maintain a high index of suspicion.

D'Agostino J: Common abdominal emergencies in children. Pediatric Emerg Med 20:139–153, 2002.

11. **What are some of the pitfalls in diagnosing appendicitis?**
The presentation of a child with appendicitis may not be "textbook." The absence of fever or anorexia, pain in an atypical location, the presence of diarrhea, prolonged symptoms, and normal laboratory values can occur in patients with appendicitis. An appendix that is located in the lateral gutter can cause flank pain and lateral abdominal tenderness; an appendix that lies toward the left may produce hypogastric tenderness; and a retrocecal appendix may cause pain elicited only on deep palpation. While vomiting occurs more commonly, diarrhea may result from direct sigmoid irritation from the adjacent low-lying pelvic appendix. Similarly, bladder or ureteral irritation may result in dysuria and pyuria.

12. **Discuss the test characteristics (e.g., sensitivity, specificity) of limited computed tomography (CT) with rectal contrast in the evaluation of children with suspected appendicitis.**
Delays in the diagnosis of appendicitis may result in increased morbidity and mortality. Limited helical CT with administration of rectal contrast material has gained popularity in recent years. Although ultrasonography has the benefit of not exposing the child to ionizing radiation, it is operator dependent and may have limited use in obese children. CT is less operator dependent than ultrasonography, may provide several alternate diagnoses, and has excellent reported test characteristics in children. The sensitivity has been reported as 97%; specificity, 99%; positive predictive value, 98%; and negative predictive value, 98%.

Mullins M, Kircher M, Ryan D, et al: Evaluation of suspected appendicitis in children using limited helical CT and colonic contrast material. AJR 176:37–41, 2001.
Pena BM, Taylor GA, Fishman SJ, Mandl KD: Costs and effectiveness of ultrasonography and limited computed tomography for diagnosing appendicitis in children. Pediatrics 106:672–676, 2000.

13. **Which patients are more likely to develop appendiceal perforation?**
Young children, those with atypical presentations, and those who present early in their clinical course are at the highest risk.

14. **What is the "Classic Triad" of intussusception? Does it occur in most patients?**
Intussusception occurs when a portion of the bowel, usually the distal ileum, telescopes into an adjacent segment of bowel. This effectively leads to intestinal obstruction followed by venous congestion and, finally, arterial insufficiency. The classic triad of pain, currant-jelly stool, and abdominal mass on palpation are present in about 20–25% of children with intussusception.

15. **In which patients should the diagnosis of intussusception be considered?**
In the classic description of intussusception, a child age 3 months to 3 years presents with the legs intermittently drawn up to the chest while crying, bloody stools, vomiting, and a sausage-shaped abdominal mass. Unfortunately, the classic presentation is not common. Many children present with lethargy or a change in mental status. The goal is to diagnose and treat intussusception prior to the evolution of "currant-jelly stools," an indicator that significant bowel ischemia has occurred.

   Klein EJ, Kapoor D, Shugerman RP: The diagnosis of intussusception. Clin Pediatr 43:343–347, 2004.
   Kuppermann N, O'Dea T, Pinckney L, Hoecker C: Predictors of intussusception in young children. Arch Pediatr Adolesc Med 154:250–255, 2000.

16. **Are plain radiographs helpful in the diagnosis of intussusception?**
Very often, plain radiography is the first imaging study performed in the evaluation of the child with possible intussusception. Early on, plain films are usually normal, but, as the disease progresses, up to 60% will show absence of air in the right upper and lower quadrants and evidence of soft tissue density. Because radiography lacks sensitivity and many false-negative results occur, normal plain films should not exclude the diagnosis of intussusception.

   Byrne AT, Goeghegan T, Govender P, et al: The imaging of intussusception. Clin Radiol 60:39–46, 2005.

17. **What other imaging modalities are commonly used in children to confirm or rule out intussusception?**
   - **Ultrasonography** has the advantage of being relatively fast, noninvasive, and without exposure to ionizing radiation. Although it may be operator dependent, in experienced hands the sensitivity and specificity are high.
   - **Contrast enema** has long been the standard for diagnosis and often treatment of intussusception. Barium or air is introduced under pressure into the bowel via a tube in the rectum during fluoroscopy. Air is safer, cheaper, more effective at reduction, and poses less risk of bowel perforation.

   Byrne AT, Goeghegan T, Govender P, et al: The imaging of intussusception. Clin Radiol 60:39–46, 2005.

18. **Are plain radiographs indicated in every child with abdominal pain?**
No. Many experts would argue against the routine use of abdominal radiographs for patients with abdominal pain. A negative x-ray rarely eliminates the concern for an underlying pathologic process. Radiographic findings, if present, are often nonspecific.

19. **What abnormalities may appear on plain radiographs in children with abdominal pain?**
The plain film should be assessed for "bones, stones, masses, and gas." An appendicolith is present in only about 10% of patients with appendicitis. Other findings in appendicitis may include diminished air, thickening of the cecal wall and mucosal folds, indistinct psoas margins with scoliosis toward the right, and obliteration of the properitoneal fat pad. Rarely, a perforated

appendix may produce pneumoperitoneum. Some renal calculi can be visualized on plain radiographs of the abdomen. The invaginating bowel of intussusception may be apparent as an intraluminal density, but the more common finding is a paucity of air in the right lower quadrant. Multiple stacked, dilated loops of bowel with air fluid levels and the absence of distal air may signify intestinal obstruction. Abdominal radiographs may show evidence of constipation, previously unsuspected.

20. **Are there any other useful radiologic studies for children with abdominal pain?**
The benefits of ultrasonography have been clearly established in some disease processes. It has become an integral component of the workup for pyloric stenosis, can be useful in evaluating the postpubertal female with possible ovarian or uterine pathology, or the child with suspected appendicitis. With the advent of spiral CT, CT scanning is gaining in popularity for detecting renal calculi and intra-abdominal infections, including appendicitis. An upper gastrointestinal series with small bowel follow-through is used to detect intestinal malrotation. Failure of the C-loop of the duodenum to cross the midline and an abnormal location of the cecum signify a malrotation diagnosis.

21. **What is the most important diagnostic "test" in cases of abdominal pain when the diagnosis is unclear?**
Serial abdominal examinations.

22. **A 17-year-old sexually-active female presents with right-upper-quadrant abdominal pain and a low-grade fever. She denies vomiting, diarrhea, dysuria, or vaginal discharge. The physical examination is remarkable for mild right-upper-quadrant tenderness without peritoneal signs. She is anicteric. The pelvic examination does not reveal discharge, cervical motion, or adnexal tenderness. What is the most likely diagnosis?**
Fitz-Hugh-Curtis syndrome occurs in 5–10% of patients with chlamydial or gonococcal pelvic inflammatory disease. It is theorized that seeding of the peritoneal cavity occurs as the organism ascends the female genital tract. It then tracks along the paracolic gutter, reaches the liver, and causes inflammation of its capsule. There have been several reported cases of perihepatitis in men, thus precipitating the emergence of alternative hypotheses for its pathophysiology: lymphatic or hematogenous spread. In affected women, the pelvic examination may be normal and cervical cultures may not isolate an organism. Hepatic aminotransferase values are normal or transiently mildly elevated. In most cases, the diagnosis is inferred as the symptoms abate with antibiotic therapy. Definitive diagnosis can only be made laparoscopically.

Peter NG, Clark LR, Jaeger JR: Fitz-Hugh-Curtis syndrome: A diagnosis to consider in women with right upper quadrant pain. Cleve Clin J Med 71:233–239, 2004.

23. **Describe the management of an acute abdominal emergency.**
The immediate management should begin with a careful assessment of the patient's airway, breathing, and circulation. Intravascular access should be obtained and fluid resuscitation initiated with normal saline or lactated Ringer's solution (20 mL/kg). Laboratory studies may be sent with blood obtained during the IV placement. Promptly administer broad-spectrum antibiotics, including anaerobic coverage, and obtain surgical consultation as early as possible.

24. **What is the most common cause of recurrent abdominal pain?**
Although numerous organic causes are possible, 90–95% of patients with recurrent abdominal pain will have functional pain. In the functional abdominal pain syndrome, the pain is generally episodic, is periumbilical, rarely occurs during sleep, and rarely is associated with eating or activities. There are no signs of systemic illness, such as fever, diarrhea, vomiting, rash, or joint pains. The child's growth and development are normal. The physical examination is usually unremarkable, with the exception of mild midabdominal tenderness without peritoneal signs.

25. **How should the diagnosis of functional abdominal pain be addressed in the emergency department (ED)?**

The diagnosis of functional abdominal pain is usually evident following the completion of the history and physical examination. Failure to mention this diagnosis early or obtaining unnecessary studies to appease an anxious family may only result in the parents' feelings that "the right" diagnostic test has yet to be performed. The parents and child should be reassured that stress-related abdominal pain is real pain and not due to the child's "faking it." They should be encouraged to continue their normal activities (e.g., school attendance) and seek psychological services. Finally, the emergency physician should provide careful instructions on the symptoms that should prompt an immediate return to the ED and should encourage follow-up with the child's primary care provider.

26. **When should a surgical consultation be obtained?**

Request the assistance of surgical colleagues when a surgical process is clearly evident or when the possibility of a surgical diagnosis cannot be ruled out. For appendicitis, consider a surgical consult when findings on two or more of the following are abnormal: history, physical examination, or laboratory studies.

KEY POINTS: PROBLEMS IN DIAGNOSING PEDIATRIC ABDOMINAL PAIN ✓

1. History may be limited; physical examination may be difficult.

2. Children may not have "classic" features of appendicitis.

3. CBC is not specific for appendicitis.

4. Plain films are often not diagnostic.

5. Differential diagnosis is extensive.

ALTERED MENTAL STATUS

Douglas S. Nelson, MD, FAAP, FACEP

1. **How can altered mental status present in an infant?**
   It may present as a combination of crying, irritability, poor feeding, or sleeping more or less than usual.

2. **What clues can I use to determine whether altered mental status is due to a toxic ingestion?**
   Suspect a toxic ingestion when no history of trauma is present, abnormal consciousness was of sudden onset, the patient was unsupervised, the patient appears to have a chaotic home situation, or the patient has a history of previous ingestions.

   Dobson JV, Webb SA: Life-threatening pediatric poisonings. J S C Med Assoc 100:327–332, 2004.

3. **What scales are in use to quantify altered mental status? Why should I use them?**
   The level of consciousness of a neurologically impaired patient may initially be evaluated by using a simple **AVPU** scale, representing four major levels of alertness: **a**lert, responsive to **v**erbal stimuli, responsive to **p**ainful stimuli, and **u**nresponsive.

   A more widely used measurement of consciousness is the Glasgow Coma Scale (GCS). Patients are graded on three areas of neurologic function: eye opening, motor responses, and verbal responsiveness. These numeric scores are added to determine the GCS score. A GCS score of 3 is the minimum score possible and represents complete unresponsiveness, while a GCS score of 15 is assigned to fully alert patients. Details of the scale are listed below:
   1. Eye opening
      - Spontaneous: 4
      - To speech: 3
      - To pain: 2
      - None: 1
   2. Best motor response
      - Obeys verbal command: 6
      - Localizes to painful stimulus: 5
      - Flexion withdrawal: 4
      - Flexion decorticate: 3
      - Extension decerebrate: 2
      - No response: 1
   3. Best verbal response*
      - Oriented; converses: 5
      - Disoriented; converses: 4
      - Inappropriate words: 3
      - Incomprehensible sounds: 2
      - No response: 1

   There are several good reasons to use a standard quantifiable mental status scale. It allows evaluation of a patient's changing neurologic status over time and the recording of this

---

* Preverbal children should receive full verbal score for crying with stimulation.

information in the medical record. The effect of medical interventions may then be more easily assessed. The use of accepted scoring systems also facilitates communication with consultants, such as neurologists and neurosurgeons.

Nelson DS: Coma and altered level of consciousness. In Fleisher G, Ludwig S (eds): Textbook of Pediatric Emergency Medicine, 5th ed. Philadelphia, Lippincott Williams & Wilkins, 2006, pp 201–212.

KEY POINTS: CLUES TO TOXIC INGESTION IN A CHILD WITH ALTERED MENTAL STATUS ✓

1. No trauma

2. Sudden onset of symptoms

3. Lack of supervision of patient

4. Chaotic home

5. Previous ingestions

4. **Which toxins not detected on most drug screens can cause abnormal mental status?**
The following toxins are associated with altered mental status and miosis: clonidine, chloral hydrate, organophosphates, and tetrahydrozoline. Mydriasis and altered mental status are found with other toxins: carbon monoxide, cyanide, methemoglobinemia, LSD, and γ-hydroxybutyrate.

5. **What do the letters *DPT*, *OPV*, *HIB*, and *MMR* stand for?**
Although these represent abbreviations for several childhood immunizations, the letters also comprise a mnemonic to recall common causes of abnormal mental status.

D = **D**ehydration	**O** = **O**ccult trauma
P = **P**oisoning	**P** = **P**ostictal or **P**ostanoxia
T = **T**rauma	**V** = **V**P shunt problem
H = **H**ypoxia or **H**yperthermia	**M** = **M**eningitis or encephalitis
I = **I**ntussusception	**M** = **M**etabolic
B = **B**rain mass	**R** = **R**eye's syndrome, other **R**arities

Schunk JE: The pediatric patient with altered level of consciousness: Remember your "immunizations." J Emerg Nurs 18:419–421, 1992.

6. **When should I consider obtaining a computed tomographic scan on a child with abnormal mental status?**
Consider computed tomography (CT) if there is any history of trauma, any focal or lateralizing signs on physical examination, or any suspicion of physical abuse.

7. **A teenager is brought to the emergency department (ED) from a party by his friends. He is comatose and has profound respiratory and neurologic depression with no history of head trauma. You send a toxicologic screen, intubate his trachea, and arrange for admission to the intensive care unit (ICU). The ICU staff obtains a CT scan, which takes an hour to accomplish. The result of the scan is normal. Upon returning from the scanner, the patient sits up, rips the endotracheal tube out of his mouth, and says he wishes to leave. His toxicology screen is normal except for a clinically insignificant amount of ethanol. What was the most likely cause of his problem?**
   At the party he drank γ-hydroxybutyrate (GHB). It is an inhibitory neurotransmitter normally found in the brain, causing central nervous system (CNS) depressant effects, but some excitatory ones as well, such as seizures. The patient may have ingested it intentionally, or it may have been surreptitiously added to an alcoholic drink.

   The CNS effects of GHB include drowsiness, ataxia, confusion, amnesia, incontinence, seizures, and coma. Behavioral manifestations can include euphoria, hallucinations, or delirium. Mydriasis and nystagmus may be present, accompanied by respiratory depression, bradycardia, and hypotension.

   Recovery from GHB intoxication is usually rapid, within several hours after ingestion. Note that routine toxicologic screens miss the presence of this drug, which should now be considered in the differential diagnosis of all teens with abnormal mental status.

   Suner S, Szlatenyi CS, Wang RY: Pediatric gamma hydroxybutyrate intoxication. Acad Emerg Med 4: 1041–1045, 1997.

8. **A 6-month-old infant is brought in by her mother after being left alone with "the boyfriend." She was well yesterday, but today will not feed and is sleepier than normal. She has no fever, congestion, vomiting, or diarrhea. The physical examination is normal except that the child seems more difficult to arouse than usual. What possible etiologies should be considered?**
   Child abuse is most likely. Also consider sepsis, intussusception, and inborn metabolic abnormalities. Pay particular attention to the fontanelle and fundi of the infant: bulging of the fontanelle or any abnormalities of the eye grounds is extremely significant. Child abuse in this scenario is most likely to take the form of a "shaken baby" injury, when the whipping motion of an infant's head causes tearing of cortical bridging veins between the dura and arachnoid veins, leading to subdural hematoma formation. These can occur bilaterally and are five to 10 times more common than epidural bleeding. Subdural hematomas may occur on a chronic basis in young abused children, and are associated with skull fractures in 30% of cases. Retinal hemorrhages are found in 75% of patients with subdural hematomas. Neuroimaging classically reveals crescent-shaped lesions between the brain and skull. Skeletal survey performed on these children typically show orthopedic injuries in various stages of healing.

   Belfer RA, Klein BL, Orr L: Use of the skeletal survey in the evaluation of child maltreatment. Am J Emerg Med 19:122–124, 2001.

9. **Magnetic resonance imaging (MRI) provides a sharper, more detailed picture of the brain than does CT. Why, then, is CT usually performed first in a patient presenting with abnormal mental status?**
   MRI scans are more costly, take longer to obtain, and are generally more difficult to arrange than CT scans. CT images show most structural lesions that may present with altered mental status, such as tumors or hemorrhage. Young children may require sedation for MRI, but not for a quick head CT.

10. **What are clues that a child may be "faking" an altered mental status?**
    Malingering should be suspected if the patient has a psychiatric history or falls down from "spells" without ever being injured. On physical examination, when you lift the patient's hand to

a position directly over his or her face and let go, the patient will not hit himself or herself in the face unless there has been an alteration in mental status. In very convincing cases, it may be necessary to perform electroencephalography to prove this suspicion.

11. **A 3-year-old is brought for evaluation one winter day because he is groggy and has had a headache for a few days. The rest of the family members are all older and have had similar although less severe symptoms. No other signs of illness, such as fever, vomiting, diarrhea, rhinorrhea, or rash, are present. No history of ingestion or head trauma is present. Physical examination reveals a well-appearing but drowsy child with very mild tachypnea. He wants to sleep if you leave him alone and is cranky when you keep him up. The examination is otherwise normal; oxygen saturation is 100% in room air. Electrolytes, complete blood count, and blood gas are obtained. What test comes back with abnormal results?**
The blood gas, which shows a carboxyhemoglobin level of 20%. This level indicates that the patient and presumably his or her family are being poisoned by carbon monoxide. This cause of abnormal mental status is seen most often in early winter, as families turn on their furnaces for the first time since the previous heating season. Treatment usually consists of administering 100% oxygen via a rebreather face mask. Severe cases, such as in children rescued from house fires, may require endotracheal intubation and hyperbaric oxygen. Pulse oximetry often reads 100% as carboxyhemoglobin is misread as oxygenated hemoglobin.

Chou KJ, Fisher JL, Silver EJ: Characteristics and outcome of children with carbon monoxide poisoning with and without smoke exposure referred for hyperbaric oxygen therapy. Pediatr Emerg Care 16:151–155, 2000.

12. **If the physical examination of a patient with altered mental status does not reveal the source of neurologic disability, what laboratory tests should I consider?**
Glucose is the most important laboratory test to check and one of the fastest and easiest. In many institutions, a rapid bedside test can be done to provide a value in minutes. Consider also a toxicologic screen, electrolytes, or head CT.

13. **What subtle signs may represent seizure activity as the cause of altered mental status?**
Suspect seizure if the patient is dazed or confused and exhibits staring, swallowing, eye blinking, lip quivering, nystagmus, and automatisms (motor actions performed without conscious intent). The degree of neurologic impairment can fluctuate over time.

Benson PJ, Klein EJ: New-onset absence status epilepsy presenting as altered mental status in a pediatric patient. Ann Emerg Med 37:402–405, 2001.

14. **What causes of abnormal mental status are particularly life-threatening?**
The list includes epidural hematoma, cerebral edema, brain neoplasms, cerebral infarctions, cerebrospinal fluid shunt malfunction, meningitis, encephalitis, toxic ingestions, carbon monoxide poisoning, hypotension, hypoxia, and sepsis.

Nelson DS: Coma and altered level of consciousness. In Fleisher G, Ludwig S (eds): Textbook of Pediatric Emergency Medicine, 5th ed. Philadelphia, Lippincott Williams & Wilkins, 2006, pp 201–212.

15. **An obese African-American patient presents with abnormal mental status, a blood glucose level > 600 mg/dl, and mild changes of bicarbonate and ketone values. You suspect the presence of what endocrine disorder?**
Type 2 diabetes is increasingly common among pediatric patients. Children with this disorder may present with a nonketotic hyperglycemic (serum glucose > 600 mg/dL) and hyperosmolar

(osmolality > 330 mOsm/L) state. In Fourtner and colleagues' series, the mean time to the return of a normal mental state was 3 days (range, 1–7 days).

Bhowmick SK, Levens KL, Rettig KR: Hyperosmolar hyperglycemic crisis: An acute life-threatening event in children and adolescents with type 2 diabetes mellitus. Endocr Pract 11:23–29, 2005.

Fourtner SH, Weinzimer SA, Levitt Katz LE: Hyperglycemic hyperosmolar non-ketotic syndrome in children with type 2 diabetes. Pediatr Diabetes 6:129–135, 2005.

16. **An 11-year-old boy is brought to the ED after awakening from sleep with headache and vomiting. He is disoriented and does not recognize his parents. Head CT, blood and cerebrospinal fluid chemistries, and toxicologic screens are normal. His mental status cleared shortly after admission. What diagnosis did the consulting neurologist make?**

Acute confusional migraine. This is an atypical type of migraine headache characterized by the sudden onset of mental status changes. These may include confusion, disorientation, dysarthria, and diminished level of consciousness. It is thought to be more common in males. Treatment consists of standard migraine medical management.

Bechtel K: Acute mental status change due to acute confusional migraine. Pediatr Emerg Care 20:238–241, 2004.

17. **A 6-year-old girl presented to the ED with diminished loss of consciousness (LOC). The prior evening, the patient had reported shortness of breath and chest pain on inspiration. In the morning, the patient was noted to be very weak and progressively less responsive to external stimuli. On physical examination, heart rate was 155 beats per minute (BPM), respiratory rate was 48 per minute, and blood pressure (BP) was 60/25 mmHg. No fever was present, nor was there any focus of infection on examination. Complete blood count and blood chemistries were normal, and room-air oxygen saturation was 98%. Mucous membranes were moist and skin turgor was normal. Lungs were clear to auscultation, and the heart had a tachycardic but regular rhythm. CT scan was normal. What problem did the patient have?**

This patient's altered mental status was due to hypotension. The cause of this abnormality was not sepsis or dehydration. This tachycardic and hypotensive patient had pericardial tamponade, despite her lack of distended neck veins or muffled heart tones. The hypotension associated with this disorder will not respond to administration of IV fluids. Pericardiocentesis is the appropriate treatment, which was performed on this patient and resulted in prompt restoration of normal mental status.

Milner D, Losek JD, Schiff J, Sicoli R: Pediatric pericardial tamponade presenting as altered mental status. Pediatr Emerg Care 19:35–37, 2003.

18. **A 4-year-old boy was brought to the ED because of sleepiness and "not acting right." He had been born prematurely and had spent several weeks in a neonatal ICU after birth. Since then, he had been doing well. He had no recent history of head trauma, fever, toxic ingestion, or illness. Review of symptoms was positive for vomiting and decreased responsiveness. Patient was afebrile, with a heart rate of 120 BPM, BP of 140/80 mmHg, and a respiratory rate of 36 per minute. The patient was difficult to arouse and cried when awake. Cerebral spinal fluid was not obtained because of concerns of increased intracranial pressure. A CT scan was ordered because of concerns of child abuse. It was read as normal, but MRI revealed subtle occipital abnormalities. After treatment, the patient's repeat MRI scan was normal. What problem caused the patient's abnormal mental status?**

The patient had hypertensive encephalopathy due to renal artery stenosis caused by an umbilical artery catheter used during their postnatal neonatal intensive care unit stay. The MRI findings were consistent with posterior leukoencephalopathy syndrome. Clinical findings may include altered mental status, seizures, headache, and blindness. Appropriate treatment of hypertension results in resolution of neurologic and MRI abnormalities.

Singhi P, Subramanian C, Jain V, et al: Reversible brain lesions in childhood hypertension. Acta Paediatr 91:1005–1007, 2002.

19. **A 12-year-old boy is brought to the ED by his parents, who are concerned by his diminished responsiveness. He has a history of sinus and ear infections. The previous evening, he had reported a headache and seemed to have a tactile fever. On the day of presentation, he is noted to be somnolent and difficult to arouse, with slower than normal reaction times. He has no focal neurologic findings, and physical examination is unremarkable. Why is he ill?**
The patient has a subdural abscess from long-standing sinusitis. Intracranial complications of sinusitis are rare but possible in childhood. When pus-filled sinuses decompress into the cranial vault, minimal facial tenderness may be present. A high index of suspicion is needed to order brain and sinus CT scans that reveal the etiology of the patient's mental status.

Giannoni C, Sulek M, Friedman EM: Intracranial complications of sinusitis: A pediatric series. Am J Rhinol 12:173–178, 1998.

CHAPTER 7

APNEA

Andrew D. DePiero, MD

1. **What defines apnea?**
   Apnea is a respiratory pause of greater than 15 seconds or any pause that is associated with cyanosis, pallor, or bradycardia.

2. **What is the difference between obstructive apnea and central apnea?**
   Obstructive apnea is related to an obstruction of the upper airway. Respiratory movements continue during attempts to relieve the obstruction. Adenotonsillar hypertrophy is a common cause. Central apnea is a dysfunction of the neurologic centers that regulate breathing. During central apnea, all respiratory efforts cease. Occasionally, both central and obstructive components are present. This is classified as mixed apnea.

3. **What is periodic breathing?**
   Periodic breathing describes a pattern of a short respiratory pause followed by an increase in respiratory rate. This occurs in cycles and is a normal pattern in infants.

4. **What are some of the pathophysiologic factors contributing to apnea in young infants?**
   - **Hypoxic drive:** In the neonate, hypoxia results in a brief increase in respiratory rate followed by depressed respiratory drive and apnea. Mild hypoxemia during sleep can cause periodic breathing or apnea, and hypoxemia during sleep may not cause arousal.
   - **Effects of feeding:** Difficulty with coordination of sucking and breathing can result in hypoxemia. The presence of an accentuated laryngeal chemoreflex can cause apnea and bradycardia if regurgitation occurs while the infant is hypoxic.
   - **Metabolic abnormalities:** Apnea can develop in newborns and young infants as the result of hypoglycemia or anemia.
   - **Mechanical factors:** Because of the pliable thoracic cage and fatigability of the diaphragmatic muscle, attempts to increase minute ventilation by increasing tidal volume can increase the work of breathing. Thus, the infant in respiratory distress is more susceptible to respiratory failure and apnea.

5. **What are some of the underlying causes of apnea?**
   - **Central nervous system:** Seizure activity, breath-holding
   - **Infection:** Meningitis, bronchiolitis (in premature infants or infants with lung or heart disease), sepsis, croup, infant botulism, pertussis
   - **Cardiac:** Dysrhythmia
   - **Gastrointestinal:** Gastroesophageal reflux
   - **Metabolic:** Hypoglycemia, inborn errors of metabolism, toxin (ingestion)
   - **Trauma:** Accidental or inflicted head or blunt abdominal injury
   - **Prematurity**

   Arens R, Gozal D, Williams JC, et al: Recurrent apparent life-threatening events during infancy: A manifestation of inborn errors of metabolism. J Pediatr 123:415–418, 1993.

   Southall DP, Plunkett CB, Banks MW, et al: Covert video recordings of life-threatening child abuse: Lessons for child protection. Pediatrics 100:735–760, 1997.

KEY POINTS: APPROACH TO THE INFANT WITH APNEA ✔

1. Determine the clinical significance of the episode.

2. Stabilize the infant if necessary.

3. Obtain detailed history from observer, emergency medical services personnel.

4. The history and physical examination should guide any diagnostic testing.

5. A period of observation and/or admission is necessary.

6. **What is sudden infant death syndrome (SIDS)? How is it diagnosed?**
   SIDS is defined as "the sudden death of an infant under 1 year of age that remains unexplained after a thorough case investigation, including performance of a complete autopsy, examination of the death scene, and review of the clinical history."

   Willinger M, James LS, Catz C: Defining the sudden infant death syndrome (SIDS): Deliberations of an expert panel convened by the National Institute of Child Health and Human Development. Pediatr Pathol 11:677–684, 1991.

7. **What is an "apparent life-threatening event" (ALTE)? Is it related to SIDS?**
   An apparent life-threatening event is a severe, apneic episode that is frightening to the observer and is characterized by change in color, muscle tone, and mental status, which may include choking. Although the cause of an apparent life-threatening event is frequently elusive, most infants who die from SIDS have not previously had such an event.

8. **What are the risk factors for SIDS? Are they the same as the risk factors for an apparent life-threatening event?**
   The risk factors for SIDS include male sex, prematurity, low birthweight, maternal smoking, lower socioeconomic status, poor prenatal care, young maternal age, higher parity, multiple gestation, and unsafe sleeping conditions. SIDS tends to peak in the winter months. These factors have not been shown to correlate well for a life-threatening event. However, there may be some association of a life-threatening event with maternal smoking. Upper respiratory tract infections are known to prolong apneic episodes during sleep.

   Kiechl-Kohlendorfer U, Hof D, Peglow UP, et al: Epidemiology of apparent life-threatening events. Arch Dis Child 90:297–300, 2005.

9. **Has the decline in the incidence of SIDS resulted in a similar decrease of apparent life-threatening events?**
   While the recommendation of prone sleeping position for babies has correlated with a significant decrease in the number of SIDS cases, the same cannot be said for life-threatening events. Several studies have concluded that the incidence of these events remains unchanged.

   Gershan WM, Besch NS, Franciosi RA: A comparison of apparent life-threatening events before and after the back to sleep campaign. West Med J 101:39–45, 2002.
   Kiechl-Kohlendorfer U, Hof D, Peglow UP, et al: Epidemiology of apparent life threatening events. Arch Dis Child 90:297–300, 2005.

10. **How should the evaluation of an infant with apnea begin?**
    The infant who requires resuscitation and stabilization must be immediately identified. Most children who have had an apneic episode do not require aggressive initial treatment. They are generally awake, alert, and breathing spontaneously by the time they arrive in the emergency

department. Nevertheless, a thorough and appropriate evaluation is essential to the identification of underlying life-threatening conditions. This process must answer two key questions:

1. Did a clinically significant episode occur?
2. What is the risk of recurrence?

11. How should the history be obtained?

It is essential to question firsthand observers of the apneic event as objectively as possible. This can be challenging considering the stressful nature of the event. Questions such as, "What did the baby look like?" "What color was she?" "Was he awake?" "Did he appear frightened?" and "Then what did you do?" may help the historian relate his or her observations to you more objectively. Information from prehospital personnel is useful as well.

12. Are there specific details that must be included in the history?

Ask these questions to ensure a thorough history:

- Where did the event take place: in the infant's crib, in another bed, in a car seat?
- How long did the episode last?
- Was the infant awake or asleep?
- Was there a change in the baby's color?
- Was there a change in tone or posture, or were there abnormal movements?
- Did the child require resuscitation, and, if so, how did he respond?
- When was the infant last fed?

13. Are there other questions that should be asked in the history?

- History of present illness: Prior to the event, was the child well? Are there symptoms of other illnesses, specifically changes in behavior, activity, and/or appetite? Does the baby have gastroesophageal reflux? Has there been a recent illness, fever, cough, or cold? Has the infant recently received an immunization?
- Past medical history: Have there been similar episodes in the past? Were there problems with pregnancy, labor, or delivery? What was the child's birthweight?
- Family history: Is there any family history of seizures, infant deaths, or serious illnesses in young family members?
- Social history: Who was watching the child at the time of the episode? Are there medications or other toxins accessible to the child?

14. Can a child with a normal physical examination have had a significant apneic episode?

Yes. After careful examination, the infant's heart rate, respiratory rate, blood pressure, pulse oximetry, and rectal temperature can be entirely normal—even though the baby "looked dead" at the time of the episode. The remaining physical examination may also be unremarkable. Therefore, you must obtain a careful history to guide further evaluation.

15. Are there physical findings that can indicate specific etiologies for an apneic episode?

Fever or hypothermia suggests the possibility of infection. Tachypnea may be the result of respiratory disease or metabolic acidosis. A young infant with cough or wheezing may have bronchiolitis. A child in shock may have sepsis or hypovolemia from an occult injury. Depressed mental status, bulging fontanelle, or papilledema are consistent with central nervous system infection or injury. An infant with dysmorphic features may have an underlying congenital abnormality as the cause of apnea.

16. What laboratory tests should be ordered?

The laboratory evaluation must be guided by the history and physical examination. An infant who has had a short choking episode and now appears entirely well may require only a careful examination with routine vital signs and a short period of observation including feeding. In contrast, a hypothermic, lethargic baby should have a full sepsis evaluation, including a lumbar puncture and possibly metabolic studies and computed tomography of the head. An arterial blood gas in an infant who required resuscitation at the scene but now appears well will undoubtedly be normal.

17. **When should an infant who has had an apneic episode be admitted to the hospital?**

If you are convinced by the history that a significant episode of apnea has occurred, admit the child for observation and further diagnostic evaluation even if no specific cause is identified. Generally, if the caretaker reports that the baby was cyanotic, hospital admission is advised. Any underlying cause of significant apnea that becomes evident will also require admission to be adequately treated.

Claudius I, Keens T: Do all infants with apparent life-threatening events need to be admitted? Pediatrics 119:679–683, 2007.

18. **When can the baby with a history of apnea be discharged from the emergency department?**

If a careful history and physical examination with appropriate laboratory studies lead you to conclude that a significant apneic episode has not occurred, the baby can often be discharged home. A period of observation, including watching the infant feed, is prudent. The seriousness of the event may not become obvious until you observe some of the features that the caretakers have described. For example, an infant with pertussis may appear well until she coughs. Arrange follow-up with the primary care provider for the next day.

19. **Should a home cardiorespiratory monitor be recommended for patients after an apparent life-threatening event?**

Home cardiorespiratory monitoring has never been proven to prevent SIDS, nor has the practice of home monitoring changed the incidence of SIDS. The Committee on Fetus and Newborn from the American Academy of Pediatrics recommends that monitoring should not be prescribed to prevent SIDS. Monitoring may be indicated for a select group of premature infants until 43 weeks after conception or until the extreme apneic and bradycardic episodes have ceased, whichever comes last.

American Academy of Pediatrics: Policy statement. Apnea, sudden infant death syndrome and home monitoring. Committee on Fetus and Newborn. Pediatrics 111:914–917, 2003.

Available at http://aappolicy.aappublications.org/cgi/content/full/pediatrics;111/4/914.

ACKNOWLEDGMENT

The author wishes to acknowledge Dr. Susan B. Torrey, who authored this chapter in the first edition of *Pediatric Emergency Medicine Secrets*.

CHAPTER 8

CHEST PAIN

Steven M. Selbst, MD, FAAP, FACEP

1. **How common is chest pain in children?**

   Chest pain is a common pediatric complaint. It is not nearly as frequent as abdominal pain or headache, but it is perhaps the third leading pain syndrome in children. Chest pain has been reported to occur in 6 of 1000 children who visit an urban pediatric emergency department (ED).

   Selbst SM, Ruddy R, Clark BJ, et al: Pediatric chest pain—a prospective study. Pediatrics 82:319–323,1988.

2. **What is the peak age for pediatric chest pain?**

   Most studies report the mean age of children with chest pain to be 12–14 years. It affects children of all ages, and half of children with chest pain are younger than 12 years of age.

3. **How does the etiology of chest pain in children differ from that in adults?**

   Children with chest pain are far less likely to have a cardiac etiology for their pain. Most children with chest pain have a self-limited, "benign" etiology.

   Massin MM, Bourguignont A, Coremans C, et al: Chest pain in pediatric patients presenting to an emergency department or to a cardiac clinic. Clin Pediatr 43:231–238, 2004.

4. **Which diagnoses are most common in children who present to an ED with chest pain?**

   In many studies, up to 45% of cases of chest pain in children are labeled "idiopathic." That is, after a careful history and physical examination, the etiology is still uncertain. When a diagnosis can be found, musculoskeletal injury is most common. Active children frequently strain chest wall muscles while carrying heavy books, exercising, or engaging in rough play. Many other children suffer chest pain from a direct blow to the chest that results in a mild contusion or, in rare cases, a rib fracture. Costochondritis accounts for about 10–20% of cases of chest pain. This musculoskeletal disorder produces tenderness over the costochondral junctions and is often bilateral. It is exaggerated by physical activity or breathing. Musculoskeletal pain is often reproducible by palpation of the chest wall or moving the arms and chest through a variety of positions. Table 8-1 lists the most common etiologies for pediatric chest pain.

   Selbst SM: Chest pain in children—consultation with the specialist. Pediatr Rev 18:169–173, 1997.

5. **How is the etiology of chest pain related to the child's age?**

   Young children are more likely to have chest pain related to a cardiorespiratory condition (cough, asthma, pneumonia, or heart disease). Children over the age of 12 years are more likely to have a psychogenic disturbance as the cause of their pain.

6. **What common gastrointestinal condition causes chest pain?**

   Gastroesophageal reflux, which is very common in children and accounts for at least 7% of pediatric chest pain. Some feel it is underdiagnosed. The pain is usually worse in the recumbent position. History may reveal that the pain is "burning" in quality and may have developed after eating spicy foods. A trial of antacids is often diagnostic and therapeutic.

TABLE 8-1. MOST COMMON CAUSES OF PEDIATRIC CHEST PAIN

Idiopathic

Musculoskeletal

    Chest wall strain

    Costochondritis

    Direct trauma

Respiratory conditions

    Asthma

    Cough

    Pneumonia

Gastrointestinal problems

    Esophagitis

    Esophageal foreign body

Psychogenic (stress related)

Cardiac pathology

    Myocarditis

KEY POINTS: MOST COMMON CAUSES OF CHILDHOOD CHEST PAIN ✔

1. Musculoskeletal pain

2. Idiopathic cause

3. Pulmonary conditions

4. Psychological cause

5. Trauma

6. Gastrointestinal problems

7. Cardiac disease

8. Sickle cell crises

7. **What is Texidor's twinge?**
In 1955, Miller and Texidor described a syndrome of left-sided chest pain that is brief (less than a 5-minute duration) and sporadic. This pain may recur frequently for a few hours in some individuals and then remain absent for several months. The pain seems to be associated with a slouched posture or bending and is not related to exercise. It is usually relieved when the individual takes a few shallow breaths, or sometimes one deep breath, and assumes a straightened posture. It is believed that the pain arises from the parietal pleura or from pressure

on an intercostal nerve, but the etiology remains unclear. Others refer to this pain syndrome as "precordial catch" or "stitch in the side."

Gumbiner CH: Precordial catch syndrome. South Med J 96:38–41, 2003.

8. **What is "slipping rib syndrome"?**
This is a rare sprain disorder caused by trauma to the costal cartilages of the eighth, ninth and tenth ribs, which do not attach to the sternum. Children with slipping rib syndrome report pain under the ribs or in the upper abdominal quadrants. They also hear a clicking or popping sound when they lift objects, flex the trunk, or even walk. It is believed that the pain is caused by one of the ribs hooking under the rib above and irritating the intercostal nerves. The pain can be duplicated and the syndrome confirmed by performing the "hooking maneuver," whereby the affected rib margin is grasped and then pulled anteriorly. Intercostal block has been tried for pain relief. Surgery to resect the involved costal cartilage may provide long-term relief, though most patients are treated satisfactorily with oral analgesics.

Mooney DP, Shorter NA: Slipping rib syndrome in childhood. J Pediatr Surg 32:1081–1082, 1997.

9. **How can ingestion of tetracycline lead to chest pain?**
Tetracycline, doxycycline, and other pill medications can cause acute esophagitis (pill-induced esophagitis). The pain is especially likely if the patient takes the medication with a minimal amount of water and then lies down. A history of esophageal dysmotility or stricture makes the pain more likely. However, many normal teenagers also report this pain. Because of the pH of the drug, doxycycline produces an acidic solution or gel as it dissolves, and thus it is caustic when it remains in the esophagus. Symptoms may be noted several days after the start of therapy with the medication, but frequently they occur after the first dose is taken.

10. **How can I diagnose pill-induced esophagitis?**
The diagnosis is made by taking a careful history. Physical examination generally is unremarkable. These medications are often taken by adolescents for treatment of acne, and since they are used long-term, teens may fail to reveal that they take the medication unless asked specifically. Some physicians prefer to perform endoscopic evaluation to document esophageal ulcers (midesophageal ulcers are most common, as the tablets are most likely to lodge in that region). Others prefer not to perform the endoscopy and, instead, discontinue use of the tetracycline medications and treat with sucralfate. This approach can be both diagnostic and therapeutic, if the patient responds well.

Palmer KM, Selbst SM, Shaffer S, et al: Pediatric chest pain induced by tetracycline ingestion. Pediatr Emerg Care 15:200–201, 1999.

11. **When should a pneumothorax be suspected in a child with chest pain?**
Suspect a pneumothorax if a child develops acute onset of sharp chest pain associated with some degree of respiratory distress. The pain is usually worsened by inspiration and may radiate to the shoulder, neck, or even the abdomen. Children with this condition do not have long-standing pain and almost all present for care within 48 hours of developing the pneumothorax. The patient will usually have dyspnea, tachycardia, and, perhaps, decreased breath sounds on the affected side, or even cyanosis. However, these signs and symptoms depend on the size of the pneumothorax and whether it is under tension (Fig. 8-1). A small pneumothorax may produce minimal findings on examination.

History of trauma may increase your suspicion of pneumothorax, but many cases occur spontaneously or with exercise or cough. In those cases, a small, unrecognized, subpleural bleb ruptures, leading to the air leak. Some underlying conditions increase the risk of "spontaneous" pneumothorax. Those with asthma, cystic fibrosis, and Marfan's syndrome are particularly

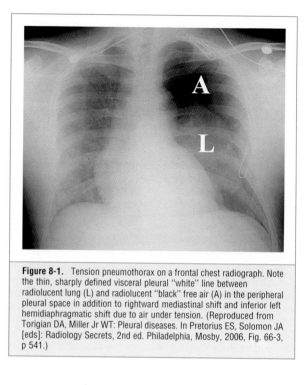

Figure 8-1. Tension pneumothorax on a frontal chest radiograph. Note the thin, sharply defined visceral pleural "white" line between radiolucent lung (L) and radiolucent "black" free air (A) in the peripheral pleural space in addition to rightward mediastinal shift and inferior left hemidiaphragmatic shift due to air under tension. (Reproduced from Torigian DA, Miller Jr WT: Pleural diseases. In Pretorius ES, Solomon JA [eds]: Radiology Secrets, 2nd ed. Philadelphia, Mosby, 2006, Fig. 66-3, p 541.)

prone to chest pain secondary to pneumothoraces. Also, several cases have been reported in teenagers who smoke crack cocaine.

Uva JL: Spontaneous pneumothoraces, pneumomediastinum, and pneumoperitoneum: Consequences of smoking crack cocaine. Pediatr Emerg Care 13:24–26, 1997.

12. **How can anxiety or emotional stress lead to chest pain in children?**
The relationship of pain to emotional stress is not quite clear. However, we assume children get headaches and abdominal pain from stress. It is reasonable to conclude that chest pain can also be related to stress. Studies have shown that stress is the cause (psychogenic pain) in about 10% of children with chest pain who present to a pediatric ED. Possible stressors include school failure, recent death or illness in the family, recent loss of friends from moving to a new city or school, and school phobia. It is important to consider stress as an etiology of chest pain in all children who present with the complaint. This should not be a diagnosis of exclusion, but if significant stress is temporally related to the pain, it is a reasonable diagnosis.

13. **Why do some adolescents who present with hyperventilation also have chest pain?**
Hyperventilation may be associated with psychogenic chest pain, and may lead to pain by producing a hypocapnic alkalosis. Prolonged hyperventilation can lead to coronary artery vasoconstriction and chest pain. Also, stomach distention due to concomitant aerophagia can occur with hyperventilation and produce chest pain. Lightheadedness, headache, and paresthesias may also be found.

Sawni A, Wright K, Ragothaman R: Hyperventilation and chest pain in an adolescent female: Index of suspicion. Clin Pediatr 43:663–666, 2004.

14. **Which children with chest pain deserve an evaluation with an electrocardiogram and/or chest radiograph?**
    1. Those with worrisome historical features:
       - Acute onset of pain
       - Chest pain associated with exercise
       - Associated syncope, dizziness, palpitations
       - History of heart disease
       - History of a condition that can affect the heart or lungs—diabetes mellitus, Kawasaki disease, Marfan's syndrome, asthma, anemia, systemic lupus erythematosus
       - History of sickle cell disease
       - Use of cocaine
       - Trauma
       - Foreign-body ingestion
       - Fever
    2. Those with an abnormal physical examination:
       - Respiratory distress
       - Decreased or abnormal breath sounds
       - Cardiac findings (murmur, rub, click, arrhythmia)
       - Fever
       - Trauma
       - Palpation of subcutaneous air

15. **Which children with chest pain do *not* need extensive evaluation with laboratory studies in the ED?**
    Those with chronic pain (and none of the worrisome features mentioned above) do not necessarily need laboratory studies. Management must be individualized, but most patients can be managed with analgesics, reassurance that cardiac disease is unlikely, and close follow-up. If the history and physical examination do not suggest an etiology for the pain, it is unlikely that laboratory tests will be helpful.

16. **Why is chest pain of acute onset more worrisome?**
    Studies have shown that children with sudden onset of pain (within 48 hours of presentation) are more likely to have an organic etiology for the pain. It is not necessarily a serious etiology, but pneumonia, asthma, trauma, and pneumothorax are more likely.

    Selbst SM, Ruddy R, Clark BJ, et al: Pediatric chest pain—a prospective study. Pediatrics 82:319–323, 1988.

17. **Why is fever associated with chest pain of concern?**
    Fever is much more likely to be associated with pneumonia, myocarditis, or pericarditis. Endocarditis is a very rare condition in otherwise healthy adolescents, but it should also be considered.

KEY POINTS: FEVER AND CHEST PAIN ✓

1. Consider pneumonia, myocarditis, pericarditis.

2. May hear decreased breath sounds (pneumonia).

3. May hear distant heart sounds (pericarditis, myocarditis).

4. Obtain a chest x-ray.

5. Consider an electrocardiogram if pneumonia is excluded.

18. **Which cardiac conditions can cause chest pain in children?**
    - **Arrhythmia:** Supraventricular tachycardia, ventricular tachycardia
    - **Infection:** Myocarditis, pericarditis
    - **Structural abnormalities:** Hypertrophic cardiomyopathy, aortic valve stenosis, anomalous coronary arteries
    - **Coronary artery disease (CAD; ischemia or infarction):** Kawasaki disease, long-standing diabetes mellitus, familial hypercholesterolemia or lipidemia

19. **How common is cardiac chest pain in children?**
    Pediatric chest pain is rarely due to cardiac pathology. Studies have found that only about 4% of children who present to a pediatric ED have a cardiac etiology for their pain, and some of these had known heart disease at the time of presentation.

20. **Which arrhythmias can possibly cause chest pain in children?**
    Consider the possibility of an arrhythmia such as supraventricular tachycardia (SVT) as a cause of chest pain in an older child who reports having palpitations. Ventricular tachycardia and premature ventricular contractions are rare in children, but may also cause sharp chest pain and an irregular cardiac rhythm. They may be found in children taking various medications or drugs such as cocaine.

21. **When should I be concerned about a cardiac infection as the cause of chest pain?**
    Children with infections such as myocarditis or pericarditis can present with chest pain and usually have fever. Those with pericarditis may report a sharp, stabbing, midsternal pain that is somewhat relieved when the patient sits up and leans forward. Distant heart sounds, neck vein distention, and a friction rub may be found. Viral myocarditis is more common and usually presents with low-grade fever and dull substernal chest pain. There is often respiratory distress as the infection progresses, and there may be muffled heart sounds or a gallop rhythm heard. Tachycardia out of proportion to the degree of fever is characteristic. Tachycardia and hypotension may be worse with standing, and this may not resolve after fluid resuscitation. A chest radiograph often reveals cardiomegaly (Fig. 8-2).

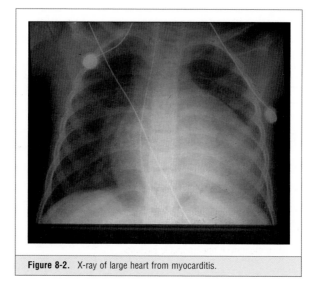

Figure 8-2. X-ray of large heart from myocarditis.

22. **Which cardiac conditions can lead to ischemia and chest pain?**
There are rare conditions that may lead to ischemic myocardial dysfunction in children. For instance, hypertrophic cardiomyopathy can cause pain, especially with exercise. Aortic valve stenosis can also cause ischemia and chest pain. Finally, those with underlying problems of the coronary arteries may develop chest pain. This is not common in children, but some with long-standing diabetes mellitus may have CAD, and children who had Kawasaki disease in the past may have persistent coronary artery aneurysms that can produce symptoms long after the initial illness.

Madhok AB, Boxer R, Green S: An adolescent with chest pain—sequela of Kawasaki disease. Pediatr Emerg Care 20:765–768, 2004.

KEY POINTS: CARDIAC CAUSES OF CHEST PAIN ✓

1. Coronary artery disease: Arteritis from Kawasaki disease, long-standing diabetes mellitus

2. Arrhythmias: SVT, premature ventricular contractions, ventricular tachycardia

3. Structural lesions: Hypertrophic cardiomyopathy, aortic valve stenosis

4. Infections: Myocarditis, pericarditis, endocarditis

23. **What are the concerns in children with Marfan's syndrome who report chest pain?**
These children may report chest pain due to rupture of an aortic aneurysm, which can be fatal. They are also at risk for spontaneous pneumothorax.

24. **Why is chest pain associated with exercise of concern?**
Mainly, young children with sudden death had preceding chest pain with exercise. Pain related to serious conditions such as myocarditis, CAD, and hypertrophic cardiomyopathy is worsened by exertion. Such patients should be referred to a cardiologist for further testing, including echocardiography, Holter monitoring, or exercise stress tests. Exercise-induced asthma is another condition in which chest pain is precipitated or worsened by exercise.

25. **What is Tietze's syndrome?**
This is a rare condition of unknown etiology that causes sternal chest pain. Physical examination may reveal tender, spindle-shaped swelling at the sternochondral junctions. The condition can last for months.

26. **Why do children with asthma report chest pain?**
Some possible etiologies include anxiety and overuse of chest wall muscles due to respiratory distress. Some have an associated pneumonia that could lead to diaphragmatic irritation. Others may develop a pneumothorax or pneumomediastinum.

27. **What etiology should be considered in an afebrile, previously well toddler, with no injury, who reports sudden midsternal chest pain?**
Foreign body in the esophagus. Many young children ingest coins, and most are asymptomatic. However, if the coin lodges in the esophagus (especially in the upper esophagus), the child may report sudden chest pain. Dysphagia may also be present. A chest radiograph or a metal detector usually confirms the diagnosis.

28. **When would you suspect hypertrophic cardiomyopathy in a child with chest pain?**
There may be a positive family history for this condition. It is generally inherited as an autosomal dominant disorder. A murmur may be heard best when the child is standing or performing a Valsalva maneuver. These positions and exercise may exaggerate the chest pain. Squatting or lying supine minimizes the obstruction and reduces the murmur. This condition is concerning because it is associated with sudden death among young athletes.

Washington RL: Sudden deaths in adolescent athletes caused by cardiac conditions. Pediatr Ann 32:751–756, 2003.

29. **Does mitral valve prolapse (MVP) cause chest pain in children?**
This is uncertain. Some postulate that MVP causes papillary muscle or left ventricular endocardial ischemia. However, in many cases, chest pain can be attributed to other causes, even in children with MVP. MVP is no more common in children with chest pain than in the general population. About 6–8% of children in the United States are believed to have MVP.

30. **Name a cutaneous condition that is associated with chest pain.**
Herpes zoster infection (Fig. 8-3). Shingles is often associated with distressing chest pain when the lesions involve a chest wall dermatome. The chest pain can sometimes precede the vesicular rash by several days.

31. **What is "devil's grip"?**
This is an unusual condition also known as *pleurodynia*. It is characterized by paroxysms of sharp pain in the abdomen or thorax. It is caused by coxsackievirus and may occur in mini-epidemics.

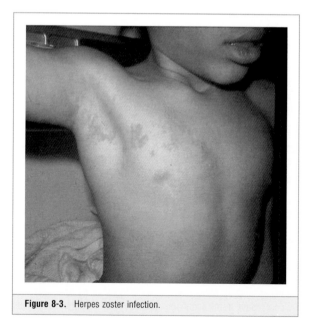

Figure 8-3. Herpes zoster infection.

32. **What are possible causes of chest pain in a teenage girl with systemic lupus erythematosus?**
These patients are at risk for pericarditis, myocarditis, endocarditis, pneumonia, pleural effusion, and myocardial ischemia if they have renal disease and hypertension.

33. **Should pulmonary embolism be considered as a cause of chest pain in a child?**
Pulmonary embolism is a rare problem in children. Consider it in a child (usually a teenage boy) with minor trauma to a lower extremity. It is very rarely reported in teenage girls who use oral contraceptives and in those who have recently had elective abortions. A patient with a pulmonary embolism usually has accompanying shortness of breath, pleuritic chest pain, fever, cough, and hemoptysis. The finding of a swollen, tender lower extremity on physical examination increases concern about venous thrombosis and a pulmonary embolism.

34. **In children with chest pain and sickle cell disease, what are the likely etiologies?**
Vaso-occlusive crises may be the cause of pain. However, consider acute chest syndrome in these patients. Pneumonia due to an encapsulated organism is also of concern. Finally, ischemia due to a heart weakened by chronic anemia is possible. All such patients deserve a chest radiograph and perhaps an electrocardiogram as part of their evaluation.

35. **Chest pain associated with a ''crunching'' sound on chest examination is found with which condition?**
Pneumomediastinum. Free mediastinal air and subcutaneous emphysema are complications of asthma exacerbation. It may also occur as a result of trauma, or spontaneously. Some children with this finding have associated dyspnea and cough. Crepitation is often noted in the suprasternal notch and may extend to the neck, axilla, and face. A chest radiograph confirms the diagnosis. The condition usually has a good outcome and resolves within a few days. Hospital admission and treatment of the underlying cause (i.e., asthma) are recommended.

Kanegaye JT: An adolescent football player with chest pain. Clin Pediatr 42:471–474, 2003.

36. **When should referral to a cardiologist be considered for a child with chest pain?**
Chest pain associated with exercise (during or immediately after) requires an evaluation by a cardiologist. If the pediatric patient has pain associated with syncope, dizziness, or palpitations, evaluation by a cardiologist is also reasonable. Furthermore, if the child has a history of underlying heart disease or cardiac arrhythmia or has a previous condition that subjects him to heart disease (i.e., long-standing diabetes mellitus, Kawasaki disease) referral to a cardiologist seems prudent. It is also recommended to have a cardiologist evaluate the child if there is a history of premature sudden death in the family or if the child has hypertension or features of Marfan's syndrome.

Owens TR: Chest pain in the adolescent. Adolesc Med State Art Rev 12:95–104, 2001.

CHAPTER 9

COUGH

Christopher King, MD, FACEP

1. **Describe the cough reflex.**

   Stimuli that induce cough can be mechanical (e.g., foreign body, dust), chemical (e.g., capsaicin, acetic acid), or inflammatory mediators (e.g., histamine, bradykinin, prostaglandin E_2).
   Such stimuli interact with cough receptors in the upper and lower airways that cause production of mediators, such as tachykinins and neurokinin A. Stimulation of the cough receptors is transmitted via the vagus nerve to the "cough center" of the brainstem (probably located in the pons). The efferent limb of the cough pathway is poorly understood, but is known to include the spinal cord from C3 to S2, spinal nerves, and the recurrent laryngeal nerve (for glottic closure). Activation of the efferent pathway causes constriction of the expiratory muscles, which produces increased airway pressure against the closed glottis. The airway also narrows slightly. When the glottis is suddenly opened, air is expelled at a high velocity, clearing the airway of secretions and foreign material.

2. **How is a cough suppressed?**

   As with respiration, cough is largely involuntary but can be suppressed voluntarily to a certain extent (cortical modulation). Opioids that suppress cough (e.g., morphine) are believed to produce this effect by acting centrally on the cough center. Inhalation of nebulized lidocaine suppresses cough by affecting cough receptors in the airway.

3. **Is the cough reflex mediated by the same pathway that produces bronchospasm?**

   It has been widely held that airway hypersensitivity (asthma/bronchospasm) and cough are manifestations of the same physiologic mechanism. By this thinking, persistent coughing, such as wheezing, is a common presentation of asthma. This view has led to the current trend of diagnosing children with persistent coughing as being asthmatic ("cough variant" asthma), even when these patients have no other evidence of bronchospasm (dyspnea, exercise intolerance, abnormal spirometry findings). However, recent evidence suggests that while airway hypersensitivity and cough receptor sensitivity can be *triggered* by the same stimuli, this probably occurs via two *different* pathways. For most children, it appears that persistent coughing results solely from increased sensitivity of cough receptors in the upper and lower airways and does not represent true asthma/bronchospasm.

   Chang AB: Cough, cough receptors, and asthma in children. Pediatr Pulmonol 28:59–70, 1999.

4. **How much coughing is normal?**

   One of the primary obstacles in studying cough in children has been that this symptom is difficult to reliably measure. Reproducibility of survey questions is poor, and, unlike the situation with asthma, there is no validated subjective cough scoring system. Fortunately, a new device that a child can wear like a Holter monitor provides an objective measurement of coughing. When this device was used with "normal" children who had no history of asthma and no respiratory illnesses in the previous 4 weeks, the mean cough frequency over 24 hours was 11.3 episodes (range, 1–34 episodes). Thus, the frequency of coughing episodes varies widely even among children without respiratory problems.

   Munyard P, Bush A: How much coughing is normal? Arch Dis Child 74:531–534, 1996.

5. **What is the most common cause of persistent cough?**
   While the differential diagnosis of persistent cough (>2 weeks) in children is relatively broad (Table 9-1), the most common cause is probably postviral or inflammatory cough, which has been variably called *nonspecific cough*, *isolated cough*, or *cough illness*. Children who develop a viral upper respiratory tract infection may continue to cough long after other viral symptoms (e.g., rhinitis, fever) have subsided. These patients have a persistent, dry cough (particularly at night), but do not have wheezing, chest tightness, dyspnea on exertion, or other symptoms of bronchospasm. This type of cough may persist for several weeks before resolving spontaneously.

   Hay AD, Wilson AD: The natural history of acute cough in children aged 0 to 4 years in primary care: A systematic review. Br J Gen Pract 52:401–409, 2002.

TABLE 9-1. DIFFERENTIAL DIAGNOSIS OF PERSISTENT COUGH BY AGE

Infancy (<1 year)

- Infection: viral, bacterial, chlamydial
- Anatomic abnormalities: tracheomalacia, vascular rings
- Cystic fibrosis
- Bronchopulmonary dysplasia (premature infants)

Preschool (1–5 years)

- Asthma
- Infection
- Foreign-body aspiration
- Cystic fibrosis

School age (5–18 years)

- Asthma
- Infection (especially mycoplasma)
- Smoking
- Psychogenic causes

---

6. **Do gastroesophageal reflux disease (GERD) and sinusitis commonly cause persistent cough?**
   No. When confounding factors such as airway hyperreactivity and atopy are removed, prospective, controlled studies among children with GERD and sinusitis who also have persistent coughing have shown no reduction in cough with treatment of these two underlying conditions. Prior studies that showed a benefit were generally anecdotal or were not placebo controlled. To date, no reliable evidence indicates that persistent cough is related to either GERD or sinusitis.

   Chang AB, Phelan PD, Sawyer SM, et al: Airway hyperresponsiveness and cough-receptor sensitivity in children with recurrent cough. Am J Respir Crit Care Med 155:1935–1939, 1997.

7. **Is cough-variant asthma underdiagnosed?**
   In fact, the opposite is more likely the case (i.e., it is probably overdiagnosed). In the past, children with persistent cough accompanied by signs of true bronchospasm such as exercise

intolerance, but *without* wheezing, often were not diagnosed with asthma. The syndrome of cough and acute exertional dyspnea was first identified in a series of adult patients in 1975, and the term *cough-variant asthma* was coined in 1979. Before that time, cough-variant asthma was certainly underdiagnosed. Now, however, the diagnosis of asthma in children with isolated cough has been widely embraced. In fact, some have suggested that recent increases in the prevalence of asthma are largely due to expanding the diagnostic criteria to include children with isolated cough. This has occurred despite evidence that most of these patients do not respond to conventional asthma therapy (see next question). It would appear that the pendulum has swung too far, and we are currently overdiagnosing and overtreating asthma in patients with simple postviral coughing.

Benedictis FM, Selvaggio D, Benedictis D: Cough, wheezing and asthma in children: Lesson from the past. Pediatr Allergy Immunol 15:386–393, 2004.

KEY POINTS: ETIOLOGY OF COUGH IN CHILDREN ✔

1. Most children with persistent coughing will have a postviral or inflammatory cough that does not respond to any standard therapies but resolves spontaneously over a period of weeks.

2. Cough variant asthma is rarely the appropriate diagnosis for a child with a persistent cough who does not have other signs of asthma (e.g., exertional dyspnea).

3. Passive cigarette or cigar smoke aggravates coughing in children.

4. Persistent coughing in a young child after a severe choking episode may represent aspiration of a foreign body into a mainstem bronchus.

8. **Do children with persistent cough respond to standard therapy for asthma?**
   Given the caveats described in the previous question, it is safe to say that children with true cough-variant asthma should respond to treatment with bronchodilators and/or steroids within hours to a few days. However, these patients represent a relatively small percentage of the children presenting to the emergency department (ED) with persistent coughing. Most will have postviral cough, which does *not* respond to conventional asthma therapy. Therefore, unless a child with persistent cough has a history that suggests a true bronchospastic etiology (severe coughing and dyspnea occurring consistently with exertion), it is not generally wise to make a de novo diagnosis of cough-variant asthma and initiate bronchodilator or steroid treatment. Conversely, if a child has been receiving conventional asthma therapy for several days to weeks and coughing has not decreased, the patient is very unlikely to have cough-variant asthma and the asthma treatments can be stopped.

   Thompson F, Masters IB, Chang AB: Persistent cough in children and the overuse of medications. J Paediatr Child Health 38:578–581, 2002.

9. **Does cough due to bronchitis respond to treatment with antibiotics?**
   Bronchitis seems to be a diagnosis in search of significance. Most clinicians use the term *bronchitis* when referring to a patient with a persistent, *productive* cough without evidence of pneumonia. Yet if the diagnostic criteria are poorly defined in adults (how much sputum? how often?), the situation with children is worse. The primary issue with children is that they do not cough up sputum; they swallow it. Consequently, diagnosing bronchitis in a child is usually difficult or impossible, since sputum production can rarely be established or quantified.

At any rate, studies in adults have shown no efficacy in treating bronchitis with antibiotics, and studies in children show no efficacy in treating persistent cough with antibiotics.

O'Brien KL, Dowell SF, Schwartz B, et al: Cough illness/bronchitis—principles of judicious use of antimicrobial agents. Pediatrics 101:178–181, 1998.

10. **Does antibiotic treatment of cough due to an upper respiratory tract infection prevent subsequent pneumonia?**
   Although most clinicians acknowledge that frequent use of antibiotics to treat viral upper respiratory tract infections is an important cause of increasing antibiotic resistance in bacteria, this practice continues to be widespread. One justification for the use of antibiotics in such cases is to provide prophylaxis against subsequent pneumonia. However, at least nine trials have assessed the utility of antibiotic prophylaxis for patients with upper respiratory tract infection, and a meta-analysis of these trials reported no effect of antibiotic treatment in preventing pneumonia.

   Dowell SF, Schwartz B, Phillips WR, et al: Appropriate use of antibiotics for URIs in children: Part II. Cough, pharyngitis, and the common cold. Am Fam Physician 58:1113–1123, 1998.
   Gadomski AM: Potential interventions for preventing pneumonia among young children: Lack of effect of antibiotic treatment for upper respiratory infections. Pediatr Infect Dis J 12:115–120, 1993.

11. **Do commonly used cough medications work?**
   In a word, no. Numerous studies have addressed this question, and the bulk of evidence indicates that the commonly used pediatric cough preparations are no more effective in suppressing cough than placebo. This includes dextromethorphan, guaifenesin, and codeine. Furthermore, many of the pediatric cough medicines also contain potentially dangerous agents such as decongestants that, if used in excessive doses, can cause cardiac arrhythmias in children. Despite these facts, we continue to spend over $2 billion annually in the United States for cough and cold preparations—another testament to the power of advertising and its influence on medicine.

   Schroeder K, Fahey T. Over-the-counter medications for acute cough in children and adults in ambulatory settings. Cochrane Database of Systematic Reviews, Vol. 2, 2005.

12. **What problem should come to mind if a toddler presents with a persistent, nagging cough after a severe choking spell?**
   This is the classic history for foreign-body aspiration. Parents of a young child who has ongoing episodes of moderate to severe coughing should be questioned about the occurrence of a choking spell. The child (who is preverbal and cannot tell what happened) typically has a small toy or bead in his or her mouth, takes a breath, and has the object enter the trachea; at this point a severe choking spell ensues. If the object is about the size of the trachea, and it cannot be expelled with coughing, the child will quickly develop signs of severe upper airway obstruction. Yet if the object is smaller than the diameter of one of the mainstem bronchi, it may lodge there so that the child recovers with only a persistent cough. A patient with normal lungs will have adequate oxygenation and ventilation despite complete occlusion of one mainstem bronchus. Expiratory chest radiographs may show decreased "deflation" of the affected lung. In a young child, or uncooperative child, bilateral decubitus x-rays may show the same finding. However, if the story is classic, it is wise to consult an otolaryngologist even if the chest radiographs are normal.

13. **What is habitual cough?**
   Habitual (or psychogenic) cough is a type of conversion reaction, in which a child responds to stressors by developing symptoms such as abdominal pain, headache, or difficulty breathing but there is no organic disease. The onset of persistent symptoms may be followed by an extensive, yet unrevealing, medical workup (e.g., multiple sets of laboratory results, multiple

computed tomographic scans). Typically, there is an issue of secondary gain—for example, obtaining increased attention, preventing parents from fighting, avoiding school—that may only be reinforced by repetitive medical tests. Habitual cough is one of the more straightforward conversion reactions to manage in the ED because unlike symptoms such as difficulty breathing or severe headache, children rarely die from cough. As such, a patient with habitual cough can often be discharged from the ED, after a specific plan for outpatient follow-up (with the child's pediatrician or possibly a pulmonologist) has been formulated, without significant doubt or worry that the child is being sent home with a potentially dangerous illness.

de Jongste JC, Shields MD: Chronic cough in children. Thorax 58:998–1003, 2003.

14. **What are the characteristics of a patient with habitual cough?**
One of the most striking aspects of this condition is the disconnect between the reaction of the parents and the reaction of the child—the parents are often extremely upset and anxious while the child appears unconcerned. Parents are commonly "at the end of their rope" and are coming to the ED for a second opinion. The child may already have had one or more normal chest radiographs or blood test results obtained by other health care providers. A patient with habitual cough is typically older (school-aged or adolescent), has missed multiple (sometimes many) days of school, is not awakened from sleep at night by the cough, and has a completely normal physical examination. Aspiration of a foreign body can generally be excluded because the patient is old enough to deny it. The cough itself will often sound like a "honk"—harsh, loud, and impossible to ignore.

Bush A: Paediatric problems of cough. Pulm Pharm Therapeutics 15:309–315, 2002.

15. **How is habitual cough managed in the ED?**
As with most other types of conversion reaction, habitual cough cannot always be diagnosed conclusively in the ED. It is generally a diagnosis of exclusion, that is, after any potentially significant conditions (e.g., pneumonia, bronchospasm, pneumothorax) have been ruled out. Sometimes this subject can be gently broached with parents, although their reaction may be very defensive ("Are you saying this is all in her head?"). Establishing rapport by demonstrating genuine concern, listening carefully, and avoiding an accusatory or judgmental tone is essential. In some situations, it may be better to leave discussion of this diagnosis to the private pediatrician or specialist (e.g., a pulmonologist).

16. **What is one thing parents should always do if their child has a persistent cough?**
They should stop smoking and forbid others from smoking in the house where the child resides.

17. **What is the strangest cause of persistent cough?**
Although this is certainly open to debate, perhaps the oddest cause of persistent cough is an eyelash stuck in the child's ear. Curiously, stimulation of the external auditory canal or the tympanic membrane by an eyelash can repetitively provoke the cough reflex in a child. Unlike other otic foreign bodies, an eyelash does not cause pain or diminish hearing and may therefore go undetected for an extended time. Furthermore, it may not be immediately obvious on otoscopy. Consequently, it is wise to carefully examine the ears of a child with persistent coughing in hopes of finding this rare and elusive, yet easily remedied, cause of a troublesome symptom.

CHAPTER 10

CRYING AND IRRITABILITY IN THE YOUNG CHILD

Robert G. Bolte, MD

1. **Why is an organized approach important to the evaluation of crying in an infant?**
   The etiology of crying in the nonverbal and frequently uncooperative infant is often obscure.
   A well-organized approach is critical because the differential diagnosis is vast, ranging from
   a normal physiologic or temperamental response to life-threatening medical or surgical
   pathology. Finding the right answer with a reasonable utilization of resources is a big part of
   the "art" of pediatrics (Table 10-1).

   > Bolte RG: Intractable crying in infancy and early childhood. In Aghababian RV (eds): Emergency Medicine:
   > The Core Curriculum. Philadelphia, Lippincott-Raven, 1998, pp 622–630.

2. **I work in an emergency department (ED) setting. Why do I have to know anything
   about colic?**
   Two reasons:
   - It's a commonly seen problem, even in an ED setting, representing a significant cause of
     parental anxiety and frustration.
   - If you know what colic *is*, then you're less likely to misdiagnose more serious problems
     assuming that they are "only colic."

3. **Describe the clinical features of the infant colic syndrome.**
   Cyclic discrete periods of intractable crying, usually on a daily basis, with onset at 1–4 weeks of age
   and spontaneous improvement by 3–4 months of age. The classic definition of infantile colic was
   first described by Wessel in 1954 as "Crying lasting more than 3 hours per day, 3 days per week, and
   continuing more than 3 weeks in infants less than 3 months of age." The crying is not relieved by
   normal parental interventions, such as feeding, burping, changing diapers, providing a pacifier, or
   rocking. Vomiting, diarrhea, or poor weight gain are *not* features of the infant colic syndrome.

   > Barr RG: Charging our understanding of infant colic. Arch Pediatr Adolesc Med 156:1172–1174, 2002.
   > Clifford TJ, Campbell MK, Speechley KN, Gorodzinsky F: Sequelae of infant colic: Evidence of transient infant
   > distress and absence of lasting effects on maternal health. Arch Pediatr Adolesc Med 156:1183–1188, 2002.

4. **Is there a "normal" amount of inconsolable crying in a young infant?**
   Brazelton's data on how much time a *normal* infant spends crying *inconsolably* shows that the
   median daily amount of inconsolable crying at 2 weeks of age is 1 hour and 45 minutes. This
   increases to 2 hours and 45 minutes at 6 weeks of age and thankfully decreases to less than
   an hour by 12 weeks of age. Inconsolable crying usually occurs in the evening (between 3 PM
   and 11 PM) when most busy parents are frantically attempting to spend precious quality time
   with their new baby. Sharing this information with prospective parents may be the most
   effective argument for birth control that you can ever deliver.

   > Brazelton TB: Crying in infancy. Pediatrics 29:579–588, 1962.

5. **Are there any effective treatments for colic?**
   There's no magic remedy, but communicating empathy is crucial. Also, providing the family with
   accurate information on "normal" amounts of inconsolable crying and when they can expect
   improvement is always of value. A behavioral-modification approach described by Taubman has been

TABLE 10-1. RELATIVELY FREQUENT SERIOUS CONDITIONS ASSOCIATED WITH INTRACTABLE CRYING THAT MUST BE EXCLUDED PRIOR TO EMERGENCY DEPARTMENT DISCHARGE

Condition	Clinical Correlates
Meningitis/encephalitis	Lethargy, vomiting, paradoxical irritability, fever
Sepsis	Lethargy, poor perfusion, fever, petechiae
Septic hip	Pain with range of motion/abnormal positioning of hip
Battered child syndrome	Bruising, bony tenderness, incompatible history
Shaken baby syndrome	Lethargy, full fontanelle, retinal hemorrhages
Intussusception	Paroxysmal abdominal pain, lethargy, bloody stool, abdominal mass; rectal examination may be abnormal
Volvulus	Bilious vomiting, abdominal tenderness
Appendicitis	Abnormal examination of abdomen
Incarcerated inguinal hernia	Abnormal examination of inguinal region
Hemolytic-uremic syndrome	Bloody diarrhea, hematuria/proteinuria, hemolytic anemia, thrombocytopenia, azotemia
Hypoxemia	Tachypnea, retractions, nasal flaring, wheezing, cyanosis
Hair encirclement	Abnormal examination of digits, genitalia, or uvula
Testicular torsion	Abnormal examination of scrotum
Supraventricular tachycardia	Heart rate >220 beats per minute

shown to be helpful. Weizman and colleagues have reported that commercially available chamomile tea (not home-grown concoctions, which are potentially dangerous) may be useful. Simethicone (Mylicon; 0.3 mL given prior to each feeding) is basically a high-grade placebo, but at least it's nontoxic. Generally avoid recommending formula changes (likely effective only in a subset of infants requiring hydrolysate formula) or medications with potentially toxic side effects, such as paregoric, dicyclomine (Bentyl), or hyoscyamine (Levsin).

Taubman B: Parental counseling compared with elimination of cow's milk or soy milk protein for the treatment of infant colic syndrome: A randomized trial. Pediatrics 81:756–761, 1988.

Weizman Z, Alkrinawi S, Goldfarb D, et al: Efficacy of herbal tea preparation in infantile colic. J Pediatr 122:650–652, 1993.

6. **What is the most common medical problem in young infants that mimics colic?**
Esophagitis (secondary to gastroesophageal reflux). This is a ubiquitous condition in young infants, and presenting symptoms often mimic colic. With both conditions, infants present to the ED during the first few months of life with intractable crying as the chief complaint. In esophagitis, there is often a history of frequent nonforceful, *nonbilious* regurgitation following feedings. The infant with an irritated esophagus may take the first few sips of the feeding avidly, but then turns away, crying in pain. Occasionally the infant with esophagitis exhibits a torticollis-like positioning of the neck (Sandifer syndrome). Treatment can be initiated with medications such as antacids or ranitidine, with follow-up by the primary medical care provider.

7. **A previously well 3-month-old presents with acute onset of intractable crying for the past 4 hours. The child is afebrile, and the general examination is normal. What is the most likely diagnosis?**
Corneal abrasion. This etiology is relatively common but easily overlooked. In a prospective study by Poole, 21% of afebrile infants younger than 6 months of age presenting to an ED with a chief complaint of crying had corneal abrasions. But you'll never diagnose it unless you first consider the possibility and then look for it by performing a corneal examination with fluorescein. Don't be misled by the lack of eye redness or discharge; most infants with this diagnosis lack these findings. A *hair tourniquet* (Fig. 10-1) could also present like this, but a meticulous physical examination (of digits, penis, clitoris, and uvula) should make that diagnosis obvious. Non-accidental trauma (child abuse) must also be considered.

Poole SR: The infant with acute, unexplained, excessive crying. Pediatrics 88:450–455, 1991.
Rittichier KK, Roback MG, Bassett KE: Are signs and symptoms associated with persistent corneal abrasions in children? Arch Pediatr Adolesc Med 154:370–374, 2000.
Sytwestrzak MS, Fischer BF, Fischer H: Recurrent clitoral tourniquet syndrome, Pediatrics 105:866, 2000.

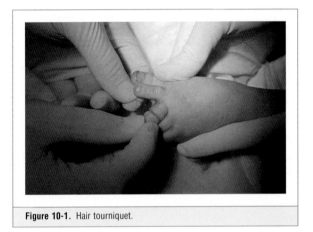

Figure 10-1. Hair tourniquet.

8. **A nontoxic-appearing 5-week-old presents with fever and crying. The mother mentions that the crying increases during diaper changes. The cerebral spinal fluid and urinalysis results appear normal, a blood culture is pending, and you've initiated parenteral antibiotics. What else should be considered?**
A septic hip. The evaluation and "processing" of the febrile child younger than 8 weeks of age can become so rote that we sometimes forget to perform a thorough physical examination, *including the hips*. A septic hip can occur in this age range and is a surgical emergency with devastating consequences if not recognized in time. The infant may exhibit "pseudo-paralysis" of the limb, with a preference for abduction and external rotation of the hip. Crying may increase at diaper changes as the parent inadvertently manipulates the hips. The peripheral white blood count is often normal. C-reactive protein and sedimentation rate are consistently elevated.

9. **An 8-month-old white female presents with crying and a history of fever. In the ED, she is febrile but nontoxic in appearance, and the general physical examination is normal. What is the most likely "treatable" diagnosis?**
Far and away, it is urinary tract infection (UTI), unless you consider viral illness "treatable." In a 1998 ED study by Shaw et al, 16% of febrile white females younger than 2 years of age

had a UTI—even if "otitis media, viral gastroenteritis, or upper respiratory infection" had been diagnosed. In the same cohort, if isolated fever was the only presenting symptom, an impressive 31% had a UTI. The rate of UTI in young Hispanic girls is probably comparable to that in whites; however, it is much lower than the rate in young African-American females.

Gorelick M, McGowan KL, Yakscoe NM, Schwartz JS: Prevalence of urinary tract infection in febrile young children in the emergency department. Pediatrics 102:e16, 1998.

10. **Are there any cardiac etiologies that present with crying as a chief complaint?**
Somewhat surprisingly, supraventricular tachycardia was the ultimate diagnosis in 4% of the afebrile infants who presented with "excessive crying" in Poole's 1991 ED study. Keep this pearl tucked away: If there is a history suggestive of paroxysmal tachycardia, remember that in the asymptomatic period, a delta wave (widened QRS with a slurred upstroke seen on 12-lead electrocardiogram) can give you the diagnosis.

Poole SR: The infant with acute, unexplained, excessive crying. Pediatrics 88:450–455, 1991.

KEY POINTS: ED EVALUATION OF THE CRYING INFANT ✓

1. An organized approach is vital to appropriate diagnosis in the ED.

2. Routine use of "screening" laboratory studies and radiographs is generally not helpful.

3. A thoughtful history and a thorough physical examination are the cornerstones of diagnosis.

4. Knowledge of the natural history of colic can be an extremely useful tool in generating a differential diagnosis.

5. Awareness of potential life-threatening etiologies with crying as a presenting symptom (e.g., meningitis, shaken baby syndrome, intussusception) is paramount.

11. **Name three relatively common, life-threatening surgical emergencies of infancy that you would expect to present with crying but in which crying sometimes is absent.**
   - **Intussusception:** Generally presents with paroxysmal irritability, vomiting, and later bloody stool. But a significant subset of patients present with *isolated lethargy*. This usually afebrile infant may be misdiagnosed as having sepsis, a toxic ingestion, or a closed head injury. Intussusception generally presents in the 2-month to 2-year age range, with a peak at 9 months of age. In the lethargic infant, always palpate for abdominal masses, and if the diagnosis is in question, include a rectal examination. You may be surprised to find blood on the examining finger.
   - **Midgut volvulus:** Although crying may be associated with this diagnosis, most infants presenting with midgut volvulus are surprisingly nontoxic and calm in appearance, with a benign abdominal examination *until* the gut begins to infarct. Eighty percent of patients present in the first 4 weeks of life, and the cardinal diagnostic sign is *bilious* vomiting. If this diagnosis is suspected, an *emergent* upper gastrointestinal study is mandatory.
   - **Shaken baby syndrome:** Although this syndrome may present with crying and irritability, many infants have a chief complaint of listlessness or lethargy. In children under 2 years of age, your threshold for computed tomography of the head should be low. Although most infants with shaken baby syndrome do *not* have external signs of trauma, *any* facial bruising

or intraoral trauma should be a major red flag. Retinal hemorrhage is generally the only physical finding (but unless the child is severely obtunded, it is problematic to diagnose). In a 1999 study by Jenny et al., physicians were most likely to miss this diagnosis if the family was white and both parents lived at home. In this same study, the most frequent misdiagnoses were viral gastroenteritis (persistent vomiting), *accidental* head trauma, rule-out sepsis, and colic.

Jenny C, Hymel KP, Ritzen A, et al: Analysis of missed cases of abusive head trauma. JAMA 281:621–626, 1999.

Reijneveld SA, van der Wal MF, Brugman E, et al; Infant crying and abuse. Lancet 364:1340–1342, 2004.

12. **Are screening laboratory and radiologic tests generally useful in the ED evaluation of the young crying child?**

    The short answer is "no." Routinely obtaining a panel of laboratory studies or x-rays as a diagnostic screen *seldom* adds to the evaluation (except for the expense). Generally the diagnosis lies in a thoughtful history and a thorough physical examination. In *selected* cases, specific laboratory tests or selected studies can certainly be of value (most commonly a catheterized urine specimen or a corneal examination with fluorescein). Sometimes the studies have critical importance (lumbar puncture in the child with meningitis, computed tomography of the head in shaken baby syndrome, air enema with intussusception, toxicology screen in methamphetamine exposure).

CHAPTER 11

DIARRHEA

Linda D. Arnold, MD

1. **What is diarrhea?**
   Diarrhea is defined as a decrease in the consistency, or an increase in the frequency, of stool. Marked variations of "normal" number, volume, and consistency of stools exist between individuals. Breastfed babies, for example, may stool more than seven times a day. An increase in stool quantity, or a frequency of more than 10 stools/day, constitutes diarrhea in infants. By age 3, stool output reaches adult norms of 100 gm/day; a high-fiber diet increases the volume. Stool output of more than 200 gm/day meets the definition of diarrhea.
   Diarrhea is caused by a disturbance of the mechanisms that regulate intestinal fluid and electrolyte transport. Nonspecific inflammation, epithelial invasion by micro-organisms, fluid or carbohydrate excess, and pharmacologic agents have all been implicated.

2. **How big a problem is diarrhea?**
   In the United States, acute gastroenteritis leads to more than 1.5 million office visits and 200,000 hospitalizations each year for children under the age of 5. It accounts for approximately 10% of all hospital admissions for this age group. Direct costs in this country have been estimated to be over $2 billion per year. Hundreds of children in the United States die each year because of resulting dehydration or systemic illness. Morbidity and mortality are greatest in infants and malnourished or immunocompromised children. Risk of dehydration is further increased in minorities, children of young single mothers, and those with a history of prematurity.

   King CK, Glass R, Bresee JS, et al: Managing acute gastroenteritis among children: Oral rehydration, maintenance, and nutritional therapy. MMWR Morb Mortal Wkly Rep 52:1–16, 2003.

3. **What role does duration of symptoms play in determining the etiology of diarrhea?**
   Diarrhea of less than 2-week duration is classified as "acute" and, in the majority of cases, results from enteric infection. Extraintestinal infections, such as urinary tract infections, otitis media, and appendicitis, can also cause diarrhea and should be ruled out. Acute diarrhea may also be the result of food-borne toxins, or the initial manifestation of milk or soy protein intolerance.

4. **What are common causes of chronic diarrhea?**
   - Chronic diarrhea in infants may be postinfectious, the result of protein intolerance or malnutrition, subsequent to metabolic disorders such as cystic fibrosis or enzyme and transport defects, or secondary to anatomic anomalies.
   - In older infants and toddlers, chronic, nonspecific "toddler's diarrhea"; protein intolerance; and postinfectious diarrhea are all common. Children in this age group frequently present with other etiologies, including giardiasis, celiac sprue, sucrase-isomaltase deficiency, and Hirschsprung's enterocolitis.
   - In school-aged children and adolescents, consider giardiasis, celiac disease, lactose intolerance, irritable bowel, and inflammatory bowel disease. Teens with chronic diarrhea should be questioned about laxative use/abuse.

5. **What clues can the history provide?**
   - Viral pathogens tend to injure the proximal small intestine. Onset of illness is generally abrupt and duration limited. These patients are more likely to be afebrile and to present with both emesis and diarrhea. Associated respiratory symptoms or rash are often seen.
   - Bacterial pathogens produce colonic inflammation, with bloody or mucoid stools, and cramping abdominal pain. Fever and tenesmus may be prominent features. Bacterial toxins may produce a watery stool.
   - Food poisoning is characterized by abrupt onset of vomiting after a meal, followed by diarrhea.
   - Foul-smelling stools suggest malabsorption.
   - An increase in flatus may be seen with *Giardia* infection or lactose intolerance.
   - Irritable bowel syndrome is characterized by cramping, as well as frequent, small-volume, liquid stools alternating with constipation; physical and emotional stress exacerbate the condition.

6. **What specific questions should I ask parents of a child with diarrhea?**
   Question parents about recent travel, pets, and possible exposure to untreated drinking water or fecally contaminated recreational waters. Ask detailed questions about duration of symptoms, oral intake, frequency of wet diapers, and weight loss to assess for degree of dehydration.

7. **What should I look for on physical examination?**
   Assess the child's hydration status carefully. Heart rate, quality of mucous membranes, capillary refill and perfusion, sunken eyes or fontanelle, and activity level all offer important clues. Plot the weight and weight/height ratios, as this may point to an underlying chronic disorder. Children with uncomplicated gastroenteritis tend to have mild diffuse abdominal tenderness and active bowel sounds. Localized tenderness, rebound tenderness, and absent or high-pitched bowel sounds indicate a possible surgical process or bowel obstruction. Palpation of a mass or a discrete loop of bowel suggests inflammatory bowel disease (IBD), intussusception, or constipation. Increased anal tone and explosive stools should raise concerns of Hirschsprung's enterocolitis, while perianal tags, fissures, or abscesses are characteristic of IBD. A "doughy" feel to the skin may be a hallmark of hypernatremic dehydration. Diarrhea associated with pallor may suggest hemolytic uremic syndrome. Children with protuberant abdomens and wasting of the buttocks and extremities should be evaluated for giardiasis, celiac sprue, and cystic fibrosis.

8. **When is diarrhea dangerous?**
   Emergency intervention is required for the child with moderate-to-severe dehydration or when a surgical etiology is suspected. Children with hypernatremic dehydration should be managed carefully, as they may develop cerebral edema if rehydration occurs too rapidly. Hirschsprung's enterocolitis has up to a 50% mortality rate: it should be treated promptly with decompression via a rectal tube, pending definitive treatment. Appendicitis, often misdiagnosed in children, may present with diarrhea secondary to cecal inflammation. When symptoms of abdominal pain, vomiting, and lethargy accompany the passage of "bloody diarrhea," intussusception should be high on the list of conditions in the differential diagnosis. Unexplained diarrhea that doesn't fit a particular pattern should raise the possibility of Munchausen syndrome by proxy in an infant or younger child and of laxative abuse in the adolescent.

9. **What is the role of daycare in childhood diarrheal disease?**
   While the average child under age 3 years has two to three episodes of diarrhea per year, the rate doubles for children in daycare. Children in this setting are at increased risk for both fecal–oral and fomite transmission of enteric pathogens. Daycare attendance has been implicated in outbreaks of rotavirus, astrovirus, shigella, campylobacter, giardia, and cryptosporidium.

10. **Name the common infectious causes of diarrhea.**
    - **Viral:** Rotavirus, Norwalk-like virus, enteric adenovirus, astrovirus, calicivirus
    - **Bacterial:** *Salmonella, Shigella, Campylobacter,* or *Yersinia* spp., *Escherichia coli, Clostridium difficile*
    - **Parasitic:** *Giardia* sp., *Cryptosporidium* sp., *Entamoeba histolytica, Strongyloides* sp., *Microsporidium* sp.

11. **What conditions may be mistaken for infectious diarrhea?**
    - Chronic nonspecific (toddler's) diarrhea
    - Sorbitol-induced diarrhea
    - Milk protein allergy
    - Lactose intolerance
    - Munchausen syndrome by proxy

12. **When is diarrhea not diarrhea?**
    Children with severe constipation can develop overflow incontinence. Encopresis involves frequent soiling with liquid stool, which leaks around a solid fecal mass. Encopretics are unaware that they are soiling because of decreased rectal tone and sensation. Physical examination often reveals stool-filled intestinal loops and impacted stool on rectal examination, while a history of "streaking" of the underpants is frequently obtained.

13. **Do the color and appearance of the stool matter?**
    Visible blood or mucus in the stool suggests an inflammatory etiology. Aside from the presence of blood, the color of the stool is generally not important. Bulky stools are seen in fat malabsorption, while watery explosive stools may indicate carbohydrate malabsorption. Parents may describe the appearance of undigested food particles in the frequent stools associated with toddler's diarrhea. These are, in fact, undigested cellulose particles that are not disintegrated in the colon.

14. **Is the odor of the stool important?**
    Carbohydrate malabsorption results in foul, watery stools that have a vinegar-like odor. The stools of a patient with fat malabsorption are bulky and foul smelling. Consider celiac disease, cystic fibrosis, pancreatic insufficiency, and bile salt malabsorption in the presence of steatorrhea. Pleasant-smelling stools simply do not exist.

15. **What foods can mimic bloody stool?**
    Children who have ingested fruit juices, gelatin, popsicles, Kool-Aid beverages, red candies, tomatoes, beets, or cranberries may have red stools. Tarry-looking stools result from the consumption of bismuth-containing antidiarrheal products, iron, black licorice, spinach, blueberries, purple grapes, chocolate, or grape juice. Nonbloody stools may test positive on fecal occult blood tests in a child who has eaten red meat, cherries, tomato skin, or iron supplements.

16. **Are there seasonal variations in the causative agents of infectious diarrhea?**
    Rotavirus, the most common cause of infectious diarrhea in infants and children, is more common during winter months in temperate climates. No seasonal variation is seen in tropical climates. Bacterial pathogens are more likely in the summer and early fall months. Undercooked meats and poorly refrigerated side dishes at picnics and cookouts are frequently implicated. Fecal contamination of recreational waters and consumption of untreated fresh water by campers may increase exposure to parasites during warmer months.

17. **Should clear liquids be given by mouth until diarrhea resolves?**
    Formula provides superior nutrition to clear liquids and should be offered throughout the course of an uncomplicated illness, if tolerated. When clear liquids are used, families should

be instructed to avoid apple juice, soda, or sports beverages. Their hypertonicity and high carbohydrate load can cause diarrhea to worsen. Use of one of the commercially available glucose electrolyte–containing solutions is preferable. Nursing mothers should not be instructed to stop breastfeeding infants or toddlers with diarrhea.

18. **Which children with diarrhea require IV hydration?**
Oral rehydration therapy (ORT) with an appropriate oral rehydration solution (ORS) is recommended for all children with uncomplicated gastroenteritis with mild-to-moderate dehydration. Though time consuming, it has been shown to be as effective as IV hydration in this group when caregivers are trained and motivated. For children with complicated illness, moderate-to-severe dehydration, shock, persistent vomiting, or mental status changes, IV hydration will be required. Personnel or caregiver limitations may lead to the need for IV hydration, in settings when ORT would otherwise be appropriate.

American Academy of Pediatrics, Provisional Committee on Quality Improvement, Subcommittee on Acute Gastroenteritis: Practice parameter: The management of acute gastroenteritis in young children. Pediatrics 97:424–435, 1996.

KEY POINTS: MANAGING FLUIDS AND NUTRITION ✓

1. Use of special or dilute formulas is generally not necessary.

2. Mothers should be encouraged to continue breastfeeding.

3. Oral rehydration with hypotonic glucose-electrolyte solutions is the therapy of choice for children with mild-to-moderate dehydration.

4. IV fluids are indicated in cases of moderate-to-severe dehydration or when oral fluids are not tolerated.

5. Rapid return to age-appropriate feeding patterns is indicated once children are rehydrated.

19. **Should children with diarrhea avoid milk products?**
A lactose-free diet is often recommended during recovery from gastroenteritis but is required only in the face of severe illness or malnutrition. Patients with severe enteritis may have damage to the brush-border membrane of the small intestine, with resulting temporary decreases in the levels of enzymes, such as lactase. Despite this, the majority of infants and children show no clinical signs of subsequent carbohydrate malabsorption when fed full-strength milk or formula. For those infants with persistent watery and explosive diarrhea, a disaccharide-free formula such as Prosobee or Isomil-DF may be useful until the gut recovers. Older children with these symptoms may benefit from avoiding lactose-containing products for a couple of weeks.

20. **What is the BRAT diet? Should children with diarrhea adhere to it?**
Bananas, rice, applesauce, and toast. Children with gastroenteritis tolerate these foods well, though limiting the diet in this way restricts calories, protein, and fat. The American Academy of Pediatrics recommends reinstituting a regular, age-appropriate diet with full-strength milk as soon as possible.

American Academy of Pediatrics, Provisional Committee on Quality Improvement, Subcommittee on Acute Gastroenteritis: Practice parameter: The management of acute gastroenteritis in young children. Pediatrics 97:424–435, 1996.

21. **What complications of infectious diarrhea should I be concerned about?**
    Both *Shigella* sp. and *E. coli* can cause seizures via high fever or toxin elaboration. *Salmonella* sp. produces bacteremia in approximately 6% of those infected; salmonella bacteremia rates of 11–45% have been reported in infants and neonates. Immunocompromised patients and those with hematologic disorders are at increased risk for developing salmonella osteomyelitis. Giardial infection, as do celiac sprue and IBD, often presents with failure to thrive. *C. difficile* overgrowth and cytotoxin release may lead to life-threatening pseudomembranous colitis. The cytotoxins elaborated by *E. coli* O157:H7 induce diffuse endothelial injury, which causes both hemolytic uremic syndrome and thrombotic thrombocytopenic purpura. Ten percent of patients with *E. coli* O157:H7 infection develop one or both of these sequelae.

22. **Should children with diarrhea be treated with antimotility agents?**
    Pharmacologic antimotility agents are generally not recommended for use in children because of limited testing and potential side effects. Bismuth-containing compounds are moderately effective in shortening the duration of acute diarrhea. They are generally safe, although salicylate absorption may occur, and bismuth encephalopathy has been reported in patients with renal insufficiency. Notably, the black stools that result are often confused with melena.

    Opiates, such as Lomotil, and synthetic opiates, such as Imodium, can cause central nervous system–induced sedation and respiratory depression. Additional complications include gastrointestinal ileus with consequent vomiting, abdominal distention, and worsening diarrhea. Gut stasis following use of these agents may lead to invasion of the bowel wall by infectious organisms, leading to worsening infection and prolonged carriage and excretion of pathogenic bacteria. Both should be avoided in infants and young children, and used with caution in older children. Especially avoid Lomotil because it contains atropine. Dysentery is an absolute contraindication to the use of these medications.

KEY POINTS: ACUTE GASTROENTERITIS ✔

1. The majority of cases of acute gastroenteritis are self-limited and require no specific therapy.

2. Morbidity and death due to diarrheal diseases in children result mostly from dehydration.

3. Infants and malnourished children have the greatest risk of sequelae from diarrheal illness.

4. Use of antidiarrheal agents is not routinely recommended for children.

5. Proper handwashing is extremely effective in preventing transmission of infectious agents.

23. **When are antibiotics indicated?**
    - Treat *Salmonella* gastroenteritis in all infants under 3 months; in bacteremic children younger than 1 year of age; and in children who are immunocompromised or asplenic or appear toxic. In older children, *Salmonella* gastroenteritis is self-limited; no clinical improvement in fever, duration, or severity occurs after antibiotic therapy (which may, in fact, *prolong* the carrier state).
    - Antibiotic resistance to *Shigella* sp. is a major problem. Therapy is recommended for the severely ill and for children with persistent symptoms. Consider treating children in daycare, as shedding is stopped within 1–2 days, reducing person-to-person transmission.
    - The same is true of *Campylobacter* enteritis. Disease is mild and self-limited, but shedding may occur for up to 7 weeks without antibiotic therapy.
    - *Yersinia* sp. requires treatment only with severe disease, bacteremia, or underlying illness.

- Antimicrobials may be administered to decrease the duration and severity of symptoms in enterotoxigenic *E. coli* (traveler's diarrhea) infections. Most experts recommend against treating children with Shiga toxin-producing *E. coli* (STEC) with antimicrobials because the risks and benefits of treatment are not known.
- Mild infections with *C. difficile* improve when antibiotics are stopped. Severe *C. difficile* colitis should be treated with oral vancomycin or metronidazole.
- *Cryptosporidium parvum* and *Giardia* sp. can both be treated with a 3-day course of nitazoxanide; *Giardia* sp. also responds to furazolidone and metronidazole. Neither food poisoning nor viral infections require antibiotics.

   Red Book. www.aapredbook.aappublications.org

24. **When should patients with diarrhea be referred to a specialist?**
   Infants or children with severe or progressive dehydration should be referred to acute care facilities for rehydration and monitoring. Referral is likewise appropriate for a patient who appears toxic or has bloody stools. When a child has a localizing examination or peritoneal signs, a surgical consultation is indicated. Patients with chronic disease or growth failure should be seen by a gastroenterologist.

25. **When is testing indicated in children with diarrhea?**
   Children with chronic diarrhea or evidence of a noninfectious cause for their diarrhea should be screened, if indicated, for conditions such as IBD, celiac disease, or carbohydrate intolerance. Giardia antigen testing, or ova and parasite samples, should be performed in children with chronic diarrhea and failure to thrive. The use of clinical and historical criteria (fever, visible blood or mucus, absence of vomiting, and stool frequency), combined with selective application of screening tests or stool cultures, offers a cost-effective means of identifying patients with bacterial pathogens. A higher index of suspicion is required for infants, as sequelae are more common. During the winter months, rotavirus stool antigen tests may be useful for infection control purposes.

26. **What is the best way to prevent diarrheal disease in children?**
   Multiple studies in both developed and developing countries, set in homes and institutions, have concluded that frequent handwashing is very effective in decreasing the frequency of diarrheal illness in children. When caregivers wash their hands with plain or antibacterial soap after defecating or changing diapers, and before preparing food, eating, and feeding children, the incidence of diarrhea decreases markedly. Likewise, studies in daycare centers show up to 50% decreases in episodes of diarrhea following training and education of children and child care providers.

   Roberts L, Jorm L, Patel M, et al: Effect of infection control measures on the frequency of diarrheal episodes in child care: A randomized, controlled trial. Pediatrics 105:743–746, 2000.

27. **What new therapies look promising in terms of managing the symptoms of diarrheal disease?**
   Probiotics such as Lactobacillus GG have gained a lot of attention for their potential role in limiting the symptoms of diarrheal disease. Several studies in children have demonstrated reduced duration of diarrhea when probiotics are used in the setting of acute viral diarrhea (particularly that caused by rotavirus), recurrent *C. difficile* diarrhea, and diarrhea related to IBD. Both inpatient and outpatient populations have been studied, and the probiotics have been successful when administered alone or when added to OLS.

   Guandalini S, Pensabene L, Zikri MA, et al: Lactobacillus GG administered in oral rehydration solution to children with acute diarrhea: A multicenter European trial. J Pediatr Gastroenterol Nutr 30:54–60, 2000.
   Rosenfeldt V, Michaelsen KF, Jakobsen M, et al: Effect of probiotic Lactobacillus strains on acute diarrhea in a cohort of nonhospitalized children attending day-care centers. Pediatr Infect Dis J 21:417–419, 2002.

CHAPTER 12

EAR PAIN

Joan E. Shook, MD, MBA

1. What is the most common cause of ear pain in the young child?

Ear pain (otalgia) is a common symptom in the pediatric emergency department (ED). While the differential diagnosis for otalgia is lengthy, the most common cause of ear pain is acute otitis media (AOM). AOM is caused by an acute bacterial (or occasionally viral) infection resulting in inflammation of the middle ear that is usually associated with pain and fever. The peak age for AOM is 3–16 months of life, but it may occur at any time.

> Arnett AM: Pain—earache. In Fleisher GR, Ludwig S, Henretig FM (eds): Textbook of Pediatric Emergency Medicine, 5th ed. Philadelphia, Lippincott Williams & Wilkins, 2006, pp 505–518.
> Elden LM, Potsic W: Otolaryngologic emergencies. In Fleisher GR, Ludwig S, Henretig FM (eds): Textbook of Pediatric Emergency Medicine, 5th ed. Philadelphia, Lippincott Williams & Wilkins, 2006, pp 1663–1678.

2. What three elements must be in place to make a diagnosis of otitis media?

- Recent, usually abrupt onset of signs and symptoms of middle ear infection (such as pain, irritability, fever, otorrhea)
- Presence of middle ear effusion
- Signs of middle ear inflammation

> American Academy of Family Physicians: Practice Guidelines: AAP, AAFP Release Guideline on Diagnosis and Management of Acute Otitis Media. www.aafp.org/afp/20040601/practice.html

3. What findings confirm the presence of a middle ear effusion?

Bulging of the tympanic membrane (TM) or limited or absent mobility of the TM with pneumatic otoscopy or air-fluid level behind the TM or otorrhea.

> American Academy of Pediatrics, Subcommittee on Otitis Media with Effusion: Otitis media with effusion. Pediatrics 113:1412–1429, 2004.
> American Academy of Family Physicians. www.aafp.org
> American Academy of Pediatrics: Diagnosis and Management of Acute Otitis Media. http://aappolicy.aappublications.org/cgi/content/full/pediatrics;113/5/1451

4. What signs or symptoms suggest middle ear inflammation?

Erythema of the TM or distinct otalgia that results in change in normal activity or sleep.

> Dolitsky JN: Otalgia. In Bluestone CD, Stool SE, Kenna MA (eds): Pediatric Otolaryngology, vol. I, 3rd ed. Philadelphia, W.B. Saunders, 1996, pp 235–241.

5. What are the most common bacterial pathogens that cause otitis media?

Streptococcus pneumoniae, Haemophilus influenzae, and *Moraxella catarrhalis* are the most common bacterial organisms that cause otitis media. While these pathogens predominate at all ages, in infants younger than 1 month of age, *Staphylococcus aureus* and gram-negative enteric bacilli account for 15–20% of the infections. The majority of *H. influenzae* organisms are nontypeable, although type B may be seen.

6. How would you treat bacterial otitis media?

Uncomplicated otitis media in the child over 1 month of age should be treated with oral antibiotics on an outpatient basis. Amoxicillin (80 mg/kg per day in two or three divided doses) is the drug of choice. Alternatives to amoxicillin include amoxicillin–clavulanic acid in a 7:1 formulation (amoxicillin, 45 mg/kg per day, in two divided doses), cefuroxime axetil, cefdinir, and cefpodoxime, or azithromycin, clarithromycin, or trimethoprim-sulfamethoxazole in the penicillin-allergic patient. If the patient is vomiting or is nonadherent with medications, a single dose of ceftriaxone (50 mg/kg) is also effective. Infants younger than 4 weeks old are usually treated with IV medications (ampicillin and gentamicin).

Elden LM, Potsic W: Otolaryngologic emergencies. In Fleisher GR, Ludwig S, Henretig FM (eds): Textbook of Pediatric Emergency Medicine, 5th ed. Philadelphia, Lippincott Williams & Wilkins, 2006, 1663–1678.

Klein JO, Bluestone CD: Otitis media. In Feigin RD, Cherry JD (eds): Textbook of Pediatric Infectious Diseases, 5th ed. Philadelphia, W.B. Saunders Co., pp 215–235, 2004.

American Academy of Pediatrics Online Learning in Otitis Media: www.aap.org/otitismedia

Klein JO: Epidemiology, pathogenesis, diagnosis and complications of acute otitis media: www.uptodateonline.com

Pelton SI: Otitis media: Re-evaluation of diagnosis and treatment in the era of antimicrobial resistance pneumococcal conjugate vaccine, and evolving morbidity. Pediatr Clin North Am 52:711–728, 2005.

7. **What analgesics are recommended for treatment of ear pain resulting from acute otitis media?**
Acetaminophen and ibuprofen are generally effective in relieving pain from otitis media. Topical therapy with Auralgan otic solution is used for children with severe pain or irritable infants. A few drops placed in the ear canal until it is filled often relieves pain promptly. Auralgan contains antipyrine, benzocaine, and glycerin.

Arnett AM: Pain-earache. In Fleisher GR, Ludwig S, Henretig FM (eds): Textbook of Pediatric Emergency Medicine, 5th ed. Philadelphia, Lippincott Williams & Wilkins, 2006, pp 505–518.

8. **What is bullous myringitis? How is the diagnosis made?**
Bullous myringitis is an infection of the TM with intensely painful bulla formation on the surface. The diagnosis is made easily by otoscopy. *S. pneumoniae* and *H. influenzae* are the most common pathogens, although *Mycoplasma* sp. has also been implicated. Antibiotic choices for this entity include azithromycin or erythromycin–sulfisoxazole (Pediazole).

Elden LM, Potsic W: Otolaryngologic emergencies. In Fleisher GR, Ludwig S (eds): Textbook of Pediatric Emergency Medicine, 5th ed. Philadelphia, Lippincott Williams & Wilkins, 2006, 1663–1678.

McCormick DP, Saeed KA, Pittman C, et al: Bullous myringitis: A case-control study. Pediatrics 112:982–986, 2003.

9. **You are evaluating a patient who presents with ear pain. On taking the history, you learn that the illness began with itchiness of the ear canal, which has become increasingly severe and evolved into pain. What is the most likely diagnosis in this child?**
This presentation is classic for otitis externa, which is also known as swimmer's ear. Otitis externa is an inflammatory process affecting the external auditory canal. It is most commonly seen during the summer because of increased swimming. Other predisposing factors include moisture retention due to a tortuous narrow canal or obstructive cerumen, loss of acidic environment due to inadequate cerumen lavage, exposure to alkaline substance, or interruption of the epithelial lining of the canal because of trauma or dermatitis.

Physical examination of these patients is significant for the pain that can be elicited by pushing on the tragus or by traction of the pinna or moving the jaw side to side. Frequently, debris or exudates line the external canal and possibly cover the TM. The most common causative organism is *Pseudomonas* sp. *Staphylococcus*, *Streptococcus*, or *Proteus* spp. may also be seen in association with *Pseudomonas*.

Dolitsky JN: Otalgia. In Bluestone CD, Stool SE, Kenna MA (eds): Pediatric Otolaryngology, vol. I, 3rd ed. Philadelphia, W.B. Saunders Co., 1996, pp 235–241.

Shah RK, Blevins N: Otalgia. Otolaryngol Clin North A 36:1137–1151, 2003.

10. **How is otitis externa treated?**

Treatment of otitis externa involves a thorough, gentle cleaning of the ear canal and instillation of an acidic solution (e.g., otic Domeboro or Vosol), a combination antibiotic–corticosteroid preparation (e.g., Cortisporin), or antibiotic drops alone (e.g., ofloxacin otic solution 0.3%, a good choice because it covers *Pseudomonas* sp. well). When severe edema of the canal does not allow instillation of the medications, a wick may be placed to facilitate medication delivery. If a wick is used, it should be removed every 24–48 hours and the external canal inspected and cleaned. Oral antibiotics are added for patients who are improving slowly with local treatment, have a concurrent middle ear infection, or are immunocompromised.

Dolitsky JN: Otalgia. In Bluestone CD, Stool SE, Kenna MA (eds): Pediatric Otolaryngology, Vol. I, 3rd ed. Philadelphia, W.B. Saunders, 1996, pp 235–241.

Shah RK, Blevins N: Otalgia. Otolaryngol Clin North Am 36:1137–1151, 2003.

11. **What is malignant otitis externa?**

It is a severe form of otitis externa that is not responsive to conventional therapy. It is caused by *P. aeruginosa* and involves the bone and marrow of the skull base and may also result in chondritis and facial nerve paralysis. Complications may include stenosis of the canal and permanent hearing loss. It is rare in children but is seen in patients with diabetes mellitus or those who are immunocompromised.

Shah RK, Blevins N: Otalgia. Otolaryngol Clin North Am 36:1137–1151, 2003.

12. **A toddler presents with bruising to the internal surface of the pinna. According to the mother, he is a very active child and falls frequently. What diagnosis should you consider?**

Bruising to the internal surface of the pinna may result from "boxing" the ear. You therefore must consider the possibility of child abuse. The unexplained presence of hemotympanum and the perforation of the TM may also suggest child abuse because they can result from a direct blow to the ear.

Licameli GR: Diagnosis and management of otalgia in the pediatric patient. Pediatr Ann 28:364–368, 1999.

Monteleone JA, Brodeur AE: Identifying, interpreting and reporting injuries. In Monteleone JA, Brodeur AE (eds): Child Maltreatment. St. Louis, GW Medical Publishing, 1994, pp 10–11.

13. **Infections at the site of ear piercing are often extremely painful and cause some concern. What organisms should you consider covering when you choose an antibiotic?**

Infections of the pinna are usually caused by *S. aureus* or *Pseudomonas* sp. Infection of the cartilage is of particular concern and should be treated aggressively with IV antibiotics.

Arnett AM: Pain-earache. In Fleisher GR, Ludwig S, Henretig FM (eds): Textbook of Pediatric Emergency Medicine, 5th ed. Philadelphia, Lippincott Williams & Wilkins, 2006, pp 505–518.

Shah RK, Blevins N: Otalgia. Otolaryngol Clin North Am 36:1137–1151, 2003.

14. **You are examining a child who came to the ED because of fever and ear pain. You notice that his ear is red and swollen and seems to be protruding from the side of his head. What diagnosis should you be entertaining?**

This child likely has mastoiditis, a relatively uncommon complication of otitis media. On physical examination the posterior auricular area is erythematous and very tender. It is important to visualize the TM because severe otitis externa also can present with postauricular erythema, swelling, and protrusion of the pinna. In mastoiditis, the TM is erythematous and bulging, while with otitis externa, the TM is usually normal. Computed tomography can help differentiate between mastoiditis and severe otitis externa when a complete physical examination is not possible.

Elden LM, Potsic W: Otolaryngologic emergencies. In Fleisher GR, Ludwig S, Henretig FM (eds): Textbook of Pediatric Emergency Medicine, 5th ed. Philadelphia, Lippincott Williams & Wilkins, 2006, pp 1663–1678.

Klein JO, Bluestone CD: Otitis media. In Feigin RD, Cherry JD (eds): Textbook of Pediatric Infectious Diseases, 5th ed. Philadelphia, W.B. Saunders Co., 2004, pp 215–235.

Klein JO: Epidemiology, pathogenesis, diagnosis and complications of acute otitis media: www.uptodateonline.com

15. **How is mastoiditis treated?**

Children with mastoiditis must be evaluated by an otolaryngologist and admitted to the hospital for IV antibiotics. Since the most common organisms in acute mastoiditis are *Staphylococcus* spp., *Streptococcus* spp., and *H. influenzae*, the patient should be treated with clindamycin or vancomycin and cefotaxime. Operative intervention may be required in children with complicated infection or evidence of abscess formation.

Klein JO, Bluestone CD: Otitis media. In Feigin RD, Cherry JD (eds): Textbook of Pediatric Infectious Diseases, 5th ed. Philadelphia, W.B. Saunders Co., 2004, pp 215–235.

16. **What are the potential complications of mastoiditis?**

Complications of mastoiditis can be intratemporal or intracranial. Intratemporal complications include facial paralysis, labyrinthitis, and Gradenigo syndrome (retro-orbital pain, otorrhea, and diplopia). Intracranial complications include meningitis; lateral sinus thrombosis; and epidural, subdural, or brain abscesses. Children with intracranial complications usually appear toxic in addition to exhibiting local findings.

Elden LM, Potsic W: Otolaryngologic emergencies. In Fleisher GR, Ludwig S, Henretig FM (eds): Textbook of Pediatric Emergency Medicine, 5th ed. Philadelphia, Lippincott Williams & Wilkins, 2006, pp 1663–1678.

Klein JO, Bluestone CD: Otitis media. In Feigin RD, Cherry JD (eds): Textbook of Pediatric Infectious Diseases, 5th ed. Philadelphia, W.B. Saunders, 2004, pp 215–235.

17. **The presence of a foreign body in the external auditory canal can cause severe pain. What is the best method for removing the foreign body?**

Occasionally a child places a foreign body in the external canal and presents with symptoms such as hearing loss or a sensation of fullness, as well as ear pain. Symptoms at presentation vary depending on the nature of the foreign material and the length of time that it has been present. Objects can be removed by using alligator forceps, curettes, right-angle hooks, Baron suction devices, or irrigation with warm water. If the foreign body is a bean or other vegetable material, do not irrigate with water because the foreign body may swell. A foreign object that is lodged tightly in the canal may require removal under sedation or even general anesthesia using an operating microscope. Canal wall lacerations are present 50% of the time after a foreign-body removal, so it is recommended that after the object is recovered, the patient be treated with topical antibiotic or steroid drops to prevent the development of otitis externa.

Bressler K, Shelton C: Ear foreign-body removal: A review of 98 consecutive cases. Laryngoscope 103:367–370, 1993.

18. **You have just examined a child who has a hearing aid battery in her external auditory canal. You have not been successful in your attempts to remove it with forceps. What should your next step be?**

Hearing aid batteries can cause extensive caustic skin and bony damage in a short period of time. Removal of this foreign object is an otologic emergency and should be performed as soon as possible after detection. If you are unable to remove the battery, an otolaryngologist should be called for removal in the operating room.

Bressler K, Shelton C: Ear foreign-body removal: A review of 98 consecutive cases. Laryngoscope 103:367–370, 1993.

KEY POINTS: EAR PAIN ✓

1. Ear pain in the child is most commonly due to acute otitis media.

2. To diagnose acute otitis media, one must demonstrate the presence of fluid in the middle ear by pneumatic otoscopy.

3. If the examination of the ear is normal, consider secondary (referred) causes of otalgia, including temporomandibular joint syndrome, dental pathology, and gastroesophageal reflux.

4. Hemotympanum is a rare finding that can result from a basilar skull fracture, barotrauma from scuba diving, a turbulent airplane flight, or a direct blow to the ear. In the absence of a history, child abuse should be entertained as an etiology.

19. **A child presents with severe ear pain of sudden onset. You determine there is a live insect, most likely a roach, moving in the ear canal. How should you manage this patient to relieve pain quickly?**
Before attempting to remove the insect, immediately place mineral oil or viscous lidocaine in the ear canal. This will "paralyze" the insect and relieve pain promptly. The foreign body can then be removed with an ear curette or by flushing the canal with water.

Leffler S, Cheney P, Tandberg D: Chemical immobilization and killing of intra-aural roaches: An in vitro comparative study. Ann Emerg Med 22:1795–1798, 1993.

Su E: External auditory canal foreign bodies. In Dieckmann RA, Fiser DH, Selbst SM (eds): Illustrated Textbook of Pediatric Emergency and Critical Care Procedures. St. Louis, Mosby, 1997, pp 712–713.

20. **Explain how swimming in the ocean can result in a ruptured TM and subsequent ear pain.**
A direct blow to the side of the face by a wave or a hand may result in rupture of the TM and severe otalgia.

Vernick DM: Ear barotrauma: www.uptodateonline.com

21. **Barotrauma as a result of flying or scuba diving may result in acute, severe otalgia with possible hearing loss and tinnitus. What findings on otoscopic evaluation are most consistent with barotrauma?**
Otoscopy usually reveals a thickened, hemorrhagic TM and a middle ear effusion. Treatment for this condition is supportive with analgesics.

Vernick DM: Ear barotrauma: www.uptodateonline.com

22. **As your patient leaves the examination room, his mother asks you whether it is safe for him to fly in an airplane even though he recently had pressure equalization tubes placed. How do you answer her?**
Children with pressure equalization tubes can fly safely because the pressure equalization in the middle ear takes place without relying on the function of the eustachian tube.

Vernick DM: Ear barotrauma: www.uptodateonline.com

23. **You are confronted with a patient who reports ear pain and yet has a normal examination of the ear. How can this phenomenon be explained?**
Otalgia can be the result of referred pain from distant sites secondary to inflammatory processes, tumors, or mechanical disturbances. Nonotogenic otalgia is most often of dental origin; however, pain that is perceived in either the external or the middle ear can be referred via cranial nerves V, VI, IX, and X and upper cervical nerves. These nerves supply the nasal sinus area, oral cavity and teeth, oropharynx, hypopharynx, larynx, and upper esophagus. Remember to search for distant sites of origin when examination of the ear is unrevealing.

Arnett AM: Pain-earache. In Fleisher GR, Ludwig S (eds): Textbook of Pediatric Emergency Medicine, 5th ed. Philadelphia, Lippincott Williams & Wilkins, 2006, pp 505–518.

Shah RK, Blevins N: Otalgia. Otolaryngol Clin North Am 36:1137–1151, 2003.

24. **Name some nonotogenic etiologies of pain in the ear. Name the nerve that carries the sensation.**
   - **Cranial nerve V:** Disturbances in the oral cavity, including stomatitis, gingivitis, trauma, and infections of the tongue; dental conditions, including eruption, impaction, trauma, caries, and abscess
   - **Cranial nerve VI:** Bell's palsy, herpes zoster, tumors
   - **Cranial nerve IX:** Tonsillitis and retropharyngeal abscess or nasopharynx, including foreign body or infection
   - **Cranial nerve X:** Lesions at the base of the tongue, trachea, larynx, and esophagus; otalgia can be a manifestation of gastroesophageal reflux in infants and children
   - **Upper cervical nerves:** Lymphadenitis, infected cysts, c-spine injuries

Arnett AM: Pain-earache. In Fleisher GR, Ludwig S, Henretig FM (eds): Textbook of Pediatric Emergency Medicine, 5th ed. Philadelphia, Lippincott Williams & Wilkins, 2006, pp 505–518.

Shah RK, Blevins N: Otalgia. Otolaryngol Clin North Am 36:1137–1151, 2003.

25. **What is Ramsay-Hunt syndrome?**
This is the eponym applied to herpes zoster otitis. Vesicles on the pinna, external auditory canal, and TM characterize the syndrome, and it is exquisitely painful. It can be complicated by hearing loss, nausea, vomiting, dizziness, facial nerve involvement, and ataxia. Treatment is with acyclovir and analgesics.

Arnett AM: Pain-earache. In Fleisher GR, Ludwig S, Henretig FM (eds): Textbook of Pediatric Emergency Medicine, 5th ed. Philadelphia, Lippincott Williams & Wilkins, 2006, pp 505–518.

Shah RK, Blevins N: Otalgia. Otolaryngol Clin North Am 36:1137–1151, 2003.

26. **Temporomandibular joint (TMJ) dysfunction is one of the most common causes of referred otalgia. How can I confirm this as a source of ear pain?**
To confirm the diagnosis of TMJ dysfunction, carefully palpate the TMJ externally by placing the fingers just anterior to the tragus and having the patient open and close the mouth. The patient will report otalgia during attempted occlusion. The pain may be caused by nerve irritation, muscle spasm, or degenerative change in the joint. TMJ dysfunction can occur in children who have bruxism, frequently clench their teeth, indulge in frequent gum chewing, or have malocclusion. Tympanometry in these patients is normal. Treatment is directed at reducing the inflammation and pain with heat therapy, soft diet, and analgesia.

Kramer II, Kramer CM: The phantom earache. Temporomandibular joint dysfunction in children. Am J Dis Child 139:943–945, 1985.

Shah RK, Blevins N: Otalgia. Otolaryngol Clin North Am 36:1137–1151, 2003.

CHAPTER 13

FEVER

Jeffrey R. Avner, MD

1. **What percentage of visits to the emergency department (ED) is for the evaluation of fever?**
   Fever is one of the most common presenting symptoms at the pediatric ED, representing 15–30% of all visits. During the first 2 years of life, a child typically has 4–6 episodes of febrile illness.

2. **What temperature is considered normal?**
   There is no single value that represents a "normal" temperature. This is largely because normal body temperature varies with age, time of day, physical activity, and environmental conditions. This individual variability limits the application of mean body temperature values derived from population studies. Thus, no single temperature should be used as the upper limit of normal. Rather, normal temperature is best described as a range of values for each individual. Although only a rough guide, some consider abnormal temperature to be >38.0–38.2°C (rectally) in an infant and 37.2–37.7°C (orally) in an older child or adult.

3. **Who is credited with the first systematic measurement of body temperature?**
   In the 1860s, German physician Carl Wunderlich used foot-long thermometers to record over 1 million axillary temperature readings from 25,000 patients. He identified 37.0°C (98.6°F) as the mean temperature of healthy adults.

4. **Does body temperature vary during the day?**
   The variation of body temperature in typical circadian rhythm becomes established by 2 years of age. Peak temperature typically occurs in late afternoon (5:00–7:00 PM), and the trough occurs in early morning (2:00–6:00 AM). Daily temperature variation ranges from 0.1°C–1.3°C.

5. **How does the body produce fever?**
   During infection, exogenous pyrogens (microbial products such as endotoxins) produced by various infectious organisms act on host inflammatory cells (especially monocytes and macrophages) to produce numerous cytokines, including endogenous pyrogens (interleukin, tumor necrosis factor, interferon). These circulating pyrogens act on the preoptic area of the anterior hypothalamus, which produces prostaglandin E_2 and causes fever.

6. **Where is the core body temperature set?**
   Core body temperature is set in the anterior hypothalamus. Variation in body temperature is detected by thermosensitive neurons in the preoptic nucleus, which then directs autonomic changes in sweat glands, blood vessels, somatic neurons, and skeletal muscles.

7. **How does the body regulate temperature?**
   Thermoregulation is controlled by a variety of physiologic and behavioral mechanisms under the direction of the hypothalamus. Elevation of body temperature occurs primarily through metabolic activity associated with increased cell metabolism, increased muscle activity, and involuntary shivering. Body temperature is decreased primarily through vasodilatation, which

thereby increases heat loss by conduction, convection, or radiation through the skin. In addition, sweating and cold preference behavior (e.g., removing clothes) help dissipate the heat.

8. **Is fever beneficial or harmful?**
Whether fever is friend or foe is a question for the ages. Fever has some physiologic benefits for the host, including an enhancement of both cellular and humoral immune responses as well as direct antimicrobial activity. On the other hand, fever makes the child uncomfortable and leads to a significant increase in metabolic activity (about 10% per degree Centigrade), which increases oxygen consumption, carbon dioxide production, and insensible water loss. Whether the benefits outweigh the metabolic costs is debatable. Regardless, the presence of fever alerts the parents and clinicians that the child is in the process of fighting disease and, as such, can serve as an invaluable diagnostic aid.

9. **What is "fever phobia"?**
Barton Schmitt coined the term in the early 1980s in reference to parents' excessive concern about low-grade fever. Nowadays, the term *fever phobia* is often used to describe heightened anxiety about the presence of fever in the child that can lead to unnecessary ED visits, laboratory testing, or empiric antibiotic treatment. Of note, both parents and providers may have "fever phobia."

Corneli HM. Beyond the fear of fever. Clin Ped Emerg Med 1:94–101, 2000.

Crocetti M, Moghbeli N, Serwint J: Fever phobia revisited: Have parental misconceptions about fever changed in 20 years? Pediatrics 107:1241–1246, 2001.

Poirer MP, Davis PH, Gonzalez-Del Rey JA, et al: Pediatric emergency department nurses' perspectives on fever in children. Pediatr Emerg Care 16:9–12, 2000.

Schmitt BD: Fever phobia: Misconceptions of parents about fevers. Am J Dis Child 134:176–181, 1980.

10. **What are the normal increases in heart rate and respiratory rate with each degree rise in body temperature?**
Fever is associated with an increase in heart rate of about 10 to 15 beats per minute and an increase in respiratory rate of about 3 to 5 breaths per minute for each rise in degree Centigrade.

11. **Does bundling cause fever in infants?**
Overbundling of young infants, especially during the summer months, is known to increase measured temperatures. If an infant is heavily bundled or in a particularly hot environment, a 30- to 60-minute period of equilibration should be followed by a repeat temperature determination. This issue is particularly important in the evaluation of young febrile infants because the height of the fever by itself is often a determinant for proceeding with an evaluation for sepsis.

12. **What are the differences in measurement among rectal, oral, and axillary temperature readings?**
The core body temperature is best measured with an esophageal or nasopharyngeal probe, but this is difficult in the setting of an ED. Therefore, rectal temperature is used as the standard measurement to indirectly measure core body temperature. Oral measurement in the sublingual pocket is estimated to be 0.5–1°C lower than rectal temperature. Axillary temperatures are imprecise, inaccurate, and insensitive and therefore of limited value.

Craig JV, Lancaster GA, Williamson PR, et al: Temperature measured at the axilla compared with rectum in children and young people: Systemic review. BMJ 320:1174–1178, 2000.

13. **Does otitis media increase tympanic membrane temperature?**
Infrared tympanic thermometry is a popular method used in EDs, and recent studies show that, at least in older children and adults, the results are reasonably accurate. Otitis media has been shown to increase tympanic temperatures only slightly, by about 0.4°C. Interestingly,

although nonobstructive cerumen does not affect tympanic thermometry, cerumen that completely obstructs the ear canal leads to underestimation of temperature.

Kelly B, Alexander D: Effect of otitis media on infrared tympanic thermometry. Clin Pediatr 30:46–48, 1991.

14. Can parents detect fever subjectively?

When parents say that their child is "burning up" with fever, they are usually correct. In general, parents are both moderately sensitive (75–85%) and specific (75–85%) in detecting the presence of fever subjectively in children. However, they may not be as accurate in estimating the height of fever. In young infants (less than 2 months old), when the height of the fever is crucial for determining management, always obtain a rectal temperature.

Hooker EA, Smith SW, Miles T, et al: Subjective assessment of fever by parents: Comparison with measurement by noncontact tympanic thermometer and calibrated rectal glass mercury thermometer. Ann Emerg Med 28:313–317, 1996.

15. When sponging a child for treatment of fever, what is the best temperature for the water?

The value of sponging to decrease temperature is controversial. Sponging uses evaporation to help cool the child. Sponging can be used in combination with an antipyretic and may take up to 20 minutes to be effective. Use tepid or lukewarm water so that the child remains comfortable and does not shiver. Never use cold water or isopropyl alcohol, as they cause excessive vasoconstriction and shivering. In addition, isopropyl alcohol can be toxic through skin absorption.

16. What did Hippocrates feel was the role of fever?

Hippocrates, the father of medicine, felt that fever helped balance the four humors (blood, yellow bile, black bile, and phlegm), which were believed to cause disease when out of balance. At the current time, this theory remains unproven!

17. Does high fever cause brain damage?

Although this concern is a cornerstone of "fever phobia" by parents, this fear is unfounded. Temperatures $< 42°C$ have not, by themselves, been associated with any serious sequelae. Deleterious effects of temperatures $> 42°C$ are based on in vitro effects on enzyme systems and not clinical studies. When brain damage does occur in association with fever, it is usually due to sequelae of the underlying disease (such as meningitis) rather than the fever itself.

18. Does fever trigger seizures?

Fever lowers the seizure threshold in children with an underlying seizure disorder and may precipitate a seizure in children (6 months to 5 years old) who are susceptible to simple febrile seizures. Fever, by itself, in the absence of predisposing factors, does not cause seizures.

19. Does teething cause fever?

Although some studies show a mild temperature elevation associated with teething, significant fever (temperature $> 38.8°C$) has never been shown to be associated with tooth emergence.

Macknin ML, Piedmonte M, Jacobs J, Skibinski C: Symptoms associated with infant teething: A prospective study. Pediatrics 105:747–752, 2000.

20. Why is the use of rubbing alcohol on children harmful?

Topical application of isopropyl alcohol can cause severe intoxication in children due to skin absorption or inhalation exposure. Furthermore, the resultant cooling effect on the skin causes peripheral vasoconstriction and limits the child's ability to dissipate internal heat.

21. **Does the response of fever to an antipyretic predict a more benign illness?**
No. Fever response to antipyretics is not clinically useful in differentiating children with serious bacterial illness from those with a more benign etiology. Most children, regardless of the underlying etiology of their fever, experience some temperature decline with antipyretics, although rarely do they become afebrile. The decision to perform additional diagnostic tests, such as a complete blood count or lumbar puncture, should be determined on clinical grounds and not based on the degree of defervescence.

22. **Is alternating acetaminophen and ibuprofen more effective for fever reduction?**
Although a common practice among pediatricians, there is currently no scientific evidence that this combination of antipyretics has greater efficacy than either agent used alone and may, in fact, increase fever phobia and potential toxicity from incorrect dosing.

    Mayoral CE, Marina RV, Rosenfeld W, Greensher J: Alternating antipyretics: Is this an alternative?. Pediatrics 105:1009–1012, 2000.

23. **What are the risk factors to consider in evaluating a febrile child?**
Children who have either immature or specific impairment of immunologic function are at higher risk of bacteremia and serious bacterial illness. Therefore, very young infants (less than 2 months), children with immune compromise (e.g., HIV infection, sickle cell disease), and children receiving immunosuppressive medication (such as chemotherapy and steroids) may require a blood culture and empiric antibiotic treatment as part of their management.

24. **Why do we treat infants less than 2 months old with fever differently than the older child?**
There are three main reasons: (1) the risk of serious bacterial illness in this age group is relatively high (approximately 10%), (2) young infants have immature immune responses that may not be able to contain infection, and (3) clinical appearance is difficult to interpret. At this age, the ability of a child to interact in an interpretable social manner is inconsistent. For example, a social smile is inconsistent, if not absent, in a 1-month-old. In a study by Baker et al, 66% of febrile infants 1–2 months of age with bacterial diseases were judged well-appearing by the ED attending physician.

    Baker MD, Bell LM, Avner JR: Outpatient management without antibiotics of fever in selected infants. N Engl J Med 329:1437–1441, 1993.

25. **What are the common pathogens that cause serious bacterial illness in febrile infants?**
In infants less than 1 month old, maternal organisms, acquired perinatally, predominate: group B streptococcus, gram-negative enteric organisms, and *Listeria*. In infants older than 6 weeks, community-acquired organisms predominate: pneumococcus, meningococcus, and *Haemophilus influenzae* type B. Infants 4–6 weeks old are infected by pathogens from either age group. Immunizations have decreased the incidence of *H. influenzae* type B and pneumococcus.

26. **What are low-risk criteria for the management of febrile infants?**
In an attempt to avoid routine hospitalization of all febrile young infants, many investigators have sought to devise clinical and laboratory criteria that would identify a subset of febrile infants at "low risk" of having bacterial disease as a cause of their fever. Three major prospective studies have established somewhat different low-risk criteria (Table 13-1).

27. **What is a "sepsis workup"?**
A "sepsis workup" is typically considered an evaluation of certain body fluids for bacterial infection. It usually includes a complete blood count; urinalysis; lumbar puncture; and cultures of blood, urine, and spinal fluid. A *"septic* workup" is a test performed with a dirty needle.

TABLE 13-1. LOW-RISK CRITERIA FOR THE MANAGEMENT OF FEBRILE INFANTS

Variable	Boston	Philadelphia	Rochester
Age (d)	28–89	29–56	0–60
Temperature (°C)	≥38	≥38.2	≥38
WBC	<20,000	<15,000	5000–15,000
Urinalysis	<10 WBC/HPF	<10 WBC/HPF & no bacteria	<10 WBC/HPF
CXR	No infiltrate	No infiltrate	Not required
CSF (WBC/μL)	<10	<8	Not required
Other		Band/total neutrophils <0.2	Absolute band count ≤1500
Sensitivity (%)	Not listed	100	92.4
Negative predictive value (%)	94.6	100	98.9

CXR = chest x-ray, CSF = cerebrospinal fluid, HPF = high-power field, WBC = white blood cell.
Data obtained from Baker MD, Bell LM, Avner JR: Outpatient management without antibiotics of fever in selected infants. N Engl J Med 329:1437–1441, 1993; Baskin MN, O'Rourke EJ, Fleisher GR: Outpatient treatment of febrile infants 28 to 89 days of age with intramuscular administration of ceftriaxone. J Pediatr 120:22–27, 1992; and Jaskiewicz JA, McCarthy CA, Richardson AC, et al: Febrile infants at low risk for serious bacterial infection—An appraisal of the Rochester Criteria and implications for management. Pediatrics 94:390–396, 1994.

28. **Do all febrile infants need a sepsis workup and admission?**
    Although there is no absolute consensus, most agree that febrile infants less than 1 month of age require an evaluation for sepsis. Many also feel that the same evaluation applies to infants 1–2 months old. However, some clinicians withhold a lumbar puncture in well-appearing febrile infants. Infants younger than 1 month and those infants at high risk should be hospitalized pending culture results. Infants 1–2 months old who are at low risk (*see* Table 13-1) for serious bacterial illness may be managed as outpatients if follow-up is assured.

    Avner JR, Baker MD: Management of fever in infants and children. Emerg Med Clin North Am 20:49–67, 2002.

    Pantell RH, Newman TB, Bernzweig, et al: Management and outcomes of care of fever in early infancy. JAMA 291:1203–1212, 2004.

29. **Do young febrile infants with respiratory syncytial virus (RSV) bronchiolitis need a sepsis workup?**
    A recent multicenter study of over 1200 infants (22% with RSV) found that febrile infants (< 60 days old) with RSV were at significantly lower risk of serious bacterial illness than RSV-negative infants; although the rate of certain infections, especially urinary tract infections, remained appreciable. However, in febrile infants less than 28 days old, the risk of serious bacterial illness remained "substantial" (about 13%) and was *not* altered by the presence of RSV infection.

    Levine DA, Platt SL, Dayan PS, et al: Risk of serious bacterial infection in young febrile infants with respiratory syncytial virus infections. Pediatrics 113:1728–1734, 2004.

KEY POINTS: THE FEBRILE INFANT ✓

1. In febrile infants less than 28 days old, the risk of serious bacterial illness is substantial (about 10%) and is not altered by the presence of RSV infection.

2. Urinary tract infection is the most common bacterial infection in febrile infants less than 2 months old.

3. For well-appearing febrile infants 4–8 weeks old, a variety of testing and management strategies are available.

30. **What is occult bacteremia?**
Occult means "mysterious" or "hidden." Bacteremia means bacteria in the blood. Simply put, occult bacteremia is unsuspected bacteria in the blood. This entity is used to describe a subset of febrile children (usually 3–36 months old) who are well-appearing and have no focus of infection but, nevertheless, have bacteremia. About 1–3% of such children in this age group have occult bacteremia. Note that the entity of occult bacteremia does *not* apply to a child who is ill-appearing or has an obvious focus of infection on physical examination.

31. **What are the common pathogens for occult bacteremia?**
The common pathogens are all encapsulated organisms. *Streptococcus pneumoniae* is responsible for 85–90% of cases, with the remainder shared among *Neisseria meningitidis*, group A streptococci, *Salmonella* sp., and *Staphylococcus aureus*. *H. influenzae* type B was a common pathogen prior to the widespread use of the HIB vaccine.

32. **How will universal pneumococcal vaccine use affect the incidence of occult bacteremia?**
The PCV-7 vaccine protects against seven of the most common serotypes involved in occult pneumococcal bacteremia. Since pneumococcal bacteremia is responsible for about 90% of cases of occult bacteremia, elimination of these serotypes will lead to a significant decline in the incidence of occult bacteremia. Some researchers suggest that the eventual occult bacteremia rate will drop to below 0.5% after vaccination.

Kaplan SL, Mason EO, Wald ER, et al: Decrease of invasive pneumococcal infections in children among 8 children's hospitals in the United States after the introduction of the 7-valent pneumococcal conjugate vaccine. Pediatrics 113;443–449, 2004.

Stoll ML, Rubin LG: Incidence of occult bacteremia among highly febrile young children in the era of the pneumococcal conjugate vaccine: A study from a Children's Hospital Emergency Department and Urgent Care Center. Arch Pediatr Adolesc Med 158:671–675, 2004.

KEY POINTS: THE FEBRILE CHILD ✓

1. Pneumococcal bacteria are responsible for about 90% of cases of occult bacteremia in children age 3–36 months.

2. The incidence of occult bacteremia is likely to decline to about 0.5% with the universal use of pneumococcal vaccination.

33. **Does the height of the fever indicate serious bacterial illness?**

    A child with a very high fever (temperature > 41.1°C) is more likely to have occult bacteremia than a child with lower fever, but is not appreciably more likely to develop serious bacterial illness. In fact, most children with serious bacterial illness, such as meningitis, have a temperature below that range. Thus, it appears that the presence or absence of fever is what is most important. This does not mean that a thorough evaluation of a child with high fever is unnecessary; rather, *any child with fever, regardless of the height of the temperature, should receive a complete evaluation*.

34. **What is the natural outcome of children with occult bacteremia?**

    Infection with *S. pneumoniae*, the most common cause of occult bacteremia, has the highest rate of spontaneous resolution. Most studies show that only a small number (4–7%) of untreated children with occult bacteremia caused by *S. pneumoniae* develop an invasive disease, such as meningitis. Invasion rates are higher for *H. influenzae* type B (7–20%) and *N. meningitidis* (25–35%). Whether empiric antibiotic therapy prevents the rare sequelae of occult bacteremia remains controversial. Clinicians should consider not only the probabilities of occult bacteremia and its progression to serious illness but also the cost of, and the value placed by parents on, the process of trying to detect these rare events.

35. **Is the peripheral white blood cell count a helpful screen for bacteremia in otherwise healthy febrile children?**

    The risk of occult bacteremia increases as the white blood cell count increases; however, since the overall incidence of occult bacteremia is very low, the positive predictive value of the white blood cell count for occult bacteremia is also fairly low, thus limiting its utility as a screening test.

    Bonsu BK, Harper MB: Identifying febrile young infants with bacteremia: Is the peripheral white blood cell count and accurate screen? Ann Emerg Med 42:216–225, 2003.

36. **Should the decision on whether to perform a lumbar puncture on a febrile child be guided by the height of the fever or the peripheral white blood cell count?**

    No! Neither of these measures is sensitive enough at any threshold to predict meningitis. The criteria for lumbar puncture should be based on history and physical examination findings rather than nonspecific laboratory tests.

37. **Why is the presence of a petechial rash in a febrile child of concern?**

    A petechial rash, especially if associated with fever, may be an early sign of infection with an invasive bacterial organism, especially *N. meningitidis*. Early identification of a child with meningococcemia is essential since the disease can progress rapidly and has high morbidity.

38. **What is the incidence of invasive bacterial disease in children with fever and petechiae?**

    The most common bacterial causes of fever and petechiae are *N. meningitidis*, *H. influenzae* type B, *S. pneumoniae*, group A streptococcus, *S. aureus*, and *Escherichia coli*. The incidence of invasive bacterial disease has been estimated to be as high as 20% in children who are hospitalized. However, in a prospective study of 411 children with fever and petechiae who presented to a hospital ED, the incidence was only 1.9%. This study, performed in the post–*H. influenzae* type B vaccine era, included children who were managed as outpatients.

    Mandl KD, Stack AM, Fleisher GR: Incidence of bacteremia in infants and children with fever and petechiae. J Pediatr 131:398–404, 1997.

39. **What evaluation is necessary in managing the child with fever and petechiae?**
If the child is ill-appearing or immunocompromised, a complete evaluation for sepsis is necessary. Hospitalization and empiric antibiotics are essential. Children who are well-appearing and have no clear cause for the petechiae should have a complete blood count and blood culture, as well as a rapid streptococcal antigen test if there is pharyngitis. Additional studies, such as coagulation tests and lumbar puncture hospitalization and need for empiric antibiotics are somewhat controversial. Management must be individualized. Most physicians admit and treat with parenteral antibiotics any child who is young (< 12 months) or has an elevated (or low) white blood cell count. For children who have normal laboratory tests, outpatient management with close follow-up is an option. The experience with outpatient antibiotic treatment in meningococcal disease is limited.

40. **How long must fever be present to be considered fever of unknown origin (FUO)?**
The definition of FUO has changed over recent years. FUO was applied to any febrile illness with unexplained, persistent temperature $> 38.5°C$ for 3 or more weeks. In light of more sophisticated diagnostic techniques, many investigators have shortened the minimum duration of fever to 5–7 days.

41. **What is the difference among intermittent fever, spiking fever, remittent fever, sustained fever, and relapsing fever?**
Lorin and Feigin provide the following useful definitions: *Intermittent* fever refers to a pattern where the temperature returns to normal at least once a day. *Hectic* or *spiking* fever has a high peak and quick defervescence. In *remittent* fever, the temperature fluctuates, but always remains elevated. *Sustained* fevers remain persistent with little fluctuation. In *relapsing* fever, the temperature may return to normal for as much as a day or more before fever returns.

   Lorin MI, Feigin RD: Fever of unknown origin. In McMillan JA (ed): Oski's Pediatrics, 3rd ed. Philadelphia, Lippincott Williams & Wilkins, 1999, pp 844–848.

42. **What is the leading cause of FUO?**
In pediatrics, almost half of the cases of FUO are due to infectious diseases (usually respiratory tract infections, followed by infections of the urinary tract, skeleton, and central nervous systems).

43. **How often does FUO have no diagnosis or resolve spontaneously?**
Almost 25% of children with FUO are either undiagnosed or have spontaneous resolution.

44. **What is the difference between fever and hyperthermia?**
Fever is caused by a rise in the hypothalamic set point, which is usually the result of the triggering of several pyrogenic cytokines. *Hyperthermia* is often used to describe a condition in which the thermoregulatory system is either dysfunctional or simply overwhelmed by a variety of internal or external factors. Hyperthermia may result from disorders of excessive heat production (exertional heatstroke, thyrotoxicosis, cocaine intoxication), disorders of diminished heat dissipation (classic heatstroke, severe dehydration, autonomic dysfunction), or disorders of hypothalamic function (cerebrovascular accidents, trauma).

45. **How do you decrease body temperature in children with heatstroke?**
Management of heatstroke begins with aggressive attempts at cooling, such as ice packs, fanning, ice water immersions, and, occasionally, cool IV fluids, until the core temperature drops below $39°C$. Avoid antipyretics and alcohol sponge baths (see question 15). Further management includes airway and cardiovascular support, IV rehydration, and pressor support if necessary.

46. **What kind of fever is associated with bizarre movements in response to disco music?**
Saturday Night Fever was first identified in the 1970s in a group of adolescents wearing unbuttoned silk shirts, flared pants, and platform shoes.

WEBSITES

1. eMedicine Health
   http://www.emedicinehealth.com/articles/10035-1.asp

2. eMedicine Health
   http://www.emedicine.com/emerg/topic377.htm

3. University of Chicago Priztker School of Medicine, Pediatrics Clerkship
   http://pedclerk.bsd.uchicago.edu/evaluationoffever.html

4. National Guideline Clearinghouse
   http://www.guideline.gov/summary/summary.aspx?ss=15&doc_id=4620&nbr=3401

CHAPTER 14

FOREIGN BODIES IN CHILDREN

Jeff E. Schunk, MD

1. **Where would you expect to find a foreign body in a child?**
   Just about anywhere. During normal play and exploration, children place objects anywhere they will fit. Common sites for children to place foreign bodies include the mouth (to be swallowed or aspirated), nose, and ears. Less commonly, objects are placed in the vagina, rectum, and urethra.

2. **Why do children hide foreign bodies in their body?**
   No one really knows. Foreign bodies are found in children of all ages. The 18-month- to 4-year-olds are particularly prone to foreign bodies. This is probably due to developmental, supervisory, and innate curiosity issues. This age group is notorious for nasal foreign bodies; aspirated foreign bodies; and impacted, nonfood, esophageal foreign bodies. Developmental issues also play a role in limiting foreign-body experience, as aspirated foreign bodies are uncommon in infants less than 6 months of age.

3. **Why is there concern about ingestion of disc batteries? How should these be managed?**
   Disc batteries may induce significant tissue injury. This is partially due to the establishment of a local electric current and may be due to content leak. Disc batteries in the esophagus should be removed promptly under direct visualization. Disc batteries in the ear and nose should also be removed promptly. If a disc battery has passed to the stomach, then expectant observation is a safe approach. Large series of disc battery ingestions failed to demonstrate significant complications; spontaneous passage once the battery is beyond the esophagus is the rule. Significant poisoning from battery contents (e.g., mercury) is usually not a concern once the battery has reached the stomach and beyond.

   Samad L, Ali M, Ramzi H: Button battery ingestion: Hazards of esophageal impaction. J Pediatr Surg 34:1527–1531, 1999.

GASTROINTESTINAL FOREIGN BODIES

4. **What are the common esophageal sites for lodgment of foreign bodies?**
   Most esophageal foreign bodies (60–70%) lodge at the level of the thoracic inlet at the cricopharyngeus muscle (Fig. 14-1). The other sites of lodgment include the lower esophageal sphincter and the level of the aortic arch. Patients with histories of congenital esophageal abnormalities or acquired strictures have objects (usually meaty foodstuffs) that impact at the area of anatomic narrowing.

   McGahren ED: Esophageal foreign bodies. Pediatr Rev 20:129–133, 1999.
   Schunk JE, Corneli H, Bolte R: Pediatric coin ingestions: A prospective study of coin location and symptoms. Am J Dis Child 143:546–548, 1989.

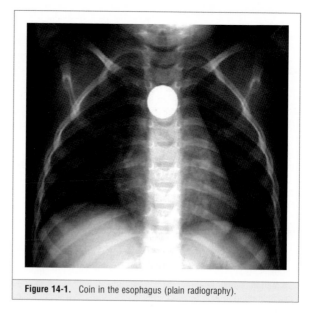

Figure 14-1. Coin in the esophagus (plain radiography).

5. **What is the most common esophageal foreign body in children?**
   Coins are the most common esophageal foreign body, and pennies the most common coin in the United States. In cultures where fish is a main food staple, fish bones are common.

6. **For a patient with a quarter in the stomach, how much time should be allowed for passage out of the stomach?**
   Some authors recommend a long period of observation (up to 6 weeks) for passage. Complications are uncommon; however, family members may not be willing to wait that long.

7. **For an ingested coin that is in the stomach or beyond, should the family check the stool to ensure safe passage?**
   There is no good reason to recommend this unless the family interest level is particularly high. If the foreign body is not found, the family may request more unnecessary x-ray studies. Blunt small objects (coins) pass the remainder of the gastrointestinal tract without complications, typically in 3–8 days. The clever physician might suggest that the family "watch for any change."

8. **How should an esophageal foreign body be removed?**
   There is no single answer; not all esophageal foreign bodies are the same, and not all operators are created equal. Local referral patterns and provincial practice guide this decision. Esophagoscopy, used at many centers, is effective for essentially all types of foreign material, and complications are rare. Typically this is performed after the child receives general anesthesia. Alternatively, flexible endoscopy can remove some foreign bodies and may not require general anesthesia.
   For blunt objects, the fluoroscopic Foley catheter technique can be used when skilled operators are available. The catheter is passed (through the nose) under fluoroscopic guidance beyond the coin; the balloon is inflated; and the object is pulled into the mouth, where it is expectorated. Alternatively, it can be pushed into the stomach. Bougienage also is used to

advance blunt objects into the stomach. The "penny pincher" technique involves an endoscopic grasping forceps within a soft rubber catheter. The catheter is advanced under fluoroscopic guidance and the grasping forceps used to retrieve the coin. These three methods should not be used for sharp objects (e.g., screws, staples, or the little "scotty dog" from the Monopoly game), or when there is associated respiratory distress or stridor. These methods without direct visualization should not be used for objects impacted more than a few days.

Gauderer MW, DeCou JM, Abrams RS, Thomason MA: The "penny pincher": A new technique for fast and safe removal of esophageal coins. J Pediatr Surg 35:276–278, 2000.

Schunk JE: Foreign body-ingestion/aspiration. In Fleisher GR, Ludwig S, Henretig FM (eds): Textbook of Pediatric Emergency Medicine, 5th ed. Philadelphia, Lippincott Williams & Wilkins, 2006, pp 307–314.

Schunk JE, Harrison AM, Corneli HM, Nixon GW: Fluoroscopic Foley catheter removal of esophageal foreign bodies in children: Experience with 415 episodes. Pediatrics 94:709–714, 1994.

Soprano JV, Mandl KD: Four strategies for the management of esophageal coins in children. Pediatr 2000;105:e5.

9. **Is there a role for observation of impacted esophageal coins?**
Many studies have shown that some (at least 30%) impacted esophageal coins pass spontaneously. If a blunt foreign body (e.g., coin) has been impacted for only a short duration, it is reasonable to allow for a short period (<1 day) for spontaneous passage as long as the child is comfortable. Repeated x-ray is needed to demonstrate that the coin has moved into the stomach.

Conners GP, Cobaugh DJ, Feinberg R, et al: Home observation for asymptomatic coin ingestion: Acceptance and outcomes. The New York State Poison Control Center Coin Ingestion Study Group. Acad Emerg Med 6:213–217, 1999.

Sharieff GQ, Brouseau TJ, Bradshaw JA, Shad JA: Acute esophageal coin ingestions: Is immediate removal necessary? Pediatr Radiol 33:859–863, 2003.

Soprano JV, Fleisher GR, Mandl KD: The spontaneous passage of esophageal coins in children. Arch Pediatr Adolesc Med 153:1073–1076, 1999.

10. **What site of esophageal impaction is most likely to pass spontaneously?**
Traditional teaching suggested that spontaneous passage of impacted esophageal foreign bodies, and particularly coins, was more likely from the lower esophageal sphincter. However, it is clear that spontaneous passage can occur from all typical (and nonpathologic) impaction sites.

Conners GP, Cobaugh DJ, Feinberg R, et al: Home observation for asymptomatic coin ingestion: Acceptance and outcomes. The New York State Poison Control Center Coin Ingestion Study Group. Acad Emerg Med 6:213–217, 1999.

Soprano JV, Fleisher GR, Mandl KD: The spontaneous passage of esophageal coins in children. Arch Pediatr Adolesc Med 153:1073–1076, 1999.

11. **Can you promote passage of an impacted blunt esophageal foreign body with medication or otherwise?**
Though some have reported successful use of medication, this information is clouded by the occurrence of spontaneous passage. A recent study found no benefit of using glucagon to induce passage of esophageal coins in children. Common sense agrees with those who advocate trial of carbonated beverage, bread, or crackers to promote passage from the esophagus, but there is no published data comparing such methods.

Mehta D, Attia M, Quintana E, Cronan K: Glucagon use for esophageal coin dislodgment in children: A prospective, double blind, placebo-controlled trial. Acad Emerg Med 8:200–203, 2001.

12. **How quickly can a disc battery injure the esophagus?**
Some reports suggest that impaction duration of less than 4–8 hours can cause mucosal injury. Removal should be emergent.

Samad L, Ali M, Ramzi H: Button battery ingestion: Hazards of esophageal impaction. J Pediatr Surg 34:1527–1531, 1999.

Sigalet D, Lees G: Tracheoesophageal injury secondary to disc battery ingestion. J Pediatr Surg 23:996–998, 1988.

13. Can other impacted blunt foreign bodies injure the esophagus?

Blunt foreign bodies are unlikely to injury the esophagus acutely. With increased duration of impaction, the mucosa grows over the object and serious complications may result. Undiagnosed, impacted blunt objects (even coins) have caused esophageal perforation, esophageal obstruction, abscess, mediastinitis, tracheoesophageal fistula, and even the potentially fatal aorto-esophageal fistula.

Katz KR, Emmens RW, Wood BP: Esophageal obstruction and abscess formation secondary to impacted eroding tiddlywink. Am J Dis Child 143:961–962, 1989.

Stuth EA, Stucke AG, Cohen RD, et al: Successful resuscitation of a child after exsanguination due to aortoesophageal fistula from undiagnosed foreign body. Anesthesiology 95:1025–1026, 2001.

14. Should sharp foreign bodies be removed from the stomach?

Most small, sharp foreign bodies (e.g., nails, pins, tacks, staples) are well tolerated. However, there is concern about the tendency for sewing needles to cause intestinal perforation. Objects that are larger than 4–5 cm may not negotiate the tighter bends in the gastrointestinal tract; consultation is recommended.

Panieri E, Bass DH: The management of ingested foreign bodies in children—a review of 663 cases. Eur J Emerg Med 2:83–87, 1995.

Schunk JE: Foreign body-ingestion/aspiration. In Fleisher GR, Ludwig S, Henretig FM (eds): Textbook of Pediatric Emergency Medicine, 5th ed. Philadelphia, Lippincott Williams & Wilkins, 2006, pp 307–314.

KEY POINTS: FOREIGN BODIES IN THE GASTROINTESTINAL TRACT ✓

1. Impacted esophageal disc batteries should be removed emergently.

2. Impacted esophageal coins may pass spontaneously.

3. An x-ray is recommended to determine the location of a swallowed coin.

4. Small, sharp objects (nails, screws, tacks, and staples) generally pass from the stomach without complications.

ASPIRATED FOREIGN BODIES

15. Classically, children with foreign bodies lodged in a bronchus or smaller airway have cough, decreased breath sounds, and new-onset wheezes. How often is this clinical constellation present?

Only about one-third of children with an aspirated foreign body have this classic triad. The longer the foreign body has been in place, the more likely this triad will be present, and the more prominent the symptoms. One study noted that 57% of children with foreign-body aspirations presented to the emergency department (ED) without symptoms, and 19% had normal physical examinations.

Losek JD: Diagnostic difficulties of foreign body aspiration in children. Am J Emerg Med 8:348–350, 1990.

Metrangolo S, Monetti C, Meneghini L, et al: Eight years' experience with foreign-body aspiration in children: What is really important for timely diagnosis? J Pediatr Surg 34:1229–1231, 1999.

16. **What do children aspirate?**

Aspirated foreign bodies vary widely, but foodstuffs predominate. Nuts (especially peanuts) are the most common, followed by raw apples and carrots, seeds, and popcorn. Radio-opaque objects account for less than 15% of the cases.

Black RE, Choi KJ, Syme WC, et al: Bronchoscopic removal of aspirated foreign bodies in children. Am J Surg 148:778–781, 1994.

17. **What signs/symptoms may be present in a child who aspirates a foreign body?**
    - Respiratory distress
    - Decreased breath sounds
    - Stridor
    - Wheezing
    - Crackles
    - Cough
    - Foreign-body sensation
    - No signs or symptoms

18. **Should all children with a proven aspirated foreign body be admitted?**

Yes. Since there are case reports of objects moving and causing acute respiratory distress or even obstruction, all children with an aspirated foreign body should be admitted until definitive removal of the foreign body.

19. **How are the signs and symptoms of an aspirated foreign body different from those of other respiratory conditions?**

Signs and symptoms of aspirated foreign bodies do not differ from those of very common conditions such as croup, asthma, bronchiolitis, and pneumonia. The history is key. In almost all instances of bronchoscopy-proven foreign-body aspiration, there is a history of choking—if only the appropriate questions are asked. For any pediatric patient with acute onset of respiratory symptoms or new onset of wheezing or coughing, a probing question regarding recent episodes of choking (especially with nuts, carrots, apples, or popcorn) detects most cases.

20. **What is the best way to diagnose an aspirated foreign body?**

Bronchoscopy is the only definitive way to diagnose airway foreign bodies. In the uncommon instances of radio-opaque objects (<15%), a plain x-ray is diagnostic. In many other instances, an inspiratory/expiratory chest x-ray will show indirect evidence of a retained foreign body: air trapping on the side of the foreign body during expiration. In equivocal cases, fluoroscopy may detect the object. However, fluoroscopy is only 70% sensitive. When there is a clear history of a choking episode involving the usual substances, with or without new symptoms or signs, the patient should undergo bronchoscopy, regardless of radiographic findings.

Black RE, Choi KJ, Syme WC, et al: Bronchoscopic removal of aspirated foreign bodies in children. Am J Surg 148:778–781, 1994.

Metrangolo S, Monetti C, Meneghini L, et al: Eight years' experience with foreign-body aspiration in children: What is really important for timely diagnosis? J Pediatr Surg 34:1229–1231, 1999.

Schunk JE: Foreign body-ingestion/aspiration. In Fleisher GR, Ludwig S (eds): Textbook of Pediatric Emergency Medicine, 5th ed. Philadelphia, Lippincott Williams & Wilkins, 2006, pp 307–314.

21. **Are some foreign bodies more concerning when aspirated?**
Of the commonly aspirated foodstuffs, nuts and other oil- or fat-containing substances present the greatest concern because they can contribute to a chemical pneumonitis. Sharp objects are uncommon, and most aspirations of radio-opaque objects tend to be inert. Some objects can be expected to dissolve without significant complications. Using candy as an example, small pieces of aspirated M&M candies are well tolerated, whereas pieces of peanut M&M candies must be removed.

22. **A teenage boy presents to the ED after a choking episode while drinking beer. He reports that he removed the pull-tab of a beer can and placed it inside the can. Then he believes he may have swallowed or aspirated the pull-tab while gulping beer. What study is best to determine the location of the pull-tab?**
Computed tomography of the chest may be needed. Plain radiographs generally do not show an aluminum pull-tab of a beer or soda can.

   Bradburn DM, Carr HF, Renwick I: Radiographs and aluminum: A pitfall for the unwary. BMJ 308:1226, 1994.

FOREIGN BODIES IN THE EAR AND NOSE

23. **What are the symptoms of a nasal foreign body?**
Children usually report a nasal foreign body to family members after experiencing minimal discomfort or airway obstruction. In many instances, the family has already tried to remove it and failed. A unilateral purulent nasal discharge (due to prolonged impaction) occurs in less than one-third of cases.

   Baker MD: Foreign bodies of the ears and nose in childhood. Pediatr Emerg Care 3:67–70, 1987.

24. **What methods are available to remove nasal foreign bodies?**
Removal with a forceps or alligator forceps under direct visualization is common. Though facilitated by a nasal speculum, this method cannot remove all nasal foreign bodies. Some objects are hard to grasp because of their shape (e.g., a small toy car wheel). Also, the mucous-laden nasal environment can hinder the process. A more reliable technique uses a small (6 Fr) Foley catheter:

   - Test the balloon (get a feel for how big with how much air or saline); deflate and lubricate (with lidocaine jelly) the catheter.
   - Pass the catheter to the posterior nasopharynx with the balloon *deflated* (usually it passes inferior to the foreign body).
   - Inflate the balloon a small amount.
   - Pull the balloon/catheter back out of the nose.
   - Note that the foreign body will come out just prior to the balloon.
   - If this technique is unsuccessful, repeat with increased balloon size.

   Additional methods to remove a nasal foreign body rely on applying positive pressure to the mouth with a bag-mask apparatus. When the patient closes the glottis, passage can be affected by occluding the uninvolved nostril. Squeeze the bag forcefully over the mouth to expel the foreign body from the nose. Alternatively, ask a parent to blow into the patient's mouth with the uninvolved nostril occluded. This is a low-cost, nonthreatening alternative.

   Backlin SA: Positive-pressure technique for nasal foreign body removal in children. Ann Emerg Med 25:554–555, 1995.
   Kadish H, Corneli HM: Removal of nasal foreign bodies in the pediatric population. Am J Emerg Med 15:54–56, 1997.

25. **What methods are available to remove ear foreign bodies?**
    For most objects, direct visualization and use of an alligator forceps is effective. Irrigation
    may recover many other foreign bodies. Do not use irrigation for vegetable matter; the foreign
    body will swell and hinder removal. Some physicians use a drop of quick-acting glue on the
    noncotton end of a cotton swab and place this against the foreign body to allow it to be pulled
    out. Care must be taken not to glue the stick or the foreign body to the patient's ear canal.

    Baker MD: Foreign bodies of the ears and nose in childhood. Pediatr Emerg Care 3:67–70, 1987.

26. **What about roaches and other insects in the external canal?**
    A moving insect in the ear canal is very painful and distressing. Lidocaine sprayed into the ear
    may encourage a hasty exit from the canal. Mineral oil placed in the canal may "drown" the
    insect and quickly relieve pain. The immobile insect can then be removed under direct
    visualization.

27. **Should children be sedated for ear or nose foreign-body removal?**
    This depends on your level of comfort, but in general, nose foreign bodies can be removed
    without sedation. However, the inner one-third of the external auditory canal is exquisitely
    sensitive, and sedation may be needed for difficult foreign bodies in the ear. Refer ear foreign
    bodies where previous attempts have created ear canal trauma, or cases where the foreign body
    is against the tympanic membrane and not amenable to irrigations.

    Bressler K, Shelton C: Ear foreign-body removal: A review of 98 consecutive cases. Laryngoscopy
    103:367–370, 1993.

CHAPTER 15

HEADACHE

Jane F. Knapp, MD, and Robert D. Schremmer, MD

1. **Do children get migraine headaches?**
   Migraine is one of the most common causes of headache in children. The reported prevalence is 3–10%. The variation in prevalence between studies is due primarily to differences in diagnostic criteria used and the age range of children studied. Of children referred to pediatric neurologists for the evaluation of headache, migraine is diagnosed in 75%.

2. **Are the international headache society (IHS) criteria for the diagnosis of migraine headache applicable to children?**
   The IHS criteria were developed primarily for the diagnosis of headache in adults. The second edition of the International Classification of Headache Disorders (ICHD-2), published in 2004, reduces the duration requirements of the headache from 4–72 hours in adults to 1–72 hours in children under age 15 years. It also acknowledges that photophobia and phonophobia must be inferred from behavior in young children. The IHS guidelines do not account for other possible symptomatic differences, including intensity and location of pain. Pediatric migraines are often bilateral. A higher incidence of photophobia or phonophobia alone also occurs, especially in younger children.

3. **List the criteria for pediatric migraine *without* aura.**
   A. At least five attacks fulfilling criteria listed for B–D
   B. Duration of 1–48 hours
   C. Headache with at least two of the following:
      - Bilateral (frontal/temporal) or unilateral location
      - Pulsatile quality
      - Headache intensity moderate or severe
      - Aggravation by routine physical activity
   D. During headache, at least one of the following occurs:
      - Nausea and/or vomiting
      - Photophobia and/or phonophobia

   Maytal J, Young M, Shechter A, Lipton RB: Pediatric migraine and the International Headache Society criteria. Neurology 48:602–607, 1997.
   Winner P, Wasiewski W, Gladstein J, et al: Multicenter prospective evaluation of proposed pediatric migraine revisions to the IHS criteria. Headache 37:545–548, 1997.

4. **List the criteria for pediatric migraine headache *with* aura.**
   A. At least two attacks fulfilling criteria listed for B
   B. At least two of the following:
      - One or more fully reversible aura symptoms, including focal cortical and/or brain stem dysfunction
      - At least one aura developing gradually over more than 4 minutes, or two or more symptoms occurring in succession
      - Headache follows less than 60 minutes after aura symptoms

5. **List some common triggers for migraine in children.**
Stress, fatigue (including lack of sleep), hunger, glare, head trauma, and certain foods containing nitrates, caffeine, tyramine, glutamate, or salt are common triggers. Eye strain, cold foods, and high altitude are less common.

6. **Do children get tension-type headaches?**
The prevalence of tension-type headaches in children and adolescents ranges from 10% to 25%, but one study reported a prevalence of 73% in Brazilian children and adolescents age 10–18 years. The ICHD-2 lists three subtypes of tension-type headaches: (1) infrequent episodic (headaches on <1 day per month), (2) frequent episodic (headaches on 1–14 days per month), and (3) chronic (headaches on ≥15 days per month). These headaches are characterized by mild to moderate pressing or tightening pain that is nonpulsatile. The pain is usually bilateral and not aggravated by routine activity. Nausea and vomiting do not occur, but phonophobia or photophobia may be present. Clinical features are the same in children and adults.
Anttila P: Tension-type headache in children and adolescents. Curr Pain Headache Rep 8:500–504, 2004.

7. **Are causes of tension-type headaches the same for adults and children?**
Pediatric tension-type headaches probably share some risk factors, but there are some differences. Analgesic overuse, psychosocial stress, psychiatric disorders, muscular tension, and oromandibular dysfunction are potential causes of tension-type headaches in adults. Analgesic overuse has not been found in children. Psychosocial stress (divorced parents, physical changes during adolescence, difficulty with peer relations, and chronic illness) are more often reported in children with tension-type headaches. Also, children with frequent episodic tension-type headaches more commonly manifest depressive symptoms. The presence of scoliosis may also precipitate tension-type headaches in some children.

8. **Can children suffer from both migraines and tension-type headaches?**
Although the ICHD-2 does not recognize a separate category of mixed migraine and tension-type headache, characteristics of both types of headache may be found in many children. In one Canadian study, one third of the patients with migraine symptoms fulfilled the IHS criteria of tension-type headaches as well. Some researchers have postulated that episodic tension-type headache and migraine may fall along the same continuum of disorder.
Sarioglu B, Erhan E, Serdaroglu G, et al: Tension-type headache in children: A clinical evaluation. Pediatr Int 45:186–189, 2003.
Seshia SS: Mixed migraine and tension-type: A common cause of recurrent headache in children. Can J Neurol Sci 31:315–318, 2004.

9. **How will I recognize the child with a brain tumor headache?**
Brain tumors are an uncommon but feared cause of headaches in children. Certain features help to distinguish a headache that is caused by a tumor (Fig. 15-1) or other intracranial mass:
- Location—occipital headaches or headaches localized to the nape of the neck
- Worsening with sneezing, coughing, or straining
- Timing—headaches that awaken the child from sleep or that are worse in the morning and improve on arising
- Positioning—headaches that worsen with body movement, especially bending forward, and improve with change in position
- Headaches associated with blurred vision
- Change over time—headaches that change in frequency, severity, or characteristics
Honig PJ, Charney EB: Children with brain tumor headaches. Am J Dis Child 136:121–124, 1982.

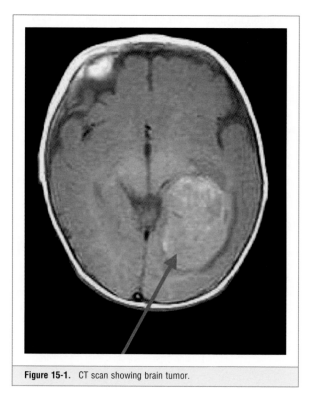

Figure 15-1. CT scan showing brain tumor.

KEY POINTS: BRAIN TUMOR HEADACHES ✓

1. Usually occipital

2. Worse with cough, sneezing

3. Worse in the early morning

4. May be worse with bending forward

5. Change in character over time

10. **Are chronic daily headaches common in children?**
    Chronic daily headaches encompass a group of headaches not specifically described by the ICHD-2, although three of the four types in a proposed classification are included in the 2004 IHS revisions:
    - **Transformed migraine:** Daily headache with average duration of 4 hours for more than a month, and a history of increased headache frequency with decreased migraine symptoms

- **Chronic tension-type headache (ICHD-2 2.3):** History of episodic tension-type headache in the past with evolution to daily headaches
- **New daily persistent headache (ICHD-2 4.8):** Acute onset of headache on more than 15 days per month lasting at least 4 hours and without history of migraine or tension-type headache in the past
- **Hemicrania continua (ICHD-2 4.7):** Unilateral, continuous headache of moderate severity known for its absolute relief with indomethacin

The prevalence of chronic daily headaches is reported to be almost 1% of children and adolescents, and as many as 30% of patients seen in pediatric neurology clinics suffer from them. They occur more commonly in females. Psychiatric comorbidity, including sleep, anxiety, and mood disorders, is high, which increases the difficulty of treatment. Transformed migraine is the most common type.

Esposito SB, Gherpelli JLD: Chronic daily headaches in children and adolescents: A study of clinical characteristics. Cephalalgia 24:476–448, 2004.

Galli F, Patron L, Russo PM, et al: Chronic daily headache in childhood and adolescence: Clinical aspects and a 4-year follow-up. Cephalalgia 24:850–858, 2004.

Seshia SS: Chronic daily headache in children and adolescents. Can J Neurol Sci 31:319–323, 2004.

11. **Describe the most important aspects of the physical examination for children with headaches.**
Pay special attention to the measurement of blood pressure to rule out hypertension, and perform a complete neurologic examination, an ocular examination including the fundi, and an assessment of linear growth and, if appropriate, head circumference. Look for signs of trauma, and examine the skin for evidence of a neurocutaneous disease. Multiple café-au-lait lesions suggest neurofibromatosis and possible intracranial tumor.

12. **What is the role of emergent neuroimaging in children with headache?**
Most headaches in children are benign. Neuroimaging is useful in identifying children with space-occupying or surgical lesions. An important concern is brain tumor, which, although rare, represents the largest group of solid neoplasms in children. Indications for neuroimaging are as follows:

- Persistent headaches of >6-month duration that have not responded to medical treatment
- Headache associated with abnormal neurologic findings, especially papilledema, nystagmus, or gait or motor abnormalities
- Persistent headaches not associated with a family history of migraine
- Headaches that awaken a child from sleep or are present immediately on awakening
- Persistent headache associated with episodes of confusion, disorientation, or vomiting
- Family history or medical history of disorders predisposing one to central nervous system (CNS) lesions (such as neurofibromatosis)
- Clinical or laboratory findings suggestive of CNS involvement

A practice parameter on the evaluation of pediatric patients with recurrent headaches written by the American Academy of Neurology discusses the issue of neuroimaging for recurrent headache. The parameter concludes that routine neuroimaging should be avoided in children with a normal neurologic examination. It should be considered, however, in patients with headache who have a history of seizures, an abnormal neurologic examination, a recent change in type of headache experienced, or characteristics implying neurologic dysfunction.

Lewis DW, Ashwal S, Dahl G, et al: Practice parameter: Evaluation of children and adolescents with recurrent headaches. Report of the Quality Standards Subcommittee of the American Academy of Neurology and the Practice Committee of the Child Neurology Society. Neurology 59:490–498, 2002.

KEY POINTS: INDICATIONS FOR COMPUTED TOMOGRAPHY IN A CHILD WITH A HEADACHE ✓

1. Headache persists >6 months

2. Persistent headache without family history of migraine

3. Abnormal neurologic examination

4. Papilledema present

5. Headache that awakens child

6. Headache associated with confusion, disorientation, vomiting

7. Family history of neurofibromatosis

13. **How should headache pain be managed acutely?**

Evidence-based guidelines similar to those published for adults for the treatment of headache do not exist. Treatment recommendations are generally based on experience, tradition, or extrapolation of information from adult studies. Most headaches in children respond to reassurance, hydration, and simple analgesics, such as acetaminophen or nonsteroidal anti-inflammatory drugs (e.g., ibuprofen).

14. **What lifestyle changes can be made to prevent headaches?**

Good nutrition can help reduce frequency of headaches. A healthy, well-balanced breakfast that includes a source of protein and minimizes excessive sugar should be eaten every day. Magnesium and vitamin B2 may reduce the frequency of migraines, so a multivitamin may be taken if the patient's diet does not have sufficient sources. Adequate hydration is also essential in the prevention of headaches. Water should be emphasized over juices and soda. Stress reduction through regular exercise and relaxation is important. Adequate, but not too much, sleep and a regular bedtime schedule are also a key to remaining headachefree.

Maizels M, Blumenfeld A, Burchette R: A combination of riboflavin, magnesium, and feverfew for migraine prophylaxis: A randomized trial. Headache 44:885–890, 2004.

Schoenen J, Jacquy J, Lenaerts M: Effectiveness of high-dose riboflavin in migraine prophylaxis. A randomized controlled trial. Neurology 50:466–470, 1998.

15. **What treatments are available for migraine headaches?**

Many children with migraines respond to over-the-counter analgesics and rest in a dark, quiet room. Sumatriptan nasal spray has been used in adolescents with migraine headaches, with results superior to placebo in one study but no significant difference in another. This treatment may be associated with taste disturbance, nausea, and somnolence. Prochlorperazine, chlorpromazine, and metoclopramide are preferred by some but may cause dystonic reactions. These reactions can be minimized by the concurrent administration of diphenhydramine. Isometheptene combines acetaminophen with a vasoconstrictor and a sedative, making it a useful agent for migraine headaches. Ergots are infrequently used for migraine in headaches because of the side effect of vomiting. Avoid narcotics or combination agents that can cause rebound headache. A practice parameter published by the American Academy of Neurology offers an evidence-based approach to treatment of acute migraine as well as prevention medications.

Barnes N, Millman G, James E: Migraine headache in children. Clin Evid 10:429–443, 2003.

Lewis D, Ashwal S, Hershey A, et al: Practice parameter: Pharmacological treatment of migraine headache in children and adolescents. Neurology 63:2215–2224, 2004.

16. **Describe therapeutic options for tension-type headaches.**

Infrequent episodic tension-type headaches can be treated with over-the-counter analgesics and do not generally come to the attention of the emergency department. For patients with frequent episodic or chronic tension-type headaches, either pharmacologic or nonpharmacologic therapies may be effective, though few studies regarding medication efficacy can be found in the literature. One preliminary study showed significant clinical improvement from daily oral amitriptyline as well as a relaxation program without medication. Biofeedback has also been shown to be an effective therapy, probably through relaxation of muscular tension in the head and neck.

Anttila P: Tension-type headache in children and adolescents. Curr Pain Headache Rep 8:500–504, 2004.

CHAPTER 16

HEMATURIA AND DYSURIA

Sandra H. Schwab, MD, and Elizabeth R. Alpern, MD, MSCE

1. **What is the definition of gross and microscopic hematuria?**
   - Gross hematuria is defined as reddish or pinkish discoloration of the urine with confirmation of red blood cells (RBCs) by microscopy. If the RBCs come from glomeruli, the acidic nature of the urine may change hemoglobin to hematin, causing the urine to appear brownish, tea-colored, or cola-colored.
   - Microscopic hematuria is normal-appearing urine that, when centrifuged, has ≥5 RBCs per high-power field on microscopy.

2. **What else, besides RBCs, can cause urine to appear red or brown?**
   Reddish or brownish discoloration of the urine from some compound other than blood is common. Myoglobinuria and porphyrinuria present with red or tea-colored urine. Several ingestions also discolor the urine. Infants may have precipitation of urate crystals that make their urine appear red or orange in the diaper.

3. **What can cause a "false-positive" urine dipstick?**
   You may encounter a positive urine dipstick, but upon microscopic examination no RBCs are seen. The dipstick is sensitive to any heme compound and will be positive for intact red blood cells as well as hemoglobin from hemolyzed RBCs and myoglobin from rhabdomyolysis. Several other oxidizing compounds, such as bleach or microbial peroxidase, can also turn the dipstick spuriously positive.

   Goldsmith DI, Novello AC: Clinical and laboratory evaluation of renal function. In Edelmann CM (ed): Pediatric Kidney Disease, 2nd ed. Boston, Little, Brown and Company, 1992, pp 461–465.
   Liao JC, Churchill BM: Pediatric urine testing. Pediatr Clin North Am 48:1425–1436, 2001.
   Liebelt EA: Hematuria. In Fleisher GR, Ludwig S, Henretig FM (eds): Textbook of Pediatric Emergency Medicine, 5th ed. Philadelphia, Lippincott Williams & Wilkins, 2006, pp 345–349.

4. **What is the most likely diagnosis of a child presenting to the emergency department (ED) with "red urine"?**
   The majority of children who visit an ED for red urine are diagnosed with urinary tract infections (UTIs) (26% with documented infections and 23% with suspected UTI or viral cystitis). Perineal irritation accounts for 11% of cases, and meatal stenosis with ulcer is found in another 7%. Hematuria is from traumatic injuries in 7% of cases; acute glomerulonephritis is diagnosed in 4%, and a rare patient may have a Wilms' tumor or other oncologic process involving the genitourinary tract.

   Even though parents or patients may assume that blood in the diaper or toilet is from urine, it may actually be from several other sources: vaginal bleeding (menses, foreign body, infection, trauma), rectal bleeding (fissure, hemorrhoid, trauma), or urethral prolapse.

   Ingelfinger JR, Davis AE, Grupe WE: Frequency and etiology of gross hematuria in a general pediatric setting. Pediatrics 59:557–561, 1977.

5. **Is there a way to determine glomerular versus nonglomerular blood in the urine?**
   See Table 16-1.

TABLE 16-1. GLOMERULAR VERSUS NONGLOMERULAR BLOOD IN THE URINE

Glomerular	Nonglomerular
Brown or tea-colored urine	Bright red or pink urine
RBC casts	Blood clots
Dysmorphic RBCs	Normal RBC morphology
Cellular casts	Blood at initiation or termination of urination
Proteinuria	

RBC = red blood cell.
Adapted from Kalia A, Travis LB: Hematuria, leukocyturia, and cylindruria. In Edelmann CM (ed): Pediatric Kidney Disease, 2nd ed. Boston, Little, Brown and Company, 1992, pp 553–563.

6. **What is the differential diagnosis of hematuria in a child?**
    See Table 16-2.

7. **How would you evaluate a child with blunt abdominal trauma for renal injury?**
    See Fig. 16-1.

TABLE 16-2. DIFFERENTIAL DIAGNOSIS OF HEMATURIA IN CHILDREN

Glomerular	Nonglomerular
Postinfectious nephritis (poststreptococcal glomerulonephritis)	Urinary tract infection
IgA nephropathy	Hemorrhagic cystitis
Hereditary nephritis (Alport syndrome)	Urethritis
Benign familial hematuria (thin basement membrane disease)	Sickle cell disease or trait
Exercise-related hematuria	Meatal stenosis
Subacute endocarditis	Nonsteroidal anti-inflammatory drugs
Ventriculoperitoneal shunt nephritis	Trauma
Hemolytic uremic syndrome	Urolithiasis
Systemic lupus erythematosus	Hypercalciuria
Henoch-Schönlein purpura	Wilms' tumor
	Polycystic kidney disease
	Urethral prolapse
	Antibiotics (penicillins, cephalosporins)
	Ureteropelvic junction obstruction
	Leukemia
	Hemophilia

Adapted from Kalia A, Travis LB: Hematuria, leukocyturia, and cylindruria. In Edelmann CM (ed): Pediatric Kidney Disease, 2nd ed. Boston, Little, Brown and Company, 1992, pp 553–563.

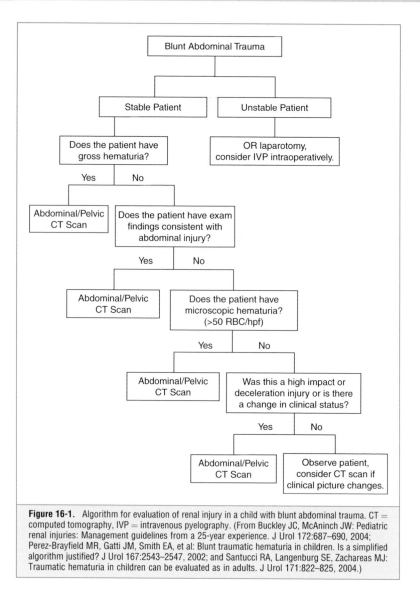

Figure 16-1. Algorithm for evaluation of renal injury in a child with blunt abdominal trauma. CT = computed tomography, IVP = intravenous pyelography. (From Buckley JC, McAninch JW: Pediatric renal injuries: Management guidelines from a 25-year experience. J Urol 172:687–690, 2004; Perez-Brayfield MR, Gatti JM, Smith EA, et al: Blunt traumatic hematuria in children. Is a simplified algorithm justified? J Urol 167:2543–2547, 2002; and Santucci RA, Langenburg SE, Zachareas MJ: Traumatic hematuria in children can be evaluated as in adults. J Urol 171:822–825, 2004.)

8. **Why are children at more risk than adults for renal injury after blunt trauma?**
    Kidneys in children are proportionally larger and have less protective perirenal fat and musculature than adult kidneys.

9. **Hypertension with hematuria is associated with which diseases?**
    Hypertension found in a patient with hematuria may indicate a renal emergency. Consider glomerulonephritis, obstructive uropathy, polycystic kidney disease, hemolytic uremic syndrome, systemic lupus erythematosus, and Wilms' tumor.

10. **Describe signs and symptoms associated with hematuria that require urgent/ emergent evaluation.**

 Children with hematuria should be evaluated with a full history, family history, and physical examination, which will allow a directed workup of the etiology. Gross hematuria should be evaluated emergently for significant renal trauma, tumor, or bleeding disorder. Hematuria accompanied by edema, proteinuria, oliguria, hypertension, or headache may portend glomerular renal disease that needs emergent evaluation. Signs and symptoms such as fever, dysuria, flank pain, abdominal pain, rash, recent sore throat, or respiratory illness are important factors that will help lead to a diagnosis. Asymptomatic isolated microscopic hematuria is found at one time or another in 1–4% of children and, in most cases, is benign. This is a diagnosis of exclusion, and referral for outpatient evaluation is indicated.

 Liebelt EA: Hematuria. In Fleisher GR, Ludwig S, Henretig FM (eds): Textbook of Pediatric Emergency Medicine, 5th ed. Philadelphia, Lippincott Williams & Wilkins, 2006, pp 345–349.

KEY POINTS: HEMATURIA ✓

1. Urinary tract infections are the most common cause of hematuria in children.

2. Distinguishing between glomerular and nonglomerular hematuria can help narrow the differential and lead to a diagnosis.

3. Any child with gross hematuria requires emergent evaluation.

4. Any child with hematuria should have a urine dipstick and microscopic urinalysis.

5. Hypercalciuria is the most common cause of pediatric urinary stones.

11. **Which laboratory tests are helpful in the evaluation of hematuria?**

 All patients with the sign or finding of hematuria should have a urine dipstick and microscopic urinalysis. Depending on the history and physical examination, further blood tests may be indicated. Hematuria with fever, flank pain, urgency, and dysuria usually indicates a urinary tract infection and should be evaluated with a urine Gram stain and culture. Complete blood count, blood urea nitrogen, and serum creatinine may be helpful in all cases except those of isolated microscopic hematuria or obvious urinary tract infection. If the child has sustained or suspected trauma, liver function tests, amylase, and lipase are also recommended. Prothrombin time and partial thromboplastin time will help diagnose any bleeding disorder. If the clinical picture indicates nephritis, then electrolytes, complement levels (C3 and C4), antistreptolysin-O or Streptozyme test, antinuclear antibody titer, hepatitis screen, and erythrocyte sedimentation rate may be helpful.

 A patient with a positive dipstick without evidence of RBCs on urine microscopic examination should be evaluated with plasma creatine kinase and urinary myoglobin concentration for rhabdomyolysis, and a bilirubin level for signs of hemolysis.

 Feld LG, Meyers KEC, Kaplan BS, Stapleton FB. Limited evaluation of microscopic hematuria in pediatrics. Pediatrics 102:E42, 1998.

 Patel HP, Bissler JJ: Hematuria in children. Pediatr Clin North Am 48:1519–1535. 2001.

12. **Describe the etiology of nephrolithiasis in children.**

 Nephrolithiasis is an increasing problem in children in the United States. Stone formation results from environmental and hereditary factors. Hypercalciuria is the most common cause of pediatric urinary stones and has many causes. Genetic syndromes, such as familial idiopathic hypercalciuria, as well as other diseases such as Bartter syndrome and distal renal tubular acidosis, lead to increased urinary calcium excretion and stone formation. Iatrogenic causes include treatment with loop diuretics and prednisone.

Other causes of stone formation include infection with urease-producing organisms (struvite or "staghorn" calculi); cystinuria; hyperoxaluria; medications such as protease inhibitors; and high-protein, low-carbohydrate diets (ketogenic diet).

Gillespie RS, Stapleton FB: Nephrolithiasis in children. Pediatr Rev 25:131–138, 2004.
Hulton SA: Evaluation of urinary tract calculi in children. Arch Dis Child 84:320–323, 2001.

13. **How do you diagnose urinary stones in children?**
Evaluation and diagnosis should begin with a complete history and physical examination, including a history of urinary infections, current medications, and a detailed family history. A urinalysis and urine culture should be obtained. Microscopic hematuria is present in >90% of children with urinary stones. Infection is commonly seen with stones, so evidence of urinary tract infection does not exclude stones. Renal ultrasonography or nonenhanced helical computed tomography (CT) are the standard methods of diagnosis; they can detect very small stones as well as underlying anatomic abnormalities or alternative diagnoses. Most stones in children are composed of radio-opaque substances and may be seen on plain abdominal radiographs (Fig. 16-2), but the small size of most stones makes this test less sensitive. Intravenous pyelography is another option, although CT has largely replaced it because of increased sensitivity and specificity.

Gillespie RS, Stapleton FB: Nephrolithiasis in children. Pediatr Rev 25:131–138, 2004.
Hulton SA: Evaluation of urinary tract calculi in children. Arch Dis Child 84:320–323, 2001.

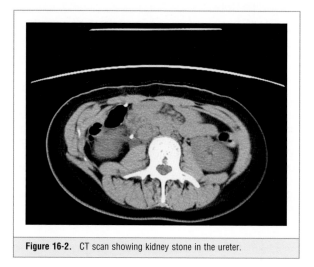

Figure 16-2. CT scan showing kidney stone in the ureter.

14. **What are the most common causes of dysuria in children?**
Dysuria (painful urination) in usually caused by irritation of the bladder or urethra. Common causes of this symptom include cystitis (viral or bacterial), urethritis (infectious, chemical, or traumatic), vaginitis, or balanitis. Children may report or exhibit perineal discomfort and parents may interpret this discomfort as dysuria in the case of pruritus from pinworms (*Enterobius vermicularis*) or in cases of sexual abuse.

Corboy JB: Pain—dysuria. In Fleisher GR, Ludwig S, Henretig FM (eds): Textbook of Pediatric Emergency Medicine, 5th ed. Philadelphia, Lippincott Williams & Wilkins, 2006, pp 499–503.

Kellogg ND, Parra JM, Menard S: Children with anogenital symptoms and signs referred for sexual abuse evaluations. Arch Pediatr Adolesc Med 152:634–641, 1998.

15. **Which systemic diseases may present with dysuria?**
Urethritis, producing dysuria, is associated with several serious systemic diseases, such as Stevens-Johnson syndrome, Reiter syndrome, and Behçet's syndrome.

Corboy JB: Pain—dysuria. In Fleisher GR, Ludwig S, Henretig FM (eds): Textbook of Pediatric Emergency Medicine, 5th ed. Philadelphia, Lippincott Williams & Wilkins, 2006, pp 499–503.

16. **Name some common causes of urethritis in children.**
Infectious urethritis in adolescents is most commonly due to *Neisseria gonorrhoeae* and *Chlamydia trachomatis*. Bubble baths, detergents, fabric softeners, and perfumed soaps are often the etiology for cases of chemical urethritis in younger children.

KEY POINTS: DYSURIA ✔

1. The most common causes of dysuria in children are urinary tract infections and urethritis.

2. Chemical urethritis is a common cause of dysuria in young children.

3. Consider diagnoses such as pinworms, systemic illness, and sexual abuse in children presenting with dysuria.

17. **A child reports dysuria but is afebrile, with no genital lesions, and has a negative urinalysis for pyuria. What are the most probable diagnoses?**
Dysuria in this child may be due to viral cystitis, chemical irritation of the urethra, pinworms, fused labia minora, idiopathic hypercalciuria, urinary tract stone, or bacterial urinary tract infection (a few children will present with negative urinalysis but positive urine cultures).

18. **What is "summer penile syndrome?"**
Summer penile syndrome is a seasonal acute hypersensitivity reaction to chigger bites on the penis. It is found in endemic areas (Southern and Midwestern United States) during the summer months. This syndrome is always accompanied by significant edema of the penis, and 33% of children present with dysuria. Chiggers are the larval form of the trombiculid mite.

Smith GA, Sharma V, Knapp JF, et al: The summer penile syndrome: Seasonal acute hypersensitivity reaction caused by chigger bites on the penis. Pediatr Emerg Care 14:116–118, 1998.

19. **What parasitic infection should be considered in a traveler or recent immigrant presenting with hematuria or dysuria?**
Urinary schistosomiasis, caused by *Schistosoma haematobium*, is a common cause of hematuria and dysuria worldwide. This worm is found mostly in sub-Saharan Africa and enters through the skin after contact with fresh water that harbors the larval form. The worms eventually migrate to the bladder mucosa, where eggs are produced and secreted in the urine. Diagnosis can be made by examination of the urine for eggs. Praziquantel is the mainstay of treatment and is curative in most cases.

Lischer GH, Sweat SD: 16-year-old boy with gross hematuria. Mayo Clin Proc 77:475–478, 2002.
Ross A, Bartley PB, Sleigh AC, et al: Schistosomiasis. N Engl J Med 346:1212–1220, 2002.

WEBSITES

1. National Kidney Foundation
   http://www.kidney.org/

2. National Kidney and Urologic Diseases Information Clearinghouse
   http://kidney.niddk.nih.gov/index.htm

CHAPTER 17

HYPERTENSION

Deirdre Fearon, MD, MA, and Susan Duffy, MD

1. **What is considered high blood pressure or hypertension in a child?**
   There's hypertension, and then there's HYPERtension. The distinction is between **significant** (>95th percentile) and **severe** (>99th percentile) hypertension. These classifications by age and sex were established by the Task Force on Blood Pressure Control in Children, updated in 2004. In addition to these classifications, the Task Force also developed standardized definitions for hypertensive urgency and hypertensive emergency. *Hypertensive urgency* refers to a severely elevated blood pressure without evidence of end-organ damage. A *hypertensive emergency* occurs when a child's blood pressure is severely elevated and the child shows evidence of end-organ damage.

   Cronan K, Kost SI: Renal and electrolyte emergencies. In Fleisher GR, Ludwig S, Henretig FM (eds): Textbook of Pediatric Emergency Medicine, 5th ed. Philadelphia, Lippincott Williams & Wilkins, 2006, pp 873–919.
   National High Blood Pressure Education Program Working Group on Hypertension Control in Children and Adolescence: The fourth report on the diagnosis, evaluation, and treatment of high blood pressure in children and adolescents. Pediatrics 114:555–576, 2004.

KEY POINTS: CLASSIFICATION OF HYPERTENSION ✔

Depending on age, height, and sex:

- Significant hypertension is >95th percentile.
- Severe hypertension is >99th percentile.
- Hypertensive urgency is >99th percentile without evidence of end-organ damage.
- Hypertensive emergency is >99th percentile with evidence of end-organ damage.

2. **If a high blood pressure is found incidentally by the triage nurse, what two questions should you ask before you get too worried?**
   - **"What size cuff did you use?"** Inappropriate cuff size can give spuriously high or low blood pressure readings. They will be falsely elevated if the cuff is too small, and low if the cuff is too big. The width of the cuff bladder should be about 40% of the circumference of the arm measured at the midpoint between the shoulder and the elbow (technically, between the acromion and the olecranon). The cuff should encircle 80–100% of the circumference of the upper arm and be about two-thirds of its length.
   - **"Will you please repeat it?"** Nonpathologic elevations in blood pressure can be caused by white coats, pain, recent activity, heat, and agitation. Ideally, a child's blood pressure should be measured after a few minutes of inactivity, as he or she sits calmly in a parent's lap.

3. **Which patients need evaluation and treatment in the emergency department (ED), and which patients can follow up with their primary physician?**
   - **Workup and treatment:** Clearly, patients with hypertensive emergencies should be treated in your department, with the initial focus on ABCs and rapidly establishing IV access. Those children experiencing hypertensive urgencies (i.e., severely elevated blood pressures without evidence of end-organ damage), should be worked up, treated, and admitted for further evaluation.
   - **Workup only:** For asymptomatic patients with *significantly* elevated blood pressure readings, a thorough history and physical examination and some screening laboratory tests should be performed. If there are no abnormalities in this workup, the patient can be discharged with close follow-up.
   - **Discharge without workup:** Patients being seen for another problem who were incidentally found to have mildly elevated blood pressures and are asymptomatic can be discharged to the care of their primary care physician. Ideally, the doctor should record several readings in a series of visits before confirming the diagnosis of hypertension (Fig. 17-1).

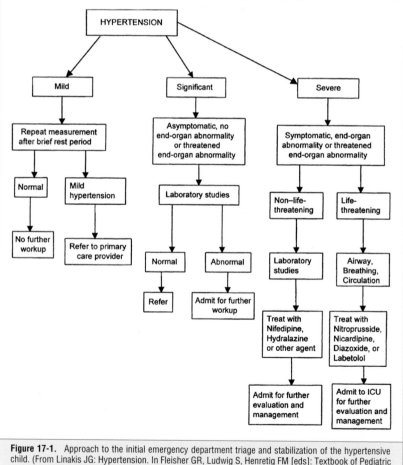

Figure 17-1. Approach to the initial emergency department triage and stabilization of the hypertensive child. (From Linakis JG: Hypertension. In Fleisher GR, Ludwig S, Henretig FM [eds]: Textbook of Pediatric Emergency Medicine, 5th ed. Philadelphia, Lippincott Williams & Wilkins, 2006, with permission.)

KEY POINTS: APPROACH TO THE HYPERTENSIVE CHILD ✓

1. Work up, treat, and admit patients with blood pressure > 99th percentile or end-organ damage.

2. Work up and discharge patients with blood pressure > 95th percentile and normal screening laboratory test results.

3. Discharge with follow-up patients with incidentally found, mildly elevated blood pressure.

4. **Name the causes of pathologic hypertension. Discuss likely causes in babies, small children, and big children.**
   In general, as the age of a child increases, the likelihood of finding a cause for hypertension decreases. A newborn infant with hypertension is most likely to have either a congenital renal anomaly or a vascular problem (e.g., a renal artery thrombosis or stenosis or coarctation of the aorta). Small children may present with these vascular or congenital causes but become more likely to have renal parenchymal disease such as pyelonephritis, glomerulonephritis, or reflux nephropathy. Big children and teenagers are most likely to have essential hypertension (including obesity), though may still present with parenchymal disease. The mnemonic **HYPERTENSION** may help you recall some of the major causes of high blood pressure:
   - **H** = **H**yperthyroidism
   - **Y** = **Why?** Cause unknown—primary hypertension
   - **P** = **P**heochromocytoma
   - **E** = **E**ats too much—obesity
   - **R** = **R**enal parenchymal disease
   - **T** = **T**hrombosis (renal artery, particularly if umbilical catheter was used as neonate)
   - **E** = **E**ndocrine (**congenital adrenal hyperplasia**, primary aldosteronism, hyperparathyroidism)
   - **N** = **N**eurologic (increased intracranial, Guillain-Barré syndrome, neurofibromatosis)
   - **S** = **S**tenosis (renal artery stenosis or coarctation of the aorta, supravalvular aortic stenosis with Williams syndrome)
   - **I** = **I**ngestion (cocaine, birth control, steroids, decongestants)
   - **O** = **O**bstetric (eclampsia)
   - **N** = **N**euroblastoma

   Linakis JG, Constantine E: Hypertension. In Fleisher GR, Ludwig S, Henretig FM (eds): Textbook of Pediatric Emergency Medicine, 5th ed. Philadelphia, Lippincott Williams & Wilkins, 2006, pp 351–358.

5. **How might a child present with hypertension?**
   Often hypertension is silent and picked up on routine physical examination. If a child does present with symptoms, they may be as vague as irritability and headache or as impressive as seizure and coma. Other possible symptoms include visual disturbances, personality changes, dizziness, nausea and vomiting, weight loss, polyuria and polydipsia, or facial nerve palsy.

6. **What historical questions are important to ask the parent of a hypertensive child?**
   - Does the child have a history of recurrent urinary tract infections? Unexplained fevers? Hematuria? Frequency? Dysuria? Any recent illness? Sore throats?
   - Did the child have an umbilical artery catheter as a neonate?
   - Does he or she have intermittent sweating, flushing, and palpitations?

- Has the child been growing well?
- Has the child suffered any recent head trauma?
- Is there a family history of hypertension, renal disease, or deafness?
- Has the child ingested anything? Decongestants? Birth control pills? Steroids? Cocaine?

7. **What physical examination findings are important with a hypertensive child?**
Carefully examine the child for evidence of end-organ damage and for possible causes of hypertension:
- **General:** Dysmorphism (e.g., Williams syndrome), overweight or underweight
- **Head, ears, eyes, nose, throat:** Evidence of head trauma, decreased visual acuity, papilledema, retinal infarcts, abnormal pupillary light reflex
- **Lungs:** Crackles (evidence of failure)
- **Heart:** Displaced point of maximal impulse, murmurs
- **Abdomen:** Bruits, hepatomegaly, renal masses
- **Extremities:** Decreased femoral pulses, discrepant four-extremity blood pressures, edema
- **Skin:** Café-au-lait spots or skin-fold freckling (neurofibromatosis), xanthomas (hyperlipidemia)
- **Neurologic:** Cranial nerve palsies, sensory-motor asymmetry

8. **What laboratory tests should you obtain in the initial workup of a patient with hypertension?**
Much information can be obtained with relatively few laboratory tests. Usually a set of electrolytes with a blood urea nitrogen and creatinine, a complete blood count, and a urine dip are enough to get started in the asymptomatic patient. In obese children, a lipid profile may be helpful, as would a urine culture in all girls and those boys with known renal disease. In patients who are symptomatic, electrocardiography and chest radiography may help you determine the degree of end-organ damage. If ultrasonography is readily available in your department, renal ultrasonography can be particularly helpful in diagnosis of a renal cause of hypertension in a baby.

KEY POINTS: LABORATORY WORKUP FOR A HYPERTENSIVE CHILD ✔

1. Urine dip (and culture if indicated)

2. Electrolytes, blood urea nitrogen, creatinine, with or without lipid profile

3. Electrocardiography and chest x-ray if patient is symptomatic

4. Renal ultrasonography if available

9. **If a child has a dangerously high blood pressure, should it be lowered to normal as quickly as possible?**
Well, sort of. It is important to normalize blood pressure to prevent further end-organ damage, but doing so too quickly can be harmful to those same organs, specifically the brain. Cerebral autoregulation maintains a relatively constant cerebral blood flow with variations in peripheral pressures. When peripheral blood pressure increases, cerebral vessels constrict. When peripheral pressure drops, those vessels dilate. There are points, however, at extremes of blood pressure, at which this system is exhausted. When the cerebral vessels are maximally constricted or dilated, the brain can no longer autoregulate. It is particularly important when

treating a hypertensive emergency to bear in mind that under hypertensive conditions, the low point at which autoregulation ceases to function is *raised* (i.e., maximal cerebral vasodilatation occurs at a higher blood pressure). Lowering the blood pressure below this point can lead to cerebral ischemia. For this reason, an elevated blood pressure should be lowered to normal as slowly as is safely possible, ideally over days rather than minutes.

10. **Discuss which medications you would use to treat hypertension in the ED.**
    Patients with hypertensive emergencies should be treated in the ED. The medicines you choose will depend on the patient's current medications, the suspected cause of the hypertension, your comfort with particular medicines, and whether the child's life is in danger. For non–life-threatening situations, nifedipine and hydralazine are both safe, effective choices. They begin to work about 10 minutes after administration and last for several hours. For immediate results in lowering a *dangerously* high blood pressure, a nitroprusside infusion will give dose-related effects that will cease within minutes of stopping the infusion. Another alternative is diazoxide, which acts within 3–5 minutes to vasodilate resistance vessels and reduce blood pressure. It is given in frequent small boluses until the desired blood pressure is reached, and lasts between 4 and 12 hours. Labetalol has rapid effects on both α- and β-adrenergic receptors; is somewhat difficult to titrate; and is contraindicated in patients with asthma, heart block, heart failure, and pheochromocytoma. Nicardipine is an effective calcium-channel blocker that acts quickly to reduce peripheral vascular resistance. Because pediatric experience with nicardipine is quite limited, it should be used with extreme caution in children. Figure 17-1 summarizes the approach to the hypertensive pediatric patient in the ED.

    Linakis JG, Constantine E: Hypertension. In Fleisher GR, Ludwig S, Henretig FM (eds): Textbook of Pediatric Emergency Medicine, 5th ed. Philadelphia, Lippincott Williams & Wilkins, 2006, pp 351–358.

KEY POINTS: MEDICAL TREATMENT OF HYPERTENSION ✔

1. Non–life-threatening: hydralazine or nifedipine

2. Life-threatening: nitroprusside

11. **Name some other classes of medications that might be useful in the treatment of a hypertensive emergency.**
    Depending on the type of end-organ damage, treatment of complications associated with severely elevated blood pressures may be necessary. For example, lorazepam for seizures, diuretics for heart failure, and appropriate intubation medications should be available when treating a child with a hypertensive emergency.

12. **An adolescent boy is brought to the ED at 5:00 AM after a night out dancing. He is euphoric and diaphoretic, and has a dry mouth. He is tachycardic and hypertensive. You consider giving him a ß-blocker, but think better of it. Why?**
    The patient has probably ingested an amphetamine-related compound, such as 3,4-methylenedioxymethamphetamine (MDMA or "ecstasy"). The cardiovascular effects of phenylethylamines are due to both α- and β-adrenergic stimulation. A β-blockade would leave α-unopposed and result in vasospasm and paradoxical hypertension. Instead, consider using nitroprusside or nifedipine.

    Albertson TE, Van Hoozen BE, Allen RP: Amphetamines. In Haddad LM, Shannon MW, Winchester JF (eds): Clinical Management of Poisoning and Drug Overdose, 3rd ed. Philadelphia, W.B. Saunders, 1998, pp 560–568.

13. A school-aged child is in your ED being evaluated for an upper respiratory tract infection. You notice he is hypertensive on repeated measurements. He is an otherwise healthy child. When asked, he admits to some leg pain after playing soccer. He has a systolic ejection murmur. His radial pulses are bounding, but you have trouble feeling his dorsalis pedis pulses. What might be the cause of his hypertension?

Coarctation of the aorta can present after infancy, with hypertension as the presenting sign. Claudication symptoms and a heart murmur may or may not be present. It is important to feel for differential upper- and lower-extremity pulses in hypertensive patients of all ages, and to check four extremity blood pressures if there is any concern about coarctation of the aorta. In normal patients, lower-extremity blood pressures are higher than upper-extremity pressures by 10–20 mmHg. In patients with coarctation of the aorta, the blood pressure in the legs is lower than that in the arms.

CHAPTER 18

JAUNDICE

James M. Callahan, MD, FAAP, FACEP

1. What is jaundice?

Jaundice, or icterus, is a yellow or green-yellow discoloration of the skin, mucous membranes, sclera, and body fluids caused by increased levels of circulating bilirubin. Jaundice is usually noticeable at serum bilirubin levels of 5 mg/dL.

2. Where does bilirubin come from?

The major source of bilirubin is the breakdown of heme pigment released from senescent erythrocytes. Bilirubin is usually cleared from the circulation by the liver and, once conjugated, is excreted in bile. Hemolysis that exceeds the liver's capacity to conjugate bilirubin or processes that impair the excretion of bile cause increased bilirubin levels.

3. Is jaundice always pathologic?

Up to two-thirds of newborns develop visible jaundice at some point in the first few weeks of life. Most of these infants have "physiologic" or "breast milk jaundice" and not a pathologic process. Exclude potentially harmful causes before deciding that these benign conditions are present. In children over 3 months of age, jaundice is almost always associated with a pathologic process.

4. How do you begin the evaluation of a patient with jaundice?

First, determine whether the jaundice is due to conjugated or unconjugated hyperbilirubinemia. *Conjugated* hyperbilirubinemia is defined as jaundice in which the direct bilirubin level is >2 mg/dL or accounts for more than 20% of the total bilirubin. *Unconjugated* hyperbilirubinemia (high indirect bilirubin level) is usually due to hemolytic processes or defects in conjugation. Conjugated hyperbilirubinemia is pathologic at any age and is usually associated with cholestatic processes due to hepatic disease or anatomic obstruction to bile flow. Further workup and treatment are guided by the determination of the type of hyperbilirubinemia. The approach also varies depending on the age of the patient (newborn versus older infant/child).

5. What are the causes of unconjugated hyperbilirubinemia in a newborn?

- Placental dysfunction
- Diabetes in mother
- Swallowed maternal blood
- Cephalohematoma or extensive bruising
- Sepsis
- Upper gastrointestinal obstruction (pyloric stenosis, duodenal web, or atresia)
- Red cell defects
- ABO, Rh, and minor blood group incompatibility
- Crigler-Najjar syndrome (defect in bilirubin conjugation)
- Lucey-Driscoll syndrome (familial benign unconjugated hyperbilirubinemia)
- Breast milk jaundice
- Physiologic jaundice

6. **What is kernicterus?**

    Kernicterus (bilirubin encephalopathy) is the most worrisome complication of neonatal unconjugated hyperbilirubinemia. At high levels, unconjugated hyperbilirubin may cross a compromised blood–brain barrier and cause lethargy, hypotonia, poor feeding, fever, seizures, and signs of increased intracranial pressure. Untreated, unrecognized, and severe cases may lead to mental retardation, cerebral palsy, and sensorineural hearing loss.

7. **Which children are at risk for kernicterus?**

    Neonates with jaundice associated with a coexisting serious condition are most likely to develop kernicterus. Children with sepsis, hypoxia or hypercarbia, brisk hemolysis (e.g., that seen with Rh incompatibility), hypoglycemia, or prematurity are most at risk. In healthy, full-term infants, kernicterus is almost never seen at unconjugated bilirubin levels < 25 mg/dL. Premature infants and those with intercurrent illnesses may experience kernicterus at lower levels. Kernicterus, though rare, still occurs, even in otherwise healthy children born at or near term.

    Ip S, Chung M, Kulig J, et al: An evidence-based review of important issues concerning neonatal hyperbilirubinemia. Pediatrics 114:e130–153, 2004.

8. **What other laboratory tests are indicated in neonates with unconjugated hyperbilirubinemia?**

    Do a complete blood count (CBC) with differential and examination of the smear, a reticulocyte count, and direct Coombs test. Seek signs of hemolysis on the CBC. The differential may indicate an infectious process. Anemia or reticulocytosis suggest blood loss or ongoing hemolysis. If the Coombs test result is positive, isoimmunization has probably occurred (because of Rh, ABO, or minor blood group incompatibility). Determine maternal and neonatal blood types (this may be known at the hospital of delivery). Hemolysis in the absence of isoimmunization suggests a red cell defect in this age group, and a G6PD assay as well as fragility testing would be useful. Unconjugated hyperbilirubinemia in the absence of hemolysis may be seen with infections (although conjugated hyperbilirubinemia is more commonly seen), and a urinalysis, Gram stain, and culture may be helpful. If these additional studies are unremarkable, the child may have breast milk jaundice or exaggerated physiologic jaundice.

    Garcia FJ, Nager AL: Jaundice as an early diagnostic sign of urinary tract in infancy. Pediatrics 109:846–851, 2002.

9. **What is breast milk jaundice?**

    Breast-fed infants are about three times as likely as formula-fed babies to have high bilirubin levels in the first week of life. In the first few days of life, this is probably due to decreased fluid and caloric intake (until their mother's milk is fully in) and decreased passage of meconium stools. Later in the first week of life, it has been proposed that lipase and nonesterified long-chain fatty acids in breast milk inhibit hepatic excretion of bilirubin, while the β-glucuronidase in breast milk increases enterohepatic circulation of bilirubin.

10. **What is physiologic jaundice? What causes it?**

    Most infants (approximately two-thirds) develop visible jaundice at some point in the first week of life. The vast majority of these children have physiologic jaundice. Many factors contribute to this "normal" hyperbilirubinemia, including a large red blood cell mass, decreased survival of red blood cells, decreased hepatic uptake of bilirubin, decreased conjugation of bilirubin in the liver, and increased enterohepatic recirculation of bilirubin. Physiologic jaundice is a diagnosis of exclusion.

11. **What are some indicators that jaundice is *not* physiologic and therefore should prompt further investigation?**

    - Jaundice in first day of life
    - Bilirubin level that increases >5mg/dL per day

- Conjugated bilirubin level > 1.5 mg/dL or > 10% of total bilirubin
- Bilirubin level > 13 mg/dL
- Jaundice beyond the first week of life
- Jaundice with hepatosplenomegaly and anemia
- Jaundice in infants who are ill-appearing

12. When is treatment indicated in neonates with unconjugated hyperbilirubinemia?
Healthy, full-term infants should be treated with phototherapy when their bilirubin level is >15 mg/dL in the first 2 days of life, or >18 mg/dL after that time. Some infants are lethargic, and the mother may report that the infant is not nursing well. Supportive measures with IV saline are often needed. If despite phototherapy the bilirubin level increases to >20 mg/dL, or if at any time the bilirubin level is >25 mg/dL, consider an exchange transfusion. Full-term infants who are ill (those with hemolysis, sepsis, hypoglycemia, acidosis, or hypoxia) and preterm infants should have phototherapy and exchange transfusions instituted at lower serum bilirubin levels. Temporary interruption of breast feeding may lead to a rapid and sustained decrease in bilirubin levels in children with breast milk jaundice.

American Academy of Pediatrics Subcommittee on Hyperbilirubinemia: Management of hyperbilirubinemia in the newborn infant 35 or more weeks of gestation. Pediatrics 114:297–316, 2004.

KEY POINTS: TREATMENT OF UNCONJUGATED HYPERBILIRUBINEMIA IN NEONATES ✔

1. Treat healthy, full-term infants with a serum bilirubin level > 15 mg/dL in the first 2 days of life or > 18 mg/dL after 2 days of age with phototherapy.
2. Treat preterm infants and infants who are ill (e.g., sepsis or other infections or hemolytic disease) at lower levels.
3. Provide infants with good supportive care.
4. Consider exchange transfusion for infants who do not respond to phototherapy or whose bilirubin level is >25 mg/dL (lower in preterm and sick infants).

---

13. Is treatment for unconjugated hyperbilirubinemia an emergency?
Yes, when the level is very high. An outside laboratory or a visiting home nurse often does a bilirubin test, and the abnormal result prompts the emergency department (ED) visit. Thus, the report may be several hours old by the time the infant presents to the ED. The bilirubin level can sometimes rise quickly to a dangerous level. Avoid unnecessary delays in evaluation and management. When the unconjugated or indirect bilirubin approaches a dangerous level, as noted above, make arrangements for prompt phototherapy. This is sometimes difficult to do in an ED setting, and some believe jaundiced infants are better managed as direct admissions to the hospital, where phototherapy can begin quickly.

Maisels MJ: Jaundice in a newborn—how to head off an urgent situation. Contemp Pediatr 22:41–54, 2005.

14. List the causes of conjugated hyperbilirubinemia in neonates.
- Sepsis
- TORCH infections (toxoplasmosis, other agents, rubella, cytomegalovirus, and herpes simplex)

- Idiopathic neonatal hepatitis
- Alagille syndrome (arteriohepatic dysplasia)
- α-1–antitrypsin deficiency
- Inborn errors of metabolism (e.g., galactosemia, tyrosinosis)
- Urinary tract infections
- Hypopituitarism
- Postshock or postasphyxia biliary sludging
- Cholestasis associated with total parenteral nutrition
- Cystic fibrosis

15. **Which laboratory tests are helpful in determining the etiology of conjugated hyperbilirubinemia in neonates?**

    Obtain CBC with differential, urinalysis, Gram stain, blood culture, and urine cultures to look for signs of sepsis or urinary tract infection. A urinalysis with increased reducing substances other than glucose suggests galactosemia, especially in a patient with hypoglycemia. Viral and toxoplasmosis titers may help establish the diagnosis of a TORCH infection. Any vesicular lesions of the skin or mucous membranes can be tested with immunofluorescence assays and cultured for herpes simplex virus. Hepatic aminotransferase levels that are markedly elevated suggest hepatitis. Sweat chloride testing (to rule out cystic fibrosis), α-1–antitrypsin phenotyping, and repeated thyroid hormone testing may be needed in some infants. Albumin and clotting studies will reflect the synthetic capabilities of the liver. Closely monitor serum glucose because infants with hepatic disease may be at risk for hypoglycemia.

KEY POINTS: APPROACH TO NEONATAL JAUNDICE ✔

1. Determine whether the jaundice is due to conjugated or unconjugated hyperbilirubinemia.

2. Conjugated hyperbilirubinemia is always due to a pathologic process in this age group and requires further diagnostic workup (including imaging studies to rule out biliary obstruction) and hospital admission.

3. Most children with unconjugated hyperbilirubinemia will have physiologic or breast milk jaundice, but the history, physical examination, and diagnostic workup must be thorough enough to exclude pathologic causes.

16. **What imaging studies are helpful?**

    Abdominal ultrasonography can evaluate the extrahepatic biliary tract, looking for choledochal cysts as well as other signs of obstruction. A radionuclide scan (DISIDA [diisopropyl iminodiacetic acid] scan) that demonstrates excretion of radionuclide into the bowel excludes biliary atresia. Absence of excretion means that biliary atresia remains a possibility and further workup (hepatic biopsy) is warranted. Early diagnosis of biliary atresia is imperative to preserve hepatic function. The above studies are generally obtained on the inpatient unit rather than in the ED.

17. **What treatment is required for neonates with conjugated hyperbilirubinemia?**

    Since conjugated hyperbilirubinemia always indicates a pathologic process, admit all infants with conjugated hyperbilirubinemia and consult with a gastroenterologist. While diagnostic testing is in progress, supportive therapy, including IV fluids and dextrose; antibiotics or antivirals if indicated (e.g., acyclovir for neonatal herpes infection); vitamin K; and clotting factor replacement may be required. Specific therapy is based on the outcome of the diagnostic evaluation and does not usually occur in the ED. Phototherapy is not helpful unless there is also a markedly elevated indirect bilirubin level.

18. **In older infants and children, can anything else be mistaken for jaundice?**
    Yes. Children who eat large amounts of yellow, orange, or red vegetables can develop a yellow discoloration of their skin. Carotene-containing vegetables can produce carotodermia, while red vegetables (e.g., tomatoes) can produce lycopenemia. Unlike jaundice, this discoloration does not affect the sclerae, and the child should be thriving and appear well.

19. **What are the causes of unconjugated hyperbilirubinemia in older infants and children?**
    Unconjugated hyperbilirubinemia after the neonatal period is due to either hemolysis or decreases in the hepatic conjugation of bilirubin. Hemolysis is seen in children with hemoglobinopathies (e.g., sickle cell disease), red blood cell defects (e.g., G6PD deficiency after exposure to an oxidant stress or children with hereditary spherocytosis or elliptocytosis), autoimmune hemolytic anemia, or Wilson's disease. Unconjugated hyperbilirubinemia in the absence of hemolysis is seen in Gilbert disease or Crigler-Najjar syndrome.

20. **What is the diagnostic approach to children with unconjugated hyperbilirubinemia?**
    Obtain a CBC with examination of the smear, reticulocyte count, and direct Coombs test. In the absence of hemolysis, there is probably a defect in hepatic uptake of albumin-bound bilirubin, as seen with Gilbert disease and Crigler-Najjar syndrome. Seek a gastroenterology consultation.
    If hemolysis is present, findings of sickle cells, spherocytes, or elliptocytes on the CBC smear may be diagnostic. Hemoglobin electrophoresis or osmotic fragility tests may confirm these diagnoses. If the Coombs test result is positive, the patient is probably experiencing autoimmune-mediated hemolysis. Hemolysis without suggestive RBC morphology and a negative Coombs test result may be seen in patients with G6PD deficiency (usually after exposure to salicylates, sulfonamides, naphthalene, etc.) or Wilson's disease (usually accompanied by psychiatric problems and physical or laboratory signs of hepatic disease).

21. **List the causes of conjugated hyperbilirubinemia in older infants and children.**
    - Viral infections (hepatitis A, B, and C; cytomegalovirus; Epstein-Barr virus)
    - Bacterial infections (sepsis, pneumonia, hepatic abscess)
    - Toxins (*Amanita* mushrooms, carbon tetrachloride and solvents, drugs)
    - Total parenteral nutrition
    - Biliary tract disease (cholelithiasis, cholecystitis, choledochal cyst, cholangitis)
    - Inflammatory disease (autoimmune chronic active hepatitis, primary sclerosing cholangitis)
    - Genetic diseases (Wilson's disease, α-1–antitrypsin deficiency, cystic fibrosis)
    - Hemochromatosis

22. **What medications can cause cholestasis leading to conjugated hyperbilirubinemia?**
    Anticonvulsants (phenobarbital, phenytoin, carbamazepine, and valproic acid); antibiotics (estolate preparations of erythromycin, tetracycline, sulfonamides, isoniazid, rifampin, ketoconazole, and griseofulvin); corticosteroids; oral contraceptives; acetaminophen;

salicylates; chlorpromazine; cimetidine; and immunosuppressants (cyclosporine, azathioprine, and methotrexate) have all been associated with cholestasis.

23. **What is the diagnostic approach to children with conjugated hyperbilirubinemia?**
    Consider biliary tract disease in patients with a predisposition to hemolysis (e.g., sickle cell disease) and in patients with severe right-upper-quadrant pain and vomiting. Cholelithiasis and other entities causing biliary tract obstruction are more likely in these patients. Abdominal ultrasonography is indicated.

    If the onset of jaundice is acute, consider toxic and infectious causes. Hepatic aminotransferase levels are usually increased in these patients. Seek history of medication use or toxic exposures. A prodrome of nonspecific symptoms and fever are more often seen with infections. Obtain viral serologic tests.

    A less acute onset and jaundice associated with signs of chronic, systemic disease should prompt investigations of possible genetic or autoimmune causes (e.g., Pi typing to rule out α-1–antitrypsin deficiency or a sweat test to exclude cystic fibrosis).

24. **When does a child with jaundice require admission to the hospital?**
    Children with dehydration, hypoglycemia, signs or laboratory findings of active biliary tract disease, severe bacterial infections, ongoing hemolysis, or signs of systemic disease should be admitted to the hospital. Any patient with indications of hepatic failure must be admitted and monitored closely. When the underlying diagnosis is uncertain, admission for continued diagnostic investigations is often warranted.

    Children without signs of hepatic failure who are able to maintain oral hydration and have laboratory evidence of intact hepatic synthetic function (normal albumin, normal prothrombin time) often can be safely discharged. Many of these patients will have viral hepatitis. If discharged, serologic tests should have been obtained and close follow-up must be ensured.

KEY POINTS: HEPATIC FAILURE IN PATIENTS WITH JAUNDICE ✓

1. In all patients with jaundice, be sure that there are no signs of hepatic failure.

2. Abnormal albumin, prothrombin time, and ammonia levels indicate hepatic failure and warrant admission, close observation, and supportive care, including treatment with vitamin K (fresh frozen plasma if there is active hemorrhage).

25. **What are the complications of severe hepatic disease (i.e., hepatic failure)?**
    Abnormal bleeding and a decreased level of consciousness are the most worrisome complications of severe hepatic disease. Decreased hepatic synthetic function leads to decreased levels of coagulation proteins and prolonged bleeding. The prothrombin time is elevated. Spontaneous hemorrhages, including intracerebral hemorrhages, may occur. Increased plasma ammonia levels and cerebral edema are associated with hepatic encephalopathy.

26. **What treatment is required for an older infant or child with jaundice?**
    The main goal is to determine the etiology of the patient's jaundice so that specific therapies can be started. While the diagnostic evaluation is proceeding, supportive treatment may involve the administration of IV fluids, vitamin K, or clotting factors as necessary; lactulose and neomycin for the treatment of hepatic encephalopathy; and possible intubation and ventilatory support in patients with a decreased level of consciousness.

CHAPTER 19

LIMP

Susanne Kost, MD, and Bambi Taylor, MD

1. **What is the most common cause of a nontraumatic acute limp in children?**
   Transient synovitis, formerly known as toxic synovitis, is the most common nontraumatic cause of limp in children. Transient synovitis is believed to be a postinfectious reactive arthritis, occurring most commonly in the hip, but occasionally in the knee or ankle. It is usually preceded by a viral respiratory or gastrointestinal illness.

2. **What is the typical clinical presentation of transient synovitis?**
   The classic patient with transient synovitis is a white boy (male–female ratio, 2:1) between 3 and 10 years old (incidence peaks at age 6) with a 1- to 2-day history of limp, reporting unilateral pain in the hip, thigh, or knee. His past medical history will include viral symptoms within the past 1–2 weeks in over half the cases. He will have little or no fever and will appear well. His examination will be remarkable for a painful hip on passive range of motion, and he will prefer to hold the hip abducted and externally rotated. Transient synovitis typically causes a lesser degree of pain and limitation of motion than septic arthritis.

3. **Can laboratory tests or imaging studies distinguish transient synovitis from septic arthritis of the hip?**
   Not always. White blood cell (WBC) counts are normal (<15,000 cells/mL) in the majority of patients with both conditions. Erythrocyte sedimentation rate (ESR) is elevated (<20 mm/h) in most patients with septic arthritis and about half of patients with transient synovitis. Fluid in the joint space on plain radiographs and ultrasound is common in both conditions. The combination of fever, non–weight-bearing, ESR > 40 mm/h, and serum WBC count > 12,000 cells/mL has a high positive predictive value for the diagnosis of septic arthritis; however, this clinical decision rule lacks consistency across institutions. When the clinician is highly suspicious of a septic joint, the definitive test is arthrocentesis.

   Kocher MS, Mandiga R, Zurakowski D, et al: Validation of a clinical prediction rule for the differentiation between septic arthritis and transient synovitis of the hip in children. J Bone Joint Surg 86A:1629–1635, 2004.

   Luhmann SJ, Jones A, Schootman M, et al: Differentiation between septic arthritis and transient synovitis of the hip in children with clinical prediction algorithms. J Bone Joint Surg 86A:956–962, 2004.

4. **Which is a better test for diagnosis and monitoring of bone and joint infections in children: C-reactive protein (CRP) or ESR?**
   CRP is more likely to be elevated at the time of presentation, peaks more quickly, and returns to normal more quickly in patients with a treated infection (within 7 days as compared to 2–3 weeks for ESR). In comparison to ESR, CRP is a better independent predictor of disease. It is a better negative predictor than a positive predictor of disease. Indeed, if the CRP is <1.0 mg/dL, the probability that the patient does not have septic arthritis is 87%.

   Levine MJ, McGuire KJ, McGowan KL, et al: Assessment of test characteristics of C-reactive protein for septic arthritis in children. J Pediatr Orthop 23:373, 2003.

5. Describe the common presentations of the following hip pathologies of children: developmental dysplasia of the hip, Legg-Calvé-Perthes disease, and slipped capital femoral epiphysis (SCFE).
    See Figure 19-1A and B. See Table 19-1.

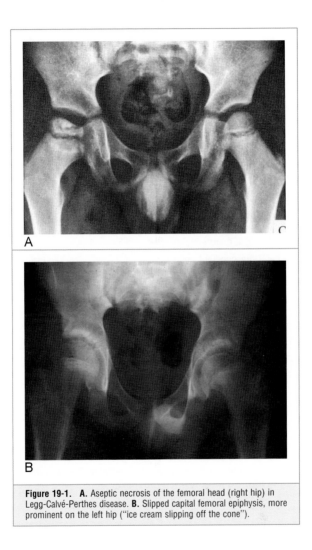

Figure 19-1. A. Aseptic necrosis of the femoral head (right hip) in Legg-Calvé-Perthes disease. **B.** Slipped capital femoral epiphysis, more prominent on the left hip ("ice cream slipping off the cone").

6. What is the likelihood of the above-hip pathologies affecting both hips?
    Developmental dysplasia of the hip is bilateral in about 20% of cases, Legg-Calvé-Perthes disease in about 20%, and SCFE in 25–80%.

TABLE 19-1.   COMMON PRESENTATIONS OF HIP DISORDERS IN CHILDREN

Variable	DDH	LCP	SCFE
Typical patient	Newborn-toddler, more common in breech positioning, F:M ratio, 9:1	Early school age, M:F ratio, 5:1	Early adolescence, obese, more common in African Americans, M:F ratio, 3:2
Pathology	Spectrum of acetabular dysplasia, hip subluxation, and hip dislocation; physiologic and mechanical factors	Avascular necrosis of the femoral head; cause unknown; associated with delayed bone age	Weakness of the femoral head physis; cause unknown (endocrinologic?)
Clinical presentation	Positive result on Barlow test in a newborn; painless limp with hip contracture in a toddler; "waddling" gait if bilateral	Hip or knee pain, insidious limp, with limitation of flexion and internal hip rotation	Can be acute (sudden severe hip or knee pain) or chronic (gradually worsening, mildly antalgic, externally rotated limp)
Best imaging test	Ultrasonography of the hips	MRI of the hips (early); plain radiography later	Plain radiographs (anteroposterior and frog lateral)

DDH = developmental dysplasia of the hip, LCP = Legg-Calvé-Perthes disease, MRI = magnetic resonance imaging, SCFE = slipped capital femoral epiphysis.
Adapted from Brancati DS, Jewell J, Omori M: Evaluation of the child with a limp. Pediatr Emerg Med Reports 9:25–36, 2004.

7. **Which endocrinopathy is associated with SCFE?**
SCFE has been associated most commonly with hypothyroidism, and more rarely with acromegaly, excess growth hormone, hypopituitarism, and hypogonadism. Hypothyroidism is especially important to consider if the SCFE occurs in a patient under the age of 10.

8. **What is the best test for distinguishing Legg-Calvé-Perthes disease (avascular necrosis of the hip) from transient synovitis?**
Tincture of time. The typical duration of transient synovitis is 1–2 weeks; Legg-Calvé-Perthes disease is chronic, with a typical course of 18–24 months. Radiographs of the hips may be helpful later in the course of the disease. Changes, best seen in the frog-leg lateral position, begin with a small, dense epiphysis and widening of the medial joint space due to cartilage hypertrophy. Later, a subchondral fracture (crescent sign) or fragmentation may be seen. As the disease progresses, reossification and healing result in deformity of the proximal femur.

9. **Describe the benefits of "special" medical imaging tests when compared to plain films in the evaluation of a limping child.**
   ■ Bone scanning is useful in detecting early Legg-Calvé-Perthes disease, osteomyelitis, stress fractures, and osteoid osteomas. Scintigraphy is 84–100% sensitive and 70–96% specific for osteomyelitis.

- Ultrasonography is helpful for diagnosing joint pathology, especially confirming the presence of an effusion and guiding aspiration.
- Computed tomography (CT) enables visualization of soft tissue as well as bone (tarsal coalition is one disorder that has been better characterized since the advent of CT).
- Magnetic resonance imaging (MRI) can distinguish living from dead bone, which is helpful in studying conditions such as Legg-Calvé-Perthes disease or avascular necrosis, and provides excellent images of the central nervous system, including spinal cord pathology. MRI also has a growing role in the evaluation of infectious processes (see Fig. 19-1).

EMedicine. Herman M: Pediatrics, limp:www.emedicine.com/emerg/topic387.htm

10. **A 4-year-old girl presents with limping secondary to knee pain, fever, and a rash. Match the following rashes to the underlying disease.**

1. Purpuric rash primarily on the lower extremities

2. Salmon-pink evanescent diffuse maculopapular rash

3. Multiple large oval papules, some with central clearing

4. Symmetric papulovesicular rash with target lesions

A. Lyme disease

B. Erythema multiforme

C. Henoch-Schönlein purpura

D. Systemic juvenile idiopathic arthritis

Answers:
1. C
2. D
3. A
4. B

11. **What is the best test for diagnosing juvenile idiopathic arthritis (previously called *juvenile rheumatoid arthritis [JIA]*) in a child with chronic limp and joint pains?**
No laboratory test is diagnostic of JIA. The diagnosis is made clinically on the basis of unexplained, persistent arthritis in one or more joints for more than 6 weeks in a child under the age of 16. The disease is subclassified into systemic arthritis, oligoarthritis ($\leq$4 joints), or polyarthritis (>4 joints), enthesitis-related arthritis, and psoriatic arthritis.

12. **In a limping child with lower-extremity joint pains who meets the clinical criteria for oligoarthritic JIA, which is a more useful serologic test: rheumatoid factor or antinuclear antibody?**
Tests for rheumatoid factor almost never have positive results in patients with oligoarthritic JIA, and will be positive in fewer than half of patients with polyarthritic JIA. On the other hand, antinuclear antibody test results are positive in about 50% of patients with oligoarthritic disease, and it serves as an important marker for increased risk of iridocyclitis.

13. **What is osteochondritis dissecans? What part of the body is most commonly involved?**
In osteochondritis dissecans, a portion of articular cartilage and underlying subchondral bone gradually separates from the surrounding tissue. The cause is unknown. The knee, specifically the lateral aspect of the medial femoral condyle or the posterior aspect of the lateral femoral condyle, is the most commonly involved site. The clinical picture is one of intermittent pain that worsens with activity; clicking or locking may also be described. Radiographs may show a delineated, dense fragment of subchondral bone separated from the rest of the affected bone by a radiolucent crescent line. The tunnel view should be added to

the anteroposterior/lateral films if this pathology is suspected. The talus, elbow, and rarely the patella can also be affected.

14. **A 2-year-old child presents with refusal to walk after jumping off of a toy box. He is tender over the distal portion of his left tibia. Plain radiographs of the lower leg are negative. What is the most likely explanation for his pain?**
The most likely reason for his pain is a nondisplaced spiral (single helix) fracture of the tibia, also known as a toddler's fracture. This type of fracture may be seen in children from the age of walking up to 5 or 6 years. Although radiographically subtle, the fracture is usually seen on the anteroposterior (AP) view, rarely on the lateral. Additional views, particularly the internal oblique, may demonstrate the fracture if it is not apparent on the AP view. Even with normal radiographs, if clinical suspicion is high, presumptive treatment with follow-up films in 10–14 days is indicated. In the absence of trauma, if occult osteomyelitis is included in the differential diagnosis, bone scintigraphy can distinguish between the two entities.

15. **An oblique view of the tibia in the previously described case reveals a subtle spiral fracture. The resident wants to consult child protective services given the spiral fracture with minimal trauma. What do you recommend?**
Unlike spiral fractures of other long bones, even with a history of minor or unobserved trauma, toddler's fractures in an ambulatory child generally do not indicate abuse, and a report is not warranted. Conversely, transverse or metaphyseal fractures of the tibia are concerning for the possibility of inflicted trauma.

KEY POINTS: LIMP ✔

1. Look beyond the leg, laboratory values, and x-rays when evaluating the limping child.
2. SCFE is an orthopedic emergency (and may present with referred knee or thigh pain).
3. Limp may be the acute presentation of a more chronic problem, abdominal or back pathology, or even systemic illness. Open physis? Think fracture before sprain.
4. Normal laboratory studies do not exclude the possibility of septic joint or osteomyelitis.

16. **What new radiologic technology may improve the accuracy of diagnosis of a toddler's fracture?**
Digital radiography. A recent study showed that the ability to manipulate images digitally increased the accuracy of both pediatric radiologists and pediatric emergency medicine physicians in the correct diagnosis of a toddler's fracture, potentially saving the patients with the initially missed diagnosis an average of $800 each on further studies.

Fahr MJ, James LP, Beck JR, et al: Digital radiography in the diagnosis of toddler's fracture. South Med J 96:234–239, 2003.

17. **A 10-year-old girl presents with limping and pain over the lateral malleolus after twisting her ankle while playing basketball. She is able to bear weight. Plain radiographs of the ankle are negative. Which is a more appropriate management plan: elastic bandage wrap, ankle-strengthening exercises, and family doctor follow-up; or plaster splint, rest, and orthopedic follow-up?**
The latter option is more appropriate in a child with open physes. The most likely site of pathology in this case is a Salter-Harris type I fracture of the distal fibula, not a sprained ligament.

18. **A 14-year-old boy presents with limp after twisting his ankle. In performing a complete ankle examination, you include palpation of the lateral aspect of the foot. Why?**
Because the peroneus brevis tendon inserts at the proximal end of the fifth metatarsal, a twisting mechanism may result in an avulsion fracture of this bone, known as a Jones fracture.

19. **A 16-year-old female competitive long-distance runner reports insidious but progressive lower-left leg pain and limp over several weeks. After a negative plain film and persistent symptoms, MRI is performed, leading to a diagnosis of stress fracture of the tibia. Why is a detailed nutritional and gynecologic history of particular importance in evaluating this patient?**
She may have a manifestation of the female athlete triad, which includes amenorrhea (or menstrual irregularity), disordered eating, and osteoporosis. Risk of stress fractures in these young female athletes is increased for multiple reasons. Concern for and treatment of this diagnosis would require a multidisciplinary approach that may not have been pursued without the appropriate history.

Brunet II M: Female athlete triad. Clin Sports Med 24:623–636, 2005.
Pepper M, Akuthota V, McCarty EC: The pathophysiology of stress fractures. Clin Sports Med 25:1–16, 2006.

20. **A school-aged or young adolescent child presents with a chronically painful flat foot. Radiographs in the past have not been helpful. What condition would you suspect, and what imaging study would be most useful in detecting it?**
Tarsal coalition. A coalition is a congenital fibrous band between the talus and calcaneus bones, or occasionally between the calcaneus and the navicular bone. Coronal CT images obtained through the posterior foot will show narrowing of the subtalar joint, sclerosis, or complete absence of joint space. "Beaking" of the talus on plain films is a clue to this condition.

21. **A 15-year-old boy has been waking up with leg pain for two weeks. Initially his symptoms were attributed to "growing pains" and were treated very successfully with aspirin, but his mother is concerned about the duration of the symptoms. What are you concerned about?**
Osteoid osteoma, the third most common benign bone tumor (after nonossifying fibroma and osteochondroma), usually presents with pain that is worse at night. The pain is dramatically relieved by salicylates, but not typically by nonsteroidal anti-inflammatory drugs. The femur or tibia is the site of 50% of these lesions, and a limp is present in more than half of those children. Classically, radiographs demonstrate a small radiolucent nidus that is smooth, regular, round or oval, and well defined, surrounded by dense sclerosis extending away from the margin with a fading edge. When the tumor is located in the proximal femur or posterior element of a vertebra, it can be particularly difficult to diagnose with plain films, in which case bone scintigraphy could support the diagnosis.

22. **Match the following potential causes of limp with the location of pain.**

1. Sever's disease	A. Patella
2. Sinding-Larsen-Johansson syndrome	B. Calcaneus
3. Osgood-Schlatter disease	C. Tibia
4. Kohler's disease	D. Metatarsal
5. Freiberg's disease	E. Navicular

These osteochondroses are a group of lesions that occur in the lower extremity in growing bones, with a clinical picture of localized pain and limp. They are presumed to be related to repetitive stress. Radiographic changes include irregularity, increase in density, or decrease in size of the affected bone.

Answers:

1. B. Sever's disease: Insertion of the Achilles tendon on the calcaneus
2. A. Sinding-Larsen-Johansson syndrome: The attachment of the patellar tendon to the inferior patellar pole
3. C. Osgood-Schlatter disease: Insertion of the patellar tendon on the proximal tibial tuberosity
4. E. Kohler's disease: The tarsal navicular
5. D. Freiberg's disease: Usually the second metatarsal head, less often in the third and fourth

23. **Which of the following conditions is not associated with limping: appendicitis, discitis, gingivitis, salpingitis, pharyngitis?**
The etiology of limp may be linked to pathology outside of the lower extremities. Inflammation in the lower abdomen or pelvis (appendicitis, salpingitis) may result in a "shuffling" gait (walking with increased hip flexion). Discitis is a subacute inflammation of the intervertebral discs, usually of the lumbar spine, which presents with progressive limp, and eventually refusal to sit or walk over a period of a few weeks. It is most common in children under the age of 5. Pharyngitis caused by group A streptococcal infection may in rare instances lead to arthralgia or arthritis in the recovery period. Though gingivitis has been implicated in problems ranging from miscarriage to heart disease, it doesn't cause limping.

24. **A 6-year-old boy presents with a 3-day history of diarrhea and a new limp. What pathogen would you expect to find in his stool?**
Salmonella enteritis and *Yersinia* infection may cause joint symptoms.

CHAPTER 20

NECK MASSES

Magdy W. Attia, MD, and Eileen C. Quintana, MD, MPH

1. **What are the important components of the medical history in a child with a neck mass?**
   The history should include:
   - Onset
   - Duration of symptoms
   - Rapidity of growth with changes in size or position
   - Pain
   - History of recent infection or trauma
   - Generalized symptoms, such as fever, weight loss, poor appetite, night sweats, or fatigue
   - History of exposure to communicable diseases
   - Travel history

2. **What are the important components of the physical examination of a child with a neck mass?**
   Observe the general appearance of the child. Screen rapidly for true emergencies. **Inspect** the patient in the neutral position to discern subtle swellings. **Palpate** the neck from behind with the patient seated or with the child on the mother's lap. Examine all masses to determine location, size, multiplicity, consistency, mobility, color, and temperature. Note other characteristics, such as tenderness, compressibility, and mobility with swallowing and with tongue protrusion. Pay special attention to associated systems, such as the chest, abdomen, and the lymphatic system, to ensure a complete examination.

   Davenport M: ABCs of general surgery in children. Lumps and swellings of the head and neck. BMJ 312:368–371, 1996.

3. **Which true emergencies are associated with neck masses?**
   True emergencies involving a neck mass include respiratory distress, vascular compromise, and cervical spinal cord compression.

4. **Describe an initial focused evaluation of a child with a neck mass.**
   Address the airway, breathing, and circulation (ABCs) appropriately. Immediately note the child's level of consciousness and work of breathing. Obtain a focused and pertinent history. Evaluate for stridor, hoarseness, dysphagia, and drooling. Perform a neurologic examination.

5. **List the etiologic classifications of neck lesions/masses.**
   See Table 20-1.

6. **List the anatomic classifications of a neck mass, with the most common masses in each category.**
   See Table 20-2.

7. **How is the workup of a child with a neck mass conducted?**
   Generally, a thorough history and physical examination lead to a provisional diagnosis and initiation of either therapy or watchful waiting. The lack of rapid resolution or the presence of

TABLE 20-1. ETIOLOGIC CLASSIFICATIONS OF NECK LESIONS AND MASSES

Congenital	Infectious	Neoplastic	Traumatic
Hemangiomas	Lymphadenitis	Lymphomas	Subcutaneous emphysema
Cystic hygromas	Soft tissue abscess	Thyroid neoplasms	Hematoma
Preauricular pits, sinuses, and cysts	Infected cysts (i.e., thyroglossal duct, branchial cleft, dermoid)	Teratoma	Cervical spine trauma
Thyroglossal duct cysts		Rhabdomyosarcoma	
Dermoid cysts		Neuroblastoma	
Cervical ribs			
Sternocleidomastoid mass			
Brachial cleft abnormalities			

TABLE 20-2. THE ANATOMIC CLASSIFICATIONS OF A NECK MASS, WITH THE MOST COMMON MASSES IN EACH CATEGORY

Midline	Lateral
Thyroglossal duct cyst	Lymphadenopathy
Lymphadenopathy	Cystic hygroma
Dermoid cyst	Branchial cleft cyst
Epidermoid cyst	Sternocleidomastoid mass
Sialadenitis	Parotitis
Ectopic thyroid tissue	Thyroid gland tumors

worrisome clinical findings should trigger the workup. The choice of the best study depends on the type of mass (solid versus cystic, benign versus malignant) and the location and extent of the lesion. Initially, ultrasonography is a good screening study; if further anatomic details are needed, contrast-enhanced computed tomography (CT) or magnetic resonance imaging (MRI) is then indicated. If signs of malignancy are present (i.e., a painless, firm, slow-growing mass in the upper third of the neck, or lymph nodes fixed to underlying tissue) or the lesion does not resolve, then surgical referral and biopsy are warranted. Consider a complete blood count, erythrocyte sedimentation rate (ESR), chest radiography, and purified protein derivative test in the early workup.

Gross E, Sichel JY: Congenital neck lesions. Surg Clin North Am 86:383–392, 2006.
Turkington JR, Paterson A, Sweeney LE, Thornbury GD: Neck masses in children. Br J Radiol 78:75–85, 2005.

8. **What are cystic hygromas? When do they usually appear?**
Cystic lymphatic malformations are believed to be formed from congenital failure of the lymphatic primordial buds to establish drainage into the venous system. This leads to the accumulation of lymphatic fluid and cyst formation, and a large neck mass. They are discrete, soft, mobile, and nontender masses most commonly found in the posterior triangle of the neck. They may be transilluminated, and usually grow in proportion to the child.
   Cystic hygromas usually appear by the end of the second year of life (80–90% of cases) during the period of active lymphatic growth; they appear less commonly at birth (10–20% of cases).

9. **What are the most common locations of cystic hygromas?**
They develop in close proximity to large veins and lymphatic ducts:
   - Lateral neck (75%)
   - Axilla (20%)
   - Mediastinum (5%)
   - Retroperitoneum (5%)
   - Pelvis (5%)
   - Groin (5%)

10. **What is the most serious complication of cystic hygroma? What are the treatments for this condition?**
Respiratory compromise, which is seen when a large mass extrinsically compresses the airway. The treatment is usually surgical excision of the lesion; however, sclerotherapy, repeated aspiration, incision and drainage, radiation therapy, and intralesional injections are other treatment modalities that have been recently recommended.
   Koch BL: Cystic malformations of the neck in children. Pediatr Radiol 35:463–477, 2005.

11. **What is the most common head and neck congenital lesion identified in infancy?**
Hemangioma. These are most noticeable after the first month of life. Females are affected three times more commonly than males.

12. **How do hemangiomas appear on physical examination?**
These masses are soft, mobile, and nontender and have a bluish or fiery red hue. Regressing hemangiomas are gray. The most common locations of hemangiomas are:
   - Face: Lips, nose, eyelids, and ears
   - Scalp

13. **Describe some of the complications of hemangiomas.**
   - Hemorrhage
   - Ulceration
   - Infection
   - Necrosis
   - Thrombocytopenia and coagulopathies: Due to platelet trapping; Kasabach-Merritt syndrome
   - Airway compromise—the child may have stridor
   - Congestive heart failure
   - Visual impairment in some periorbital hemangiomas

14. **What are the treatments for hemangiomas?**
The treatment of hemangiomas is observation; most hemangiomas resolve spontaneously. Other treatment modalities include compression garments, steroids, chemotherapy, radiation therapy, and laser therapy. Surgical excision is reserved for rapidly growing lesions compromising vision, hearing, or the airway.
   Connor SE, Flis C, Langdon JD: Vascular masses of the head and neck. Clin Radiol 60:856–868, 2005.

15. **What is the origin of branchial cleft cysts?**
These develop from malformations of the branchial arches (first through fourth). Most of them arise from the second branchial cleft.

16. **How does a child with a branchial cleft sinus or cyst present?**
Generally, the child presents with a single, painless, cystic lesion deep to the anterior, upper one third of the sternocleidomastoid. The lesion is movable, smooth, tense, and nontranslucent, and occasionally has clear mucoid drainage from a small opening along the anterior border of the sternocleidomastoid muscle. Sometimes the tract is palpable.

17. **What is the most common complication of branchial cysts?**
Infection is the most common complication, and usually responds well to antibiotics and warm soaks. The definitive treatment is complete excision of the cyst and tract.

KEY POINTS: BRANCHIAL CLEFT CYSTS ✓

Usually a single painless cystic lesion

May become infected, thus red and tender

Found on the lateral neck, at the anterior upper third of sternocleidomastoid

Treat infection with antibiotics and surgical excision

18. **Compare dermoid and epidermoid cysts.**
See Table 20-3.

TABLE 20-3.	COMPARISON BETWEEN DERMOID AND EPIDERMOID CYSTS	
Features	Dermoid Cyst	Epidermoid Cyst
Origins	Congenital	Traumatic or inflammatory
	Inclusion of embryonic epidermis within embryonal fusion planes	Follicular infundibulum of the hair shaft
Location	Head and neck: lateral to the supraorbital palpebral ridge, midline face, especially nasal bridge or neck	Head and neck: lateral to the supraorbital palpebral ridge, midline face, especially nasal bridge or neck
Contents	Lined by epithelium and contain sebaceous glands, hair follicles, connective tissues, and papillae	Lined by epithelium, does not contain cutaneous appendages but rather keratinized cellular debris
Treatment	Surgical excision	Surgical excision

19. **How is radiologic imaging helpful in management of a dermoid cyst?**
Either MRI or CT may be used to evaluate a dermoid cyst prior to complete excision because dermoid cysts occasionally have intracranial extension.

20. **What is a thyroglossal duct cyst?**
This common congenital neck mass is due to a ductal ectodermal remnant that never obliterated. Remember, a thyroglossal duct cyst has no external opening because the tract does not reach the skin surface.

21. **How does a thyroglossal duct cyst present clinically?**
This is commonly noted in a child 2–10 years old, as a midline cystic structure, immediately adjacent to the hyoid bone, at or about the level of the thyroid cartilage. Some may be sublingual (3%) or suprasternal (7%). A thyroglossal duct cyst is a soft, smooth, nontender (unless infected) mass that can be noted when the child swallows or with tongue protrusion.

22. **Describe the workup of a child with a thyroglossal duct cyst.**
The diagnosis is often made on clinical grounds alone. Ultrasonography, CT, or MRI may be indicated in unusual clinical presentations. CT provides better visualization of lesions adjacent to the hyoid bone. Radioisotope scanning is used for detecting ectopic thyroid tissue within thyroglossal ducts. Postoperative thyroid function tests may be indicated to determine whether thyroid replacement therapy is needed.

KEY POINTS: THYROGLOSSAL DUCT CYSTS ✓

Midline swelling, usually near the thyroid cartilage

Moves when the child swallows or protrudes the tongue

Diagnosis is made clinically

23. **Is cervical lymphadenopathy common in childhood?**
Yes, cervical lymphadenopathy is common during the middle years of childhood but is seldom pathologic. Children usually present with an indolent, nontender, dominant node in the jugular chain that persists over several months. Systemic symptoms are rare. Although laboratory studies are not usually indicated, most children have a normal blood count and normal chest radiograph, and if the node is biopsied it shows reactive hyperplasia.

24. **Is a supraclavicular lymph node more concerning?**
Supraclavicular adenopathy in any age group should be considered pathologic until proven otherwise. Swelling of these nodes may be the first sign of occult thoracic or abdominal pathology, such as malignancy (lymphoma). Initiate a workup including a chest x-ray and consultation with a surgeon immediately.

25. **What is the most common cause of acute cervical lymph node enlargement?**
Infection:
- **Viral:** Severe viral pharyngitis can cause cervical lymph nodes to enlarge acutely, usually bilaterally. Infections of the upper respiratory tract can lead to lymph node enlargement. Agents include influenza A and B viruses, Epstein-Barr virus, rhinovirus, enterovirus, and adenovirus.
- **Bacterial:** Acute suppurative cervical lymphadenitis secondary to bacterial infection is another cause for cervical lymph node enlargement. Common bacterial pathogens include *Staphylococcus aureus*, group A β-hemolytic streptococci, *Streptococcus pneumoniae* (rarely), anaerobes from mouth flora, and *Bartonella henselae* (cat scratch disease).

26. **How does a child with acute suppurative cervical lymphadenitis present?**
Acute suppurative cervical lymphadenitis often presents after upper respiratory tract infection, pharyngitis, or tonsillitis, with rapid, unilateral enlargement of multiple adjacent lymph nodes. Marked tenderness, warmth, and erythema are often seen. Fever, irritability, and toxic appearance are more common in the younger child. Spontaneous purulent drainage may occur if the infection is untreated.

27. **How is acute suppurative cervical lymphadenitis best treated?**
The initial treatment consists of oral antibiotics and warm soaks to the neck. If the child is young and toxic, admission is warranted for IV antibiotic therapy and close observation. If fluctuance is identified, drainage by surgical incision or ultrasonography-guided needle aspiration is recommended for both therapeutic and diagnostic purposes.

28. **What is the differential diagnosis of subacute or chronic cervical lymphadenitis?**
This condition refers to a child with a large, minimally tender, mildly inflamed, and nonfluctuant cervical lymph node that appears slowly over several weeks with no associated prodrome or systemic illness. Elements of the differential diagnosis are the following:
   - Reactive response to a nonspecific infection (bacterial or viral)
   - Cat scratch disease
   - Infectious mononucleosis
   - *Mycobacterium tuberculosis:* typical or atypical
   - Toxoplasmosis
   - Cytomegalovirus
   - HIV infection
   - Sarcoidosis
   - Histoplasmosis
   - Actinomycosis
   - Malignancy

29. **What is the workup for a child with subacute or chronic cervical lymphadenitis?**
   - Perform a complete history and physical examination.
   - Note the child's overall general appearance.
   - Assess the number, size, and location of lymph nodes.
   - Palpate for any organomegaly.
   - Consider laboratory studies, including complete blood count with differential, ESR, chest x-ray, and a purified protein derivative test.
   - Begin antibiotics to cover staphylococcus and streptococcus.
   - Arrange for the patient to be followed closely by his or her primary care physician.

30. **When should a child with chronic lymphadenopathy be referred for biopsy?**
Referral is warranted if the condition does not respond to treatment or a lymph node persists or enlarges despite adequate antibiotic therapy (of a few weeks duration).

31. **Describe the clinical picture of cat scratch disease.**
Children with cat scratch disease may give a history of a scratch by a kitten or only exposure to a kitten. Cat scratch disease is a common infectious disease in all ages groups. Kittens, in particular, are the reservoir for this disease. Although most children do not recall the scratch, a papule at the primary inoculation "scratch site" and regional lymphadenopathy usually develop in 1–2 weeks. A positive result on a cat scratch disease antigen skin test (not recommended) or demonstration of micro-organism (*B. henselae*) by silver stain from an aspirated node is confirmatory. If cat scratch disease is suspected, the best initial test is the *B. henselae* IgM enzyme immunoassay. If the test result is negative, consider polymerase chain reaction for *Bartonella* by using the biopsy tissue.

32. **What is the treatment for cat scratch disease?**
Cat scratch disease is self-limited; resolution is expected in 6–8 weeks. Initial treatment may consist of warm compresses and analgesics. Treatment should be reserved for those with systemic symptoms or severe local reaction. However, many physicians start antibiotics, such as trimethoprim-sulfamethoxazole or azithromycin, upon clinical suspicion.

KEY POINTS: CAT SCRATCH DISEASE ✓

1. Most patients do not recall a cat scratch.

2. Kittens are usually the reservoir.

3. Lymphadenopathy develops 1–2 weeks after the scratch.

4. *B. henselae* IgM enzyme immunoassay is the best test.

5. Treat with observation or trimethoprim-sulfamethoxazole or azithromycin.

33. **Describe the most common neoplasm of the neck based on age.**
Approximately 5% of all neoplastic lesions occur in the head and neck region.
- In preschool-age children: neuroblastoma, non-Hodgkin's lymphoma, rhabdomyosarcoma, and Hodgkin's lymphoma are most common.
- In school-age children: lymphomas, either non-Hodgkin's or Hodgkin's, thyroid carcinoma, and rhabdomyosarcoma are more likely.
- In adolescents: Hodgkin's lymphoma predominates.

34. **When should a neoplastic lesion in the neck be suspected? What evaluation is necessary?**
A neoplastic lesion presents as a painless, firm, fixed cervical mass. Other presenting signs and symptoms are unilateral ptosis, nasal obstruction, or otorrhea. A detailed history and physical examination, complete blood count with differential, renal and liver profiles, chest x-ray, or CT/MRI are sometimes obtained in the emergency department. An urgent referral to a surgeon or oncologist is recommended for further studies, such as a bone marrow examination.

CHAPTER 21

PEDIATRIC RASHES

Ronald I. Paul, MD

1. **Name five bioterrorism agents that may have skin manifestations.**
See Table 21-1.

> O'Brien KK, Higdon ML, Halverson JJ: Recognition and management of bioterrorism infections. Am Fam Physician 67:1927–1934, 2003.
> eMedicine: Dermatologic Aspects of Bioterrorism Agents. Available at www.emedicine.com/derm/topic905.htm#section~viral_agents.

TABLE 21-1. BIOTERRORISM AGENTS THAT MAY HAVE SKIN MANIFESTATIONS	
Agent	**Skin Findings**
Smallpox	Maculopapular rash on face, forearms, and mucous membranes that becomes vesicular/pustular within 48 hours
Anthrax	Painless pruritic papule on skin that develops into a painless, ulcerated black eschar within a few days
Tularemia	Painful maculopapular lesion that ulcerates; associated with papular painful inflamed regional lymph nodes
Plague	Acutely swollen lymph nodes called buboes
Viral hemorrhagic fever	Maculopapular rash on trunk followed by mucosal bleeding

2. **What are four skin findings associated with syphilis?**
See Table 21-2.

> Sexually Transmitted Disease. Syphilis pictures. Available at http://herpes-coldsores.com/std/syphilis_pictures.htm.

TABLE 21-2. SKIN FINDINGS ASSOCIATED WITH SYPHILIS	
Chancre	Painless ulcer of skin and mucous membranes at site of inoculation
Rash	Maculopapular rash of secondary syphilis frequently involving palms and soles
Condyloma lata	Cauliflower-appearing warts on penis, labia, or rectum
Gumma	Painless pink to dusky red nodules of various sizes that may necrose or ulcerate

3. **How does perianal streptococcal dermatitis manifest?**
Perianal streptococcal infection usually occurs in children between 6 months and 10 years of age. It presents as sharply circumscribed superficial perianal erythema. In some patients, the rash is bright red with a wet surface, while in others it is dry and pink. Fever is generally absent, and delays in culturing, diagnosing, and initiating therapy are common.

Herbst RA: Perineal streptococcal dermatitis/disease: Recognition and management. Am J Clin Dermatol 4:555–560, 2003.

4. **An atopic child with chronic eczema suddenly develops a painful, vesicular eruption in previous areas of eczema. What is the most likely diagnosis?**
Eczema herpeticum, caused by the herpes simplex virus, is a vesicular eruption concentrated in areas of eczematous skin. Children with eczema herpeticum often become seriously ill with high fever because the disease can be complicated by secondary bacterial infections and viremia, leading to multiple organ involvement with meningitis and encephalitis. Treatment with IV acyclovir is necessary for children with extensive or rapidly progressing involvement.

Wollenberg A, Wetzel S, Burgdorf HC, et al: Viral infections in atopic dermatitis: Pathogenic aspects and clinical management. J Allergy Clin Immunol 112:667–674, 2003.

5. **What are the clinical features of measles?**
Measles, caused by an RNA virus in the paramyxovirus family, has almost been eradicated in the United States. Epidemics were seen most recently in the early 1990s, and sporadic cases still occur among travelers and immigrants. It is an acute disease characterized by fever, cough, coryza, conjunctivitis, and an erythematous maculopapular rash that begins on the forehead and behind the ears, spreading to the face, neck, torso, and extremities. Koplik spots, bright red punctae with central white flecks on the buccal mucosa near the second molars, are seen early in the disease course and are pathognomonic for measles.

American Academy of Pediatrics: Measles. In Pickering LK, Baker CJ, Long SS, et al (eds): Red Book: 2006 Report of the Committee on Infection Diseases, 27th ed. Elk Grove Village IL, American Academy of Pediatrics, 2006, pp 441–452.

6. **Differentiate between erythema multiforme (EM), Stevens-Johnson syndrome (SJS), and toxic epidermal necrolysis (TEN).**
EM is now thought to be a separate process from SJS and TEN. It is an erythematous maculopapular rash, characterized by target lesions that may coalesce and develop annular or serpiginous borders. The course is brief and usually resolves within 2 weeks, although recurrences are common.

SJS and TEN are now thought to represent a spectrum of the same disease. They are severe drug eruptions, and TEN has a mortality rate of around 30%. SJS is characterized by febrile erosive stomatitis, ocular involvement, and a diffuse rash of discrete dark red macules, sometimes with a necrotic center. TEN involves extensive loss of epidermis due to necrosis that leaves the skin surface looking scalded.

Bachot N, Roujeau JC: Differential diagnosis of severe cutaneous drug eruptions. Am J Clin Dermatol 4:561–572, 2003.
Roujeau JC: Stevens-Johnson syndrome and toxic epidermal necrolysis are severity variants of the same disease which differs from erythema multiforme. J Dermatol 24:726–729, 1997.

7. **How does the rash of Rocky Mountain spotted fever change over time?**
The rash is initially erythematous and macular, but later becomes more papular and, frequently, petechial. The rash first appears on the wrists and ankles, spreading centrally within hours to involve the proximal extremities and trunk. The palms and soles are usually involved.

8. **A child helps his mother cut limes before going outside to play and then returns with inflamed hands that quickly develop hyperpigmentation. What is the name of the rash and the causative agent?**
This condition is a type of toxic photoreaction called phytophotodermatitis. It is caused when the skin comes into contact with psoralen, a photosensitizing agent, and then immediately with sunlight. Psoralens can be found in some perfumes, plants, grasses, fruits, and vegetables. Limes, celery, and parsley are examples of foods that contain psoralens.

   Bergeson PS, Weiss JC. Picture of the month. Phytophotodermatitis. Arch Pediatr Adolesc Med 154:201–202, 2000.

9. **What are the typical features of pityriasis rosea?**
Seen primarily in adolescents, pityriasis rosea begins in 80% of patients with a large, oval, solitary lesion known as a *herald patch* somewhere on the trunk or upper thighs. This is followed by an eruption of smaller, oval, and slightly raised papules that are pink to brown and have peripheral scales. The lesions are described as having a Christmas tree pattern on the back and involve mostly the truncal areas (Fig. 21-1), usually sparing the face, scalp, and distal extremities. Eruption is prolonged and can last 4–8 weeks.

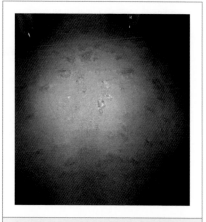

Figure 21-1. Large herald patch of pityriasis rosea near the axilla, with numerous secondary oval lesions that follow skin lines.

10. **List key features that help differentiate the purpuric rash of Henoch-Schönlein purpura from more serious infectious purpuric rashes, such as purpura fulminans.**
See Table 21-3.

TABLE 21-3. HENOCH–SCHÖNLEIN PURPURA VS. PURPURA FULMINANS	
Henoch-Schönlein Purpura	**Purpura Fulminans**
■ Distribution usually limited to extremities, appearing most commonly on lower legs, buttocks, and occasionally upper extremities. In infants, facial involvement may be seen.	■ Distribution of purpura is widespread.
	■ Associated features include lethargy, hypoventilation, and shock.
■ Associated features include arthralgias, abdominal pain, and hematuria.	■ Children appear ill, with varying degrees of toxicity.
■ Children appear well except for painful joints and abdominal pain.	■ Thrombocytopenia is present, and coagulation test results are abnormal.
■ Platelet count and results of other coagulation tests are normal.	

11. **What are five skin manifestations that may be seen in Kawasaki syndrome?**
    1. Dry, cracked erythematous lips
    2. Erythematous polymorphic truncal rash that may be scarlatiniform or morbilliform
    3. Red, swollen hands and feet
    4. Peeling around nails and fingers
    5. Desquamating perineal rash

    Yamamoto LG: Kawasaki disease. Pediatr Emerg Care 19:422–424, 2003.

12. **What are some skin findings that may be mistaken for child abuse?**
    See Table 21-4.

    Mudd SS, Findlay JS: The cutaneous manifestations and common mimickers of physical child abuse.
    J Pediatr Health Care 18:123–129, 2004.

TABLE 21-4. SKIN FINDINGS THAT MAY BE MISTAKEN FOR CHILD ABUSE	
Lichens sclerosis	Indurated and shiny atrophic plaques found in vulvar and perianal areas
Mongolian spots	Hyperpigmented areas commonly seen over sacrum
Coining	Asian folk remedy of rubbing coin or spoon on back and trunk to rid body of "bad winds"
Accidental ecchymoses	Normal childhood bruises found over bony prominences, such as shins, knees, forearms, elbows, foreheads, and chins

13. **How does scabies manifest in infants?**
    Scabies in infants and young toddlers may be more eczematous and less typical than in adults. In addition to the characteristic burrows on the hands and feet, young infants may present with diffuse dermatitis on the trunk, face, neck, and scalp. The axilla, diaper area, palms, and soles are frequent sites of distribution. Since infants are not able to scratch the intensely pruritic lesions, they may become irritable and sleep poorly.

    Peterson CM, Eichenfield LF: Scabies. Pediatr Ann 25:97–100, 1996.

KEY POINTS: SCABIES IN INFANCY ✓

1. Infant is often irritable.

2. Lesions may appear more eczematous than in older children.

3. Characteristic burrows are seen on the hands and feet.

4. Axillae, groin, palms, and soles are often involved.

5. Dermatitis may be present on trunk, face, neck, and scalp.

14. **What are the cutaneous manifestations of disseminated gonococcemia?**

    The skin lesions associated with disseminated gonococcemia are often located on the extremities and may overlie the involved joints. Small macules appear initially and progress to papules. These tender lesions may develop a small vesicle and then a gray umbilicated center. A diagnosis can be established with a Gram stain or culture of the skin lesion.

15. **Is poison ivy contagious?**

    A common misconception among families and school officials is that the rash of poison ivy is contagious. This belief occurs because of the vesicles and weepy bullae that develop in some individuals. Once the skin, clothes, and fingernails are cleaned of the sap from this treacherous plant, the rash will not spread beyond the areas already exposed. Contributing to this misconception is the fact that areas with minimal contamination can develop 5–10 days after the heavily contaminated areas appear. The bottom line is the child should go back to school!

16. **Should topical agents be used to treat poison ivy?**

    Unfortunately, good studies have shown that topical hydrocortisone and antihistamines have no more effect on poison ivy than do bland, soothing lotions, such as calamine. Supportive care includes baths, cool compresses, and calamine lotion for mild cases. Systemic oral steroids almost always bring the acute dermatitis under control and are appropriate for moderate to severe cases. Oral antihistamines may also be helpful.

17. **What is a pyogenic granuloma?**

    A pyogenic granuloma is a rapidly growing vascular proliferation that develops at the site of an obvious or unnoticed trauma (Fig. 21-2). Despite its name, this lesion is not infectious. Patients usually present to the emergency department with spontaneous bleeding, or after local minor trauma. Acute bleeding can be controlled with prolonged pressure or silver nitrate sticks. Ultimately, treatment consists of electrodesiccation and curettage.

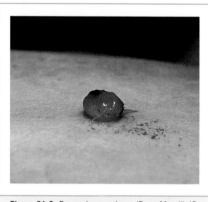

Figure 21-2. Pyogenic granuloma.(From Morelli JG: Vascular neoplasms. In Fitzpatrick JE, Morelli JG [eds]: Dermatology Secrets in Color, 3rd ed. Philadelphia, Mosby, 2007, Fig. 42-7, p. 351.)

18. **How do the following two newborn rashes differ: transient pustular melanosis and erythema toxicum neonatorum?**

    Transient pustular melanosis is a benign newborn rash consisting of superficial vesiculopustular lesions that are present at birth. The lesions rupture easily with the first bath, leaving a collarette of fine, white scales and brown, hyperpigmented macules. Lesions fade within several weeks to months and are asymptomatic. Erythema toxicum neonatorum is a benign, self-limited eruption that usually appears between the first 3–4 days of life and sometimes as late as the 10th. The lesions begin as blotchy erythema that develops into pale yellow or white papules or pustules. Individual lesions last an average of 2 days, and cytologic examination, if needed to differentiate from other rashes, reveals clusters of eosinophils and neutrophils and an absence of bacteria.

Wagner A: Distinguishing vesicular and pustular disorders in the neonate. Curr Opin Pediatr 9:396–405, 1997.

19. **What is the appropriate treatment for a herpetic whitlow?**
    Herpetic whitlow is a localized herpes simplex infection consisting of singular or multiple vesicular lesions on the distal fingers or toes. The first episode may accompany herpetic gingivostomatitis. Treatment consists of local care for mild cases, while those with severe lesions may benefit from oral acyclovir. Avoid incision and drainage, which can prolong recovery and worsen the condition.

    Feder HM Jr, Long SS: Herpetic whitlow. Epidemiology, clinical characteristics, diagnosis and treatment. Am J Dis Child 137:861–863, 1983.

    e-Medicine: Herpetic whitlow: www.emedicine.com/emerg/topic754.htm

20. **What condition is associated with recurrent pustules on the feet of infants?**
    Infantile acropustulosis consists of 7- to 10-day episodes of pruritic pustules and papulovesicles on the hands and feet of infants. The age of onset is usually between 2 and 10 months, and the condition resolves by 2 to 3 years of age. Treatment with mid- to high-potency topical corticosteroids is effective.

    Dromy R, Raz A, Metzker A: Infantile acropustulosis. Pediatr Dermatol 8:284–287, 1991.

21. **A diaper rash consisting of diffuse papular, scaly, and fissuring eruptions does not respond to anti-inflammatory or antifungal agents. What is a potential serious cause?**
    This may be one of the skin manifestations of histiocytosis X, which is a disorder characterized by proliferation of Langerhans histiocytes in the skin and other organ systems. Consider a biopsy to confirm the diagnosis or absence of histiocytosis X when a difficult-to-treat diaper rash does not improve with standard therapy.

22. **What is Nikolsky's sign?**
    It is a vulnerability of the skin such that apparently normal epidermis can be rubbed off with slight trauma. It may be seen in epidermal blistering diseases, such as scalded skin syndrome and pemphigus vulgaris.

23. **How long do patients with erythema infectiosum (fifth disease) need isolation?**
    This infection is caused by parvovirus B19. For most patients with typical presentation of a "slapped cheek" and a lacelike rash on arms and legs, no isolation is needed at the time of diagnosis. By the time the rash becomes clinically obvious, these patients are unlikely to be infectious. The rash usually resolves within 3–5 days of onset.

    American Academy of Pediatrics. Parvovirus B19. In: Pickering LK, Baker CJ, Long SS, et al (eds). Red Book: 2006 Report of the Committee on Infectious Diseases, 27th ed. Elk Grove Village, IL, American Academy of Pediatrics, 2006, pp 484–487.

24. **What are the similarities and differences between granuloma annulare and tinea corporis?**
    Both are characterized by circular plaques consisting of a ring of papules around a depressed center. Granuloma annulare is a ring of *nonscaling*, skin-colored or red papules that are most commonly seen on the dorsal surface of the hands and feet. They are asymptomatic and resolve spontaneously after a few months to a year. Tinea corporis is a common, superficial fungal infection consisting of lesions with *scaly* inflammatory borders that appear anywhere on the body. There may be multiple lesions.

25. **What causes roseola? What are the usual features?**
    Roseola infantum (exanthem subitum) is an acute febrile illness that primarily affects young children between the ages of 6 and 36 months. Most cases are now thought to be caused

by human herpesvirus 6 and human herpesvirus 7. After 3 or more days of high fever, the patient abruptly defervesces, and an erythematous, morbilliform rash with discrete rose-pink macules appears. The rash begins first on the trunk and then spreads rapidly to the extremities, neck, and face. By this time, the rash is bothering the parents more than the patient.

American Academy of Pediatrics: Human herpes virus 6 (including roseola) and 7. In: Pickering LK, Baker CJ, Long SS, et al (eds). Red Book: 2006 Report of the Committee on Infectious Diseases, 27th ed. Elk Grove Village, IL, American Academy of Pediatrics, 2006, pp 441–452.

26. **What are the usual findings in Gianotti-Crosti syndrome?**
This self-limiting condition is characterized by symmetric erythematous papules that are primarily found on the extremities but often involve the cheeks and buttocks. Also known as papular acrodermatitis, the rash may last 2–8 weeks, and may become recurrent. Although first identified in Europe in children with hepatitis B, it is seen in the United States primarily in association with other viruses, including Epstein-Barr virus, cytomegalovirus, and coxsackie virus A16.

Weston WL, Lane AJ, Morelli JG: Viral infections. Color Textbook of Pediatric Dermatology, 2nd ed. St. Louis, Mosby, 1996, pp 97–130.

27. **A toddler presents with several small, round, erythematous, and inflamed macules in a straight column down the middle of his chest and abdomen. What is the most likely etiology?**
One of the most common causes of contact dermatitis in children is allergy to nickel. Infants present with skin lesions corresponding to the location of snaps on their pajamas or other garments. Avoidance of the offending object by an undershirt or nonsnap clothes, and application of a mild topical steroid, will solve the problem.

28. **Which organisms cause bullous and nonbullous impetigo?**
- Bullous impetigo involves vesicles and is usually caused by toxin-producing strains of *Staphylococcus aureus*.
- Nonbullous impetigo consists of small vesicles or pustules that rupture and then develop honey-colored, crusting lesions. It is mostly caused by group A streptococcus.

29. **What are the dermal manifestations of zinc deficiency?**
Dietary deficiency or inadequate absorption of zinc leads to acrodermatitis enteropathica. It is characterized by erythema, crusting, and fissuring of the perioral skin and cheeks. The diaper area may develop a diffusely erythematous rash with a sharply marginated border on the abdomen. Psoriasiform lesions may develop around the anus and on the buttocks and feet. Treatment with dietary zinc supplementation provides dramatic resolution of all dermal and systemic symptoms.

Perafan-Riveros C, Franca LF, Alves AC, et al: Acrodermatitis enteropathica: Case report and review of the literature. Pediatr Dermatol 19:426–431, 2002.

30. **Contrast and compare smallpox with chickenpox.**
See Table 21-5.

Koenig KL, Boatright C: Derm and doom: The common rashes of chemical and biological terrorism. Critic Decis Emerg Med 17:1–7, 2003.

TABLE 21-5. SMALLPOX VS. CHICKENPOX

Characteristic	Smallpox	Chickenpox
History	Febrile with systematic symptoms for several days prior to rash	Mild fever with minimal symptoms for 1–2 days prior to rash
Severity	Very ill from start	Not severely ill unless complications develop
Lesions	Hard circumscribed pustules	Vesicles on an erythematous base
Distribution	Face and distal extremities, involving palms and soles	Face and trunk, with no involvement of palms or soles
Lesion development	Slow, with all lesions at same stage of development	Rapid, with lesions at different stages

KEY POINTS: BIOTERRORISM AGENTS WITH DERMATOLOGIC FINDINGS ✓

1. Smallpox

2. Anthrax

3. Tularemia

4. Plague

5. Hemorrhagic viral fevers

31. **Describe and name the skin finding associated with Lyme disease.**

    Erythema chronicum migrans (ECM) develops 4–20 days after a tick bite in 60–70% of patients who have contracted Lyme disease (Fig 21-3). The first sign may be a red papule at the site of the tick bite. An annular ring with a flat border slowly grows while clearing develops in the center. Some patients develop multiple secondary annular rings, days after the primary lesion appears.

    Weston WL, Lane AJ, Morelli JG: Bacterial infections (pyodermas) and spirochetal infections of the skin. Color Textbook of Pediatric Dermatology, 2nd ed. St. Louis, Mosby, 1996, pp 50–69.

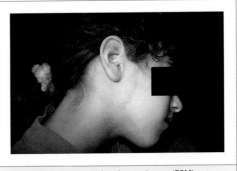

Figure 21-3. Erythema chronicum migrans (ECM) developed after patient contracted Lyme disease.

32. **What is the typical skin finding following a bite from the brown recluse spider?**
    Loxosceles recluse spiders are often found in old buildings and produce a number of toxins in their venom. A hemorrhagic painful blister may initially appear. Over several days a dry gangrenous eschar will develop.

    Swanson DL, Vetter RS: Bites of brown recluse spiders and suspected necrotic arachnidism. N Engl J Med 352:700–707, 2005.

    Vetter R: Identifying and misidentifying the brown recluse spider. Dermatology Online Journal. Available at http://dermatology.cdlib.org/DOJvol5num2/special/recluse.html.

33. **What does the term *morbilliform* mean?**
    Morbilliform literally means "measles-like." Eruptions that are generalized, discrete red to pink macules are referred to as being morbilliform. These include rashes in association with several viral infections, including rubella, enterovirus, adenovirus, roseola, parvovirus, and Epstein-Barr virus.

34. **A 7-year-old child presents with five café-au-lait spots that are 2–4 mm in diameter. Does this child have neurofibromatosis?**
    The diagnostic criteria for neurofibromatosis type 1 include six or more café-au-lait spots greater than 5 mm in diameter in prepubertal children and greater than 15 mm in older children.

    Listernick R, Charrow J: Neurofibromatosis-1 in childhood. Adv Dermatol 20:75–115, 2004.

35. **What common skin features are present in children with scarlet fever?**
    - Flushed face with perioral pallor
    - Diffuse, blanching, erythematous rash that has a sandpaper consistency, with accentuation in the axillae and groin
    - Pastia's lines in the flexural surface of the elbows.
    - Desquamation as the acute phase of illness resolves

36. **How can you distinguish irritant contact diaper rash from candidal diaper dermatitis?**
    - Generic diaper rash is caused by contact of the skin with urine or feces in the moist, closed environment created by a diaper. Red papules or patches appear on the prominent surfaces of the diapered areas, especially in areas of overlapping skin folds and skin directly adjacent to the plastic parts of the diaper or elastic.
    - Candidal diaper dermatitis comes from the gut flora, *Candida albicans*. Features of this infectious rash consist of perianal erythema and maceration spreading to produce moist, bright red, confluent plaques in the diaper area, especially in the intertriginous folds. Satellite lesions are common.

CHAPTER 22

RED EYE

Kathy Palmer, MD

1. **What are the dangerous associated features of a "red eye"?**
   - Severe ocular pain
   - Photophobia
   - Persistent blurred vision
   - Proptosis
   - Irregular corneal light reflection
   - Worsening signs after 3 days of pharmacologic treatment
   - Corneal epithelial defect or opacity
   - Pupil unreactive to direct light
   - Ciliary flush
   - Reduced ocular movements
   - Compromised host: neonate, immunosuppressed patient, and contact lens wearer

2. **What is included in the differential diagnosis for a red eye in a pediatric patient?**
   - Abnormalities of the lids or lashes
   - Conjunctivitis (allergic, bacterial, viral, or chemical)
   - Periorbital or orbital cellulitis
   - Corneal abrasion (trauma)
   - Chemical burn
   - Subconjunctival hemorrhage
   - Contact lens–related problems
   - Ocular inflammation from systemic disease (uveitis, episcleritis)
   - Neoplasms
   - Foreign body

   Levin AV: Eye—red. In Fleisher GR, Ludwig S, Henretig FM (eds): Textbook of Pediatric Emergency Medicine, 5th ed. Philadelphia, Lippincott Williams & Wilkins, 2006, pp 267–271.

3. **What systemic conditions are associated with red eyes?**
   Collagen vascular disorders, juvenile rheumatoid arthritis, infectious diseases (varicella, measles, mumps, otitis media), Kawasaki disease, inflammatory bowel disease, cystic fibrosis, Stevens-Johnson syndrome.

   Levin AV: Eye—Red. In Fleisher GR, Ludwig S, Henretig FM (eds): Textbook of Pediatric Emergency Medicine, 5th ed. Philadelphia, Lippincott Williams & Wilkins, 2006, pp 267–271.

4. **Describe the characteristics of bacterial conjunctivitis.**
   Mucopurulent discharge that involves one eye and usually spreads to the second eye associated with injection of the bulbar conjunctiva. *Haemophilus influenzae*, *Streptococcus pneumoniae*, and staphylococci are the most common pathogens. Treat with topical antibiotic drops every 4–6 hours or ointment three times daily for younger children. Trimethoprim sulfate and polymyxin B sulfate (Polytrim) is a good choice because it provides broad-spectrum coverage and is well tolerated (minimal stinging with application).

   Wright KW: Pediatric "pink eye." In Pediatric Ophthalmology for Pediatricians. Baltimore, Williams & Wilkins, 1999, pp 165–193.

5. **What is epidemic keratoconjunctivitis (EKC)?**

   EKC is a specific type of viral conjunctivitis caused by adenovirus types 8, 19, and 37. It usually affects older children and adolescents. Physical examination findings include severe bilateral conjunctivitis with conjunctival hyperemia, watery discharge, eyelid swelling, petechial conjunctival hemorrhages, pseudomembrane along the conjunctiva, and preauricular adenopathy. One third of patients develop corneal inflammation (keratitis) associated with severe photophobia. EKC is extremely contagious, and patients may need to be isolated for as long as 2 weeks. Because of the risk for keratitis, refer all patients with EKC to an ophthalmologist.

   Wright KW: Pediatric "pink eye." In Pediatric Ophthalmology for Pediatricians. Baltimore, Williams & Wilkins, 1999, pp 165–193.

6. **How do a stye and a chalazion differ?**

   A **stye** or external hordeolum is an inflammation of the ciliary follicles or accessory glands of the anterior lid margin. A **chalazion** or internal hordeolum is an inflammation of the meibomian glands and involves deeper eyelid tissues than does a stye. Both conditions cause painful focal tenderness of an eyelid and are treated with warm compresses. If they fail to resolve after several months, refer the patient to an ophthalmologist.

   Levin AV: Ophthalmic emergencies. In Fleisher GR, Ludwig S, Henretig FM (eds): Textbook of Pediatric Emergency Medicine, 5th ed. Philadelphia, Lippincott Williams & Wilkins, 2006, pp 1653–1661.

7. **What is blepharitis? How is it treated?**

   Blepharitis is an inflammation of the eyelids. **Anterior** blepharitis affects the skin, cilia follicles, or accessory glands of the eyelids. **Posterior** blepharitis is an infection of the meibomian sebaceous glands. Clinical findings include swollen, erythematous lid margins with crusting, a gritty or burning sensation of the eyes, and mild conjunctival injection. Scrubbing the eyelid margins with diluted baby shampoo and applying bacitracin or erythromycin ointment are done to treat anterior disease. Posterior disease is treated with eyelid hygiene and oral antibiotics.

   Wright KW: Pediatric "pink eye." In Pediatric Ophthalmology for Pediatricians. Baltimore, Williams & Wilkins, 1999, pp 165–193.

8. **What is the most common cause of conjunctivitis in the newborn period?**

   Red, watery eyes in an infant who is only a few hours old is almost always a chemical conjunctivitis secondary to the use of topical prophylaxis (1% silver nitrate, 1% tetracycline ointment, or 0.5% erythromycin ointment) for ophthalmia neonatorum. True neonatal conjunctivitis rarely presents prior to 48 hours of age. The infectious organisms associated with neonatal conjunctivitis include *Neisseria gonorrhoeae* (onset, 2–4 days of age), staphylococci or streptococci (onset, 4–7 days of age), chlamydia (onset, 4–10 days of age), haemophilus (onset, 5–10 days of age), and herpes simplex virus type II (onset, 6 days–2 weeks).

   Wright KW: Pediatric "pink eye." In Pediatric Ophthalmology for Pediatricians. Baltimore, Williams & Wilkins, 1999, pp 165–193.

9. **List the differential diagnosis of red, teary eyes in a newborn.**
   - Neonatal conjunctivitis
   - Congenital glaucoma
   - Dacryocystitis
   - Endophthalmitis

   Wright KW: Pediatric "pink eye." In Pediatric Ophthalmology for Pediatricians. Baltimore, Williams & Wilkins, 1999, pp 165–193.

10. **What is endophthalmitis?**

Endophthalmitis is a devastating intraocular infection that can be either bacterial or fungal in origin. It can be caused by traumatic intraocular introduction of organisms or result from hematogenous spread. The prognosis is poor, even with high-dose antimicrobial therapy and vitrectomy to remove the infection.

Wright KW: Ocular inflammation and uveitis. In Pediatric Ophthalmology for Pediatricians. Baltimore, Williams & Wilkins, 1999, pp 195–211.

11. **Describe the clinical features of gonococcal conjunctivitis.**

This condition usually occurs in infants at least 48 hours old, and even earlier in infants born to mothers with prolonged rupture of membranes. Physical examination findings include unilateral or bilateral, purulent conjunctivitis with copious discharge and lid edema. The onset of the disease is often hyperacute. *N. gonorrhoeae* infection can cause corneal ulceration or perforation. Gram stain of conjunctival scrapings reveals gram-negative intracellular diplococci. Treat with topical erythromycin and IV cefotaxime. Ophthalmology consultation is required. If left untreated, gonococcal conjunctivitis can lead to septicemia and meningitis.

Wright KW: Pediatric "pink eye." In Pediatric Ophthalmology for Pediatricians. Baltimore, Williams & Wilkins, 1999, pp 165–193.

12. **Which groups of patients are most often diagnosed with gonococcal conjunctivitis?**

Neonates and sexually active adolescents.

13. **When are systemic antibiotics indicated in neonatal conjunctivitis?**

Systemic antibiotics are used in chlamydial and gonococcal disease to control the risk of systemic involvement.

14. **What is dacryocystitis?**

This is an inflammation of the lacrimal sac in patients with an obstructed nasolacrimal passage. It causes erythema and swelling of the medial lower lid, excessive tearing, and mucopurulent discharge. It is found commonly in infants with a blocked nasolacrimal duct or in older patients with chronic sinusitis or facial trauma. It is treated with oral and topical antibiotics.

Wright KW: Pediatric "pink eye." In Pediatric Ophthalmology for Pediatricians. Baltimore, Williams & Wilkins, 1999, pp 165–193.

15. **What are the classic signs of orbital cellulitis?**

Orbital cellulitis is an infection of the tissues posterior to the orbital septum. Erythema and edema of the eyelids, decreased eye movement, proptosis, decreased vision, and papilledema are the classic signs of this infection.

16. **List the causes of orbital cellulitis.**

Most common is sinusitis invading the orbit. It can also occur as sequelae of an orbital fracture, a skin or lacrimal sac infection, hematogenous spread of organisms seeding the orbit, or even an ascending dental infection.

Greenberg MF: The red eye in childhood. Pediatr Clin North Am 50:105–124, 2003.

17. **What other noninfectious conditions can mimic the physical findings of orbital cellulitis?**

- Orbital tumors (rhabdomyosarcomas, lymphangiomas, neuroblastomas)
- Orbital pseudotumor (an autoimmune process)

- Graves' disease
- Ruptured dermoid cyst

18. **Do all patients with orbital cellulitis require hospital admission?**
Yes, orbital cellulitis is a potentially vision- or life-threatening condition.

   Greenberg MF: The red eye in childhood. Pediatr Clin North Am 50:105–124, 2003.

19. **What are the potential complications of orbital cellulitis?**
Vision loss, meningitis, cavernous sinus thrombosis, brain abscess, and death.

20. **What are the causative organisms for orbital cellulitis?**
In younger children (< 8 years old), infections are most often caused by a single organism, either staphylococcus or streptococcus. In older children, infections can include multiple bacterial strains and even anaerobes. Mucormycosis and aspergillosis can be seen in immunocompromised hosts. These guidelines should be used to select initial empiric antimicrobial coverage.

   Greenberg MF: The red eye in childhood. Pediatr Clin North Am 50:105–124, 2003.

21. **How is orbital cellulitis treated?**
With IV antibiotics, many cases can be managed medically but others require surgical drainage. Computed tomography should be performed to look for evidence of abscess formation and sinusitis, which are most often the inciting process. Urgent ophthalmologic consultation is indicated once the diagnosis of orbital cellulitis is considered. If operative drainage is necessary, an otolaryngologist often consults in conjunction with the ophthalmologist to drain the sinuses.

   Greenberg MF: The red eye in childhood. Pediatr Clin North Am 50:105–124, 2003.

22. **Which cases of orbital cellulitis are more likely to require surgical intervention and drainage?**
Infections in older children and adults and those resulting from an extension of frontal sinusitis. Infections extending from ethmoid sinus disease are often amenable to medical management.

   Greenberg MF: The red eye in childhood. Pediatr Clin North Am 50:105–124, 2003.

23. **What is periorbital cellulitis?**
Periorbital or preseptal cellulitis is an infection of the tissues of the eyelids that does *not* involve the posterior orbit. Periorbital cellulitis is associated with predominantly unilateral swelling, erythema, and tenderness of the eyelids but normal visual acuity and eye motility. Computed tomography is often useful in distinguishing between periorbital and orbital cellulitis, especially when severe eyelid edema precludes an adequate eye examination to ensure normal eye motility.

   Levin AV: Ophthalmic emergencies. In Fleisher GR, Ludwig S (eds): Textbook of Pediatric Emergency Medicine, 5th ed. Philadelphia, Lippincott Williams & Wilkins, 2006, pp 1653–1661.

24. **What problems can lead to the development of preseptal cellulitis?**
- Eyelid trauma
- Impetigo
- Dacryocystitis (infection of the tear sac)
- Infections of the oil glands or hair follicles on the lid margins

   Greenberg MF: The red eye in childhood. Pediatr Clin North Am 50:105–124, 2003.

25. **Which conditions can mimic periorbital cellulitis?**
- Insect bites (punctum can often be seen with direct ophthalmoscope)
- Contact dermatitis (poison ivy)

- Allergic reactions (usually bilateral swelling)
- Underlying sinusitis
- Severe conjunctivitis (adenoviral or chlamydial and gonococcal)
- Eyelid tumors (capillary hemangiomas and nevus flammeus hemangiomas)

26. **Do all patients with periorbital cellulitis require hospitalization?**
No. Children beyond infancy who are otherwise healthy and have no signs of systemic infection may be treated with intramuscular or oral antibiotics as outpatients. They require close follow-up for at least 24–48 hours. Patients who demonstrate no improvement or worsening disease should be admitted for IV therapy.

Levin AV: Ophthalmic emergencies. In Fleisher GR, Ludwig S (eds): Textbook of Pediatric Emergency Medicine, 5th ed. Philadelphia, Lippincott Williams & Wilkins, 2006, pp 1653–1661.

27. **How should you treat a red eye in a contact lens wearer?**
A red eye in a contact lens wearer may signify a sight-threatening condition (infection or a breakdown of corneal epithelium). Remove the contact lens and refer the patient for urgent ophthalmologic examination (within 12 hours). Do not treat empirically with antibiotics; it will prevent the ophthalmologist from obtaining an accurate culture.

Levin AV: Eye—red. In Fleisher GR, Ludwig S (eds): Textbook of Pediatric Emergency Medicine, 5th ed. Philadelphia, Lippincott Williams & Wilkins, 2006, pp 267–271.

KEY POINTS: RED EYE ✔

1. Red, watery eyes in an infant less than 24–48 hours of age are almost exclusively due to chemical conjunctivitis from topical antibiotics used to prevent ophthalmia neonatorum.

2. A red eye in a contact lens wearer is an emergent problem requiring consultation with an ophthalmologist.

3. Orbital cellulitis is a potentially vision- or life-threatening condition that requires hospital admission and emergent consultation with an ophthalmologist.

4. Orbital cellulitis in children younger than 8 years is often amenable to medical therapy; infections in older children often require surgical intervention.

5. Many systemic conditions are associated with "red eyes."

28. **What are the common causes of conjunctivitis?**
Infectious (viral, bacterial, or chlamydial), allergic or seasonal, and chemical.

Greenberg MF: The red eye in childhood. Pediatr Clin North Am 50:105–124, 2003.

29. **Describe the different types of allergic conjunctivitis.**
- **Seasonal allergic conjunctivitis** (hay fever) is associated with itchy, tearing eyes, and relatively minor eye irritation. Chemosis (a blisterlike swelling of the bulbar conjunctivae) is sometimes present. Conjunctival scrapings reveal increased mast cells and eosinophils. Treatment includes topical antihistamines and mast cell–stabilizing agents.
- **Vernal conjunctivitis** is an allergic condition associated with severe itching, tearing, and mucous production and giant papillae of the upper tarsal conjunctiva. Some patients have corneal involvement (keratitis) secondary to scraping by the enlarged papillae. Treatment includes topical antihistamines and mast cell stabilizers. Topical steroids are reserved for the

most severe cases, and an ophthalmologist should supervise use. Of affected patients, 20% have permanent vision loss from keratitis.

- **Giant papillary conjunctivitis** is similar to vernal conjunctivitis but is secondary to soft contact lens use. It represents a sensitization to components of the lenses and/or cleaning solutions. Treatment includes topical mast cell stabilizers and temporary discontinuation of contact lens use.

  Wright KW: Pediatric "pink eye." In Pediatric Ophthalmology for Pediatricians. Baltimore, Williams & Wilkins, 1999, pp 165–193.

30. **Describe the different types of antiallergy eye drops available for treating ocular allergies.**
    - Ketorolac (a nonsteroidal anti-inflammatory eye drop: may cause stinging on installation)
    - Levocabastine (antihistamine)
    - Lodoxamide and cromolyn sodium (mast cell stabilizers)
    - Olopatadine (antihistamine and mast cell stabilizer)
    - Nedocromil and pemirolast (mast cell stabilizers that inhibit eosinophil activation and chemotaxis)
    - Ketotifen and azelastine (antihistamine, mast cell stabilizing, and eosinophil chemotaxis–inhibiting effects)

    Greenberg MF: The red eye in childhood. Pediatr Clin North Am 50:105–124, 2003.

31. **What are the characteristics of herpes simplex keratoconjunctivitis?**
    The ocular involvement with herpes simplex virus is characterized by an episode of primary ocular herpes (skin eruption with multiple vesicles) that lasts for 2–3 weeks, followed later by recurrent corneal disease. The recurrences are almost always **unilateral** and associated with **preauricular adenopathy**. A **dendritic pattern** of corneal defects is a classic sign of recurrent herpes simplex keratitis. Viral replication causes punctate, dendritic, or geographic epithelial defects. Treatment is topical antivirals, usually Viroptic 1% every 2 hours while awake. Corticosteroids are contraindicated because they diminish the body's immune response. The cumulative effect of repeated infections can lead to corneal clouding and vision loss.

    Wright KW: Pediatric "pink eye." In Pediatric Ophthalmology for Pediatricians. Baltimore, Williams & Wilkins, 1999, pp 165–193.

CHAPTER 23

SCROTAL PAIN

Joel A. Fein, MD, MPH

1. **Do infants and toddlers get testicular torsion?**
   Neonates most frequently have *extravaginal* torsion (twisting above the tunica vaginalis), which usually occurs in utero and is more often associated with a nonviable testicle despite early discovery. *Intravaginal* testicular torsion (twisting of the spermatic cord within the tunica vaginalis) is most common in the second decade of life and is rare before the age of 10 years. Nevertheless, boys of any age with acute scrotal pain and swelling require prompt attention, probably radiologic evaluation, and possible surgical evaluation.

   Pinto KJ, Noe HN, Jerkins GR: Management of neonatal testicular torsion. J Urol 158:1196–1197, 1997.
   Stone KT, Kass EJ, Cacciarelli AA, Gibson DP: Management of suspected antenatal torsion: What is the best strategy? J Urol 153:782–784, 1995.

2. **What are some of the important factors in the patient's history that suggest testicular torsion?**
   Boys with testicular torsion will frequently report relatively sudden onset of unilateral scrotal pain, and they also may have nausea or vomiting. They may report that they had this pain on prior occasions, but that information does not argue against acute testicular torsion. Fever and painful voiding are uncommon. A history of trauma does not preclude, and can even predispose the patient to, torsion. It is important to recognize that the child with scrotal pathology often reports lower abdominal or groin pain. The patient reporting abdominal pain should always have a genital examination performed. Conversely, it is important to examine the abdomen of all patients with scrotal pain to evaluate peritoneal inflammation, intestinal obstruction, and abdominal masses.

   Kamaledeen S, Surana R: Intermittent testicular pain: Fix the testes. BJU Int 91:406–408, 2003.
   Lewis AG, Bukowski TP, Jarvis PD, et al: Evaluation of acute scrotum in the emergency department. J Pediatr Surg 30:277–282, 1995.
   Seng YJ, Moissinac K: Trauma induced testicular torsion: A reminder for the unwary. Emerg Med J 17:381–382, 2000.

3. **What is the "bell clapper deformity"?**
   Normally, the testicle is fixed to the posterior wall of the scrotum. Although it is almost impossible to detect this on physical examination, the majority of patients with testicular torsion have a congenital condition called the *bell clapper deformity,* whereby the tunica vaginalis completely envelopes the testicle. This allows the testicle and spermatic cord to twist in relation to the tunica vaginalis, compressing the vessels and nerves within. Although the deformity is bilateral, symptoms usually occur unilaterally. The left testicle is more commonly affected because the left spermatic cord is usually longer than the right.

4. **What is manual detorsion?**
   In general, the prognosis is excellent if the testis is detorsed within 3 hours of symptom onset. Manual detorsion in the emergency setting can allow the testicle to remain viable until emergency surgery can be performed. Although the testicle can twist in either direction, it more commonly twists medially, toward the contralateral thigh. In the manual detorsion procedure, one holds the affected testicle between thumb and forefinger and untwists 360 degrees toward

the ipsilateral thigh (Fig. 23-1). If relief is noted, the testicle should be rotated another 360° or more, since the usual twist is 720°. The direction can be reversed if more pain or swelling occurs after the initial maneuver. The trick is not to be shy or reserved while performing this procedure; it will hurt while it is being done, but if done correctly will greatly relieve symptoms almost immediately. Sedation and analgesia may be warranted to facilitate the detorsion procedure. Surgical correction (bilateral orchiopexy) is still necessary after this maneuver; however, the emergency detorsion procedure can help salvage the affected testicle.

Cattolica EV: Preoperative manual detorsion of the torsed spermatic cord. J Urol 133:803–805, 1985.

Sessions AE, Rabinowitz R, Hulbert WC, et al: Testicular torsion: Direction, degree, duration and disinformation. J Urol 169:663–665, 2003.

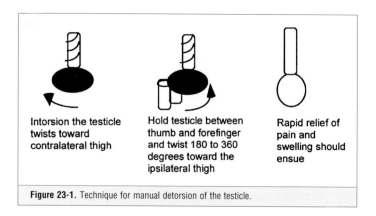

Intorsion the testicle twists toward contralateral thigh

Hold testicle between thumb and forefinger and twist 180 to 360 degrees toward the ipsilateral thigh

Rapid relief of pain and swelling should ensue

Figure 23-1. Technique for manual detorsion of the testicle.

5. **How long will a torsed testicle be viable after the onset of pain?**
   Timing is crucial in the diagnosis and management of testicular torsion. In general, the prognosis is excellent if the testis is detorsed within 3 hours of symptom onset. Almost 100% of testes detorsed 3 hours after onset of symptoms will be viable. About 75% of testes detorsed after 8 hours, 10–20% of testes detorsed after 12 hours, and 0% of testes detorsed after 24 hours will be viable.

6. **What is torsion of the appendix testis?**
   There are many appendages to the testis that are not functional but can certainly cause problems for younger children. The testicular appendix that is located on the superior pole of the testis is the most common appendage to twist on its pedicle and compromise vascular supply. This causes pain and swelling of the scrotum, albeit less so than testicular torsion. This occurs most often in school-aged children and early adolescents, and rarely in those over the age of 20 years. Nausea and vomiting are rare, and on physical examination the cremasteric reflex should be brisk unless swelling is severe. The diagnosis is more easily made if tenderness is located on the anterior and/or lateral pole of the testicle, or there is a "blue dot sign," which signifies the appearance of a hemorrhagic appendix testis visible through the scrotal wall. If the diagnosis can be secured, torsion of the appendix testis is treated with oral analgesics and bedrest. The appendix will likely autoamputate, with no known sequelae.

Kadish HA, Bolte RG: A retrospective review of pediatric patients with epididymitis, testicular torsion, and torsion of testicular appendages. Pediatrics 102:73–76, 1998.

> ## KEY POINTS: DIFFERENTIATING TESTICULAR TORSION AND TORSION OF APPENDIX TESTIS ✓
>
> **Testicular torsion**
>
> 1. Most commonly seen in mid to late adolescence.
>
> 2. Pain is sudden onset, located in the entire testicle.
>
> 3. Cremasteric reflex is absent.
>
> **Torsion of appendix testis**
>
> 1. Most commonly seen in children and early adolescence.
>
> 2. Pain can be more gradual, located in a specific area of the testicle.
>
> 3. Cremasteric reflex is brisk.

7. **What is the difference between epididymitis and orchitis, other than one being easier to spell?**

   Epididymitis is most often caused by infection. If the inflammation spreads to the testicles, the resulting epididymo-orchitis can be difficult to differentiate from primary orchitis. There are, however, some distinguishing features that can guide diagnosis. Fever, nausea, and vomiting are uncommon in patients with epididymitis. Conversely, orchitis is almost always due to a viral infection, and accompanies the other signs and symptoms of the specific virus, such as mumps. A history of urinary tract infections, penile discharge, or urologic abnormalities indicates the need for a workup for infectious causes of scrotal swelling. Epididymitis causes tenderness posteriorly and superiorly within the scrotum, whereas orchitis usually causes diffuse and often bilateral tenderness. Epididymitis can be due to *Chlamydia trachomatis* or *Neisseria gonorrhea*; however, prepubertal patients may be infected with gram-negative bacteria, such as *Pseudomonas* sp., *Escherichia coli*, or enterococci. The urinalysis is positive for white blood cells in less than one-third of patients with epididymitis and even less frequently in patients with orchitis.

   Fein JA: Pathology in the privates: Acute scrotal swelling in children and adolescents. Pediatr Emerg Med Report 2:47–56, 1997.

8. **Are there any rare entities causing scrotal pain or swelling that would be impressive to mention on rounds?**

   Some of the childhood vasculitides can cause scrotal swelling, including Henoch-Schönlein purpura (HSP), Kawasaki disease, and familial Mediterranean fever (FMF). Scrotal involvement occurs in approximately 30% of patients with HSP. Genital involvement usually follows the skin, joint, and intestinal symptoms by several days, and lasts up to 1 week. Surgical management is rarely necessary, but testicular torsion has rarely been noted to occur during the course of HSP.

   Children with Kawasaki disease may report mild to moderate scrotal pain. The perineal rash involves the scrotal walls rather than the testicle, and usually accompanies the acute phase of the illness. Some patients with Kawasaki disease may have swelling of the epididymis as well.

   In contrast to children with Kawasaki disease and HSP, children with FMF may report scrotal pain even before the final diagnosis is recognized. FMF is a genetic disease that affects Sephardic Jews, Turks, Armenians, and Middle Eastern Arabs. The illness is characterized by acute attacks of serositis, as well as the possibility of renal amyloidosis. Although rare in this disease, granulocytic infiltration can cause inflammation of the spermatic cord or the epididymis. Children report gradual onset of unilateral, red, painful scrotal swelling. They have fever, leukocytosis, and an elevated sedimentation rate.

Eshel G, Vinograd I, Barr J, Zemer D: Acute scrotal pain complicating familial Mediterranean fever in children. Br J Surg 81:894–896, 1994.

Hara Y, Tajiri T, Matsuura K, Hasegawa A: Acute scrotum caused by Henoch-Schönlein purpura. Int J Urol 11:578–580, 2004.

9. **How can I differentiate among the variety of painless scrotal masses?**
The most common painless scrotal masses are inguinal hernia, hydrocele, varicocele, spermatocele, and testicular tumor. Table 23-1 describes the features of each of these entities.

Skoog SJ: Benign and malignant pediatric scrotal masses. Pediatr Clin North Am 44:1229-1250, 1997.

TABLE 23-1. FEATURES OF PAINLESS SCROTAL MASSES			
Feature	History	Physical Examination	Management
Inguinal hernia	Increases with Valsalva maneuver; painful only when incarcerated or strangulated	Mass in groin or scrotum; palpable at internal inguinal ring; bowel feels "sausage- shaped"	Assess for obstruction; Trendelenburg position, ice packs, analgesia, muscle relaxation
Varicocele (dilated veins of pampiniform plexus due to incompetent valves located along spermatic cord)	15% prevalence in adolescence; left > right; if found on the right, consider tumor, situs inversus, or renal vein thrombosis	Decreases when supine; "wormy" vessels around the cord	Surgical ligation of internal spermatic vein only if causing testicular atrophy
Spermatocele (sperm-containing cysts of the epididymis or efferent duct system)	Postpubertal males; painless	Nontender, small, cystic nodule located posterior or superior to testicle	Surgical intervention only if painful or unusually large
Neoplasm	15–35 years old; incidence increased if undescended, worse if intra-abdominal; painless unless bleeding into tumor	Hard mass, smooth or irregular, adherent to testicle; gynecomastia or other paraneoplastic phenomena from β-human chorionic gonadotropin or estrogen	Orchiectomy and investigation of preaortic lymph node involvement

10. **Someday, somehow, every male will be kicked in the testicles. When do I worry about the patient who has this chief complaint?**

Traumatic injuries to the testicle include, in order of increasing severity, contusion, hematoma, rupture, and dislocation. Physical examination should focus on the severity of swelling, the presence of both testicles inside the scrotal sac, and the relative size of each testicle. In general, the patient who has suffered recent scrotal trauma and who continues to report pain while in the emergency department setting deserves further evaluation. Similarly, patients with massive swelling of one or both sides of the scrotum require urgent urologic consultation. In general, these patients will require ultrasonography or surgical exploration to rule out testicle-threatening lesions. Ultrasonographic findings of testicular rupture may be subtle, and normal findings do not rule out this diagnosis. Patients in whom the pain resolves quickly and the physical examination is normal may be referred for follow-up, but need not undergo radiologic or surgical evaluation in the acute setting.

All males who suffer abdominal or pelvic trauma should undergo genital examination for concomitant injury. Absence of a testicle within the scrotum is concerning because patients with undescended testicles are at a higher risk for more severe testicular damage after blunt abdominal trauma.

Finally, it is important to remember that testicular torsion may follow minor trauma to the region, and this diagnosis must be considered for any patient with testicular pain regardless of the preceding history.

Micallef M, Ahmad I, Ramesh N, et al: Ultrasound features of blunt testicular injury. Injury 32:23–26, 2001.

Mulhall JP, Gabram SG, Jacobs LM: Emergency management of blunt testicular trauma. Acad Emerg Med 2:639–643, 1995

KEY POINTS: MOST COMMON CAUSES OF SCROTAL PAIN IN CHILDREN ✓

Older children and adolescents

1. Testicular torsion

2. Epididymitis

3. Orchitis

4. Scrotal trauma

Infants and young children

1. Torsion of the appendix testis

2. Incarcerated hernia

3. Vasculitis (Kawasaki disease, Henoch-Schönlein purpura)

CHAPTER 24

SORE THROAT

Magdy W. Attia, MD, and Yamini Durani, MD

1. **How do you define acute pharyngitis, tonsillitis, and pharyngotonsillitis?**
   Acute pharyngitis is an infection of the tonsils or the pharynx. *Pharyngitis*, *tonsillitis*, and *pharyngotonsillitis* are interchangeable terms often used to describe the clinical diagnosis of sore throat regardless of the etiology.

2. **What is the incidence of pharyngitis in children?**
   The exact incidence of pharyngitis is not known. It is, however, the second most common diagnosis in children 1–15 years of age in the ambulatory setting.

3. **What is the most common etiology for pharyngitis?**
   Viral agents account for most cases of pharyngitis seen in children as well as adults (70–80%). These include:
   - Rhinoviruses
   - Epstein-Barr virus
   - Parainfluenza viruses
   - Influenza A and B
   - HIV
   - Adenovirus
   - Herpes simplex virus types 1 and 2
   - Enteroviruses
   - Cytomegalovirus

4. **How can I distinguish throat infections caused by these viruses?**
   The signs and symptoms often overlap between different causes of throat infection. Some helpful diagnostic clues are as follows:
   - When pharyngitis is associated with conjunctivitis, the diagnosis of pharyngoconjunctival fever secondary to *adenovirus* is highly likely.
   - The presence of ulcerative lesions on an erythematous base on the posterior palate is associated with *coxsackie A virus*, a condition known as herpangina. Another variant of coxsackie pharyngitis is hand, foot, and mouth disease. Small vesiculopustular lesions or shallow ulcers are seen on the soft palate, palms, and soles.
   - The association of significant cervical or generalized adenopathy and hepatosplenomegaly is highly suspicious for infectious mononucleosis due to *Epstein-Barr virus* or, less commonly, *cytomegalovirus*.

5. **Which bacterial pharyngitis is the most common?**
   Streptococcus pyogenes, also known as group A β-hemolytic streptococcus (GABHS), is the most common bacterium causing pharyngitis in children. It is implicated in as many as 20–30% of all cases of pharyngitis in children. Other bacterial causes of sore throats (group C β-hemolytic streptococci, group G β-hemolytic streptococci, *Mycoplasma pneumoniae*, *Neisseria gonorrhoeae*) are much less common and almost irrelevant to everyday practice.

6. **Why is it important for clinicians to diagnose and treat GABHS pharyngitis?**
   Antibiotic treatment of GABHS pharyngitis prevents rheumatic fever and suppurative complications. In addition, early treatment of GABHS pharyngitis shortens the course of the disease and reduces transmission to contacts.

7. **Can rheumatic fever occur after a skin GABHS infection or after non-GABHS pharyngitis?**
   No. It is only known to occur after GABHS pharyngitis.

8. **List the suppurative complications of GABHS.**
   These include peritonsillar cellulitis or abscess (quinsy), retropharyngeal abscess, cervical adenitis, otitis media, and sinusitis.

9. **What are other important complications of GABHS infections? Does treatment of GABHS prevent these complications?**
   Poststreptococcal glomerulonephritis (GN) is one of the complications of GABHS. Treating GABHS infection does not prevent poststreptococcal GN. Poststreptococcal GN can occur following non-GABHS, particularly groups C and D. Toxin-mediated diseases, such as scarlet fever and toxic shock syndrome, are also important complications of GABHS infection.

KEY POINTS: TREATMENT OF STREP THROAT ✔

1. Shortens the course of the disease

2. Prevents suppurative complications

3. Prevents rheumatic fever

4. Reduces transmission to contacts

5. Does not prevent poststreptococcal glomerulonephritis

---

10. **What are the clinical features of GABHS pharyngitis?**
    - Sudden onset of fever and sore throat in a school-aged child. Fever is often low grade or absent.
    - Scarlatiniform rash—an erythematous, fine, sandpaper-like exanthem that generally appears in axillary and inguinal folds before it is generalized. It is pathognomonic for GABHS infection.
    - Headache, vague abdominal pain, nausea, vomiting, and halitosis may be present.
    - The pharynx is erythematous, and the tonsils are enlarged. Tonsillar exudate, palatine petechiae, and nasal excoriation may be noticed. Nasal excoriation is rare but more common in the younger child.
    - Significant submandibular lymphadenopathy is usually present.
    - Absence of cough or coryza is characteristic.

    Attia MW, Zaoutis, T, Klein JD, Meier FA: Performance of a predictive model for streptococcal pharyngitis in children. Arch Pediatr Adolesc Med 155:687–691, 2001.

11. **True or False: GABHS pharyngitis is usually obvious and easy to diagnose clinically.**
   False. Initially, signs and symptoms are often absent because of the child's early presentation to clinicians. GABHS and viral pharyngitis have many overlapping clinical features and are often difficult to distinguish from one another.

12. **Are some of the signs and symptoms more reliable than others in diagnosing strep throat?**
   Yes. Scarlatiniform rash, large and tender submandibular lymph nodes, and the absence of coryza are more reliable than fever and tonsillar exudates. The latter two features are more common and reliable in adults.

   Del Mar CB: A clinical prediction model did well in diagnosing pediatric group A beta-hemolytic streptococcal pharyngitis. ACP J Club 136:37, 2002.

13. **What laboratory tests are available to diagnose GABHS infections? What are their advantages and disadvantages?**
   Throat culture is considered the gold standard for diagnosing GABHS pharyngitis, though it has limitations. Throat culture has a relatively high incidence of false-negative results (10–20%). Also, a positive throat culture for GABHS without serologic evidence does not distinguish between carrier state and an acute infection. Finally, cultures may take 24–48 hours of incubation to detect GABHS which may delay diagnosis and care.
   Alternative tests include serologic testing (ASO, anti-Dnase) and rapid antigen tests. Serologic testing is impractical in the acute evaluation of suspected GABHS pharyngitis. Rapid antigen tests by a reference laboratory method are highly specific, but the sensitivity varies (60–90%) depending on the practice. Hence, the American Academy of Pediatrics recommends use of rapid antigen tests only in conjunction with throat cultures.
   Currently under investigation is a new rapid real-time polymerase chain reaction test to detect GABHS pharyngitis with potentially high sensitivity and specificity.

14. **What is the carriage rate of GABHS in healthy children?**
   10–20% of healthy children have a positive throat culture for GABHS while they are asymptomatic (i.e., carriers).

15. **What is the antibiotic of choice for treating GABHS sore throat?**
   Penicillin is the mainstay of treatment for GABHS pharyngitis. Resistance to penicillin has never been documented. It is least expensive and has a proven efficacy. Oral penicillin V or a penicillin derivative such as amoxicillin is most often used (because liquid penicillin has an unpleasant taste). The recommended dose is 40 mg/kg/day for 10 days. While the symptoms improve rapidly, it is crucial to complete the entire 10-day period of therapy. If compliance is in question, intramuscular benzathine penicillin G (0.6–1.2 million units) is the alternative. Erythromycin, cephalosporins, and clindamycin are excellent alternate choices for penicillin-allergic patients.

16. **Do GABHS carriers need to be treated with antibiotics?**
   Carriers do not usually need to be treated. Up to 20% of school-aged children may be carriers of GABHS. They are at low risk for disease transmission or development of suppurative and nonsuppurative complications.

   Bisno AL, Gerber MA, Gwaltney JM, et al: Practice guidelines for the diagnosis and management of group A streptococcal pharyngitis. Clin Infect Dis 35:113–125, 2002.
   Gerber MA: Diagnosis and treatment of pharyngitis in children. Pediatr Clin North Am 52:729–747, 2005.

17. Should sore throat secondary to non-GABHS be treated?
There is not enough evidence in the literature to answer this question, and there are currently no clear recommendations on the necessity of treating these infections. In one report, children with group G β-hemolytic streptococci seem to have improved more quickly with oral penicillin. Group C is usually seen in older adolescents and young adults and is generally a milder illness than GABHS pharyngitis.

KEY POINTS: GABHS PHARYNGITIS ✓

1. Accounts for 20–30% of pharyngitis in children

2. Presents with sore throat, red pharynx, tender submandibular lymph nodes

3. Absence of cough, coryza is characteristic

4. Penicillin or amoxicillin—still the drugs of choice for treatment

18. What is the current recommendation for tonsillectomy in patients with recurrent pharyngitis?
Tonsillectomy should be considered in patients with three or more episodes of pharyngitis per year for 3 consecutive years, or five episodes per year in 2 consecutive years, or seven episodes in 1 year despite adequate medical therapy.

   Paradise JL, Bluestone CD, Colborn DK, et al: Tonsillectomy and adenotonsillectomy for recurrent throat infection in moderately affected children. Pediatrics 110:7–11, 2002.

19. True or False: tonsillectomy affects the incidence and the course of pharyngitis.
False. The presence or absence of the tonsils has no bearing on the overall incidence or the course of the disease. However, after tonsillectomy, the frequency of streptococcal pharyngitis diminishes for 1–2 years, after which the incidence returns to that of the general population.

20. Are steroids helpful in treating pharyngitis?
Recent evidence suggests that a single dose of oral dexamethasone (Decadron) decreases time to onset of pain relief and recovery only in patients with moderate to severe pharyngitis. The greatest benefit was noted in patients with viral pharyngitis compared to those with bacterial pharyngitis.

   Olympia RP, Khine H, Avner JR: Effectiveness of oral dexamethasone in the treatment of moderate to severe pharyngitis in children. Arch Pediatr Adolesc 159:278–282, 2005.

21. How soon can children with GABHS pharyngitis return to school or child care?
The American Academy of Pediatrics and recent studies recommend that children receive a full 24 hours of antibiotics before returning to school or child care.

   American Academy of Pediatrics: Group A streptococcal infections. In Pickering L (ed): 2006 Redbook. Report of the Committee on Infectious Diseases, 27th ed. Elk Grove Village, IL, American Academy of Pediatrics, 2006, pp 610–620.

22. How can recurrent episodes of rheumatic fever be prevented?
If GABHS pharyngitis develops in a patient who has already had rheumatic fever in the past, he or she is at high risk for recurrent rheumatic fever. GABHS pharyngitis should therefore be prevented in any patient who has previously had rheumatic fever by administering continuous

antibiotic prophylaxis. In most cases, intramuscular benzathine penicillin G every 4 weeks is preferred.

23. **Can GABHS pharyngitis occur in children < 3 years of age?**
Yes. Although it is a much more prevalent disease in school-aged children, it is a common myth that GABHS pharyngitis does not occur in younger children. Studies have reported disease rates between 5% and 25% in this age group. Rheumatic fever is very rare in these young children.

CHAPTER 25

STIFF NECK

Nicholas Tsarouhas, MD, and Marla J. Friedman, DO

1. **What is the pathophysiology of meningismus?**
   Flexion of the neck stretches the inflamed nerve roots and meninges of the cervical region. The patient's protective muscle spasm manifests as neck stiffness, or meningismus.

2. **Is meningismus usually seen in neonates with meningitis?**
   Neonates rarely manifest meningismus or nuchal rigidity. The most common symptoms of meningitis in young infants are fever, lethargy, irritability, and poor feeding.

   Pong A, Bradley JS: Bacterial meningitis and the newborn infant. Infect Dis Clin North Am 13:711–733, 1999.

3. **At what age is meningismus or nuchal rigidity reliable in evaluation of children for meningitis?**
   While this is controversial, most experts feel that after 18–24 months this finding becomes more useful. It may be a late finding in meningitis in younger infants.

4. **What are Kernig's and Brudzinski's signs?**
   These are physical examination maneuvers to evaluate for the presence of meningeal inflammation. Kernig's sign refers to extension of the patient's leg causes neck pain and flexion. Brudzinski's sign involves flexion of the patient's neck and produces flexion at the knees and hips.

5. **What are the indications for lumbar puncture (LP) in a child with stiff neck?**
   Consider performing an LP to rule out meningitis in any febrile child with a stiff neck and no other obvious source of infection. This is especially important in children who are not well appearing.

   Ostenbrink R, Moons KGM, Theunissen, CCW, et al: Signs of meningeal irritation at the emergency department: How often bacterial meningitis? Pediatr Emerg Care 17:161–164, 2001.

6. **What are the contraindications to doing an LP?**
   LP may be dangerous in an unstable, critically ill child. "Curling" the young patient into position for the LP may limit ventilation and lead to respiratory arrest in an already compromised infant. If the child is unstable, draw a blood culture and administer antibiotics. Defer the LP until the child is more stable. Other contraindications to LP include increased intracranial pressure and lumbosacral cutaneous infection.

   Cronan K, Wiley J: Lumbar puncture. In Henretig FM, King C (eds): Textbook of Pediatric Emergency Procedures. Baltimore, Williams & Wilkins, 1997, p 542.

7. **Describe some possible complications of LP.**
   While complications are rare, they do occur. Examples include hematomas, persistent cerebrospinal fluid (CSF) leaks, radiculopathies, nerve injuries, epidermoid cysts, post-LP headache, and infection. Headaches after LP in children are uncommon because a small needle is used for the procedure and minimal CSF leak occurs. Life-threatening and extremely rare complications include herniation, respiratory arrest, and cardiac arrest.

   Cronan K, Wiley J: Lumbar puncture. In Henretig FM, King C (eds): Textbook of Pediatric Emergency Procedures. Baltimore, Williams & Wilkins, 1997, p 542.

8. **What other spinal infections may present with a stiff neck?**
Osteomyelitis, epidural abscess, and discitis may occur in the cervical region. Focal spine tenderness in the presence of fever should raise suspicion for these infections. Conventional radiography is sometimes helpful, but radionuclide bone scanning or magnetic resonance imaging are more diagnostic.

9. **Which serious deep neck infection can present with stiff neck?**
Retropharyngeal abscess. Retropharyngeal infections (cellulitis, adenitis, abscess) can develop in the potential space between the anterior border of the cervical vertebrae and the posterior wall of the esophagus. These infections generally occur in infants and toddlers and are rarely seen in children older than 5 years. They are usually caused by group A streptococcus, *Staphylococcus aureus*, or anaerobes. These ill-appearing children may present with fever, respiratory distress, drooling, difficulty swallowing, stridor, or meningismus. Obtain a lateral neck radiograph to investigate for widening of the upper cervical prevertebral tissues. Computed tomography is confirmatory. Management includes IV antibiotics and, sometimes, surgical drainage.

   Harries PG: Retropharyngeal abscess and acute torticollis. J Laryngol Otol 111:1183–1185, 1997.

10. **What are the most common causes of torticollis in well-appearing, *afebrile* children?**
Minor irritation, muscle spasm, and awkward sleep malposition are quite common in young children. The onset is usually sudden, often occurring after waking from sleep. These children have no history of fever or trauma, and should have a completely normal neurologic examination. Supportive care and analgesics/anti-inflammatories are usually the only therapies indicated.

11. **What are some common causes of stiff neck in well-appearing, *febrile* children?**
Cervical adenitis. A large, tender node can often be visualized and palpated in the examination of a child with a stiff neck. Most are febrile. Group A streptococcus or *S. aureus* are the most likely organisms responsible, but *Bartonella henselae* (cat scratch disease), and mycobacterial disease should also be considered. Pharyngitis/tonsillitis and upper respiratory tract infections may also be associated with stiff neck.

KEY POINTS: COMMON INFECTIOUS CAUSES OF STIFF NECK ✔

1. **Meningitis:** Ill appearance, irritability, lethargy; fever; neck held stiffly or pain with flexion

2. **Tonsillitis/pharyngitis:** Red, inflamed tonsils, but not always exudative; consider peritonsillar abscess

3. **Cervical adenitis:** Single, enlarged, tender cervical node; fever common, but not universal

4. **Viral myositis/myalgia:** Cervical muscles diffusely tender to palpation; other viral symptoms present

5. **Upper respiratory tract infection:** Similar to viral myositis, with prominent upper respiratory tract symptoms

12. **Define torticollis.**

Torticollis, which is derived from the Latin *tortus*, meaning "twisted," and *collum*, meaning "neck," is a characteristic tilting of the head to one side secondary to some underlying disorder. The child with torticollis may or may not have pain, and usually holds the head tilted to one side with the chin rotated in the opposite direction. There is unilateral neck muscle contraction. This condition can be due to a variety of causes, including minor trauma.

Kahn ML, Davidson R, Drummond DS: Acquired torticollis in children. Orthop Rev 20:667–674, 1991.

13. **What common pulmonary condition may be associated with torticollis?**

Upper lobe pneumonia, which causes referred pain to the neck. It is sometimes difficult to distinguish this from meningitis as both conditions can cause fever, meningismus, and ill appearance.

14. **Which gastroenterologic condition may be associated with torticollis?**

Sandifer syndrome, which is characterized by intermittent torticollis, opisthotonus, and irritability. This is caused by severe gastroesophageal reflux with esophagitis in infants. Many infants with this condition exhibit failure to thrive.

15. **What is the most common oncologic cause of torticollis in children?**

Posterior fossa tumors. In addition to head tilt, torticollis, or stiff neck, children with these tumors may present with headache, early-morning vomiting, clumsiness, ataxia, strabismus, visual changes, or papilledema.

Gupta AK, Roy DR, Conlan ES, et al: Torticollis secondary to posterior fossa tumors. J Pediatr Orthop 16:505–507, 1996.

16. **What is the most common form of torticollis in infancy?**

Congenital muscular torticollis (also called sternocleidomastoid [SCM] tumor of infancy or pseudotumor of infancy). This usually presents in the first 2 weeks of life as a unilateral, hard, immobile, and fusiform swelling in the inferior aspect of the SCM muscle. The infant's head is tilted toward the affected side. The etiology is controversial. The most common explanation implicates birth trauma with resultant hematoma formation followed by muscle contracture. Another theory postulates that intrauterine abnormal fetal position causes unilateral shortening of the SCM muscle. Passive stretching of the involved muscle is usually curative; recalcitrant cases may require surgical release ($< 5\%$ of all cases). Intramuscular injections with botulinum toxin have also been employed.

Cheng JCY, Tang SP, Chen TMK: Sternocleidomastoid pseudotumor and congenital muscular torticollis in infants: A prospective study of 510 cases. J Pediatr 134:712–716, 1999.
Robin NH: Congenital muscular torticollis. Pediatr Rev 17:374–375, 1996.

17. **Define paroxysmal infantile torticollis.**

This is a benign, self-limited condition characterized by intermittent episodes of torticollis that last for minutes to hours and may recur for weeks to months. Onset is usually in the first few months of life. It usually remits by 2–3 years of age. These episodes are associated with pallor, vomiting, agitation, or lethargy. The etiology is unknown.

18. **Which congenital syndrome is identified by the triad of short neck (brevicollis), limited neck motion, and low occipital hair line?**

Klippel-Feil syndrome. This is a skeletal malformation characterized by the fusion of a variable number of cervical vertebrae. It may also be associated with other bony anomalies and significant scoliosis. These children may have anomalies of multiple organ systems as well. The cause is unknown.

Jones KL: Klippel-Feil syndrome. In Smith's Recognizable Patterns of Human Malformation, 5th ed. Philadelphia, WB Saunders, 1997.

19. **What is Sprengel's deformity?**
This is a congenital failure of the scapula to descend to its correct position. In its most severe form, the scapula is connected by bone to the C-spine and limits neck motion.

> Ballock RT, Song KM: The prevalence of nonmuscular causes of torticollis in children. J Pediatr Orthop 16:500–504, 1996.

20. **What are the first priorities in managing a trauma victim with a stiff neck?**
While maintaining in-line stabilization of the C-spine, ensure adequacy of the airway. The physical examination should then focus on the presence of neurologic deficits (weakness, paresthesias, bowel or bladder dysfunction). If neurologic deficits are present, obtain emergent neurosurgical consultation.

> Kupperman N: Neck stiffness. In Fleisher GR, Ludwig S, Henretig FM (eds): Textbook of Pediatirc Emergency Medicine, 5th ed. Philadelphia, Lippincott Williams & Wilkins, 2005, pp 437–447.

21. **Which initial radiographs should be obtained in the trauma victim with neck pain?**
The routine initial views include an anterior-posterior cervical spine film, lateral cervical spine, and an open-mouth odontoid view.

> Swischuk LE: Injured neck with mild pain. Pediatr Emerg Care 12:241–242, 1996.

22. **If the initial radiographs are inconclusive, which other images may be helpful?**
Flexion/extension views of the cervical spine may be useful in the patient who reports pain yet has no abnormality noted on the initial films. If plain radiographs are still inconclusive, computed tomography of the cervical spine is indicated next. If focal neurologic findings are present, spinal magnetic resonance imaging is indicated.

23. **What is the most common anatomic abnormality identified in cases of traumatic torticollis?**
Atlantoaxial rotary subluxation. The ligamentous laxity of the pediatric cervical spine predisposes children to this condition, which is often seen after only a minor injury such as a fall from a low height. These patients report stiff neck with pain but have no neurologic deficits. Plain films of the cervical spine may reveal asymmetry of the odontoid relative to the atlas. Computed tomography, ideally with three-dimensional reconstructions or done dynamically, is confirmatory. In most cases, soft collar, rest, and anti-inflammatory agents or analgesics are curative. Severe cases, however, may require traction or surgery.

> Muñiz AE, Belfer RA: Atlantoaxial rotary subluxation in children. Pediatr Emerg Care 15:25–29, 1999.

24. **Is atlantoaxial subluxation always a result of trauma?**
No, atlantoaxial subluxation may result from ligamentous laxity following an infection or inflammatory process. It may be associated with rheumatoid arthritis, systemic lupus erythematosus, or tonsillitis/pharyngitis, and it may follow an otolaryngologic procedure (e.g., tonsillectomy, adenoidectomy). This is called Grisel's syndrome. Children with Down and Marfan syndromes are particularly susceptible to this subluxation, secondary to the laxity of the transverse ligament of the atlas.

> Chipparini L, Zorzi G, De Simone T, et al: Persistent fixed torticollis due to atlanto-axial rotatory fixation. Neuropediatrics 36:45–49, 2005.

25. **Are there other injuries to consider in a child with a stiff neck after a minor fall?**
Some children with a clavicle fracture may hold their neck to one side and limit movement because of pain and sternocleidomastoid muscle spasm. Always remember to examine/palpate the clavicles of a child who has sustained a fall.

26. **What is the name given to drug-induced torticollis?**
Dystonic reaction. This is characterized by muscle spasm and abnormal postures, and it most commonly affects the eyes, face, neck, and throat. Patients with dystonic reactions may present

with nuchal rigidity, opisthotonus, trismus, oculogyric crisis, or cogwheel rigidity. These patients are awake and often very distraught over their condition. The torticollis is caused by increased cholinergic activity and change in dopaminergic activity in the basal ganglia, which are responsible for muscle tone.

27. **Which drugs most commonly cause dystonic reactions in children?**
    Metoclopramide (Reglan) and phenothiazines such as prochlorperazine (Compazine). These reactions are dose-related and usually begin within 2–5 days of initiating therapy.

28. **How are dystonic reactions treated?**
    IV diphenhydramine (Benadryl) at a dose of 1 mg/kg usually terminates the reaction. Oral diphenhydramine should be continued for several days after discharge from the emergency department. Benztropine mesylate (Cogentin) is an alternate therapy. Of course, the offending drug should be discontinued.

29. **What arachnid envenomation may be associated with torticollis?**
    The bite of *Lactrodectus mactans*, the dreaded black widow spider, is a neurotoxic envenomation that causes muscle pain and sometimes nuchal rigidity. There is little to no local reaction at the site of the bite. Black widow spider bites are the leading cause of death from spider bites in the United States.

30. **Summarize the extensive differential diagnosis of stiff neck in children.**
    See Table 25-1.

TABLE 25-1. CAUSES OF STIFF NECK	
Infectious	
Meningitis*	Brain/epidural abscess
Encephalitis	Septic arthritis/osteomyelitis
Epiglottitis	Discitis
Retropharyngeal abscess	Viral myositis/myalgia*
Tonsillitis/pharyngitis*	Upper respiratory infection*
Cervical adenitis*	Pneumonia (upper lobe)
Otitis media	Mastoiditis
Traumatic	
Muscle contusion/spasm*	Subarachnoid hemorrhage
Atlantoaxial rotary subluxation	Epidural hematoma
Congenital muscular torticollis*	Spinal cord injury
C-spine fracture	Clavicle fracture*
Congenital	
Benign paroxysmal torticollis	Skeletal malformation (Klippel-Feil syndrome, Sprengel's deformity)
Congenital muscular torticollis*	
Atlantoaxial instability (Down syndrome)	Arnold-Chiari malformation

Continued

TABLE 25-1.   CAUSES OF STIFF NECK—CONT'D

Toxic

Dystonic reaction*   Black widow spider bite

Oncologic

Posterior fossa tumors   Lymphoma

Benign tumors of the head and neck   Meningeal leukemia

Miscellaneous

Migraine   Spasmus nutans

Sandifer syndrome   Syringomyelia

Collagen vascular disease (juvenile rheuma-   Pseudotumor cerebri
   toid arthritis, ankylosing spondylitis)   Psychogenic

*Denotes most common causes of stiff neck.

CHAPTER 26

STRIDOR

Susanne Kost, MD

1. **What are the four primary diagnostic considerations in a febrile child with acute stridor?**
   - Croup
   - Epiglottitis
   - Retropharyngeal abscess
   - Bacterial tracheitis

   Table 26-1 illustrates clinical criteria helpful in distinguishing among the four.

TABLE 26-1. CLINICAL CRITERIA HELPFUL IN DISTINGUISHING AMONG THE FOUR PRIMARY DIAGNOSES IN A FEBRILE CHILD WITH ACUTE STRIDOR

Criteria	Croup	Epiglottitis	Retropharyngeal Abscess	Bacterial Tracheitis
Anatomy	Subglottic	Supraglottic	Retropharyngeal nodes	Trachea
Etiology	Viral: parainfluenza	Bacterial*	Bacterial: oral flora	Bacterial: *Staphylococcus aureus*
Age range	6 mo–3 y	Any, sporadic	6 mo–4 y	Any, sporadic
Onset	1–3 d	Hours (prodrome—days)	1–3 d	3–5 d
Toxicity	Mild–moderate	Marked	Marked	Marked
Drooling	No	Yes	Yes	No
Hoarseness	Yes	No	No	No
Cough	Barky	No	No	Yes, painful
White blood cell count	Normal	Elevated	Elevated	Elevated
X-ray	"Steeple" sign (anteroposterior)	"Thumb" sign (lateral)	Widened soft tissues[†]	"Shaggy" trachea

*HIB now accounts for <25% of cases; other causes include staphylococci; streptococci; and in immunosuppressed patients, *Candida* species and herpes simplex virus.
[†]Expiratory film may also show significant widening; best test is computed tomography of neck.

2. **What is the most common cause of stridor in the pediatric population?**
   Laryngotracheobronchitis (croup) accounts for >90% of all emergency department visits for stridor in the pediatric population. The key features of croup include barky cough, stridor, and hoarseness, usually preceded by symptoms of a mild upper respiratory tract infection. Croup is most common in older infants and toddlers, though it is not uncommon in school-aged children.

   eMedicine: Stridor. Available at www.emedicine.com/ped/topic2159.htm.

3. **Name three animal sounds to which the croup cough has been compared.**
   The bark of a seal or sea lion, the bark of a dog, and the honking of a goose.

4. **What is meant by the term *spasmodic croup*?**
   Spasmodic croup, also known as laryngismus stridulus, is a variant of croup that lacks the typical viral prodrome (low-grade fever, runny nose). Symptoms start suddenly, often in the middle of the night, and resolve quickly. Symptoms may recur for several nights in a row. The etiology of spasmodic croup is unclear. Since the diagnosis can be made only upon resolution of the symptoms, the distinction between viral and spasmodic croup during initial presentation lacks clinical relevance.

5. **What is the characteristic radiographic finding in a patient with croup? In epiglottitis?**
   The classic radiographic finding in croup is the "steeple sign," a narrowing of the laryngotracheal air column just below the vocal cords on an anterior-posterior view (Fig. 26-1). Another finding includes "ballooning" (distention) of the hypopharynx during inspiration, seen on a lateral view. The steeple sign has been show to lack sensitivity and specificity. The primary reason for obtaining radiographs in children with suspected croup should be to evaluate the possibility of other causes of stridor in atypical cases. The classic finding in epiglottitis is the "thumb sign," referring to the lateral view of the swollen epiglottis resembling a lateral view of one's thumb (Fig. 26-2). The thumb sign is also subjective, and

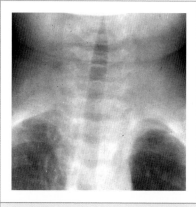

Figure 26-1. Radiographic view of the steeple sign.

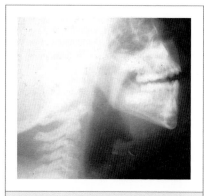

Figure 26-2. Radiographic view of the thumb sign.

radiographs alone should not be used to diagnose epiglottitis. If clinical suspicion is high, imaging should be deferred in favor of direct visualization of the airway under controlled circumstances.

6. **Which bacterial infection of the upper airway most closely clinically mimics croup: Epiglottitis, bacterial tracheitis, or retropharyngeal abscess?**
The clinical presentation of bacterial tracheitis is nearly indistinguishable from that of severe croup. In fact, croup caused by parainfluenza and influenza type A may lead to bacterial superinfection in some cases. Bacterial tracheitis presents with symptoms of stridor, fever, and toxicity generally worsening over a 3- to 7-day period. Racemic epinephrine and steroids are not effective, and many patients will require intubation and surgical debridement of the membranous tracheal exudates. The most common organism has generally been reported to be *Staphylococcus aureus*, though *Moraxella catarrhalis* infection is also prevalent and potentially more severe.

    Salamone FN, Bobbitt DB, Myer CM, et al: Bacterial tracheitis reexamined: Is there a less severe manifestation? Otolaryngol Head Neck Surg 131:871–876, 2004.

7. **Why are retropharyngeal abscesses uncommon in children over the age of 5 years?**
A retropharyngeal abscess generally occurs in infants and toddlers, typically under the age of 4 years. The abscess is caused by seeding of the retropharyngeal nodes with bacteria, usually oral pathogens. After the age of 4, the retropharyngeal nodes atrophy.

8. **What is stertor? How does it differ from stridor?**
Stertor is the noise most aptly described as snoring. It refers to the low-pitched vibratory noise made when airflow is obstructed in the nose and soft tissues of the pharynx; stridor is higher pitched and refers to the noise of turbulent airflow through the larynx and trachea. Thus, a snoring patient is stertorous, and a "croupy" patient is stridulous (not stridorous!).

9. **What is the most common cause of congenital stridor?**
Laryngomalacia is the most common cause of stridor in infants. It is generally benign and resolves spontaneously as the child grows. The exact cause is unknown, though anatomically one finds one or more supraglottic abnormalities, including a long epiglottis that prolapses posteriorly, bulky arytenoids that prolapse anteriorly, or shortened aryepiglottic folds.

    Manning SC, Inglis AF, Mouzakes J, et al: Laryngeal anatomic differences in pediatric patients with severe laryngomalacia. Arch Otolaryngol Head Neck Surg 131:340–343, 2005.

10. **What is the best test for diagnosing laryngomalacia?**
Clinical clues to the diagnosis of laryngomalacia include stridor that improves with prone positioning and worsens with crying. Airway fluoroscopy is suggestive of the diagnosis, but the gold standard for diagnosis is direct laryngoscopy in an awake, upright, spontaneously breathing infant. Direct laryngoscopy also rules out other less common causes of congenital stridor, including vocal cord paralysis and laryngeal webs and cysts.

KEY POINTS: DIAGNOSING LARYNGOMALACIA ✔

1. Clinical diagnosis

2. Airway fluoroscopy

3. Direct laryngoscopy

11. **Where in the airway is the likely site of pathology in a patient with stridor that is loudest in the expiratory phase?**
Expiratory stridor suggests tracheal pathology. The differential diagnosis includes complete tracheal rings, primary tracheomalacia (faulty tracheal development), and secondary tracheomalacia (associated with external compression). External compression may be caused by vascular abnormalities or mediastinal masses, such as thymic cysts, cystic hygroma, thyroid hyperplasia, or mediastinal tumor.

KEY POINTS: CLINICAL CLUES TO THE ETIOLOGY OF STRIDOR ✔

1. Hoarseness in the presence of stridor indicates vocal cord inflammation and is reassuring for the lack of supraglottic pathology, such as epiglottitis or retropharyngeal abscess.

2. Conversely, drooling with stridor is concerning for supraglottic obstruction.

3. Inspiratory stridor suggests an extrathoracic lesion (e.g., laryngeal, nasal, pharyngeal).

4. Expiratory stridor implies an intrathoracic lesion (e.g., tracheal, bronchial).

5. Biphasic stridor may represent subglottic or glottic pathology.

12. **What are the three most common vascular anomalies associated with tracheal compression?**
    - Double aortic arch (the most common anomaly, where two arches encircle the trachea and esophagus)
    - Pulmonary sling (aberrant left pulmonary artery arising from the right pulmonary artery, passing between the trachea and esophagus)
    - Aberrant innominate artery (arising from aortic arch or left carotid, causing pressure on the anterior tracheal wall)

    Kussman BD, Geva T, McGowan FX: Cardiovascular causes of airway compression. Paediatr Anaesth 14:60–74, 2004.

13. **A toddler born to an adolescent mother gradually develops hoarseness over a few-month period and presents with an acute exacerbation of stridor. What important pathologic condition must be considered?**
Recurrent respiratory papillomatosis, caused by certain strains of the human papilloma virus (HPV), may cause significant airway obstruction preceded by an indolent history of hoarseness, chronic or intermittent coughing spells, or poor feeding. HPV is very common in sexually active

females, with adolescent prevalence rates ranging from 20% to 40%, and about 1% of infants born to mothers with vaginal condyloma will develop recurrent respiratory papillomatosis. Treatment includes both surgical (laser) and medical (antiviral) modalities.

Wiatrak BJ: Overview of recurrent respiratory papillomatosis. Curr Opin Otolaryngol Head Neck Surg 11:433–441, 2003.

14. **In a child who presents with stridor following a suspected foreign-body aspiration, where in the airway is the object likely to be found? What percentage of foreign bodies will be found in this location?**
In two large retrospective studies of foreign body aspiration, stridor was reported as a symptom only when the object was located in the *trachea*. Conversely, the percentage of patients with tracheal foreign bodies reported as stridulous ranged from 15% to 50%. Of all respiratory foreign bodies, 10–15% were found in the trachea. Interestingly, tracheal foreign bodies resulted in normal radiographs in 50–80% of the cases, a higher percentage of normal radiographs when compared with foreign bodies in the lower respiratory tract.

Metrangolo S, Moneti C, Meneghini, et al: Eight years' experience with foreign body aspiration in children: What is really important for a timely diagnosis? J Pediatr Surg 34:1229–1231, 1999.

Zerella JT, Dimler M, McGill LC, Pippus KJ: Foreign body aspiration in children: Value of radiography and complications of bronchoscopy. J Pediatr Surg 33:1651–1654, 1998.

15. **Parents of an asymptomatic 2-year-old report that he coughed and choked while playing with small plastic blocks, but they are resistant to unnecessary bronchoscopy. What is the best diagnostic test?**
Computed tomography (CT). Three-dimensional postprocessing of spiral CT images allows virtual views of the airway similar to those seen with endoscopy. CT has been shown to be accurate, and may be useful in both showing the exact location of a foreign body prior to bronchoscopy and ruling out a foreign body in patients with a low level of suspicion.

Kosucu P, Ahmetoglu A, Kormaz I, et al: Low-dose MDCT and virtual bronchoscopy in pediatric patients with foreign body aspiration. Am J Roentgenol 183:1771–1777, 2004.

16. **Name five causes of stridor that are not directly related to the anatomy of the upper airway.**
   - **Allergic:** Anaphylaxis or hereditary angioedema
   - **Cardiac:** Vascular rings; surgical injury to recurrent laryngeal nerve
   - **Gastrointestinal:** Extraesophageal reflux
   - **Neurologic:** Arnold-Chiari malformation with brainstem compression
   - **Psychiatric:** Paradoxical vocal cord adduction

17. **What electrolyte abnormality has been associated with stridor?**
Hypocalcemia may be associated with laryngospasm and stridor, in addition to tetany and the characteristic Chvostek's and Trousseau's signs.

CHAPTER 27

SYNCOPE

James M. Callahan, MD, FAAP, FACEP

1. **What is syncope?**

   Syncope is a sudden, brief, and transient loss of consciousness and muscle tone due to a reversible impairment in cerebral perfusion or substrate delivery (oxygen or glucose). Unconsciousness usually lasts no longer than 1–2 minutes. Patients or their families may say they fainted, passed out, or blacked out.

2. **How common is syncope in the pediatric age group?**

   Syncope is relatively common. The overall incidence is 0.5–1.0% in children and adolescents. In younger children, incidence does not differ by sex. Syncope is more common in adolescents, with 15–50% of all adolescents experiencing at least one episode of syncope by adulthood (not all of these patients will present to medical care). In adolescence, twice as many females as males have syncope. In one series, syncope accounted for about 0.1% of all visits to an urban pediatric emergency department (ED), with a presenting age range of 21 months to 21 years (mean age, 12.7 years).

   Pratt JL, Fleisher GR: Syncope in children and adolescents. Pediatr Emerg Care 5:80–82, 1989.
   Weitlin W, Ganzeboom KS, Saul JP: Reflex syncope in children and adolescents. Heart 90:1094–1100, 2004.

3. **Is syncope serious in children?**

   Most cases of syncope in children are due to benign etiologies. One-third to as many as 80% of cases are **simple neurocardiogenic or vasodepressor (vasovagal) episodes**. In the adult population, only 5% of episodes are vasodepressor events, and one-quarter are due to a cardiac etiology. Even so, syncope may be due to a life-threatening condition in children and adolescents. Up to 25% of pediatric and adolescent patients with sudden death have had at least one prior episode of syncope.

   Massin MM, Bourguignont A, Coremans C, et al: Syncope in pediatric patients presenting to an emergency department. J Pediatr 145:223–228, 2004.
   Pratt JL, Fleisher GR: Syncope in children and adolescents. Pediatr Emerg Care 5:80–82, 1989.

4. **What are the common causes of syncope in children and adolescents?**

   Up to half of patients have experienced a simple vasodepressor episode. Other disorders of autonomic control, including orthostatic hypotension (20% of cases in one series), breath-holding spells, situational syncope (e.g., tussive syncope, micturition syncope), and hyperventilation, are also common. Hysterical faints (pseudosyncope) are common in adolescents.

5. **Name the potentially life-threatening causes of syncope in children and adolescents.**
   - Cardiac arrhythmias
   - Structural heart disease
   - Seizures
   - Subarachnoid hemorrhage
   - Carbon monoxide poisoning
   - Medications and ingestions

KEY POINTS: POTENTIALLY FATAL CAUSES OF SYNCOPE IN CHILDREN AND ADOLESCENTS ✓

1. Cardiac arrhythmias (especially long QT causing ventricular tachycardia)

2. Structural heart disease (e.g., hypertrophic cardiomyopathy and aberrant coronary arteries)

3. Seizures

4. Subarachnoid hemorrhage

5. Carbon monoxide poisoning

6. Medications and ingestions

6. **How is the etiology of a syncopal event usually determined?**
   The history and physical examination are enough to suggest the most likely cause of syncope in the vast majority of patients. Even so, remember that tachyarrhythmias often present in much the same way as vasodepressor syncope. All patients presenting with syncope should have electrocardiography.

7. **What historical factors help to separate benign from serious causes of syncope?**
   Patients with vasodepressor syncope usually experience a prodrome and often faint after a precipitating event (e.g., pain, fright, startle). The patient can usually describe dizziness or lightheadedness, nausea, warmth, and a visual gray-out, often with tunnel vision, before fainting. They often have time to lower themselves slowly or brace themselves against something, and associated injuries such as lacerations or large hematomas are rare. Vasodepressor syncope usually occurs in a standing position.
   Syncope that occurs with associated injuries, with exertion, when the patient is supine, or in infancy, or syncope that recurs is more likely due to a serious, underlying disorder.

   Strieper MJ: Distinguishing benign syncope from life-threatening cardiac causes of syncope. Semin Pediatr Neurol 12:32–38, 2005.

8. **What is the goal of the evaluation of syncope in the ED?**
   It has been said that "Syncope and death are the same—except that in one you wake up." The goal of the ED evaluation is to identify the rare pediatric patient with a serious underlying disorder, while realizing that the majority of patients have probably suffered a vasodepressor episode (a diagnosis of exclusion). Extensive workups are rarely required, usually nondiagnostic, and often expensive.

   Steinberg LA, Knilans TK: Syncope in children: Diagnostic tests have a high cost and low yield. J Pediatr 146:355–358, 2005.

9. **Are there diagnostic tests that *every* patient with syncope should undergo in the ED?**
   A thorough history (including family history and social history) and physical examination are the most important parts of the ED evaluation. Measure orthostatic blood pressures and complete cardiac and neurologic examinations on every patient. Screen all patients with electrocardiography (ECG), looking for signs of hypertrophy or abnormal conduction times (e.g., long QT syndrome). Other diagnostic testing is guided by the results of the history, physical examination, and ECG (see question 17). When there are diagnostic questions after this initial workup, or when syncope recurs, referrals for specialized testing (echocardiography, tilt-table testing, Holter or event-recorder monitoring, or stress testing) may be made.

KEY POINTS: INITIAL WORKUP FOR ALL PEDIATRIC PATIENTS WITH SYNCOPE ✓

1. Complete history, including family history of syncope, sudden death, cardiac diseases, and sensorineural hearing loss

2. Thorough physical examination, including complete cardiac examination with orthostatic vital signs and complete neurologic examination

3. Electrocardiography

10. **How are episodes of vasodepressor syncope and seizures different?**
The description of the syncopal event and surrounding circumstances may help distinguish between the two. With vasodepressor syncope, the patient is usually unconscious for only a matter of seconds, and incontinence is rare. Once awake, there may be some mild fatigue, but a true postictal period with decreased responsiveness and marked confusion is absent. Tonic-clonic movements usually occur near the end of a syncopal episode and last for only a few seconds, while they often are more persistent and last for at least a few minutes in patients with seizures. If the nature of the event is uncertain, electroencephalography may be helpful. It will be normal in patients with vasodepressor syncope and frequently abnormal—even in an interictal period—in patients with seizures.

11. **What is the proposed pathophysiology of vasodepressor syncope?**
It is thought that a prolonged upright position leads to venous pooling in the lower extremities, causing a decreased left ventricular volume. In response to this and possibly a precipitating event, there is a catecholamine surge that causes increased contractility and a strong contraction against a relatively empty ventricle. Cardiac vagal fibers in the ventricular wall are activated and stimulate the medulla oblongata, causing a sympathetic withdrawal with or without vagal stimulation. This sequence is known as the Bezold-Jarisch reflex. These events produce bradycardia as well as a profound loss in systemic vascular resistance, decreased cerebral perfusion, and syncope. The term *vasodepressor syncope* is more accurate than *vasovagal syncope* because it has been shown that vagal activity may contribute to these events but is not necessary for them to occur.

Batra AS, Hohn AR: Palpitations, syncope and sudden cardiac death in children: Who's at risk? Pediatr Rev 24:269–275, 2003.

Wieling W, Ganzeboom KS, Saul JP: Reflex syncope in children and adolescents. Heart 90:1094–1100, 2004.

12. **What are breath-holding spells?**
Breath-holding spells are a common cause of syncope in infants and toddlers, probably related to developmental differences in autonomic control. Classically, two types are described. In *cyanotic* breath-holding spells, some provocation produces crying. The child develops a sustained expiration and becomes silent. Deepening cyanosis, a loss of muscle tone, and, often, opisthotonus occur. There may be a brief period of tonic-clonic movement at the event's conclusion. The child then makes an inspiratory gasp, normal respirations resume, and the child slowly awakens.

With *pallid* breath-holding spells, there is usually the abrupt onset of pallor and loss of consciousness after one to two cries. Opisthotonus is followed by relaxation and gradual awakening. In one series, 17% of children with pallid breath-holding spells went on to have vasodepressor syncope in later life.

Breath-holding spells associated with unconsciousness are seen in up to 5% of all children. Onset of spells is usually in the first year of life and almost always by age 2. These are benign events that resolve spontaneously, and the spells cease occurring in 50% of children by age 4, 90% by age 6, and > 99% by age 8.

13. **What types of syncope are associated with orthostatic changes?**
Orthostatic hypotension may be due to dehydration or anemia. **Micturition syncope, syncope with defecation**, and **syncope occurring during menses** are all related to orthostatic changes. A variety of medications (prescribed; accidentally or intentionally ingested) may cause orthostasis, including antihypertensives, antidepressants, phenothiazines, sedatives, and diuretics. Tussive syncope (seen in patients with pertussis and severe asthma) results when coughing, respiratory spasm, and the Valsalva maneuver cause increased intrapleural pressure, decreased venous return, and decreased left ventricular filling.

14. **What arrhythmias may produce syncope in children and adolescents?**
Ventricular tachycardia, although rare, is a potentially life-threatening cause of syncope. Supraventricular tachycardia may cause presyncopal symptoms, but rarely true syncope. Congenital complete heart block may not become symptomatic until later childhood or adolescence. Complete heart block may also be acquired (e.g., in patients with untreated Lyme disease). Patients with structural heart disease and those who have had previous surgery to repair congenital heart disease are at increased risk of arrhythmias. Paroxysmal episodes of ventricular tachycardia may occur in the setting of a long QT interval.

15. **How is the diagnosis of long QT syndrome made?**
Long QT syndrome is diagnosed by finding a long QT interval on the patient's ECG. The QT interval must be corrected (QTc) for the patient's heart rate by using Bazett's formula:

$$QTc = (QT/\sqrt{RR'})$$

The QTc should be <0.45 seconds in infants under 6 months of age, <0.44 seconds in children, and <0.425 seconds in adolescents. Occasionally, a patient's QTc may only become long with exertion, and exercise testing may be required to make the diagnosis.

16. **What are the familial forms of long QT syndrome?**
Long QT syndrome is associated with sensorineural hearing loss and autosomal recessive inheritance in the Jervell and Lange-Nielsen syndrome, and with autosomal dominant inheritance and normal hearing in the Romano-Ward syndrome. Family history of recurrent syncope, tachyarrhythmias, seizures, sudden death, and hearing loss should be ascertained.

Friedman MJ, Mull CC, Sharieff GQ, Tsarouhas NT: Prolonged QT syndrome in children: An uncommon but potentially fatal entity. J Emerg Med 24:173–179, 2003.

17. **If a diagnosis of long QT syndrome is made, what should be done?**
Patients with long QT have a mortality rate of up to 70% if not treated. Immediate cardiology consultation is required. β-blockers are the usual medical treatment for this disease. Disposition often includes admission for further monitoring. Advise family members to have ECGs to investigate for the familial forms of this syndrome. A long QT interval may be acquired in the setting of electrolyte abnormalities (e.g., hypocalcemia) and may be due to certain medications.

18. **Name the medications and other drugs that may be associated with tachyarrhythmias.**
   - Nonsedating antihistamines (terfenadine and astemizole)[*]
   - Cisapride
   - Tricyclic antidepressants

*Especially when taken with macrolide antibiotics, metronidazole, or ketoconazole; of note, these medications are no longer available in the United States.

- Cocaine (including crack)
- Carbamazepine (usually in overdose only)
- Amphetamines
- Inhalants (especially Freon)

19. **Are there other causes of syncope that are cardiac in nature?**

    Structural heart disease may cause episodes of syncope or sudden death. Hypertrophic cardiomyopathy (idiopathic hypertrophic subaortic stenosis) is associated with a thickened left ventricular wall, especially along the septum in the subaortic outflow tract. With exertion and increased contractility, outflow tract obstruction and syncope occur. **Hypertrophic cardiomyopathy** is the most common autopsy-proven cause of death in young athletes.

    An aberrant coronary artery that courses between the aorta and pulmonary artery also can be associated with exertional syncope, due to ischemia resulting in arrhythmias. Other rare causes that result in ventricular outflow obstruction include valvular aortic stenosis, atrial myxoma, and primary pulmonary hypertension. Dilated cardiomyopathies can be associated with arrhythmias or pump failure.

20. **Other than seizures, are there other central nervous system events that may precipitate syncope?**

    Syncope may be a presenting symptom of **atypical migraines**. Often there is a history of an aura and headaches. Nausea and vomiting are common. Pain is frequently unilateral and may be throbbing in nature. Basilar artery migraines may affect equilibrium and the patient's vision. A family history of migraines can help make the diagnosis.

    Spontaneous subarachnoid hemorrhage is rare in children but may present with severe, thunderclap headache (worst of the patient's life) and a period of syncope.

21. **What metabolic derangements can cause syncope?**

    Hypoglycemia can cause syncope. This is rare in children after infancy, except those receiving insulin. A decreased level of consciousness due to hypoglycemia usually does not resolve spontaneously. Fasting, which leads to increased counter-regulatory hormones (including catecholamines), may play a role in vasodepressor syncope. Carbon monoxide poisoning, anemia, dehydration, and pregnancy may also be associated with syncope.

22. **How does a patient with pseudosyncope (hysterical faints) present?**

    Hysterical faints are usually seen in adolescents. They typically occur in front of an audience, with an absence of physical findings. There is often eye fluttering behind half-closed eye lids. Self-protective behaviors are preserved (e.g., patients will not allow their own hand to fall and hit their face). Social history often reveals marked stress at home, in school, or in other social situations.

23. **What is the treatment for the most common causes of syncope (vasodepressor and orthostatic)?**

    The most effective treatment for vasodepressor and orthostatic causes of syncope is to ensure adequate fluid intake. Older children and adolescents should drink at least 64 ounces of noncaffeinated fluids daily. The patient should drink enough so that their urine remains pale and clear. Small amounts of salty food may also help to maintain intravascular volume. Counsel patients to lie down when they have prodromal symptoms to prevent episodes of syncope. Patients who continue to have episodes of syncope should be referred for tilt-table testing and possible pharmacologic therapy.

24. **Which patients with syncope require referral to a cardiologist or neurologist?**

    Patients who have syncope with exertion, syncope associated with chest pain, arrhythmias, or palpitations; syncope that recurs or does not respond to usual therapies; and syncope accompanied by an abnormal cardiac history, physical examination, or ECG should be referred to a cardiologist. Patients who have a family history of sudden death or who have atypical episodes of syncope should also be referred. Focal neurologic findings, other neurologic abnormalities, or a history that is consistent with the presentation of a seizure should be seen by a neurologist as soon as possible.

Delgado CA: Syncope. In Fleisher GR, Ludwig S, Henretig FM (eds): Textbook of Pediatric Emergency Medicine, 5th ed. Philadelphia, Lippincott Williams & Wilkins, 2006, pp 649–655.

25. What findings in patients with syncope require admission?
Admit patients to the hospital who have cardiovascular disease or an abnormal cardiac examination, patients with serious ECG abnormalities (e.g., long QTc or complete heart block), patients with syncope and chest pain, and patients with cyanotic spells, apnea, or focal neurologic findings. Patients with toxic ingestions, focal neurologic findings, and orthostatic hypotension that doesn't respond to IV fluids should also be admitted for observation, further diagnostic testing, and treatment.

Delgado CA: Syncope. In Fleisher GR, Ludwig S, Henretig FM (eds): Textbook of Pediatric Emergency Medicine, 5th ed. Philadelphia, Lippincott Williams & Wilkins, 2006, pp 649–655.

CHAPTER 28

VAGINAL BLEEDING/DISCHARGE

Jane M. Lavelle, MD

1. What is the average age at menarche? Describe the normal menstrual cycle.

The average age at menarche is 12.7 years, with a normal range of 11–14 years. Typically, it occurs approximately 2 years after thelarche and 1 year after peak height velocity.

One menstrual cycle is the time between the onset of one menses to the onset of another. Normal cycle length varies (21–45 days in teens), lasts from 2–8 days, and results in an average blood loss of 30–40 mL. Clinically, the menstrual cycle is usually defined by the ovarian cycle, which includes the follicular, ovulatory, and luteal phases.

During the follicular phase (7–22 days), low levels of estradiol and progesterone result in elevated gonadotropin-releasing hormone levels and, thus, rises in both follicle-stimulating hormone (FSH) and luteinizing hormone (LH). FSH stimulates the maturation of one follicle, while LH stimulates the theca cells to produce androgens, which are converted to estrogens that stimulate proliferation of the endothelium. As estradiol levels rise, FSH levels begin to fall. During the ovulatory phase, a preovulatory estradiol surge causes an LH surge, resulting in release of the ovum. During the luteal phase, the corpus luteum produces large amounts of progesterone and estrogen, resulting in development of the secretory endometrium. If fertilization does not occur, involution of the corpus luteum occurs, and there is loss of estrogen and progesterone. Sloughing of the endometrium follows, and increased levels of FSH lead to a new cycle.

Adams Hillard PJ, Dietch HR: Menstrual disorders in the college age female. Pediatr Clin North Am 52:179–198, 2005.

Gordon CM, Neinstein LS: Normal menstrual physiology. In Neinstein LS (ed). Adolescent Health Care: A Practical Guide, 4th ed. Baltimore, Williams & Wilkins, 2002, pp 947–952.

2. What is dysfunctional uterine bleeding (DUB)?

DUB is excessive menstrual bleeding occurring during the menses or outside the normal intervals in the absence of underlying structural abnormalities. An orderly sequence of hormonal and endometrial events is responsible for the regular and limited bleeding that occurs in adult women. In adolescents, the most common cause of DUB results from anovulatory menstrual cycles due to "immaturity" of the hypothalamic–pituitary–ovary axis, with lack of normal negative feedback. During anovulatory cycles, estrogen levels are increased without increasing FSH responsible for subsequent fall in the estrogen level. Lack of progesterone normally produced by the corpus luteum, which stabilizes the endometrium, results in sporadic growth and slough of the endometrium. In adolescents, it may be more useful to think of this as anovulatory uterine bleeding because this term reflects the most common etiology in adolescents.

Adams Hillard PJ, Dietch HR: Menstrual disorders in the college age female. Pediatr Clin North Am 52:179–198, 2005.

Mitan LA, Slap GB: Dysfunctional uterine bleeding. In Neinstein LS (ed). Adolescent Health Care: A Practical Guide, 4th ed. Baltimore, Williams & Wilkins, Baltimore, 2002, pp 966–972.

3. **List the causes of abnormal vaginal bleeding in the adolescent female.**

Although anovulation is the most common cause of dysfunctional vaginal bleeding in the adolescent, it remains a diagnosis of exclusion. The diseases listed in Table 28-1 must be considered when excessive vaginal bleeding is present.

TABLE 28-1. CAUSES OF ABNORMAL BLEEDING IN THE ADOLESCENT FEMALE

Life-threatening: Ectopic pregnancy, vaginal/cervical laceration

Common: Anovulation, sexually transmitted infections, pregnancy/complications of pregnancy, hormonal contraception

Complete Differential Diagnosis by Category

Pregnancy-related	*Systemic Disease*	*Genital Tract*
Pregnancy	Coagulation abnormalities	Sexually transmitted diseases
Ectopic pregnancy	Von Willebrand's disease	
Threatened abortion	Idiopathic thrombocytopenic purpura	Trauma
Spontaneous abortion		Tumor
Hydatidiform mole	Renal failure	Foreign body
Endocrine	Liver failure	Malignancy
Anovulation	Systemic lupus erythematosus	Endometriosis
Polycystic ovary syndrome	Malignancies	Myoma, polyp
Hypothyroidism/ hyperthyroidism	*Drugs*	
Cushing's disease	Hormonal contraceptives	
Addison's disease	Anticonvulsants	
Premature ovarian failure	Anticoagulants	
Ovarian tumor	Chemotherapeutic agents	

4. **How should a clinician evaluate a patient to determine a source of vaginal bleeding?**

After a careful physical examination, include a pelvic examination to evaluate the source of the bleeding and any pathology. Screens for sexually transmitted diseases (STDs), a pregnancy test, and a serum hemoglobin are useful. In the young teenager who is not sexually active and has mild symptoms, a pelvic examination may be deferred. As always, follow-up is an important part of patient care.

Adams Hillard PJ, Dietch HR: Menstrual disorders in the college age female. Pediatr Clin North Am 52:179–198, 2005.

Mitan LA, Slap GB: Dysfunctional uterine bleeding. In Neinstein LS (ed): Adolescent Health Care: A Practical Guide, 4th ed. Baltimore, Williams & Wilkins, 2002, pp 966–972.

5. **What are the recommended therapies for dysfunctional uterine bleeding?**

Patients with DUB present with a wide spectrum of severity of illness. Therapy is aimed at stopping the bleeding by converting the endometrium to the secretory state so that sloughing can occur under controlled conditions, correcting the anemia, restoring normal cyclic bleeding, and preventing recurrence and long-term sequelae of anovulation.

A combination of estrogen and progesterone is needed in patients with active bleeding. Any pill combining 35 or 50 μg of ethinyl estradiol or mestranol and a progestin can be used. Progestin only may be used in patients who are not actively bleeding (Table 28-2).

In patients with severe bleeding, attention to the ABCs is necessary with IV access and fluid/blood resuscitation. All patients with active bleeding, low hemoglobin, and change in vital signs require admission for treatment. Evaluation should include coagulation studies. Bleeding usually stops after 24 hours of treatment. Combination pills with a higher dose of estrogen (50 μg of ethinyl estradiol) are the first-line therapy. IV estrogen is reserved for use in unstable patients; pulmonary embolism is associated with this therapy. In patients for whom estrogen is contraindicated, progesterone regimens can be tried. If this fails, other therapies include aminocaproic acid, desmopressin, or surgical curettage.

Mitan LA, Slap GB: Dysfunctional uterine bleeding. In Neinstein LS (ed). Adolescent Health Care: A Practical Guide, 4th ed. Baltimore, Williams & Wilkins, 2002, pp 966–972.

Slap BG: Menstrual disorders in adolescence. Best Prac Res Clin Obstet Gynaecol 17:75–92, 2003.

Strickland JL, Wall JW: Abnormal uterine bleeding in adolescents. Obstet Gynecol Clin North Am 30:321–335, 2003.

TABLE 28-2. THERAPIES FOR DYSFUNCTIONAL UTERINE BLEEDING

Severity	Hemoglobin Level (g/dL)	Therapy
Mild	>12	Menstrual calendar Iron therapy Follow-up 3–6 months
Moderate	10–12, not bleeding	Low-dose OCP or progestin only Iron therapy Follow-up 3–6 months
	<10, not bleeding	Low-dose OCP or progestin only Iron therapy Follow-up 3–6 months
	<10, bleeding	High-dose OCP 1 pill four times daily for 4 days 1 pill three times daily for 3 days 1 pill twice daily for 2 weeks
Severe	<7, hemodynamic symptoms	IV conjugated estrogen and/or high-dose OCP Iron therapy Follow-up 3–6 months

OCP = oral contraceptive pill (combination of estrogen, progesterone, and suggested minimum of 30 μg ethinyl estradiol). Antiemetics are usually needed when higher dose of estrogen is given.

6. **What is primary dysmenorrhea?**
Primary dysmenorrhea is painful menses without associated pelvic disease that typically appears 6–24 months following menarche. Dysmenorrhea typically occurs with ovulatory cycles, which become more frequent as the hypothalamic–pituitary–ovarian axis matures. Two years after menarche, 20–50% of teens have ovulatory cycles. Typical symptoms include

crampy, lower abdominal pain beginning a few days before or at the start of the menstrual cycle and last for 1–3 days. Associated symptoms include fatigue, back pain, headache, nausea, vomiting, and diarrhea.

7. **What causes dysmenorrhea, and how frequently does it occur?**
Dysmenorrhea is caused by prostaglandin E_2 and $F_{2\alpha}$. These are produced in higher concentrations in ovulatory cycles during the secretory phase. Locally, prostaglandins cause myometrial contraction; however, when they enter the systemic circulation they can cause fatigue, headache, dizziness, nausea, vomiting, diarrhea, and back pain. Prostaglandin $F_{2\alpha}$ causes uterine contractions, vasoconstriction, and ischemia. Prostaglandin E_2 causes platelet disaggregation and vasodilation.

8. **How common is dysmenorrhea?**
It occurs very commonly during adolescence. Half to three-quarters of teens experience dysmenorrhea that affects their daily activities. Fifteen percent of teens describe severe symptoms that incapacitate them for 1–3 days during each menstrual cycle. However, only 15% of teens seek medical care for menstrual pain.

Banikarim C, Middleman AB: Primary dysmenorrhea in adolescents. UpToDate, version 13.3, 2005. www.utdol.com.

Braverman PK, Neinstein LS: Dysmenorrhea and premenstrual syndrome. In Neinstein LS (ed): Adolescent Health Care: A Practical Guide, 4th ed, Baltimore, Williams & Wilkins, 2002, pp 952–963.

9. **What is the treatment for primary dysmenorrhea?**
Nonsteroidal anti-inflammatory drugs (NSAIDs) are first-line therapy for dysmenorrhea; a majority (70–80%) of patients experience relief with their use. Ibuprofen, naproxen, and naproxen sodium have all been used successfully. The patient should begin the medication at the onset of the premenstrual symptoms or at the onset of menses and continue this for 1–3 days as needed to control symptoms. The patient should use the chosen NSAID for four cycles until treatment failure is considered. A second NSAID can be tried at that time. Mefenamic acid competes with prostaglandin-binding sites, antagonizes existing prostaglandin, and inhibits prostaglandin synthesis and thus may be more effective than other NSAIDs.

If the patient continues with symptoms despite NSAID use, a 3- to 6-month course of oral contraceptive therapy may alleviate dysmenorrhea. Ovulation is suppressed, as are prostaglandin production and menstrual flow.

Patients should be followed closely. If they do not respond to the described therapies, a re-evaluation seeking secondary causes is indicated.

Banikarim C, Middleman AB: Primary dysmenorrhea in adolescents. UpToDate, version 13.3, 2005. Available at www.utdol.com.

Braverman PK, Neinstein LS: Dysmenorrhea and premenstrual syndrome. In Neinstein LS (ed): Adolescent Health Care: A Practical Guide, 4th ed. Baltimore, Williams & Wilkins, pp 952–963.

10. **What are the causes of secondary dysmenorrhea?**

Other Gynecologic Disorders	Nongynecologic Disorders
Endometriosis	Inflammatory bowel disease
Pelvic inflammatory disease	Irritable bowel syndrome
Pelvic adhesions	Ureteropelvic junction obstruction
Ovarian cysts, mass	Renal stone
Polyps, fibroids	Cystitis
Congenital obstructive Müllerian malformations	Psychogenic disorder

KEY POINTS: VAGINAL BLEEDING ✔

1. Anovulation due to immaturity of the hypothalamic–pituitary–ovarian axis is the most common cause of dysfunctional uterine bleeding in the adolescent patient.

2. Dysmenorrhea is common in adolescents and begins 6–24 months after menarche, when ovulatory cycles occur with more frequency. It is associated with significant morbidity.

11. **What is the approach to a patient with secondary dysmenorrhea?**
Teens who present 6–12 months after menarche, who are <20 years of age, and who describe pain with menses can be treated and followed for resolution of symptoms. A pelvic examination is not necessary in young teens who are not sexually active. Pelvic examination, laboratory testing, and imaging are reserved for patients who have atypical symptoms; have signs, symptoms, or risk factors for other diseases; or do not respond to therapy.

   Banikarim C, Middleman AB: Primary dysmenorrhea in adolescents. UpToDate, version 13.3, 2005. Available at www.utdol.com.
   Braverman PK, Neinstein LS. Dysmenorrhea and premenstrual syndrome. In Neinstein LS (ed): Adolescent Health Care: A Practical Guide, 4th ed. Baltimore, Williams & Wilkins, 2002, pp 952–963.

12. **When should the pregnancy test be included in a workup?**
Unfortunately, teenage pregnancy continues to be a common occurrence; thus, physicians caring for teens should always include pregnancy in the differential diagnosis of many chief complaints, and they should have a low threshold for performing a pregnancy test. Fortunately, these tests have become very sensitive and specific and are quick and relatively inexpensive.
   The most commonly used tests rely on enzyme-linked immunosorbent assay (ELISA) for the detection of the β–human chorionic gonadotropin (hCG) subunit. The level of β-hCG secreted by the trophoblast doubles every other day during the first 6 weeks of pregnancy. By the time it reaches 1000–2000 mIU/mL, a gestational sac can be seen via vaginal ultrasound. Urine ELISA detects β-hCG levels of 30–50 mIU/ml and is typically positive within 7 days of implantation. Thus, the result of this test is positive at the time of the missed menses. Practically, if the teen is concerned about pregnancy, and the urine test result is negative, she should return the following week for a repeat test.

   Neinstein LS, Farmer M: Teenage pregnancy. In Neinstein LS (eds): Adolescent Health Care: A Practical Guide, 4th ed. Baltimore, Williams & Wilkins, Baltimore, 2002, pp 809–833.

13. **What is the differential diagnosis of vaginitis in young women?**
Vaginal discharge, foul odor, itching and irritation of the vulva, and dyspareunia characterize vaginitis. The most common causes include infections due to *Trichomonas vaginalis*, *Candida albicans*, and *Gardnerella vaginalis*. Vaginal discharge can also occur with cervicitis due to *Neisseria gonorrhoeae* or *Chlamydia trachomatis*. Noninfectious causes include foreign body (tampon), trauma, allergies, chemical irritants, and poor hygiene. Etiology of vaginitis is determined by physical examination, the vaginal pH, the whiff test, saline, and potassium hydroxide (KOH) microscopy, and cervical cultures for gonorrhea and chlamydia.

   Centers for Disease Control and Prevention: Sexually transmitted diseases treatment guidelines 2002. MMWR Morb Mortal Wkly Rep 51:1–80, 2002.

14. **How is the diagnosis of cervicitis made?**
Most young women with cervicitis are asymptomatic. Some, however, may present with abnormal vaginal discharge or bleeding, dysuria, frequency, dyspareunia, or bleeding with

intercourse. On pelvic examination, the cervix appears inflamed, and mucopurulent discharge is visible. Often, increased friability leads to bleeding. Causes of cervicitis include *Chlamydia trachomatis, N. gonorrhoeae, T. vaginalis, Candida albicans,* and herpes simplex virus. Thus, evaluation should include a wet mount, a KOH prep, and diagnostic tests for *Chlamydia trachomatis* and *N. gonorrhoeae.* A significant number of patients do not have laboratory evidence of *Chlamydia trachomatis* and *N. gonorrhoeae* infection.

15. **What are the recommended treatment and follow-up for cervicitis?**
    Treatment at the time of the examination depends on the level of clinical suspicion, as well as reliability of follow-up of the patient. Currently, unless cervicitis is known to be caused by one of the organisms above, therapy should cover both *Chlamydia trachomatis* and *N. gonorrhoeae.* Recently, quinolone-resistant *N. gonorrhoeae* has increased; ceftriaxone and cefixime are excellent alternatives.
    The following are acceptable treatments for *Chlamydia trachomatis*:
    - Azithromycin, 1 gm orally
    - Doxycycline, 100 mg orally twice daily for 7 days
    - Erythromycin, base 500 mg orally four times daily for 7 days
    The following are acceptable treatments for *N. gonorrhoeae*:
    - Ciprofloxacin, 500 mg orally, single dose
    - Ceftriaxone, 125 mg via intramuscular or IV route, single dose
    Because these treatment regimens are so successful, "test of cure" or reculture is not routinely recommended. Some adolescent specialists consider screening at 2–3 months, as the rate of reinfection is high. As always, the patient's sexual partners within the preceding 2 months should be evaluated and treated.

    Centers for Disease Control and Prevention: Sexually transmitted diseases treatment guidelines 2002. MMWR Morb Mortal Wkly Rep 51:1–80, 2002.

16. **What is pelvic inflammatory disease (PID)?**
    PID is a polymicrobial infection of the upper genital tract in postpubertal women caused by a sexually transmitted disease. This disease presents with a broad spectrum of clinical manifestations, making an accurate diagnosis challenging. Further, many teens have mild or subtle symptoms. Clinical diagnosis is imprecise; in symptomatic patients salpingitis can be demonstrated by laparoscopy 65–95% of cases. There is no single historical finding, physical examination finding, or laboratory test that is sensitive and specific for the diagnosis. Many cases of PID are missed. Common symptoms include crampy, lower abdominal pain; abnormal vaginal discharge/bleeding; anorexia/vomiting; fever; diarrhea; dysuria; and dyspareunia. Important parts of the differential diagnosis include ectopic pregnancy, ovarian torsion, appendicitis, threatened abortion, and endometriosis.

17. **How is the diagnosis of PID made?**
    In 2002, the Centers for Disease Control and Prevention guidelines changed the criteria for the diagnosis of PID in an effort to capture and treat more patients with mild disease in order to reduce long-term sequelae. The minimum criteria for diagnosis are uterine/adnexal tenderness and/or cervical motion tenderness. All patients who have minimum criteria should be empirically treated unless another diagnosis is present. Additional criteria include oral temperature > 38.3° C, abnormal cervical or vaginal mucopurulent discharge, presence of white blood cells on saline microscopy of vaginal secretions, elevated erythrocyte sedimentation rate, elevated C-reactive protein level, and laboratory evidence of *Chlamydia trachomatis* or *N. gonorrhoeae* infection.

    Centers for Disease Control and Prevention: Sexually transmitted diseases treatment guidelines 2002. MMWR Morb Mortal Wkly Rep 51:1–80, 2002.
    Pletcher JR, Slap GB: Pelvic inflammatory disease. In Neinstein LS (ed): Adolescent Health Care: A Practical Guide, 4th ed. Baltimore, Williams & Wilkins, 2002, pp 1161–1170.

18. **What is the treatment for PID? When is hospitalization necessary?**

Regimens for the treatment of PID have been developed to cover the polymicrobial nature of the disease. Thus, therapy must be effective against *N. gonorrhoeae* and *Chlamydia trachomatis* as well as anaerobes, *Streptococcus* sp., gram-negative enterics, and *Mycoplasma* sp. Consider hospitalization in the following instances: pregnancy, unclear diagnosis, vomiting, peritoneal signs, the young teenager (age < 15 years), tubo-ovarian abscess present or suspected, failed outpatient treatment, or patient's inability to follow the outpatient regimen. Ideally, patients should take their medications, rest, and avoid intercourse. Treatment of all sexual partners within the preceding 2 months is indicated. Follow-up is needed at 48–72 hours.

The following represent acceptable treatment regimens for PID:

Parenteral Therapy

- Cefoxitin, 2 gm via IV route every 6 hours, or cefotetan, 2 gm via IV route every 12 hours (continued 24 hours after clinical improvement), *plus* doxycycline, 100 mg twice daily for 14 days
- Clindamycin, 900 mg via IV route every 8 hours, *plus* gentamicin, 2 mg/kg body weight for first dose, then 1.5 mg/kg every 8 hours
- Ofloxacin, 400 mg via IV route every 12 hours, *with or without* metronidazole, 500 mg via IV route every 8 hours
- Ampicillin/sulbactam, 3 gm via IV route every 6 hours, *plus* doxycycline, 100 mg orally twice daily

Oral Therapy

- Levofloxacin, 500 mg once daily, *with or without* metronidazole, 500 mg twice daily for 14 days
- Ofloxacin, 400 mg twice daily for 14 days, *with or without* metronidazole, 500 mg twice daily for 14 days
- Ceftriaxone, one 125-mg dose via intramuscular route, *plus* doxycycline, 100 mg twice daily for 14 days

Centers for Disease Control and Prevention: Sexually transmitted diseases treatment guidelines 2002. MMWR Morb Mortal Wkly Rep 51:1–80, 2002.

Pletcher JR, Slap GB: Pelvic inflammatory disease. In Neinstein LS (ed): Adolescent Health Care: A Practical Guide, 4th ed. Baltimore, Williams & Wilkins, Baltimore, 2002, pp 1161–1170.

KEY POINTS: SEXUALLY TRANSMITTED INFECTIONS ✔

1. Adolescents between the ages of 15 and 19 years have the highest rate of sexually transmitted infections (STIs).

2. Consider STIs when evaluating teens with lower abdominal pain, vaginal discharge/discomfort, dysuria, or abnormal menstrual bleeding.

3. Sexually transmitted infections are rarely found in prepubertal children who are victims of sexual abuse.

4. Routine vaginal cultures for STIs are not indicated in prepubertal children who are victims of sexual abuse.

19. **What diagnostic tests should be considered when evaluating an adolescent with a suspected sexually transmitted infection?**

The development of Food and Drug Administration–approved nucleic acid amplification tests (NAATs) for *N. gonorrhoeae* and *Chlamydia trachomatis* has revolutionized the ability to screen at-risk populations as well as to identify infection in symptomatic patients. The sensitivity of these tests range from 85% to 100%. The specificity is 99%. Because these tests can be done by using urine, NAAT offers the most noninvasive method for screening and diagnosing sexually transmitted infections. These tests can be used on cervical, urethral, or vaginal swab specimens and can be incorporated into the annual evaluation of adolescents. In many circumstances, a careful sexual history and physical examination, review of symptoms, along with the NAATs, can replace routine pelvic examinations. In the teen with suspected PID, the pelvic examination can be limited to the bimanual examination.

The following laboratory tests may be helpful in the evaluation of postpubertal females with vaginal discharge/discomfort or suspected PID:

- **N. gonorrhoeae, Chlamydia trachomatis:** "Dirty" urine specimen for NAAT
- **Bacterial vaginosis:** Gram stain for clue cells, whiff test, vaginal pH
- **Trichomonas vaginalis:** Wet prep (sensitivity, 60–70%); antigen detection (sensitivity, 79–99%)
- **Candidiasis (based on clinical symptoms):** 10% KOH or Gram stain on vaginal swab for pseudohyphae; culture
- **Herpes simplex virus 2 (HSV-2) (based on clinical symptoms, examination):** Direct fluorescent antibody on scrapings from base of unroofed vesicle (sensitivity decreases with healing); culture (sensitivity decreases with healing); serologic type-specific IgG-based assays (rapid blood test, specific for HSV-2)
- Urinalysis and urine culture
- Gram stain on blind vaginal swab for white blood cell detection
- Urine hCG (affects therapy choices)
- Hepatitis B serology (based on clinical symptoms, examination)
- Syphilis serology (based on clinical symptoms, examination)
- **HIV:** Testing in the emergency department (ED) setting is not optimal; refer patient to anonymous testing site, adolescent clinic
- **Suspected PID:** Complete blood count, C-reactive protein, erythrocyte sedimentation rate

Centers for Disease Control and Prevention: Sexually transmitted diseases treatment guidelines 2002. MMWR Morb Mortal Wkly Rep 51:1–80, 2002.

Pletcher JR, Slap GB: Pelvic inflammatory disease. In Neinstein LS (ed): Adolescent Health Care: A Practical Guide, 4th ed. Baltimore, Williams & Wilkins, 2002, pp 1161–1170.

20. **What is Fitz-Hugh-Curtis syndrome?**

Fitz-Hugh-Curtis syndrome, or perihepatitis, results from salpingitis in 5–20% of patients. Inflammatory exudate travels up the paracolic gutter of the abdominal cavity and settles around the liver capsule. The hallmark of this disease is acute right-upper-quadrant pain and tenderness. The patient may also have splinting, anorexia, vomiting, or fever. Other important diagnoses to consider include pneumonia, pulmonary embolus, hepatitis, and gall bladder disease. It is not unusual for the patient to have silent pelvic infection. Liver function test results should be minimally elevated. The treatment regimens for PID are appropriate for these patients.

Pletcher JR, Slap GB: Pelvic inflammatory disease. In Neinstein LS (ed): Adolescent Health Care: A Practical Guide, 4th ed. Baltimore, Williams & Wilkins, Baltimore, 2002, pp 1161–1170.

21. **List the causes of vaginal discharge in the prepubertal girl.**

The complaint of vaginal discharge in young girls presenting to the ED is not uncommon. Remember that a very small number of these children are victims of sexual abuse, and that in most a variety of infectious and noninfectious causes is possible. The most common etiology is "nonspecific vaginitis," which is vaginitis without an identifiable cause. This is attributed to poor hygiene, tight-fitting clothes, soaps, creams, and bubble baths. Pathogens include group A β-hemolytic streptococcus, *Haemophilus influenzae, Staphylococcus aureus, Moraxella catarrhalis, Streptococcus pneumoniae, Neisseria meningitidis, Shigella* sp., and *Yersinia enterolitica.* Respiratory pathogens (*Streptococcus pneumoniae* and *Streptococcus pyogenes*), enteric organisms (*Shigella* sp.), and sexually transmitted diseases can also be associated with vaginitis. The most common cause of bloody vaginal discharge is a foreign body. Other causes to consider include pinworms, trauma, urethral prolapse, atopic dermatitis, lichen sclerosis, and scabies.

Emans SJ: Vulvovaginal problems in the prepubertal child. In Emans SJ, Laufer MR, Goldstein DP (eds): Pediatric and Adolescent Gynecology, 5th ed. Philadelphia, Lippincott Williams & Wilkins, 2005, pp 83–119.

22. **What treatment is recommended for vaginal discharge in a prepubertal girl?**
Therapy includes sitz baths, good hygiene, and removal of any irritants.

23. **When should you consider vaginal cultures in the prepubertal girl?**
It is helpful to culture patients with vaginal symptoms when an abnormal discharge is present upon physical examination. Routine cultures in the evaluation of children who are potential victims of sexual abuse are not indicated. The rate of STDs in prepubertal children as a result of sexual abuse is only 1–3%. Additionally, children with an STD can usually be identified by the presence of abnormal genital findings, such as discharge and inflammation. Therefore, although the decision to obtain vaginal cultures for *N. gonorrhoeae* and *Chlamydia trachomatis* in the evaluation of children suspected of being sexually abused must be made on an individual case basis, general recommendations include the following: in the presence of vaginal discharge, genital symptoms, evidence of acute injury, or history of stranger abduction. Currently, culture techniques are the only acceptable method to identify and document an STD in prepubertal children. Rapid tests, such as ligase chain reaction or direct fluorescent antibody, should not be used solely.

Emans SJ: Vulvovaginal problems in the prepubertal child. In Emans SJ, Laufer MR, Goldstein DP (eds): Pediatric and Adolescent Gynecology, 5th ed. Philadelphia, Lippincott Williams & Wilkins, 2005, pp 83–119.
Leder MR, Emans SJ: Sexual abuse in the child and adolescent. In Emans SJ, Laufer MR, Goldstein DP (eds): Pediatric and Adolescent Gynecology, 5th ed. Philadelphia, Lippincott Williams & Wilkins, 2005, pp 939–975.

24. **What are the symptoms and signs of ectopic pregnancy?**
This diagnosis must be entertained in any postpubertal female with abdominal pain, especially when vaginal bleeding is present. Classically, patients present with abdominal pain, with or without vaginal bleeding in the face of either missed menses or irregular vaginal bleeding. As the pregnancy progresses, pain becomes more severe, and signs of peritoneal irritation develop with rupture, vaginal bleeding and hemodynamic compromise. More commonly, however, patients present with abnormal vaginal bleeding and a smaller than expected uterus. Importantly, remember that 50% of patients are asymptomatic. The differential diagnosis includes PID, spontaneous/threatened abortion, ovarian torsion, ovarian or corpus luteal cyst, and appendicitis. A negative urine pregnancy test result rules out the presence of an ectopic pregnancy.

25. **What is the initial approach to a patient with suspected ectopic pregnancy?**
Attention to the ABCs is important in these patients because they are at risk for severe hemorrhage. Immediate gynecologic consultation is mandatory. Stable patients with positive results on a β-hCG and a closed cervical os can be followed with serial quantitative β-hCG determination and transvaginal ultrasound. Several protocols for the care of these patients exist in the literature.

Sowter MC, Farquhar CM: Ectopic pregnancy: An update. Curr Opin Obstet Gynecol 16:289–293, 2004.

26. **What is bacterial vaginosis?**

Bacterial vaginosis is the most common cause of vaginitis. This condition results from replacement of the normal *Lactobacillus* spp. with overgrowth of facultative anaerobes, including *Gardnerella vaginalis*, *Prevotella* sp., *Mobiluncus* spp., and *Mycoplasma hominis* Sexual transmission of this infection has not been substantiated, but the condition is more common in women who have had multiple partners and rare in women who are not sexually active. Partner treatment does not affect recurrence of infection. Bacterial vaginosis is associated with an increased risk for premature labor, premature rupture of membranes, and postpartum or postprocedure endometritis or PID. It remains unproven whether treatment reduces these risks.

The clinical diagnosis is made when patients have three of the four following criteria: (1) presence of a homogenous, gray-white discharge; (2) vaginal pH > 4.5; (3) clue cells present on Gram stain of vaginal fluid (epithelial cells studded with many small bacteria, producing a fuzzy border; offers a "clue" to the diagnosis); and (4) malodorous, fishy smell before or after exposure to 10% KOH. Culture for *Gardnerella vaginalis* has very poor specificity because it is present in many women who do not have bacterial vaginosis.

27. **What is the treatment for bacterial vaginosis?**

All symptomatic women should be treated. Treatment options include metronidazole, 500 mg twice daily for 7 days; clindamycin cream 2%, one full applicator once a day at bedtime for 7 days; metronidazole gel 0.75%, one full applicator twice daily for 5 days; or clindamycin, 300 mg twice daily for 7 days. The recurrence rate 1 month after therapy is 20%; accordingly, patients should be instructed to return if symptoms reappear. The addition of vaginal lactobacilli suppositories to metronidazole regimens is currently under investigation.

Centers for Disease Control and Prevention: Sexually transmitted diseases treatment guidelines 2002. MMWR Morb Mortal Wkly Rep 51:1–80, 2002.

Okun N, Gronau KA, Hannah ME: Antibiotics for bacterial vaginosis or *Trichomonas vaginalis* in pregnancy: A systematic review. Obstet Gynecol 105:857–868, 2005.

28. **What are genital ulcers? What causes them?**

Genital ulcers are lesions characterized by disruption of the epithelium/mucosa with associated inflammation. Infections associated with ulcers include herpes simplex virus (HSV), syphilis, and chancroid. HSV is, by far, the most common cause of genital ulcers. Grouped vesicles on an erythematous base that rupture and leave a shallow, painful ulcer are typical in HSV infection. Patients often have pain and paresthesias preceding the appearance of the ulcers. During primary infection, 16–24 lesions are present and systemic symptoms may be present for 2–3 days. Lesions resolve in 2–4 weeks.

Noninfectious causes of genital ulcers include inflammatory bowel disease, Behçet's disease, fixed drug eruptions, trauma, and neoplasms.

Centers for Disease Control and Prevention: Sexually transmitted diseases treatment guidelines 2002. MMWR Morb Mortal Wkly Rep 51:1–80, 2002.

29. **How are genital ulcers caused by HSV treated?**

In addition to analgesia and hygiene, one of the following therapies should be given: acyclovir, 400 mg three times daily; famciclovir, 250 mg three times daily; or valacyclovir, 1 gm twice daily for 7–10 days. For recurrent infection, treatment must be initiated within 1 day of the onset of lesions, so patients should be given a prescription with instructions to begin treatment when symptoms and lesions appear. Recommended regimens include acyclovir, 400 mg three times daily; acyclovir, 500 mg twice daily; famciclovir, 125 mg twice daily; or valacyclovir, 500 mg twice daily for 5 days. Daily suppression, with acyclovir, 400 mg twice daily, or famciclovir, 250 mg twice daily, is indicated in patients with more than six recurrences in 1 year. Patients who are immunocompromised, or who have severe or disseminated infection, such as hepatitis, pneumonia, encephalitis, or meningitis, require systemic acyclovir therapy.

Centers for Disease Control and Prevention: Sexually transmitted diseases treatment guidelines 2002. MMWR Morb Mortal Wkly Rep 51:1–80, 2002.

30. **Describe the genital ulcers caused by syphilis and chancroid. How are they treated?**

The ulcer or chancre of primary syphilis is typically painless and solitary, with smooth margins and a clean indurated base with a serous exudate. The diagnosis of syphilis is confirmed by a positive result on a rapid plasma reagin test. Treatment for primary syphilis is one intramuscular 2.5-μU dose of benzathine penicillin G. Patients should be re-evaluated at 6 and 12 months.

Chancroid, a much less common etiology, results in one or several painful ulcers with irregular margins and deep undermined edges. These ulcers can become quite large. If evaluation for HSV and syphilis is negative, the patient should be treated for chancroid with one 1-gm dose of azithromycin; one 250-mg intramuscular dose of ceftriaxone; ciprofloxacin, 500 mg twice daily for 3 days; or erythromycin base, 500 mg four times daily for 7 days.

Centers for Disease Control and Prevention: Sexually transmitted diseases treatment guidelines 2002. MMWR Morb Mortal Wkly Rep 51:1–80, 2002.

HELPFUL WEBSITES

1. American Social Health Association
   www.ashastd.org

2. Child Trends
   http://childtrends.org

3. Centers for Disease Control and Prevention: Sexually Transmitted Diseases
   www.cdc.gov/std/

CHAPTER 29

VOMITING

Martha S. Wright, MD

1. **What is the pathophysiology of vomiting?**
   True vomiting is the forceful elimination of gastrointestinal contents through the mouth or nose. Vomiting is caused by coordinated diaphragmatic and abdominal contractions in conjunction with pyloric constriction and gastroesophageal relaxation. This motor activity occurs in response to stimulation of the medullary "vomiting center" by impulses from a variety of anatomic locations. Sources of these impulses include the pelvic and abdominal viscera, the heart, the peritoneum, the labyrinth, and the "chemoreceptor trigger zone," an area on the floor of the fourth ventricle that is sensitive to circulating drugs, toxins, and metabolic derangements.

2. **What is the clinical difference between vomiting and "spitting up"?**
   It is important to differentiate vomiting from "spitting up" because the causes of spitting up are rarely serious while vomiting may indicate a potentially life-threatening condition. Spitting up is characterized by effortless regurgitation of stomach or esophageal contents and in most infants and children is due to gastroesophageal reflux or overfeeding. Vomiting, on the other hand, is forceful, may be accompanied by retching, and is frequently associated with autonomic symptoms, such as salivation, pallor, sweating, tachycardia, and mydriasis.

KEY POINTS: FORCEFUL VOMITING ✓

1. Effortless regurgitation is usually caused by non–life-threatening conditions.

2. Forceful vomiting may be associated with more serious conditions, such as gastrointestinal obstruction, metabolic disease, or toxic ingestions.

3. **What is the differential diagnosis of vomiting in the pediatric patient?**
   Vomiting may be caused by abnormalities in a variety of organ systems. When preschool-aged patients report "vomicking," they help us to remember the wide-ranging differential diagnosis with the following mnemonic:
   - **V** = **V**estibular: labyrinthine disorders, otitis media
   - **O** = **O**bstruction: malrotation, volvulus, adhesions, intussusception, obstipation, pyloric stenosis, incarcerated hernia, intestinal atresias, annular pancreas, duodenal hematoma
   - **M** = **M**etabolic: diabetic ketoacidosis, inborn errors of metabolism (e.g., urea cycle defects, carbohydrate or amino acid metabolic defects), congenital adrenal hyperplasia, Reye's syndrome
   - **I** = **I**nfection/Inflammation: gastrointestinal (appendicitis, hepatitis, pancreatitis, cholecystitis, gastroenteritis, gastritis, necrotizing enterocolitis) or extragastrointestinal (upper respiratory tract infections, sinusitis, pharyngitis, pneumonia, sepsis, cystitis, asthma)

- **C** = **C**entral nervous system disease: increased intracranial pressure (brain tumor, intracranial hematoma, cerebral edema), hydrocephalus, meningitis, pseudotumor cerebri, concussion, migraine, ventriculoperitoneal shunt malfunction
- **K** = **K**idney disease: acute renal failure, chronic renal failure, pyelonephritis, renal calculi, renal tubular acidosis, obstructive uropathy
- **I** = **I**ntentional: eating disorders, rumination
- **N** = **N**asty drugs/poisons: chemotherapeutics, ipecac, iron, salicylates, organophosphates, theophylline, alcohols, lead and other heavy metals, poisonous mushrooms
- **G** = Other **GI/GU/GYN** causes (**GI [gastrointestinal]:** gastroesophageal reflux, formula intolerance, peptic ulcer disease, cyclic vomiting syndrome; **GU [genitourinary]:** testicular torsion, epididymitis; **GYN [gynecologic]:** dysmenorrhea, ovarian torsion, pregnancy, pelvic inflammatory disease)

Furnival RA: Vomiting. In Harwood-Nuss A, Linden CH, Luten RC, et al (eds): The Clinical Practice of Emergency Medicine, 2nd ed. Philadelphia, Lippincott-Raven, 1996, pp 1265–1267.

4. **The differential diagnosis for vomiting depends on the age of the pediatric patient. What are the life-threatening causes of vomiting in the different pediatric age groups?**
See Table 29-1.

Burton BK: Inborn errors of metabolism in infancy: A guide to diagnosis. Pediatrics 102:E69, 1998.
Stevens M, Henretig FM: Vomiting. In Fleisher GR, Ludwig S, Henretig FM, et al (eds): Textbook of Pediatric Emergency Medicine, 5th ed. Baltimore, Williams & Wilkins, 2006, pp 682–683.

TABLE 29-1. LIFE-THREATENING CAUSES OF VOMITING BY AGE	
Age	**Cause**
Neonate	GI obstruction
	▪ Congenital intestinal obstruction
	▪ Atresias
	▪ Malrotation with volvulus
	Renal
	▪ Obstructive uropathy
	▪ Uremia
	Trauma
	▪ Shaken baby syndrome with subdural hematoma
	▪ Abdominal trauma
	Metabolic
	▪ Inborn metabolic errors
	▪ Congenital adrenal hyperplasia
	Infectious
	▪ Sepsis
	▪ Meningitis
	▪ Severe gastroenteritis
	▪ Necrotizing enterocolitis
	Neurologic
	▪ Hydrocephalus

TABLE 29-1. LIFE-THREATENING CAUSES OF VOMITING BY AGE—CONT'D

Age	Cause
Older infant/toddler	GI obstruction ■ Pyloric stenosis ■ Intussusception ■ Incarcerated hernia ■ Malrotation with volvulus Renal ■ Uremia Trauma ■ Shaken baby syndrome with subdural hematoma ■ Abdominal trauma Infectious ■ Sepsis ■ Meningitis ■ Severe gastroenteritis Neurologic ■ Hydrocephalus ■ Mass lesion Toxic ingestions
Older child/adolescent	GI obstruction ■ Malrotation with volvulus ■ Small bowel obstruction Renal ■ Uremia Infectious ■ Meningitis Metabolic ■ Diabetic ketoacidosis ■ Reye's syndrome Neurologic ■ Intracranial mass lesion (e.g. tumor, hematoma) Toxic ingestions Inflammatory ■ Appendicitis

GI = gastrointestinal.

5. **What are the most common causes of vomiting in the different pediatric age groups?**
See Table 29-2.

Stevens M, Henretig FM: Vomiting. In Fleisher GR, Ludwig S, Henretig FM, et al (eds): Textbook of Pediatric Emergency Medicine, 5th ed. Baltimore, Williams & Wilkins, 2006, p 683.

TABLE 29-2. COMMON CAUSES OF VOMITING BY AGE	
Age	Causes
Neonates	GI
	■ GE reflux
	■ Congenital GI obstruction (intestinal atresias, malrotation)
	■ Milk-protein allergy
	Infectious
	■ Sepsis/meningitis
Older infant/toddler	GI
	■ GE reflux
	■ Gastroenteritis
	■ Milk-protein allergy
	■ Incarcerated hernia
	■ Pyloric stenosis
	■ Intussusception
	Infectious
	■ Otitis media
	■ Urinary tract infection
	Toxic ingestion
Older child/adolescent	GI
	■ Gastroenteritis
	■ Appendicitis
	Infectious
	■ Urinary tract infection
	Metabolic
	■ Diabetic ketoacidosis
	Toxic ingestion
	Other
	■ Eating disorder

GE = gastroesophageal; GI = gastrointestinal.

6. **What should be the first steps in evaluating the infant or child with vomiting?**
In the stable child who does not require resuscitation, evaluation of the infant or child with vomiting should begin with a careful history and physical examination. There is little value in screening laboratory or radiologic tests in most infants and children who have uncomplicated gastroenteritis. The information gathered will help to identify any acute needs the child may have, quantify the degree of dehydration caused by the vomiting, and allow the clinician to focus the differential diagnosis.

7. **What information should be obtained in the history of a child who is vomiting?**
Useful historical information includes:
- Appearance of the emesis
- Duration, frequency, and forcefulness of vomiting
- Presence of other gastrointestinal symptoms (e.g., abdominal pain, diarrhea, constipation)
- Presence of other nongastrointestinal symptoms (e.g., headache, neck stiffness, fever, polydipsia/polyphagia/polyuria, dysuria, respiratory symptoms, vaginal discharge, menstrual history, vertigo)

8. **What clinical clues can be obtained from the appearance of the vomitus?**
When obtaining a history from a patient with vomiting, details about the appearance of the vomitus can help pinpoint the location of the problem.

Appearance	Source/Cause
Undigested food	Esophageal lesion or reflux
Digested food, milk curds	Stomach, proximal to pylorus
Yellow-green, bilious	Obstruction distal to ampulla of Vater or retrograde peristalsis during retching causing gastroduodenal reflux
Feculent	Distal obstruction, colonic stasis
Blood	Lesion proximal to ligament of Treitz
Bright red blood	Esophagus or stomach above the cardia minimal contact of blood with gastric secretions
Brown, "coffee grounds"	Gastric bleeding or swallowed blood mixed with gastric secretions
Mucus	Upper respiratory tract, gastric mucous hypersecretion

Orenstein SR, Peters JM: Vomiting and regurgitation. In Kliegman RM, Greenbaum LA, Lye PS (eds): Practical Strategies in Pediatric Diagnosis and Therapy. Philadelphia, WB Saunders, 2004, pp 291–321.
Sadow KB, Atabaki SM, Johns CM, et al: Bilious emesis in the pediatric emergency department: Etiology and outcome. Clin Pediatr 41:475–479, 2002.

KEY POINTS: BILIOUS EMESIS ✔

1. All infants and children with bilious emesis should be presumed to have a bowel obstruction until proven otherwise.

2. Only 10–38% of infants and children evaluated in the emergency department (ED) with yellow-green emesis are found to have a surgical emergency.

9. **What information should be obtained during the physical examination of a child with vomiting?**

The physical examination should initially focus on adequacy of perfusion and cardiovascular stability. Then, measures that indicate degree of dehydration should be assessed. The presence of two of the following four findings (dry mucous membranes, absent tears, abnormal lethargy or restlessness, and capillary refill time > 2 seconds) are associated with at least 5% dehydration; the presence of three or more is associated with 5% dehydration or greater. The remainder of the examination should comprehensively assess the abdomen as well as the respiratory, cardiac, and neurologic systems.

Gorelick MH, Shaw KN, Murphy KO: Validity and reliability of clinical signs in the diagnosis of dehydration in children. Pediatrics 99:e6, 1997.

10. **What laboratory tests are indicated in the child with vomiting?**

Laboratory testing in the child with vomiting should be guided by the history and physical examination. In children with significant dehydration or those whose initial assessments suggest causes other than uncomplicated gastroenteritis, carefully selected laboratory tests can provide useful clues or confirm diagnoses (Table 29-3).

Liebelt EL: Clinical and laboratory evaluation and management of children with vomiting, diarrhea and dehydration. Curr Opin Pediatr 10:461–469, 1998.

Orenstein SR, Peters JM: Vomiting and regurgitation. In Kliegman RM, Greenbaum LA, Lye PS (eds): Practical Strategies in Pediatric Diagnosis and Therapy. Philadelphia, WB Saunders, 2004, pp 291–321.

TABLE 29-3. LABORATORY TESTING IN PEDIATRIC PATIENTS WITH VOMITING	
Test	**Diagnostic Utility**
Serum electrolytes	Sodium
	Elevated in hypernatremic dehydration
	Decreased in hyponatremic dehydration, adrenal insufficiency
	Potassium
	Elevated in renal failure, adrenal insufficiency
	Decreased in pyloric stenosis
	Chloride
	Decreased in pyloric stenosis, bulimia
	Bicarbonate
	Elevated in significant or chronic vomiting (e.g., bulimia), pyloric stenosis
	Decreased in inborn metabolic errors, renal tubular acidosis, other causes of metabolic acidosis (sepsis, uremia, toxic ingestions, shock, acute gastroenteritis with dehydration)
	Glucose
	Elevated in diabetic ketoacidosis
	Decreased in inborn metabolic errors, starvation, toxic ingestion
Serum blood urea nitrogen/creatinine	Elevated in dehydration, renal failure
White blood count	Elevated in serious bacterial infection
Urinalysis	Specific gravity: elevated in dehydration
	Glucose with or without ketones: present in diabetes, diabetic ketoacidosis

TABLE 29-3. LABORATORY TESTING IN PEDIATRIC PATIENTS WITH VOMITING— CONT'D

Test	Diagnostic Utility
	Ketones: elevated in starvation, dehydration, inborn metabolic error Red blood cells: renal calculi, nephritis, UTI White blood cells: UTI
Urine pregnancy test	Pregnancy
Amylase, lipase	Elevated in pancreatitis
Aminotransferases	Elevated in hepatitis

UTI = urinary tract infection.

11. **When are radiographic tests indicated in the pediatric patient with vomiting?**
    Radiographic tests may help differentiate causes of vomiting that require surgical intervention from those that do not. Plain radiographs of the abdomen are an appropriate initial study in this clinical situation. A plain abdominal film together with an upright film (or cross-table lateral view in the nonambulatory patient) may demonstrate distended bowel loops or air-fluid levels consistent with obstruction. A plain radiograph may also demonstrate abnormal calcifications, such as renal or biliary stones or fecaliths. Free air may be observed on the upright/cross-table film in the case of hollow viscus perforation. Basilar infiltrates caused by lower-lobe pneumonias may be noted serendipitously on an abdominal film, although chest radiography would be the better diagnostic test for pulmonary pathology.

12. **Which radiographic tests are most useful when further evaluating specific causes of vomiting that may require surgical intervention?**
    See Table 29-4.

    Heller RM, Hermanz-Schulman M: Applications of new imaging modalities to the evaluation of common pediatric conditions. J Pediatr 135:632–639, 1999.

TABLE 29-4. RADIOGRAPHIC STUDIES FOR EVALUATING THE CHILD WITH VOMITING

Clinical Concern	Radiographic Study of Choice
Appendicitis	Abdominal ultrasonography and/or abdominal CT with or without rectal contrast
Intussusception	Abdominal ultrasonography, contrast enema
Malrotation, intestinal atresias	Upper GI series
Pyloric stenosis	Abdominal ultrasound or upper GI series
Renal calculi	Abdominal CT without contrast
Ovarian or uterine pathology	Pelvic ultrasonography
Pancreatic pathology	Abdominal CT with IV and oral contrast
Duodenal hematoma/other intestinal pathology	Abdominal CT with IV and oral contrast
Abdominal mass	Abdominal CT with IV and oral contrast

CT = computed tomography; GI = gastrointestinal.

13. **What treatment is indicated for the infant or child with vomiting?**

Treatment of the infant or child with vomiting is focused first on treating dehydration or maintaining adequate hydration and then on treating the specific cause of the vomiting, when indicated. Dehydration can be treated effectively by either rapid IV rehydration using isotonic crystalloid solution or by appropriately supervised oral rehydration with a suitable rehydration solution. Because most vomiting in children is self-limited or resolves when the underlying cause is treated, antiemetics are not routinely advised, except in specific clinical circumstances (e.g., vomiting from chemotherapy or in the cyclic vomiting syndrome). In children who require ED rehydration during an acute gastrointestinal illness associated with vomiting, randomized controlled trials have demonstrated reductions in emesis and the need for hospitalization with the use of the 5-HT$_3$ receptor antagonist, ondansetron.

Freedman SB, Adler M, Seshadri R, Powell EC: Oral ondansetron for gastroenteritis in a pediatric emergency department. N Engl J Med 354:1698–1705, 2006.

Reeves JJ, Shannon MW, Fleisher GR: Ondansetron decreases vomiting associated with acute gastroenteritis: A randomized controlled trial. Pediatrics 109: e62, 2002.

Reid SR, Bonadio WA: Outpatient rapid intravenous rehydration to correct dehydration and resolve vomiting in children with acute gastroenteritis. Ann Emerg Med 28:318–323, 1996.

KEY POINTS: PYLORIC STENOSIS ✓

1. A high index of suspicion for pyloric stenosis is necessary in young infants who present with vomiting because the characteristic physical examination and laboratory findings may not be present early in the course.

2. Infants with pyloric stenosis always have nonbilious vomiting.

14. **A 6-week-old infant presents with vomiting. What are the important historical findings that will help in distinguishing pyloric stenosis from gastroesophageal reflux?**

The typical history of an infant with pyloric stenosis is that of nonbilious vomiting beginning around 2 weeks of age that worsens in force and volume over the next several weeks. As the degree of obstruction increases, the vomiting becomes projectile and typically occurs during or soon after feeding. Most commonly seen in first-born infants, pyloric stenosis affects males five times more often than females. By contrast, gastroesophageal reflux typically presents soon after birth and is characterized by effortless, nonprogressive spitting up, frequently occurring with burping or within 30–60 minutes after feeding. In most cases, the infant with gastroesophageal reflux will thrive despite the parent's impression that "he's been vomiting everything since birth."

KEY POINTS: INTUSSUSCEPTION ✓

1. The classic triad of intermittent crampy pain, vomiting, and currant jelly stool is seen in only 10–20% of children with intussusception.

2. Intussusception should be considered in any infant or toddler with unexplained lethargy.

15. **What are the important physical examination and laboratory findings that will help distinguish pyloric stenosis from gastroesophageal reflux?**
If the vomiting has progressed significantly, the physical examination in an infant with pyloric stenosis may reveal a fussy, hungry infant who sucks vigorously unless weakened by dehydration. Peristaltic waves may be visible on inspection of the abdomen, and an olive-shaped mass (the hypertrophied pylorus) may be palpable in the subxiphoid region. The classic electrolyte abnormalities noted in pyloric stenosis are hypochloremia, hypokalemia, and metabolic alkalosis.

Papadakis K, Chen EA, Luks FI, et al: The changing presentation of pyloric stenosis. Am J Emerg Med 17:67–69, 1999.

16. **A 12-month-old infant presents with vomiting and intermittent abdominal pain. How will you differentiate gastroenteritis from intussusception in this patient?**
The classic patient with intussusception is between 3 months and 2 years of age and presents with the triad of episodic cramping abdominal pain, vomiting, and bloody ("currant jelly") stools. The pain typically lasts 5–10 minutes and is associated with crouching or drawing legs up, after which the infant may appear well or be lethargic. A tender mass may be palpated in the right upper quadrant, and in 75% of patients the stool will be positive for occult blood or grossly bloody. Early intussusception may be confused with gastroenteritis, although the latter is most often characterized initially by vomiting that progresses to diarrhea, fever, and nonspecific abdominal pain or cramping pain with defecation.

Harrington L, Connolly B, Hu X, et al: Ultrasonographic and clinical predictors of intussusception. J Pediatr 132:836–839, 1998.

17. **An 8-year-old boy presents with headache and vomiting. How will you distinguish vomiting caused by an intracranial mass lesion from that associated with migraine headaches?**
After headache, vomiting is the second most commonly noted symptom in children with intracranial mass lesions. However, vomiting is not likely to be the only abnormality. In >90% of children with vomiting from an intracranial mass, other neurologic or ocular abnormalities will be present. Vomiting that accompanies brain tumors is commonly seen in the mornings, is usually effortless (although it may become projectile), and is not particularly associated with meals or abdominal pain. The vomiting may persist intermittently for weeks. Vomiting associated with migraine headaches is typically associated with infrequent, severe, diffuse headaches that resolve with sleep or when the cephalgia is treated.

Squires RH: Intracranial tumors. Vomiting as a presenting sign. A gastroenterologist's perspective. Clin Pediatr (Phila) 28:351–354, 1989.

ANAPHYLAXIS

Linda D. Arnold, MD

CHAPTER 30

1. **What is anaphylaxis?**

   Anaphylaxis is an acute, systemic allergic reaction with varied mechanisms and clinical presentations. Signs and symptoms develop rapidly as mast cells and basophils release potent biologically active mediators. The acute constellation of symptoms results from the effect of these mediators on multiple target organs, including the skin, the respiratory and gastrointestinal tracts, and the cardiovascular system. Severity can vary from mild to life-threatening or fatal; more severe reactions are characterized by respiratory insufficiency and hemodynamic compromise. "Classic" anaphylaxis refers to IgE-mediated hypersensitivity responses, though other immunopathogenic mechanisms exist.

2. **How common is anaphylaxis?**

   Although frequency and causes vary with the population studied, most estimates of prevalence fall just below 1%. In the United States, food allergies are the most common cause of anaphylaxis, accounting for 30,000 emergency department (ED) visits, 2000 hospitalizations, and 150–200 deaths each year. Among children under age 4 years, 6–8% have documented food allergies, with the rates dropping to 2% after age 10. One percent of people in the United States are allergic to peanuts, tree nuts, or both. Hypersensitivity reactions account for one third of all adverse drug reactions. Serious systemic reactions to hymenoptera stings occur in 0.4–0.8% children and 3% of adults, resulting in approximately 50 deaths each year.

   Sampson HA: Anaphylaxis and emergency treatment. Pediatrics 111:1601–1608, 2003.
   Ellis AK, Day JH: Clinical reactivity to insect stings. Curr Opin Allergy Clin Immunol 5:349–354, 2005.

3. **How dangerous is anaphylaxis?**

   Anaphylaxis often occurs outside of the hospital setting, with case fatality rates of 0.7%. The median time to respiratory or cardiac arrest in fatal cases of anaphylaxis is 5 minutes for reactions to medications or contrast material, 15 minutes for reactions to insect venom, and 30 minutes for reactions to food. Fatal reactions are frequently the first reactions for most sting, medication, and contrast deaths. Most ingestions are inadvertent, and reactions to aerosolized fish and shellfish in restaurants have been reported. The majority of allergic reactions for children take place in school or daycare. In the rare instances when written management plans exist, they are implemented only 75% of the time.

   Sicherer SH, Furlong TJ, DeSimone J, et al: The US peanut and tree nut allergy registry: Characteristics of reactions in schools and day care. J Pediatr 138:560–565, 2001.

4. **What are common causes of anaphylaxis?**

   Food allergies are the leading cause of anaphylaxis for children presenting to EDs in the United States, accounting for a third to a half of such visits. Allergies to peanuts, tree nuts, shellfish, cow's milk, eggs, soy, and wheat are most common. Peanuts and tree nuts alone are responsible for 90% of all food anaphylactic events, with commercial catering implicated in the majority of nut-related reactions.

Among antibiotics, cephalosporins, sulfonamides, and penicillins are most frequently implicated. Insect stings and allergen immunotherapy are also important causes of anaphylaxis. Anaphylaxis to immunizations is rare.

5. **What are some of the causes of anaphylaxis related to medical treatment?**
   - Neuromuscular blockers (succinylcholine, vecuronium, atracurium) account for 60% of episodes of anaphylaxis related to medical treatment.
   - Latex, antibiotics, induction agents (barbiturates, etomidate, propofol) and narcotics (fentanyl, meperidine, morphine) are also important causes.
   - Colloids, opioids, radiocontrast media, and blood products are implicated less than 10% of the time.

   The incidence of latex allergy has leveled off, probably because of increased awareness and the use of latex-free and low-powder gloves. Reactions are more common in atopic individuals, health care workers, and patients with a history of genitourinary surgeries or long-term bladder catheterizations.

   Lieberman P: Anaphylactic reactions during surgical and medical procedures. J Allergy Clin Immunol 110:S64–S69, 2002.

6. **Is there a way to predict who is at risk for more severe anaphylactic reactions?**
   Most deaths from anaphylaxis due to food occur in adolescents and young adults. Patients with poorly controlled asthma and those with a history of previous anaphylaxis are at greater risk. Reactions to peanuts, tree nuts, fish, and shellfish are the most severe, with peanuts and tree nuts responsible for 94% of deaths. The severity of previous episodes does not predict the severity of future reactions, as antigen doses may vary. Large local reactions to stings are not predictive of anaphylaxis to insect venom. Many fatal or near-fatal reactions to foods and insect venom occur in children who have not required previous urgent medical intervention.

   Bock SA, Munoz-Furlong A, Sampson HA: Fatalities due to anaphylactic reactions to food. J Allergy Clin Immunol 108:861–866, 2001.

KEY POINTS: RISK FACTORS FOR SEVERE ANAPHYLAXIS

1. Adolescent or young adult
2. History of previous severe reaction
3. Peanuts, tree nuts, fish, or shellfish as inciting agent
4. Asthma, especially if poorly controlled
5. Taking β-blockers

7. **What are anaphylactoid reactions? How do they differ from anaphylaxis?**
   Anaphylactoid reactions result from non–IgE-mediated degranulation of mast cells or basophils. They are clinically indistinguishable from anaphylaxis, and the treatment is identical. Examples include reactions to nonsteroidal anti-inflammatory drugs (NSAIDs), radiocontrast media, blood products, and exercise.

8. **What are the clinical manifestations of anaphylaxis?**
   Anaphylaxis is characterized by the abrupt onset of symptoms minutes to hours after an ingestion or exposure (Table 30-1). The timing, sequence, and severity of symptoms vary. The shorter the interval between the exposure and the symptoms, the more likely the reaction is to be severe.
   - The oral cavity and throat are affected first, with a tingling or pruritic sensation and edema of the lips or mucosa. Laryngeal and epiglottic edema may develop.
   - Gastrointestinal signs follow and include nausea, vomiting, and colicky pain.
   - Skin symptoms and signs, which may be absent in up to 30% of severe reactions, include flushing, pruritus, and urticaria. The urticaria may be localized or diffuse.
   - Respiratory symptoms, such as stridor or wheezing, may develop in more severe reactions.
   - Dizziness and altered mental status are associated with hypotension, resulting from effects on the cardiovascular system.

TABLE 30-1. CLINICAL SIGNS AND SYMPTOMS OF ANAPHYLAXIS
Oropharyngeal: metallic taste, pruritus, and/or edema of lips, tongue, palate or uvula
Otorhinolaryngologic: congestion, rhinorrhea, pruritus, sneezing, throat tightness, hoarseness, dysphagia
Dermatologic: erythema, pruritus, urticaria, angioedema, morbilliform rash
Gastrointestinal: nausea, colicky abdominal pain, vomiting, diarrhea
Respiratory: cough, shortness of breath, dyspnea, chest tightness, stridor, wheezing
Cardiovascular: faintness, tachycardia, syncope, chest pain, hypotension
Neurologic: headache, mental status changes
General: anxiety, sense of impending doom

9. **What is the differential diagnosis of anaphylaxis?**
   Anaphylaxis must be ruled out first since failure to identify it can have serious consequences for the patient. The differential diagnosis includes:
   - **Scombroid poisoning:** Develops within a half hour of eating spoiled fish; urticaria, nausea, headache, and dizziness occur.
   - **Physical urticaria:** Examples include cold urticaria and cholinergic urticaria.
   - **Near-fatal asthma exacerbations:** Can present with bronchospasm and stridor but usually without a rash.
   - **Angioedema:** The hereditary form is difficult to distinguish from early anaphylaxis.
   - **Panic disorder:** Can present with functional stridor but none of the other symptoms.

   2005 American Heart Association Guidelines for Cardiopulmonary Resuscitation and Emergency Cardiovascular Care. Part 10.6: Anaphylaxis.

10. **How should anaphylaxis be managed?**
    See Table 30-2. The extent and severity of symptoms should be rapidly assessed, with a focus on airway, oxygenation, cardiac output, circulation, and tissue perfusion. A history of any confounding medications should be obtained.
    Administer epinephrine promptly and repeat as necessary. Place patients in a supine position, with legs elevated, to improve venous return and help maintain adequate blood pressure. When hypotension is present, aggressively support the circulation with intravenous crystalloids. Supportive care should include oxygen and bronchodilators for wheezing. Steroids and antihistamines are often administered but have no effect on acute symptoms.

TABLE 30-2. ACUTE MANAGEMENT OF ANAPHYLAXIS
Rapid assessment of ABCs
Place patient in supine position, with legs elevated
Supplemental oxygen and airway management
Epinephrine IM or IV, as indicated
IV fluids for hypotension
Albuterol for bronchospasm
Consider H_1 and H_2 antagonists
Consider IV or PO steroids
Monitor for a minimum of 4 hours for signs of a biphasic reaction

11. **What are the most common errors in the management of anaphylaxis?**
Studies suggest that anaphylaxis is under-recognized and undertreated in both prehospital and ED settings. Delays in initial treatment of anaphylaxis are associated with worse outcomes and higher fatality rates. The more advanced the reaction, the less likely it is to reverse with epinephrine. Failure to administer epinephrine, delayed administration, and errors in dosing and route of administration are all common. Notably, multiple studies have shown that few physicians can demonstrate proper use of an EpiPen, and even fewer have a placebo to demonstrate use to patients and families.

Sampson HA, Munoz-Furlong BA, Bock A, et al: Symposium on the definition and management of anaphylaxis: Summary report. J Allergy Clin Immunol 115:584–591, 2005.

12. **How can severity be determined?**
As a general rule, the rapid onset of symptoms following allergen exposure suggests a more severe or life-threatening reaction. Many different grading systems exist, ranking severity on the basis of the organ systems involved and the presence of respiratory symptoms and hypotension. Reactions that are confined to the skin are classified as mild. Urticaria and angioedema alone are not correlated with hypoxia or hypotension. Moderate reactions are characterized by diaphoresis, throat tightness or respiratory features, and abdominal pain or vomiting. Neurologic changes signify a severe reaction. The presence of airway obstruction in conjunction with cardiovascular symptoms is an ominous sign.

Brown SG: Clinical features and severity grading of anaphylaxis. J Allergy Clin Immunol 114:371–376, 2004.

13. **What are the most common causes of death?**
Most deaths are caused by respiratory arrest or cardiovascular collapse. Severe bronchospasm and upper airway swelling can both lead to asphyxia. Increased vascular permeability can result in transfer of up to 50% of the intravascular fluid into the extravascular space within 10 minutes. Concomitant vasodilation leads to mixed distributive/hypovolemic shock, which may be refractory to aggressive fluid resuscitation and pressor support, particularly in patients taking β-blockers. Direct mediator effects on the myocardium are associated clinically with myocardial ischemia, conduction defects, atrial and ventricular arrhythmias, and T-wave abnormalities.

14. **How does epinephrine work in anaphylactic reactions?**
    Epinephrine is a direct-acting sympathomimetic with complex pharmacologic effects on many target organs. Vasoconstriction, with subsequent reversal of peripheral vasodilation and increases in peripheral vascular resistance, is the primary α effect. β effects include prevention of further mediator release, bronchodilation via smooth muscle relaxation, and increases in heart rate and contractility via direct effects on the myocardium. Clinically, these effects decrease the cutaneous signs of angioedema and urticaria. More importantly, they lead to improvements in cardiovascular function by increasing blood pressure and enhancing coronary blood flow.

KEY POINTS: EPINEPHRINE ✓

1. Most important medication in the treatment of anaphylaxis

2. Reverses bronchospasm by relaxing bronchial smooth muscle

3. Increases blood pressure via peripheral vasoconstriction

4. Increases heart rate and contractility

5. Delays in administration are associated with higher fatality rates

15. **How should epinephrine be administered?**
    Epinephrine should be administered by intramuscular injection at a dose of 0.01 mL/kg body weight of the 1:1000 solution (maximum dose, 0.5 mL). The anterolateral thigh is the preferred injection site because of superior vascularity compared with the deltoid muscle. Doses can be repeated every 5 minutes, as needed. Epinephrine should not be given subcutaneously, as slow absorption by this route leads to extreme delays in peak plasma concentration. IV epinephrine may be required for refractory anaphylaxis; it should be diluted and administered slowly, to minimize the risk of adverse cardiac effects.

16. **When should bronchodilators be used in anaphylaxis?**
    Use intermittent or continuous aerosolized β-adrenergic agents (e.g., albuterol) when wheezing is present.

17. **Are H_1 and H_2 blockers effective in relieving symptoms of anaphylaxis?**
    Histamine is an important mediator in anaphylaxis, producing symptoms of pruritis, rhinorrhea, tachycardia, bronchospasm, headache, flushing, and hypotension. Histamine levels peak early and transiently during anaphylaxis, while the onset of activity for oral diphenhydramine occurs up to an hour after administration. IV diphenhydramine has a faster onset of action, but, it too, is likely of little benefit for all but limited cutaneous reactions. H1 antihistamines may work better in combination with H2 blockers, such as ranitidine or cimetidine, although they have not been shown to reduce the release of mediators, fail to relieve upper airway edema or hypotension, and have little to no role in relieving respiratory or gastrointestinal symptoms.

Simons FE: First-aid treatment of anaphylaxis to food: focus on epinephrine. J Allergy Clin Immunol 113(5):837–844, 2004.

18. **Do steroids have a role in treatment?**
Steroids have no immediate effect in the acute management of anaphylaxis but may help to modulate late-phase responses. Many experts recommend giving prednisone (1–2 mg/kg orally) for mild to moderate reactions, and methylprednisolone (2 mg/kg via IV route) for severe allergic reactions. Despite the lack of supporting evidence, oral steroids are often prescribed for 48–72 hours after the initial episode. Table 30-3 summarizes the drugs used to treat anaphylaxis.

TABLE 30-3. MEDICATIONS USED TO TREAT ANAPHYLAXIS	
Epinephrine:	0.01 mg/kg (1:1000) IM in the anterolateral thigh (max 0.5 mg); repeat q 5 min as needed; 0.01–1.0 µg/kg/min (1:10,000) IV infusion for refractory hypotension
Albuterol:	Intermittent or continuous nebulized solution for bronchospasm
Diphenhydramine:	1 mg/kg PO, IM, or IV (max 75 mg)
Ranitidine:	1–2 mg/kg PO or IV (max 75 mg)
Cimetidine:	5–10 mg/kg PO, IM, or IV (max 300 mg)
Prednisone:	1–2 mg/kg PO (max 75 mg)
Methylprednisolone:	1–2 mg/kg IV (max 125 mg)
Glucagon:	5–15 µg/min IV infusion for refractory hypotension
Dopamine:	2–20 µg/kg/min IV infusion for refractory hypotension

19. **Are laboratory tests ever helpful?**
In a word: no. Though histamine levels rise dramatically in the setting of acute anaphylaxis, it is only for a few minutes, and special collection techniques are required for measurement. During reactions due to drugs and bee stings, plasma tryptase levels become elevated within an hour, and stay elevated for up to 12 hours. Tryptase is stable at room temperature and post mortem (i.e., levels may be helpful retrospectively in establishing a cause of sudden death). Notably, tryptase levels are not elevated in food-related anaphylaxis.

20. **What are some unusual causes of anaphylaxis in children?**
- **Exercise-induced anaphylaxis** develops when exercise follows the ingestion of a specific food to which an individual is sensitive. Symptoms may appear up to 4 hours after exercise stops. Generalized itching and flushing herald the onset of upper respiratory tract obstruction and hypotension. Management includes prompt cessation of exercise and administration of epinephrine. Vascular and airway support should be provided, if indicated. Antihistamines are partially effective at preventing exercise-induced anaphylaxis. Other measures include avoiding exercise 4–6 hours after eating and avoidance of aspirin and NSAIDs prior to exercise, as they may potentiate the reaction.
- **Cold urticaria** is an acute reaction to cold temperatures. When generalized such as in an immersion in a cold body of water, an anaphylactic reaction can be precipitated.

Hosey RG, Carek PJ, Goo A: Exercise-induced anaphylaxis and urticaria. Am Fam Phys 64:1367–1372, 2001.

Stevenson M, Ruddy R: Asthma and allergic emergencies. In Fleisher G, Ludwig S, Henretig F (eds): The Textbook of Pediatric Emergency Medicine, 5th ed. Lippincott Williams & Wilkins, Philadelphia, 2006, pp 1077–1081.

21. **What are biphasic anaphylactic reactions?**

Classically, anaphylaxis is monophasic, with complete resolution within 2 hours of treatment. Biphasic reactions occur in 6–20% of patients, with recurrence of symptoms 2–72 hours after initial complete resolution, without a new exposure. Management may be complicated by a poor response to epinephrine and by severe bronchospasm, which is refractory to β-agonists. The likelihood of a biphasic reaction cannot be predicted on the basis of the severity of the initial episode, though more epinephrine may have been required to alleviate the initial symptoms. Prompt administration of epinephrine during the initial episode is associated with decreased occurrence of biphasic reactions, while steroids have no effect.

Shimamoto SR, Bock SA: Update on the clinical features of food-induced anaphylaxis. Curr Opin Allergy Clin Immunol 2:211–216, 2002.

22. **How long should therapy for anaphylaxis be continued?**

Duration of therapy depends on the severity of the anaphylactic reaction. Therapy with antihistamines or steroids, if initiated, is commonly continued for 48–72 hours after the exposure.

23. **Which patients with an anaphylactic reaction should be admitted?**

Children presenting with allergic reactions should be observed at least 4 hours for progression of symptoms or biphasic response. Those who have had a mild reaction, responded quickly to therapy, and can be closely monitored at home can then be discharged with detailed instructions about signs and symptoms of recurrence. Children who present with severe reactions, have a history of severe reactions, or are judged to be unable to return if symptoms recur should be admitted to the hospital or an extended-stay unit for observation.

24. **Will children "outgrow" their sensitivities?**

Conventional wisdom is that food allergies associated with milder symptoms, such as egg, milk, and soybean, are often outgrown. Persistent sensitivity is more common in allergies to peanuts, tree nuts, fish and shellfish, though recent studies suggest that up to a third of children may "outgrow" their peanut allergies. Tolerance to peanuts is more likely to develop in those whose initial presentations were milder. Despite this, parents should remain vigilant. Half of children with peanut allergy may experience life-threatening symptoms with repeat exposures—even when symptoms with the initial exposure were mild.

Kemp SF, Lockey RF: Anaphylaxis: A review of causes and mechanisms. J Allergy Clin Immunol 110:341–348, 2002.

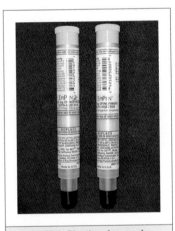

Figure 30-1. Directions for use of EpiPen or EpiPen Jr. (1) Unscrew yellow or green cap and remove autoinjector from case. (2) Form a fist around the unit, with black tip pointing downward. (3) Pull off the gray safety cap with other hand. (4) Firmly jab unit, at a 90 degree angle, into anterolateral thigh. (5) After a click is heard, hold firmly in place for 10 seconds. (6) Remove unit and massage area for 10 seconds. (7) Call 911 and seek immediate medical attention.

25. **Who should be discharged with EpiPens? What instructions should be given for their use?**

Prescribe autoinjectable epinephrine (Fig. 30-1) for children who have had an anaphylactic reaction and who have a history of wheezing, a personal or family history of a severe reaction, or an allergy to peanuts, tree nuts, fish or shellfish. Train parents to administer intramuscular epinephrine during an acute event when a child experiences worrisome symptoms or has a history of severe anaphylaxis to that agent. The threshold should be lower if nonmedical people are with the child; the reaction is from peanuts, nuts, or seafood; or when the reaction occurs in a location that is more than 15 minutes from a medical facility. After epinephrine administration, the child should be taken to the hospital immediately. Doses may be repeated every 15–20 minutes as needed.

26. **What is the optimal dosing for EpiPens?**
Autoinjectable epinephrine comes in just two unit doses. The EpiPen Jr. contains 0.15 mg of epinephrine, ideal for a 15-kg child. EpiPen contains 0.3 mg of epinephrine, dosed for those who weigh 30 kg or more. In practice, the EpiPen Jr. is generally prescribed for children between 10 and 20 kg and the EpiPen for those who weigh more than 28 kg. For those in between, the dosage should be based on the assessed risk of a severe anaphylactic reaction, taking both history and specific agents into account. For children under 10 kg, parents should be taught to draw a weight-based dose of epinephrine up into a syringe, with the knowledge that this process takes longer and is prone to more errors.

Free EpiPen training videos and demonstration sets are available for parents and child care workers who are in need of hands-on experience.

Kim JS, Sinacore JM, Pongracic JA: Parental use of EpiPen for children with food allergies. J Allergy Clin Immunol 116:164–168, 2005.

Simons FER, Chan ES, Gu X, et al: Epinephrine for the out-of-hospital (first aid) treatment of anaphylaxis in infants: Is the ampule/syringe/needle method practical? J Allergy Clin Immunol 108:1040–1044, 2001.

27. **What other discharge instructions should be given?**
All patients must be discharged with a friend or family member who has been instructed to watch for signs and symptoms of a biphasic reaction. Include a written emergency action plan, to be accessible at all times, with a detailed treatment plan, including medications prescribed and indications for their usage. Provide education on allergen avoidance, particularly with respect to cross-contamination of food during processing in factories and preparation in restaurants. Educational resources are helpful in this regard. A referral to an allergist should be made or strongly recommended.

KEY POINTS: DISCHARGE INSTRUCTIONS FOLLOWING ANAPHYLAXIS ✓

1. Instruct a family member to watch for signs of a biphasic reaction.
2. Outline a specific management plan for future reactions, including names and doses of medications.
3. Provide education on allergen avoidance.
4. Prescribe autoinjectable epinephrine for patients at risk of a severe reaction, and demonstrate its usage prior to discharge.
5. Refer to an allergist.

HELPFUL WEBSITES

1. The Food Allergy & Anaphylaxis Network
   www.foodallergy.org

2. The National Agricultural Library: Allergies
   www.nal.usda.gov/fnic
   http://fnic.nal.usda.gov

CHAPTER 31

CARDIAC EMERGENCIES

Sarah W. Alander, MD, and James Edward Hulse III, MD

1. **What are the new pediatric advanced life support (PALS) recommendations regarding the use of endotracheal tube resuscitation medications?**

   The IV or intraosseous (IO) route of administration is preferred. The endotracheal tube (ETT) doses of resuscitation medications are not listed in the updated advanced cardiac life support algorithm for pulseless arrest. They may be used if IV or IO access is not obtained. The thinking is that drugs administered into the trachea result in a lower blood concentration than the same dose given via the IV route. Lower epinephrine concentrations may produce transient β-adrenergic effects, leading to hypotension and reduced coronary artery perfusion pressure.

   American Heart Association: Currents in Emergency Cardiovascular Care. 16:2005–2006. Available at www.americanheart.org/downloadable/heart/1132621842912Winter2005.pdf.

2. **If ETT resuscitation medications are used, how does the technique differ compared with the previous PALS recommendations?**

   The recommended dose should be diluted in water or normal saline and injected *directly* into the ETT. Previously, health care providers were urged to pass a catheter beyond the tip of the tracheal tube to inject the drugs.

   American Heart Association: Currents in Emergency Cardiovascular Care. 16:2005–2006. Available at www.americanheart.org/presenter.jhtml?identifier=3012268.

3. **Is high-dose epinephrine still recommended in pediatric cardiac arrest?**

   The 2005 American Heart Association recommendation is as follows: Use a standard dose of epinephrine (0.01 mg/kg body weight via IV/IO route) for the first and subsequent doses. There is no survival benefit from use of high-dose epinephrine, and it may be harmful, particularly in patients with asphyxia.

   American Heart Association: Currents in Emergency Cardiovascular Care. 16:2005–2006. Available at www.americanheart.org/presenter.jhtml?identifier=3012268.

4. **What is bradycardia? When is it a significant threat to the health and well-being of patients?**

   The definition of bradycardia is a heart rate less than 80 beats per minute in newborns and less than 60 beats per minute in infants and children. It is significant when it results in symptoms of shock such as hypotension, acidosis, lethargy, and coma.

5. **What are indications for emergency or urgent intervention in a patient with bradycardia?**

   Intervention is necessary in the bradycardic patient with a history of syncope or with symptoms of poor perfusion (decreased capillary refill, hypotension, and altered consciousness).

6. **What are the initial steps in treatment for a patient with hemodynamically compromising bradycardia?**

   Assess the airway. Remove any foreign body from the airway, if present, and reposition the patient (jaw-thrust maneuver). After securing a patent airway, assist respiration with 100%

oxygen, and perform chest compressions for heart rate < 80 beats per minute in newborns, < 60 beats per minute in infants and children. Give atropine (0.002 mg/kg via IV route, with 0.1 mg as minimum dose and 0.5 mg as maximum dose) or epinephrine (1:10,000, 0.01 mg/kg via IV route). Recall that both atropine and epinephrine can be given via IV, IO, or endotracheal route. However, IV and IO routes are preferred.

7. **What criteria are considered absolute indications for implantation of a permanent pacemaker for rate support?**
   Patients with a history of syncope or symptoms related to bradycardia should not be released from the emergency department (ED) until close cardiology follow-up has been arranged. Absolute indications for permanent pacemaker include the following:
   - Complete heart block with history of syncope or symptoms
   - Heart block after repaired congenital heart disease
   - Heart block in an infant with associated congenital heart disease
   - Heart block in an infant younger than 6 months of age with a sustained heart rate less than 55 beats per minute

KEY POINTS: CAUSES OF BRADYCARDIA IN CHILDREN ✔

1. Noncardiac: Hypoxemia (most common), central nervous system insult, sepsis, hypothermia, poisoning, anorexia nervosa, hypothyroidism
2. Cardiac: Cardiomyopathy, complete heart block, sick sinus syndrome

8. **Give the corrected QT criteria for determining prolongation of the QT interval for differences between children and adults and between males and females.**
   Corrected QT is the calculation of QT measured/RR interval.
   - In children and infants, the maximum normal corrected QT interval (QTc) is 440 msec.
   - In adolescent and adult males, it is 450 msec.
   - In adolescent and adult females, it is 460 msec.

   Case CL: Diagnosis and treatment of pediatric arrhythmias. Pediatr Clin North Am 46:347–354, 1999.

9. **List the associated electrocardiographic findings that may be useful clues to help establish the diagnosis of long QT syndrome.**
   - Torsades de pointes
   - Intermittent T-wave inversions (T-wave alternans)
   - Notched T waves
   - Low heart rate for age

10. **What history in a patient presenting with sudden and unexpected syncope would make you consider familial long QT syndrome?**
    - History of sudden unexplained death in an immediate family member under the age of 30
    - Definite family history of long QT syndrome or familial deafness
    - An episode of syncope precipitated by sudden stress or startle

11. **What is the first treatment for patients with known familial long QT syndrome?**
    First-line treatment is a β-blocker, such as propanolol (2–4 mg/kg/day). In adolescents, a once-daily dose of long-acting propanolol can be used. Treatment should be instituted regardless of presence or absence of symptoms.

12. **List several reasons for an abnormally long QTc interval that is not due to familial long QT syndrome.**
    - Electrolyte disturbances such as hypomagnesemia, hypocalcemia, hypokalemia
    - Central nervous system insult (increased intracranial pressure, hypoxia)
    - Anorexia nervosa or liquid protein diets
    - Many drug ingestions

13. **What is the most common arrhythmia in childhood?**
    Supraventricular tachycardia.

14. **What is the usual heart rate for infants and children with supraventricular tachycardia (SVT)?**
    Infants with SVT have heart rates of 220–230 beats per minute. Heart rates of older children are 150–250 beats per minute.

15. **What is the most likely presentation for children with SVT?**
    Older children may report chest pain, palpitations, or dizziness. Infants may present with tachypnea, irritability or lethargy, poor perfusion, and other signs of congestive heart failure.

16. **What are the preferred vagal maneuvers used to convert SVT to normal sinus rhythm in infants and children?**
    - Consider vagal maneuvers if the patient is stable and without symptoms.
    - Application of a bag of ice with water to the face for 15–30 seconds is effective in 30–60% of patients.
    - In infants, rectal stimulation with a thermometer may be effective.
    - In children, the Valsalva maneuver via bearing down for 15–20 seconds provides vagal stimulation.
    - Orbital pressure and carotid massage are *not* recommended in children.

    Kugler JD, Danford DA: Management of infants, children, and adolescents with paroxysmal supraventricular tachycardia. J Pediatr 129:324, 1996.

17. **Which medication is the treatment of choice for SVT?**
    Adenosine (0.1 mg/kg) given as a rapid IV bolus, followed by an immediate bolus of saline, 5 mL. This prevents metabolism of adenosine by red blood cells before it reaches the heart. Double the dose of adenosine if conversion is unsuccessful. Adenosine has been reported to terminate atrioventricular reentrant tachycardia in 85–90% of cases. SVT recurs soon after termination in 25–30% of cases.

    Losek JD, Endom E, Dietrich A, et al: Adenosine and pediatric supraventricular tachycardia in the emergency department: Multicenter study and review. Ann Emerg Med 33:185, 1999.

18. **Which initial steps should be performed in the management of a pediatric patient presenting with an excessively fast heart rate?**
    As with all emergencies, establish ABCs first. Then perform synchronized cardioversion for the hemodynamically compromised patient. If the patient appears stable, obtain a brief history directed toward the underlying cause, such as dehydration or blood loss, febrile illness, and exposure to toxins or drug overdose. Obtain an electrocardiogram (ECG) and IV access. Assess the ECG for wide versus narrow tachycardia, rate for age, and rhythm. Remember that infants and children tolerate much more rapid rates than adolescents and adults.

19. **Describe the appropriate treatment of a patient presenting with hemodynamic compromise (unconsciousness, shock, and disorientation) due to excessively fast rhythm (either wide or narrow complex tachycardia).**
Maintain a patent airway, assist breathing with 100% oxygen, and treat with synchronized cardioversion with an initial energy dose of 0.5–1 J/kg. If this is not effective, increase the dose to 2 J/kg.

20. **Give the initial rhythm differential diagnosis for patients presenting with sustained wide complex tachycardia.**
Unlike in adults, the definition of wide QRS is not always a duration longer than 100 msec. The normal QRS duration increases with age. The infant or small child may have a widened QRS complex (abnormal ventricular activation) *without* duration longer than 100 msec.
   Regardless of the patient's level of consciousness, consider ventricular tachycardia (VT) first in the patient with wide complex tachycardia. Other causes include SVT with bundle-branch block or SVT with aberrant conduction.

21. **Describe the initial treatment/assessment plans for a patient presenting with sustained wide complex tachycardia not associated with hemodynamic compromise.**
Assess ABCs. Consider VT first, and give amiodarone, 5 mg/kg over 20–60 minutes, *or* procainamide, 15 mg/kg via IV route over 30–60 minutes, *or* lidocaine, 1 mg/kg via IV bolus.

   American Heart Association: Handbook of Emergency Cardiovascular Care For Healthcare Providers. Dallas, TX, American Heart Association, 2006.

KEY POINTS: WIDE COMPLEX TACHYCARDIA ✔

1. Causes may be VT, SVT with bundle-branch block, or SVT with aberrant conduction.

2. Assume VT, regardless of clinical status of patient, and give lidocaine.

22. **Define congestive heart failure. List signs and symptoms in infants or small children.**
Congestive heart failure is the pathophysiologic state in which the heart is unable to pump enough blood to meet metabolic demands. The primary symptoms in infants are tachycardia (heart rate > 160 beats per minute) and respiratory distress, indicated by tachypnea and grunting. The infant may have hepatomegaly and decreased capillary refill as well. Older children have tachycardia with heart rate > 100 beats per minute, extra heart sounds (S_3 and S_4), and decreased capillary refill. They may also have peripheral edema and ascites.

23. **What are the most likely causes of heart failure in neonates presenting to the ED?**
Structural congenital heart disease is the most likely cause of heart failure in the neonate. In the first week of life, transposition of the great vessels or total anomalous pulmonary venous return are the most likely causes. Between weeks 1 and 4, critical aortic stenosis or pulmonary stenosis or preductal coarctation of the aorta is the most likely cause.

   Lee C, Mason LJ: Pediatric cardiac emergencies. Anesth Clin North Am 19:287–308, 2001.

24. **What is the clinical presentation of the neonate with congestive heart failure?**
Congestive heart failure in the very young infant is easily confused with sepsis, meningitis, pneumonia, or bronchiolitis. Affected infants have a history of poor feeding, grunting, tachypnea, tachycardia, pulmonary rales, or rhonchi. Presence of hepatomegaly, weak or absent peripheral pulses, and cardiomegaly on chest radiograph help to distinguish heart failure from other illnesses. Echocardiography confirms the diagnosis.

25. **What is the initial ED management of the neonate with congestive heart failure?**
Secure the airway and ventilate. Administer oxygen to maintain SaO_2 at 75–80%.
Obtain IV access and administer prostaglandin E_1 (0.05 µg/kg/min) to reopen the ductus arteriosus.

26. **Describe the difference between "digoxin effect" and "digoxin toxicity"—both clinically and in terms of ECG findings.**
The patient who is therapeutic while receiving digoxin may show ST segments that are depressed and concave upward. The QT interval is shortened, and the PR interval is increased. Heart rate decreases. The patient with significant digoxin toxicity may present with nausea and vomiting. The ECG may show profound sinus bradycardia, atrioventricular block, or tachyarrhythmia (junctional tachycardia).

27. **List the expected ECG findings or clinical manifestations of patients who have received overdoses of the following medications:**
   - **β-blockers:** Bradycardia, increased PR interval
   - **Calcium-channel blockers:** Bradycardia, prolonged atrioventricular node conduction or block
   - **Tricyclic antidepressants:** Tachycardia, prolonged QRS, decreased atrioventricular conduction time, VT, ventricular fibrillation, torsades de pointes
   - **Phenothiazines:** QTc prolongation, torsades de pointes
   - **Type 1A antiarrhythmic medications (quinidine, procainamide, disopyramide):** Prolongation of QT interval, torsades de pointes, and ventricular tachycardia
   - **Amiodarone:** Atrioventricular block, sinus node dysfunction (marked bradycardia), torsades de pointes

   Clancy C: Electrocardiographic evaluation of the poisoned or overdosed patient. In Goldfrank LR, Flomenbaum NE, Lewin NA, et al (eds): Goldfrank's Toxicologic Emergencies, 6th ed. Stamford, CT, Appleton and Lange, 2002, pp 105–128.

28. **What potential long-term cardiac toxicity is likely in a patient who has a history of previously treated cancer?**
Cardiomyopathy has been described in patients who have been treated with anthracyclines such as doxorubicin and daunomycin. Pericarditis may be seen in patients who have had mediastinal radiation.

29. **List some of the late complications after the Fontan operation that may be encountered in the ED.**
   - **Supraventricular arrhythmias:** Atrial flutter, atrioventricular reentry tachycardia, atrial ectopic tachycardia, pleural effusions
   - **Thromboembolic complications:** Cerebrovascular accident, inferior or superior vena cava syndrome, pulmonary embolus

- Protein-losing enteropathy
- Pulmonary arteriovenous fistulas

    Tsai W, Klein B: The postoperative cardiac patient. Clin Pediatr Emerg Med 6:216–221, 2005.

30. **Describe the ECG changes seen at varying levels of hyperkalemia.**
    K^+ 5–6 mEq/L: Peaked T waves
    K^+ > 6 mEq/L: ORS widening
    K^+ > 7 mEq/L: Increased P-R interval
    K^+ 8–9 mEq/L: Disappearance of P waves and irregular ventricular rate
    K^+ 12–14 mEq/L: Ventricular fibrillation or asystole

    Gewitz M, Woolf P: Cardiac emergencies. In Fleisher G, Ludwig S, Henretig F (eds): The Textbook of Pediatric Emergency Medicine, 5th ed. Philadelphia, Lippincott Williams & Wilkins, 2006, p. 744.

31. **What is the most common cause of chest pain in children?**
    Parents often fear chest pain as a sign of cardiac disease. Fortunately, most chest pain in children is noncardiac in origin. The most common causes are idiopathic chest pain, musculoskeletal, costochondritis, asthma, gastroesophageal reflux and esophagitis, pneumonia, and pneumothorax.

32. **What are cardiac causes of chest pain in children?**
    Obstructive hypertrophic cardiomyopathy, aortic stenosis, pericarditis, arrhythmias, coronary insufficiency, and mitral valve prolapse can all cause chest pain.

33. **What are the cutaneous criteria of rheumatic fever?**
    Erythema marginatum and subcutaneous nodules. Erythema marginatum appears on the trunk and proximal extremities and is evanescent. It is described as a lacy rash and is not pruritic. Subcutaneous nodules are found over extensor aspects of joints, such as the elbows. They are firm and mobile.

34. **How does a child with myocarditis present?**
    The manifestations of myocarditis are very nonspecific; the affected child often presents with symptoms of congestive heart failure. Also consider the diagnosis of myocarditis in a child with unexplained tachypnea and tachycardia or a new onset of sustained arrhythmia. A low-grade fever is often present. Some children report chest pain, or possibly back pain.

35. **What are the ECG findings of myocarditis?**
    The ECG findings are nonspecific, adding to the diagnostic dilemma. Delayed atrioventricular conduction (AV block), prolongation of QTc, decreased amplitude of the T wave, low QRS amplitude (5 mm or less in all six limb leads), arrhythmias, or ectopic beats may all be seen in the patient with myocarditis.

36. **Describe the two murmurs that may be heard in a patient with tetralogy of Fallot.**
    Classically, tetralogy of Fallot consists of pulmonic stenosis, ventricular septal defect (VSD), dextroposition of the aorta, and right ventricular hypertrophy. The two murmurs are of pulmonic stenosis and VSD. The VSD murmur is generally early to holosystolic, harsh, and heard best at the lower left sternal border. The pulmonic stenosis murmur is a high-pitched, systolic ejection murmur that is best heard at the upper left sternal border and radiates to the left infraclavicular area. It is a crescendo-decrescendo type.

37. **What is a hypercyanotic, or "tet," spell?**

   A "tet" spell is an episode of cyanosis that occurs in the infant or small child with uncorrected tetralogy of Fallot. Such spells can occur in both acyanotic patients ("pink tets") and in patients who are consistently cyanotic. The underlying problem is a decrease in pulmonary blood flow, probably due to a spasm of the infundibular muscle, thus obstructing the right ventricular outflow tract. The spells occur most often in the morning after awakening, may be precipitated by activity and are heralded by the infant becoming fussy. As the hypoxemia worsens, the infant may become lethargic or unconscious.

38. **How should a tet spell be managed initially?**

   Place the infant in knee-chest position, either prone with the knees brought up under the abdomen or held against an adult's chest with the knees drawn up. Administer oxygen and give morphine sulfate (0.1–0.2 mg/kg via intramuscular or subcutaneous route).

39. **What is the mechanism of action of morphine in alleviating a tet spell?**

   Morphine may help either because of its negative inotropic effect on the infundibular myocardium or by breaking the cycle of agitation that leads to an increased oxygen requirement.

40. **When should echocardiography be performed in a patient with suspected Kawasaki disease?**

   An echocardiogram should be obtained as soon as Kawasaki disease is suspected. It may help to confirm the disease; if the disease is certain, it allows a baseline evaluation of cardiac function.

   Newburger JW, Takahashi M, Gerber MA, et al: Diagnosis, treatment, and long-term management of Kawasaki disease: A statement for health professionals from the Committee on Rheumatic Fever, Endocarditis, and Kawasaki Disease, Council on Cardiovascular Disease in the Young, American Heart Association. Circulation 110:2747, 2004.

41. **What are the cardiac complications of Kawasaki disease?**

   - Coronary artery aneurysm (major complication)
   - Decreased myocardial contractility
   - Pericardial effusion
   - Mild valvular disease
   - Coronary arteritis

   Sundel R: Clinical manifestations and diagnosis of Kawasaki's disease, 2006. Available at www.uptodate.com.

42. **What are the cardiac conditions causing sudden death in young athletes?**

   - Hypertrophic cardiomyopathy
   - Coronary artery anomalies
   - Myocarditis
   - Aortic rupture (Marfan syndrome)
   - Commotio cordis
   - Arrhythmogenic right ventricular hypertrophy

   Maron BJ, Shirani J, Poliac LC, et al: Sudden death in young competitive athletes. Clinical, demographic, and pathological profiles. JAMA 276:199–204, 1996.

43. **What is the most common cause of sudden cardiac death in the pediatric population?**

Hypertrophic cardiomyopathy is the most common cause of sudden cardiac death in children and adolescents, accounting for about half of the 500 annual deaths. There currently are no guidelines for screening of athletes, although the ECG will be abnormal in 75–95% of cases.

Berger S, Kugler J, Thomas J, et al: Sudden cardiac death in children and adolescents: Introduction and overview. Pediatr Clin North Am 51:1201–1210, 2004.

44. **What are the common ECG findings in children with hypertrophic cardiomyopathy?**

The ECG shows left ventricular hypertrophy in most patients with hypertrophic cardiomyopathy. Echocardiography provides definitive diagnosis.

CHAPTER 32

CENTRAL NERVOUS SYSTEM EMERGENCIES

Nanette C. Dudley, MD

1. **Describe the physical findings in Bell's palsy.**
   Bell's palsy refers to peripheral facial nerve weakness on one side of the face, including inability to wrinkle the forehead on the affected side, inability to close the affected eye, and flattening of the affected nasolabial fold. Bell's palsy may also involve hyperacusis in the affected ear (noises sound excessively loud) because the site of injury is thought to be in the facial canal and may involve other branches of C7—including those to the stapedius muscle, which dampens sound waves.

2. **What is the definition of status epilepticus?**
   Seizures that are continuous for 30 minutes or longer or that are repetitive with the patient not regaining consciousness are defined as status epilepticus.

   Tharp BR: Clinical features and complications of status epilepticus in children, 2006. Available at www.uptodate.com.

3. **What is Todd's paralysis?**
   Todd's paralysis refers to paresis or paralysis of one or more areas of the body that is transient, usually disappearing within 24 hours following a seizure.

4. **A child is having an acute seizure. You know that IV access will not be possible quickly. What are your options?**
   - Rectal diazepam
   - Intranasal midazolam
   - Buccal midazolam
   - Intraosseous access (any medication listed in Table 32-1 can be given through an intraosseous line)

   Wiznitzer M: Buccal midazolam for seizures. Lancet 366:182–183, 2005.

5. **List the drugs commonly used to stop seizures acutely in the emergency department (ED).**
   See Table 32-1.

6. **Describe the characteristics of absence (petit mal) seizures.**
   Absence seizures usually develop in school-age children before puberty. The seizures are characteristically of abrupt onset with a brief loss of consciousness. Most are less than 30 seconds in duration. Children may appear to be staring or may have eye blinking or rhythmic nodding. The child does not fall, although he or she may drop things. These seizures are often easily precipitated by having the child hyperventilate.

7. **What are infantile spasms?**
   Infantile spasms are characteristic seizures usually beginning when a baby is 4–7 months old. The seizures are usually of sudden onset and generalized, with bilateral and symmetric contraction of the muscles in the neck, trunk, and extremities. The initial contraction typically lasts < 2 seconds and is then followed by a sustained contraction of 2–10 seconds. Patients

TABLE 32-1. DRUGS COMMONLY USED TO STOP SEIZURES IN THE EMERGENCY DEPARTMENT

Drug	Dose	Route	Maximum Dose
Lorazepam	0.05–0.1 mg/kg	IV	4 mg
Diazepam	0.05–0.3 mg/kg	IV	10 mg
	0.5 mg/kg	PR	
Midazolam	0.05–0.3 mg/kg	IV/IM	10 mg
	0.2 mg/kg	IN	
Phenytoin	15–20 mg/kg	IV	1000 mg
Fosphenytoin	15–20 PE/kg	IV	1000 mg
Phenobarbital	15–20 mg/kg	IV, IM	1000 mg

The latter three drugs have a longer onset of action (10–20 min) and are better second-line therapy. IM = intramuscular, IN = intranasal, PE = phenytoin sodium equivalents, PR = per rectum. (From Gorelick MH, Blackwell CD: Neurologic emergencies. In Fleisher GR, Ludwig S, Henretig FM [eds]: Textbook of Pediatric Emergency Medicine, 5th ed. Philadelphia, Lippincott Williams & Wilkins, 2006, pp 759–781.)

with infantile spasms have a poor developmental prognosis, and 65–90% are developmentally delayed at the time of diagnosis.

Glaze DG: Management and prognosis of infantile spasms, 2006. Available at www.uptodate.com.

8. **A 16-year-old boy presents after an early-morning generalized tonic clonic seizure. On history, he describes occasional, brief, jerking movements in the morning that make teeth brushing and hair combing difficult. These jerking movements resolve and do not recur later in the day. What does this symptom pattern suggest?**
Juvenile myoclonic epilepsy most commonly presents between 12 and 18 years of age with brief, bilateral flexor jerking movements of the arms. The seizures can be precipitated by sleep deprivation, alcohol ingestion, and awakening from sleep. Patients may have generalized tonic clonic seizures but are normal neurologically.

Yu KT: Approach to the child with seizures. In Osborn LM, Dewitt TG, First LR, Zenel JA (eds): Pediatrics. St. Louis, Elsevier Mosby, 2005, pp 752–756.

9. **How are seizures distinguished from breath-holding spells?**
Involuntary muscular contractions occur in both, although they are more prominent with seizures. In breath-holding spells, these contractions are due to transient cerebral hypoperfusion. With breath-holding spells, a precipitating event causes the child to cry or be angry or frustrated, and thus hold his or her breath or perform the Valsalva maneuver. Seizures usually do not have an obvious precipitating event. Breath-holding spells are usually brief, and may feature a short period of sleepiness afterwards. Seizures may be brief, but suspicion for a seizure disorder occurs when the episode lasts > 1 minute or if the postictal period is prolonged. Finally, breath-holding spells usually occur in children 6 months to 4 years of age; episodes outside these limits are more suspicious for seizures.

10. **What are the indications for urgent computed tomography (CT) after a seizure?**
    - Postictal focal neurologic deficits not quickly resolving
    - Signs of increased intracranial pressure
    - More than a transient change in level of consciousness
    - Posttraumatic seizures (not impact seizures)

    Magnetic resonance imaging (MRI) is the preferred study in all cases but is usually not immediately available in the emergency setting. Patient stability may also be a factor, as CT is typically faster and often does not require sedation.

    Hirtz D, Ashwal S, Berg A, et al: Practice parameter: Evaluating a first nonfebrile seizure in children. Neurology 55:616–623, 2000.

11. **What are the indications for nonurgent MRI after a seizure?**
    - Focal features of the seizure
    - Cognitive or motor impairment of unknown etiology
    - Changes in seizure character, neurologic examination, or electroencephalogram
    - Age < 1 year

    MRI testing for the preceding indications avoids unnecessary radiation exposure from CT.

    Hirtz D, Ashwal S, Berg A, et al: Practice parameter: Evaluating a first nonfebrile seizure in children. Neurology 55:616–623, 2000.

12. **What is the incidence of febrile seizures? When do they occur?**
    About 3–4% of all children have a febrile seizure; most occur in children between the ages of 6 months and 5 years.

    American Academy of Pediatrics. Available at www.aap.org/patiented/febrileseizures.htm.

13. **What makes a febrile seizure "simple" or "complex"?**
    A **simple febrile seizure** has all of the following characteristics:
    - The seizure is brief (< 15 minutes).
    - The seizure is generalized.
    - The child appears well shortly after the seizure stops.

    A **complex febrile seizure** has at least one of the following characteristics:
    - The seizure is prolonged (> 15 minutes).
    - The seizure is focal.
    - The child has two or more seizures in one day.

14. **What is the recurrence risk for a febrile seizure?**
    Approximately 30%. This number varies by age at onset of first febrile seizure.

15. **Is the risk of recurrence increased if the initial febrile seizure is complex?**
    No. Children at greater risk of recurrence may have one or more of the following features:
    - Young age at onset
    - History of febrile seizures in a first-degree relative
    - Lack of hyperpyrexia in the ED
    - Brief duration between the onset of fever and the initial seizure

    Berg AT, Shinnar S, Darefsky AS, et al: Predictors of recurrent febrile seizures. A prospective cohort study. Arch Pediatr Adolesc Med 151:371–378, 1997.

16. **Is the risk of epilepsy increased in children with febrile seizures?**
    Yes, but to a small degree. The risk of epilepsy in the general population of children without febrile seizures is 0.5%, which increases to 2–4% in children with febrile seizures. If there is

a family history of epilepsy, and if the child has a neurologic disorder or developmental delay, then the risk of a subsequent afebrile seizure increases to 10%.

Waruiru C, Appleton R: Febrile seizures: An update. Arch Dis Child 89:751–756, 2004.

17. **What tests should be performed on children after a simple febrile seizure?**
There is no need for brain imaging studies or electroencephalography after a simple febrile seizure. Laboratory testing or radiography should be performed as appropriate for the diagnosis and management of the cause of the fever.

American Academy of Pediatrics, Provisional Committee on Quality Improvement, Subcommittee on Febrile Seizures: Practice Parameter: The neurodiagnostic evaluation of the child with a first simple febrile seizure. Pediatrics 97:769–772, 1996.

18. **When should you consider a lumbar puncture in a child with a febrile seizure?**
   - History concerning for meningitis
   - Cranky, irritable child who is difficult to console
   - Meningeal signs or bulging fontanelle
   - Young age, making evaluation difficult (generally < 12 months of age)
   - Prolonged or serial seizures (particularly if postictal state is prolonged)
   - Pretreatment with antibiotics

American Academy of Pediatrics, Provisional Committee on Quality Improvement, Subcommittee on Febrile Seizures: Practice Parameter: The neurodiagnostic evaluation of the child with a first simple febrile seizure. Pediatrics 97:769–772, 1996.

19. **In a child with suspected meningitis, what are some contraindications to performing an immediate lumbar puncture?**
   - Focal neurologic findings on examination
   - Evidence of spinal cord trauma
   - Infection in the tissues near the puncture site
   - Focal seizures
   - Coma
   - Papilledema
   - Severe coagulation defects (not corrected)
   - Cardiopulmonary instability
   In these cases, antibiotic therapy may be initiated presumptively and lumbar puncture delayed.

Cronan K, Wiley J: Lumbar puncture. In Henretig F, King C (eds): The Textbook of Pediatric Emergency Medicine Procedures. Philadelphia, Lippincott Williams & Wilkins, 2008, p 507.

20. **What is an impact seizure?**
An impact seizure is a brief, generalized seizure occurring immediately at the time of injury. The seizure activity is thought to be due to traumatic depolarization of neurons on impact, and these children do not have a higher incidence of epilepsy.

21. **How is a hyponatremic seizure managed?**
Hyponatremic seizures are often managed with hypertonic saline to transiently raise plasma sodium levels by 5–10 mEq to stop the seizure. The dose is 2–4 mL/kg body weight of 3% sodium chloride (0.5 mEq/mL), given rapidly and intravenously.

22. **What are some differentiating features of Guillain-Barré syndrome and transverse myelopathy?**
See Table 32-2.

KEY POINTS: SEIZURES ✓

1. Many common seizure types have characteristic presentations that can be identified with the initial history and physical examination.

2. Immediate testing or imaging is not always indicated after a seizure.

3. Workup after a febrile seizure should be directed to the cause of the fever.

4. When IV access is unavailable, absorption of benzodiazepines by the mucous membranes of the nose, buccal mucosa, or rectum may terminate the seizure.

TABLE 32-2. GUILLAIN-BARRÉ SYNDROME VS. TRANVERSE MYELOPATHY

Symptom	Guillain-Barré Syndrome	Tranverse Myelopathy
Early pain/paresthesias	+	+
Progressive symmetrical weakness	Arms and legs	Legs
Bilateral facial weakness	+	−
Areflexia	+	+
Autonomic dysfunction	+	−
Sensory level*	−	+
Abnormal rectal tone	−	+

*A level below which the patient has absence of sensation.
(From Gorelick MH, Blackwell CD: Neurologic emergencies. In Fleisher GR, Ludwig S, Henretig FM [eds]: Textbook of Pediatric Emergency Medicine, 5th ed. Philadelphia, Lippincott William & Wilkins, 2006, pp 759–781.)

23. **What is the Miller Fisher variant of Guillain-Barré syndrome?**
Ophthalmoplegia, areflexia, and ataxia.

24. **What simple grooming measure should be performed on any patient with acute onset of ascending paralysis?**
Combing the hair. Tick paralysis can present very similarly to Guillain-Barré syndrome, although the rate of progression is faster and tick paralysis is accompanied by ataxia (not present in Guillain-Barré syndrome). Removal of the tick can bring about rapid improvement, and the tick is often found serendipitously.

Felz MW, Smith CD, Swift TR: A six-year-old girl with tick paralysis. N Engl J Med 342:90–94, 2000.

25. **A 2-month-old baby with a history of hypotonia presents in acute respiratory distress. He has abdominal respirations and appears to be tiring out. In preparing for intubation, what skeletal muscle relaxant is relatively contraindicated?**
Succinylcholine. In children with undiagnosed skeletal myopathy, concern is raised about the use of succinylcholine and the potential for ventricular dysrhythmias and cardiac arrest from hyperkalemia.

26. **What is the initial symptom seen in infantile botulism?**
Infantile botulism commonly presents with constipation for days to weeks before lethargy, feeding difficulties, diminished reflexes, weakness, hypotonia, and diminished gag reflex appear.

27. **How is the diagnosis of infant botulism made?**
The diagnosis is largely clinical and relies on the elimination of other causes of lethargy and weakness. *Clostridium botulinum* toxin may be identified in the stool. Brief, small, abundant motor action potentials are characteristic on electromyogram.

American Academy of Pediatrics: Clostridial infections. In Pickering LK (ed): 2003 Red Book: Report of the Committee on Infectious Diseases, 26th ed. Elk Grove Village, IL, American Academy of Pediatrics, 2006, pp 257–260.

28. **Which antibiotics should be avoided in infant botulism?**
The aminoglycosides, because they may potentiate the neuromuscular blockade and lead to respiratory arrest.

29. **How would you differentiate a migraine headache from that due to pseudotumor cerebri?**
Both conditions present with headache, although headache due to pseudotumor cerebri may be worse in the morning, while migraine symptoms are often relieved by sleep. Nausea, vomiting, and visual problems may also occur with both, and the neurologic examination may be normal. However, **papilledema** is seen in most cases of pseudotumor cerebri and is not present in migraine. Perform CT or MRI to rule out other causes of elevated intracranial pressure. If imaging does not demonstrate a mass lesion, perform a lumbar puncture to measure opening pressure, which will be elevated in pseudotumor cerebri.

30. **Describe the weakness in myasthenia gravis.**
Bilateral ptosis and ophthalmoplegia are the most common manifestations of myasthenia gravis. The weakness is variable, and the specific muscles affected may vary from examination to examination. Those with generalized weakness may report a history of worsening throughout the day or with continued activity. In the ED, easy fatigability of muscle strength may be demonstrated.

Gorelick MH, Blackwell CD: Neurologic emergencies. In Fleisher GR, Ludwig S, Henretig FM (eds): Textbook of Pediatric Emergency Medicine, 5th ed. Philadelphia, Lippincott Williams & Wilkins, 2006, pp 759–781.

31. **Which electrolyte abnormality is responsible for periodic paralysis?**
Periodic paralysis can be due to hypokalemia or hyperkalemia. Paralytic episodes may occur after strenuous exercise. Persistent weakness is possible.

32. **Acute cerebellar ataxia is most commonly attributed to which viral illness?**
Varicella. Acute cerebellar ataxia typically occurs within 10 days of a viral illness and is felt to be a parainfectious or postinfectious phenomenon. The onset of ataxia is acute, and nystagmus and slurred speech can occur, but most children are otherwise normal. Recovery typically takes a few weeks, and residual neurologic deficits are possible.

33. **What is "milkmaid's hand"?**
Milkmaid's hand is found in patients with chorea. The child cannot maintain a continuous grasp when asked to squeeze the examiner's fingers, but instead performs intermittent squeezing as if he or she were "milking" the finger. These low-amplitude, jerking movements are characteristic of chorea.

34. **What is the most common cause of acquired chorea in children?**
Sydenham's chorea, which is a manifestation of rheumatic fever.

35. **In uncal (unilateral transtentorial) herniation, is pupillary dilation present on the same side as the increased intracranial pressure or the opposite side?**
The pupil dilates on the same side where the temporal lobe causes the uncus to bulge into the tentorial notch.

36. **Why does the pupil dilate in uncal herniation?**
Direct pressure on the oculomotor nerve (cranial nerve III) causes the ipsilateral pupil to dilate.

37. **How do brain abscesses occur?**
- From direct extension from chronic infection in the sinuses, ears, or dental structures
- Following acute infections such as meningitis
- Hematogenously from endocarditis or congenital heart disease (particularly with right-to-left shunting)
- Following penetrating brain injury or neurosurgery

38. **Why is the diagnosis of sphenoid sinusitis often difficult?**
The sphenoid sinuses are located posterior to the ethmoid sinuses, and the usual physical examination techniques, such as percussion and transillumination, are not useful. Headache is usually severe, but can mimic migraine and is often located on top of the head, behind the eyes or at the back of the neck. Painful paresthesias may occur in the trigeminal nerve distribution. Eighty percent of pediatric patients with intracranial complications of sinusitis have sphenoid involvement.

Saitoh A, Beall B, Nizet V: Fulminant bacterial meningitis complicating sphenoid sinusitis. Pediatr Emerg Care 19:415–417, 2003.

39. **What are the neurologic complications of sinusitis?**
- Orbital cellulitis
- Ophthalmoplegia
- Cavernous sinus thrombosis
- Intracranial empyema or abscess
- Meningitis

40. **Where are pediatric brain tumors most commonly located?**
Posterior fossa tumors account for 50% of brain tumors in children of all ages, and are the most common location for brain tumors in children ages 1–8 years. This explains why gait disturbances are common in children with brain tumors.

41. **Brain tumors in children commonly present with which ocular nerve palsy?**
The sixth nerve (abducens) is commonly affected in children with posterior fossa brain tumors. In some, the inability to perform lateral rectus motion may be the sole manifestation of the tumor. The sixth nerve lies close to the cerebellum, fourth ventricle, and pons, which may explain its involvement in childhood brain tumors.

Rheingold SR, Lange BJ: Oncologic emergencies. In Fleisher GR, Ludwig S, Henretig FM (eds): Textbook of Pediatric Emergency Medicine, 5th ed. Philadelphia, Lippincott Williams & Wilkins, 2006, pp 1239–1274.

42. **What is acute demyelinating encephalomyelitis (ADEM)?**

ADEM is an inflammatory demyelinating disease that presents in children and young adults. It is an uncommon illness usually occurring in the winter and spring. In many cases it follows an upper respiratory tract infection. Children present with multifocal neurologic signs. Symptoms last for 2–4 weeks.

Murthy SN, Faden HS, Cohen ME, Bakshi R: Acute disseminated encephalomyelitis in children. Pediatrics 110:e21, 2002.

KEY POINTS: INTRACRANIAL PRESSURE ✓

1. A careful cranial nerve examination may be the clue to a mass lesion in the brain.

2. The presence of papilledema should prompt an imaging study of the brain.

3. A dilated unilateral pupil after head injury is concerning for herniation.

4. Headache from sinusitis may not be focused directly over the sinuses.

43. **What is the differential diagnosis of ADEM?**
    - Multiple sclerosis
    - Optic neuritis
    - Transverse myelitis
    - Devic's syndrome

CHAPTER 33

ENDOCRINE DISORDERS

Robert E. Sapien, MD, FAAP

1. **Why are children susceptible to hypoglycemia? What glucose level is considered hypoglycemia? How do you correct it?**
   Children are susceptible because:
   - Glycogen stores are small.
   - Glucose utilization is high because of increased metabolic demands.
   - Fewer gluconeogenesis precursors are generated because of less fat and muscle mass.
   - A child's developing brain needs a constant source of substrate.

   The level at which to treat is controversial, but most clinicians treat at a level < 60 mg/dL. The treatment for infants is typically at a level < 40 mg/dL. Treat infants with D10W (10% dextrose in water), 2–4 mL/kg body weight; for 1- to 8-year-olds, D25W (25% dextrose in water), 2–4 mL/kg; older children and adolescents, D50W (50% dextrose in water) ampule.

   Reid SR, Losek JD: Hypoglycemia in infants and children. Pediatr Emerg Med Rep 5:23–30, 2000.

2. **At what point should diagnostic tests for hypoglycemia be obtained? What would they be?**
   The tests should be obtained at first presentation of the hypoglycemic child to the emergency department (ED) (at triage)—but only if they can be obtained quickly. A bedside glucose test is essential because a delay in treatment can be neurologically devastating. A diagnostic workup is indicated for infants and children in whom the hypoglycemia has no explanation (i.e., oral hypoglycemic ingestion, sepsis, poor intake, anorexia in a diabetic child who received insulin). The tests include plasma glucose, electrolytes, lactate, pyruvate, keto hydroxybutyrate, acetoacetate, insulin, glucagon, cortisol, growth hormone, free fatty acids, alanine, glycerol, and urinalysis, including reducing substances.

KEY POINTS: HYPOGLYCEMIA ✓

1. Rapid identification is essential.

2. Children are susceptible because of small glycogen stores and high glucose utilization.

3. Treat hypoglycemia as follows: for infants (glucose level < 40 mg/dL), D10W, 2–4 mL/kg; for 1- to 8-year-olds (glucose level < 60 mg/dL), D25W, 2–4 mL/kg; for older children and adolescents, D50W ampule.

3. **What is the most common cause of hyperthyroidism in children?**
   Graves' disease is the most common etiology. Children at risk include females (female to male ratio, 5:1), those with familial autoimmune diseases (e.g., diabetes, adrenal insufficiency), and those from families with a history of thyroid disease.

   Sills IN: Hyperthyroidism. Pediatr Rev 15:417–420, 1994.
   McKeown NJ, Tews MC, Gossain VV, Shah S: Hyperthyroidism. Emerg Med Clin North Am 23:649–667, 2005.

4. **Presenting symptoms of hyperthyroidism are commonly attributed to which other body systems or disorders?**
   Symptoms from hyperthyroidism are commonly confused with other conditions. For example, cardiac disorders (palpitations, sinus tachycardia) and psychological problems (school difficulties, labile emotions, hyperactivity) mimic hyperthyroidism.

   Sills IN: Hyperthyroidism. Pediatr Rev 15:417–420, 1994.
   McKeown NJ, Tews MC, Gossain VV, Shah S: Hyperthyroidism. Emerg Med Clin North Am 23:649–667, 2005.

5. **What is thyroid storm? What is the treatment?**
   The symptoms may be nonspecific (fever, tachycardia, agitation, nausea, vomiting), making the diagnosis difficult unless there is a clear hyperthyroid history. The three systems most affected include the cardiovascular, gastrointestinal, and central nervous systems. Supportive care is the first step in management (oxygen, IV fluids, acetaminophen for fever). This should be followed by an IV β-blocker for the cardiac effects, and routine hyperthyroid treatments (propylthiouracil, iodine) in high doses.

   Sills IN: Hyperthyroidism. Pediatr Rev 15:417–420, 1994.
   McKeown NJ, Tews MC, Gossain VV, Shah S: Hyperthyroidism. Emerg Med Clin North Am 23:649–667, 2005.

6. **If congenital hypothyroidism is missed in the neonatal period, when will signs/symptoms present?**
   Patients will present with symptoms at 6–12 weeks of age. The first signs and symptoms are constipation, a large posterior fontanel, poor feeding, jaundice, and hypothermia.

   Fisher DA: Hypothyroidism. Pediatr Rev 15:227–232, 1994.
   Foley TP: Hypothyroidism. Pediatr Rev 25:94–99, 2004.

7. **How do the adrenal glands respond to stress? What are examples of such body stressors? What do children with adrenal insufficiency and children taking long-term exogenous glucocorticoid therapy have in common?**
   The adrenal glands respond to stress by secreting increased amounts of glucocorticoids and mineralocorticoids. Physiologic stresses include surgery, trauma, and infection. All of these children require stress dose replacement of glucocorticoids and mineralocorticoids because their adrenal glands cannot respond to such stressors.

   Oberlin JM, Rogers WM, Fenton CL: Endocrine emergencies: Recognizing signs and symptoms. Pediatr Ann 34:870–877, 2005.
   Spahn JD, Kamada AK: Special considerations in the use of glucocorticoids in children. Pediatr Rev 16:266–272, 1995.

8. **What signs and symptoms are likely in children with acute adrenal insufficiency?**
   Signs and symptoms are due to failure of the adrenals to respond to a stress, and they are fairly nonspecific. They include dehydration with hypovolemic shock, hypoglycemia, hyponatremia, hyperkalemia, fever, abdominal pain, and lethargy.

   Kappy MS, Bajaj L: Recognition and treatment of endocrine/metabolic emergencies in children. Part I. Adv Pediatr 49:245–272, 2002.
   Oberlin JM, Rogers WM, Fenton CL: Endocrine emergencies: Recognizing signs and symptoms. Pediatr Ann 34:870–877, 2005.

9. **What is the emergency treatment for acute adrenal insufficiency?**
   Much of the initial stabilization is supportive care. The treatment includes:
   - Fluid resuscitation with normal saline (500 mL/m^2) for shock and dehydration
   - Correction of the hypoglycemia with D25W

- Hydrocortisone, 2–3 mg/kg via IV route
- Correction of the hyperkalemia (sodium polystyrene sulfonate, glucose/insulin, calcium gluconate, sodium bicarbonate)
- Monitoring of vital signs, cardiac rhythm, perfusion, glucose, and electrolytes

August GP: Treatment of adrenocortical insufficiency. Pediatr Rev 18:59–62, 1997.

Kappy MS, Bajaj L: Recognition and treatment of endocrine/metabolic emergencies in children. Part I. Arch Pediatr 49:245–272, 2002.

10. What is the most common cause of amenorrhea in adolescents?

Pregnancy is the most common cause. Other causes include oral contraceptive use, pituitary infarctions, uterine synechiae in postpartum adolescents, outflow obstruction (imperforate hymen, vaginal or uterine agenesis), and hypoestrogenic states (anorexia, athletics).

Braverman PK, Sondeimer SJ: Menstrual disorders. Pediatr Rev 18:17–25, 1997.

Hillard PJ, Deitch HR: Menstrual disorders of the college age female. Pediatr Clin North Am 52:179–107, 2005.

11. What endocrine conditions are associated with dysfunctional uterine bleeding?

Dysfunctional uterine bleeding is associated with immaturity of the hypothalamic–pituitary axis, prolactinomas, thyroid tumors, type 2 diabetes, and adrenal hyperplasia or tumors.

12. Why is it difficult to make the diagnosis of type 1 diabetes in early childhood?

The diagnosis is difficult to make because the classic symptoms of polydipsia and polyuria are not easily discernible. The very young, therefore, are more likely to present with diabetic ketoacidosis (DKA) initially.

Mallare JT, Cordice CC, Ryan BA, et al: Identifying risk factors for the development of diabetic ketoacidosis in new onset type 1 diabetes mellitus. Clin Pediatr 42:591–597, 2003.

Plotnick L: Insulin-dependent diabetes mellitus. Pediatr Rev 15:137–148, 1994.

13. What questions or clinical findings may help you consider type 1 diabetes in your differential diagnosis?

Type 1 diabetes should be ruled out in children who are clinically dehydrated yet continue with urine output. Information regarding the number of wet diapers per day, nocturnal incontinence, or leaving the classroom often to urinate may help you hone in on the diagnosis. Children with weight loss and a history of vague abdominal pain should be considered as possibly having type 1 diabetes.

14. What are acute complications of type 1 diabetes?

DKA and hypoglycemia are common, recurrent, critical issues that can occur. They are related to socioeconomic factors, psychiatric problems, blood glucose control, duration of the disease, and the child's age.

Kappy MS, Bajaj L: Recognition and treatment of endocrine/metabolic emergencies in children. Part I. Arch Pediatr 49:245–272, 2002.

Rewers A, Chase P, Mackensie T, et al: Predictors of acute complications in children with type 1 diabetes. JAMA 287:2511–2518, 2002.

15. What usually leads to DKA?

Insulin underutilization is the usual factor leading to DKA. As DKA starts, the child usually is anorexic and nauseated, and begins to vomit. Parents or the patient may stop administering insulin even though the child is hyperglycemic, hence worsening the condition. Acute infections (viral gastroenteritis, appendicitis, bacterial infection), psychologically stressful situations, medical nonadherence, and inflammatory processes can also lead to DKA. Signs and symptoms include dehydration, abdominal pain, tachypnea, nausea, vomiting, listlessness, coma, fruity odor, ketonuria(emia), hyperglycemia(uria), measured hyponatremia and intravascular hyperkalemia (despite total body depletion).

Wolfson AB (ed): Clinical Practice of Emergency Medicine, 4th ed. Philadelphia, Lippincott Williams & Wilkins, 2005.

16. **Is there only one level of DKA severity?**
No. DKA can be mild, moderate, or severe. Mild DKA is merely hyperglycemia with ketosis as demonstrated by urinalysis. Children with mild DKA have normal mental status and respiratory status. They are good candidates for outpatient therapy as long as they can keep themselves hydrated orally.

	pH	HCO_3
Moderate	7.2–7.3	15
Severe	7.1	10

The degree of DKA is *not* dependent on the extent of hyperglycemia. The glucose level is always elevated with DKA, but there is a common misconception that the glucose has to be *severely* elevated for DKA to exist.

17. **Of what do children and adolescents with type 1 diabetes die?**
Children with type 1 diabetes in DKA die of cerebral edema (60–80% mortality rate), which is the final pathway in over half of hospital deaths and 30% of home deaths. Cerebral edema is unpredictable and probably multifactorial. It seems to be associated with high initial blood urea nitrogen level, lower partial pressure of arterial carbon dioxide, more severe acidosis (lower bicarbonate and pH), administration of bicarbonate, and inadequate increase in serum sodium concentration. Rates of fluid or sodium administration do not affect the risk of cerebral edema.

Edge JA, Adams M, Dunger DB: Causes of death in children with insulin-dependent diabetes 1990–96. Arch Dis Child 81:318–323, 1999.
Glaser N, Barnett MB, McCaslin I, et al: Risk factors for cerebral edema in children with diabetic ketoacidosis N Engl J Med 344:264–269, 2001.
Wolfson AB (ed): Clinical Practice of Emergency Medicine, 4th ed. Philadelphia, Lippincott Williams & Wilkins, 2005.

18. **Is there a standard treatment for DKA?**
There are many protocols for DKA management. In fact, agreement is lacking among specialists (pediatric intensivists, endocrinologists, and emergency physicians). Keeping to a standard treatment protocol helps ensure consistent care. The key issues are fluid replacement, acid correction, and glucose and electrolyte adjustment. Attention to all of these is necessary in the approach to the child with DKA.

Initially, fluid replacement with an isotonic solution (normal saline) at 5–10 mL/kg in the first hour is recommended. Fluid deficits are replaced over the subsequent 24–48 hours (if 10% dehydration is assumed, then 100 mL/kg) in addition to maintenance fluids. With hydration, the glucose level usually begins to fall, and the acidosis begins to correct as the serum ketones metabolize, producing bicarbonate. Careful monitoring of potassium, sodium, and phosphate is also indicated. There is total-body potassium depletion, which is initially masked, and extracellular potassium levels are generally normal to high. As the acidosis corrects, potassium moves intracellularly, and the serum potassium level begins to fall, more accurately reflecting the total-body depletion.

Insulin may be administered as an IV drip (0.05–0.1 U/kg/h), but this should be done carefully as hydration also lowers glucose levels. Subcutaneous insulin administration is not the route of choice in DKA. Glucose should be decreased no faster than 50–100 mg/dL/h. Add dextrose when the serum level is 300 gm/dL, but do not discontinue the insulin. The insulin also helps drive potassium intracellularly, compounding the hypokalemia. Bicarbonate administration increases the risk of cerebral edema and has not been shown to improve outcomes.

Glaser NS, Kuppermann N, Yee CKJ: Variation in the management of pediatric diabetic ketoacidosis by specialty training. Arch Pediatr Adolesc Med 151:1125–1132, 1997.

Green SM, Rothrock SG, Ho JD, et al: Failure of adjunctive bicarbonate to improve outcome in severe pediatric diabetic ketoacidosis. Ann Emerg Med 31:41–48, 1998.

Wolfson, AB (ed): Clinical Practice of Emergency Medicine, 4th ed. Philadelphia, Lippincott Williams & Wilkins, 2005.

19. **How is time a factor in the treatment of DKA?**

A philosophy to follow in treating a child with DKA is to remember that there are many aspects of DKA, which took time to develop. Taking sufficient time to correct them avoids many of the complications of treatment. With judicious fluid resuscitation, careful monitoring, and frequent reassessment, you should see steady improvement. Do not expect or strive for drastic, rapid improvement. Treatment should be judged as successful if the child does not further deteriorate and the clinical state steadily improves (lower respiratory rate, more alert mental status, and electrolytes approaching normal).

Lavin N: Manual of Endocrinology and Metabolism, 2nd ed. Boston, Little, Brown & Company, 1994.

Sperling MA: Pediatric Endocrinology. Philadelphia, W.B. Saunders, 2002.

20. **What signs and symptoms should make you consider the diagnosis of type 2 diabetes mellitus?**

Obesity (over 85% of patients are overweight); acanthosis nigricans (seen in over 85% of patients), a sign of insulin resistance; nonketotic hyperglycemia; glycosuria; weight loss (less common than with type 1 diabetes); polyuria and polydipsia (less common than with type 1 diabetes); rarely DKA; and ketonuria in 25% of patients. Type 2 diabetes mellitus is becoming more prevalent among children between 10 and 21 years old.

Nesmith JD: Type 2 diabetes mellitus in children and adolescents. Pediatr Rev 22:147–152, 2001.

American Diabetes Association. Available at www.diabetes.org.

21. **What is the probable abnormality in type 2 diabetes mellitus?**

The probable abnormality is insulin resistance. This develops over a long period of time and results in a hyperinsulinemic condition. It can lead to dysfunctional uterine bleeding, hypertension, polycystic ovary disease, and acanthosis nigricans. The islets of Langerhans eventually become unable to maintain this level of insulin production, which leads to a relative insulin deficiency and hence hyperglycemia.

Nesmith JD: Type 2 diabetes mellitus in children and adolescents. Pediatr Rev 22:147–152, 2001.

KEY POINTS: DIABETES MELLITUS ✔

1. Children in DKA need skillful correction of electrolyte, metabolic, and glucose abnormalities as well as careful clinical monitoring and reassessment.

2. For children in DKA, try to reduce glucose level at a rate of 50–100 mg/dL/h.

3. When treating DKA, add glucose when the serum level is < 300 mg/dL, but do not discontinue insulin.

22. **True or false: DKA is the only acute metabolic abnormality that occurs in children with type 2 diabetes mellitus.**
False. There are reported deaths from hyperglycemic hyperosmolar states. A hyperglycemic hyperosmolar state is described as hyperglycemia with glucose level > 600 mg/dL, small ketonuria, low or no ketonemia, stupor/coma, serum carbon dioxide level > 15 mmol/L, and serum osmols > 320 mOsm/kg. Just as in DKA, cerebral edema is a grave complication that can occur from the hyperglycemic, hyperosmolar state of type 2 diabetes.

> Morales AE, Rosenbloom AL: Death caused by hyperglycemic hyperosmolar state at the onset of type 2 diabetes. J Pediatr 144:270–273, 2004.
> American Diabetes Association. Available at www.diabetes.org.

23. **Can a child be dehydrated yet still produce copious amounts of urine?**
Yes, this is common with diabetes insipidus. Dilute urine produced by an otherwise clinically dehydrated child, polydipsia, polyuria, fever, irritability, poor feeding and weight gain, constipation, and hypernatremia are presenting signs and symptoms of diabetes insipidus. In severe presentations, weak pulse, poor skin turgor, seizure, and hypotension may also occur.

> Saborio P, Tipton GA, Chan JCM: Diabetes insipidus. Pediatr Rev 21:122–129, 2000.

24. **Congenital hypothyroidism is familiar to pediatricians, but can newborns be hyperthyroid?**
Indeed they can. In fact, substantial mortality is associated with neonatal thyrotoxicosis. Neonatal thyrotoxicosis presents in the first 2 weeks of life in infants born to hyperthyroid mothers. Symptoms include irritability, sweating, weight loss, poor feeding, vomiting, and diarrhea. Signs are typical of hyperthyroidism, such as exophthalmos, goiter, hyperthermia, tachycardia, jaundice, hepatomegaly, and even cardiac failure.

> Wolfson AB (ed): Clinical Practice of Emergency Medicine, 4th ed. Philadelphia, Lippincott Williams & Wilkins, 2005.

25. **What endocrine comorbidities might be present with childhood obesity?**
The prevalence of childhood obesity is skyrocketing among our youth and stresses all body systems. Obesity contributes and may even lead to several endocrine abnormalities. They include advanced physical maturation, type 2 diabetes, and polycystic ovary disease. Polycystic ovary disease probably is a result of insulin resistance and elevated levels of androgens leading to obesity, infertility, hirsutism, and menstrual dysfunction are common.

> Perkin RM: The epidemic of pediatric obesity: Clinical implications for the ED physician. Pediatr Emerg Med Rep 9:65–80, 2004.

26. **What is the most common form of congenital adrenal hyperplasia presenting in infancy? What is the incidence of this type?**
The most common form of congenital adrenal hyperplasia (CAH) during infancy is 21-hydroxylase deficiency. It accounts for 90% of all cases. Clinical salt wasting develops in 30–70% of patients. The incidence of this type of CAH is 1 in 15,000 live births.

27. **When does a child with salt-losing CAH generally present to the ED?**
The infant generally presents around 2 weeks of life. Symptoms are usually nonspecific, consisting of poor feeding, lethargy, irritability, vomiting, and poor weight gain. A general examination should be done, as well as a thorough evaluation of the genitals.

28. **In the ED, what are the most urgent laboratory studies to perform if CAH is suspected?**
Check serum electrolytes and glucose. In salt-losing CAH, hyperkalemia and hyponatremia are typically seen; the glucose level can be normal or low. Metabolic acidosis is usually present. Infants with CAH tolerate hyperkalemia better than do other infants and children.

29. **How is this type of CAH treated in the ED?**

If dehydration is present, volume expansion with normal saline should begin promptly. Hydrocortisone, 25 mg, should be given immediately via IV bolus. If hypoglycemia is present, a dextrose bolus will be necessary. Hyperkalemia needs to be addressed.

Agus MSD: Endocrine emergencies. In Fleisher G, Ludwig S, Henretig F, et al (eds). The Textbook of Pediatric Emergency Medicine, 5th ed. Philadelphia, Lippincott Williams & Wilkins, 2006, pp 1167–1192.

30. **What are the most common symptoms of pheochromocytoma?**

Headache, palpitations, and excessive sweating. The headache is usually pounding and severe, and palpitations may be associated with tachycardia. Other symptoms include tremor, fatigue, chest or abdominal pain, and flushing.

CHAPTER 34

FLUIDS AND ELECTROLYTES

Kathy N. Shaw, MD, MSCE

1. **How do you estimate the extent of dehydration in children?**
   Since serial weights on the same scale are rarely available in the emergency department (ED) setting, rely on the physical examination to estimate the degree of fluid loss (Table 34-1).

TABLE 34-1. CLINICAL FINDINGS OF DEHYDRATION

Signs and Symptoms	None or Mild	Degree of Impairment	
		Moderate	Severe
General condition, infants	Thirsty; alert; restless	Lethargic or drowsy	Limp; cold, cyanotic extremities; may be comatose
General condition, older children	Thirsty; alert; restless	Alert; postural dizziness	Apprehensive; cold, cyanotic extremities; muscle cramps
Quality of radial pulse	Normal	Thready or weak	Feeble or impalpable
Quality of respiration	Normal	Deep	Deep and rapid
Skin elasticity	Pinch retracts immediately	Pinch retracts slowly	Pinch retracts very slowly (>2 sec)
Eyes	Normal	Sunken	Very sunken
Tears	Present	Absent	Absent
Mucous membranes	Moist	Dry	Very dry
Urine output (by report of parent)	Normal	Reduced	None passed in many hours

Adapted from World Health Organization: The Treatment of Diarrhea: A Manual for Physicians and Other Senior Health Workers, 3rd ed. Washington, DC, Division of Diarrheal and Acute Respiratory Disease Control, World Health Organization. WHO/CDD/SER/80.2, 1995.

2. **What are the most reliable clinical examination findings that help you predict how dry a child has become?**
   An abnormal capillary refill time is probably the most reliable sign for predicting 5% dehydration in children. However, a combination of examination signs is better than any individual sign. The presence of two or more of the following four clinical measures seems most reliable in predicting dehydration:
   - "Ill" general appearance
   - Lack of tears

- Capillary refill time at the fingertip > 2 seconds
- Dry mucous membranes

  Gorelick MH, Shaw KN, Murphy KO: Validity and reliability of clinical signs in the diagnosis of dehydration in children. Pediatrics 99:e6, 1997.

  Steiner MJ, DeWalt DA, Byerley JS: Is this child dehydrated? JAMA 291:2746–2754, 2004.

3. **How does the extent of dehydration translate into fluid lost?**
   For each kilogram of weight loss, 1 L of fluid was lost. Using weight obtained in the ED and your estimate of the percentage dehydration, you can calculate the "well" or rehydrated weight. The difference between the estimated well weight and current weight is converted into liters or cubic centimeters. For example, a 9-kg, ill-appearing baby presents with dry mucous membranes, crying with no tears, and a capillary refill time of > 2 seconds. She is estimated to have lost 10% of her body weight (severe dehydration).

$$\text{Calculated well weight} = x$$

$$x = \frac{current\ weight}{1 - \text{dehydration percent}}$$

$$x = \frac{current\ weight}{1 - 10\%}$$

$$x = \frac{9\,\text{kg}}{0.9}$$

$$x = 10\,\text{kg}$$

$$\text{Weight lost} = 10\,\text{kg} - 9\text{ kg} = 1\,\text{kg} = 1\,\text{L}$$

4. **How much fluid and what type do you use for a "bolus" to begin IV hydration?**
   The first objective in treating a child with dehydration is to restore intravascular volume and treat shock. Isotonic fluid, such as normal saline or Ringer's lactate, should be used. Give boluses of 20 mL/kg, and reassess the child. The goal is to restore blood pressure, reduce heart rate, restore perfusion to the tissues (return of capillary refill < 2 seconds), improve mental status or general appearance, and produce urine. If initial fluid boluses > 60 mL/kg are needed, reconsider the diagnosis and management plan.

5. **Should 5% dextrose in water be used as a fluid bolus for dehydration?**
   No, 5% dextrose in water (D5W) should not be used to treat dehydration. Only isotonic crystalloid fluid should be used for treatment of dehydration in pediatrics. Giving dextrose along with a large fluid bolus can lead to hyperglycemia.

6. **Are there any children who should not receive a rapid fluid bolus?**
   Children with diabetic ketoacidosis or hypernatremic dehydration (serum sodium level > 150 mEq/dL) who are in a hyperosmolar state require slower and more cautious fluid resuscitation. Clearly, uncompensated shock (hypotension) must be treated rapidly, but 10-mL/kg boluses of normal saline should be used and the child reassessed after each bolus. Also administer fluids more cautiously to children in cardiogenic shock (heart failure).

7. **What stock should be used after the initial IV bolus or if the child is not dehydrated?**
   Generally, D5¼ normal saline (NS) or D5½ NS, with 10 mEq potassium chloride/L added if the child has urinated. Use D5½ NS in children who have had < 20 mL/kg NS boluses or who have hyponatremic dehydration (serum sodium level < 130 mEq/dL). Children with burns, pyloric stenosis with hypochloremia, and diabetic ketoacidosis are usually kept on a normal saline infusion in the ED.

8. **At what rate should fluids run on a child who has orders to receive nothing by mouth? How is this maintenance rate adjusted for the dehydrated child?**
All children who are unable to drink should receive maintenance fluids, and if they are dehydrated, the rate is higher to replace some of the remaining fluid deficit. Calculate all rates by using the child's well or rehydrated weight. Increase rates above maintenance if the child is febrile or has increased insensible or gastrointestinal losses.

$$\text{Maintenance rate} = 4 \text{ mL/kg/h for the first 10 kg}$$
$$+ 2 \text{ mL/kg/h for the second 10 kg}$$
$$+ 1 \text{ mL/kg/h for each kg over 20}$$

Example: Maintenance rate for a 16-kg child: 40 mL/h (first 10 kg) + 6 kg × 2 mL = 12 mL/h (next 6 kg) or 52 mL/h (if the child is febrile, add 10% more, or 55–60 mL/h). To determine the rate for the dehydrated child, half of the total fluid deficit (minus the fluid boluses already given) is added to the maintenance rate for the first 8 hours. The other half of the deficit is added to the maintenance rate over the next 16 hours (hopefully outside of the ED!). For children with hypertonic dehydration, the remaining fluid deficit after initial boluses is replaced evenly over the next 48 hours.
Example: A 9-kg dehydrated baby was given 400 mL of NS (40 mL/kg) as an initial fluid bolus. The fluid deficit was 1000 mL. Half of the deficit is 500 ML. Since 400 mL was already given, 100 mL of the deficit should be added to the maintenance rate over the next 8 hours. Thus, 100 mL/8 h = 12.5 mL/hr should be added to the maintenance rate of 40 mL/hr (based on 10-kg "well" weight), or 52 mL/hr of D5¼ NS should be ordered.

Shaw KN, Spandorfer P: Dehydration. In Fleisher GR, Ludwig S, Henretig FM (eds): Textbook of Pediatric Emergency Medicine, 5th ed. Philadelphia, Lippincott Williams & Wilkins, 2006, pp 233–238.

KEY POINTS: DEHYDRATION ✔

1. The first objective in treating a child with severe dehydration is to restore intravascular volume and treat shock, regardless of etiology.

2. In all children receiving IV fluids, the serial electrolytes and urine output should be monitored and fluid rates adjusted on the basis of the child's hydration status, urine output, and presence or absence of increased ADH.

3. Compared with IV therapy, oral rehydration therapy is effective in treating dehydration in most children, has fewer complications, and may be faster.

9. **Will use of hypotonic maintenance solutions cause dangerous hyponatremia?**
Most children admitted with fever and volume depletion require free water. However, some children are at risk for secretion of antidiuretic hormone (ADH), which may cause retention of free water and hyponatremia. Conditions that have been associated with this state include bronchiolitis, meningitis, pneumonia, and postoperative pain or nausea. These children may require fluid restriction. In all children receiving IV fluids, the serial electrolytes and urine output are monitored and fluid rates adjusted on the basis of the child's hydration status, urine output, and presence or absence of increased ADH. Keeping children on isotonic parenteral maintenance solution may cause hypernatremia and may not replace insensible water loss; evidence to support its safety is lacking.

Hatherill M: Rubbing salt in the wound. Arch Dis Child 89:414–418, 2004.

Moritz ML, Ayus JC: Prevention of hospital-acquired hyponatraemia: A case for using isotonic saline. Pediatrics 111:227–230, 2003.

10. **Which children may be treated with oral rehydration?**
Strongly consider oral rehydration in all children with mild or moderate dehydration who do not have uncompensated shock, severe vomiting, high stool output of >20 mL/kg/h, or poor adherence. It is very effective in treating dehydration and has a low failure rate.

Centers for Disease Control and Prevention: Managing acute gastroenteritis in children. MMWR Morb Mortal Recomm Rep 52:1–16, 2003.

11. **Then why aren't more children treated orally rather than with IV fluids?**
Oral rehydration therapy takes time, one-to-one care, and patience. Many parents bring the child to the ED because they want a "quick fix." Nevertheless, recent studies have shown that oral rehydration therapy is as effective as IV rehydration and may require less time with a lower complication rate.

Atherly-John YC, Cunningham SJ, Crain EF: A randomized trial of oral vs intravenous rehydration in a pediatric emergency department. Arch Pediatr Adolesc Med 156:1240–1243, 2002.

Spandorfer PR, Alessandrini EA, Joffe MD, et al: Oral versus intravenous rehydration of moderately dehydrated children: A randomized, controlled trial. Pediatrics 115:295–301, 2005.

12. **How do you calculate the fluid and amount to give for oral rehydration?**
The fluid deficit is calculated based on the estimate of the degree of dehydration, and *the entire deficit is given by mouth over 4 hours*. The parent is asked to offer a small amount of fluid every 5–10 minutes. For mild to moderate dehydration, give 1 mL/kg of an oral electrolyte solution every 5 minutes. For moderate to severe dehydration, give 2 mL/kg by mouth every 5 minutes.

Example: A 9-kg dehydrated baby with an estimated "well" weight of 10 kg has a fluid deficit of 1000 mL. We ask the mother to give 60 mL every 15 minutes (2 ounces in a bottle) or to insert via syringe 20 mL (2 mL/kg) into the baby's mouth every 5 minutes for the next 4 hours (1000 mL/4 h = 250 mL/h; 250 mL/60 minutes = ~4 mL/minute).

13. **What type of fluid should be used for oral rehydration?**
Use an oral rehydration solution. These have the correct proportion of dextrose and salt to allow for maximal absorption of electrolytes. Although solutions with higher concentrations of sodium (75–90 mEq/dL) are recommended initially (Rehydralyte [manufactured by Ross], ORS packets [Jaianas]), solutions with lower sodium content (40–60 mEq/dl) may be used and are more readily available (Pedialyte [Ross], Infalyte [Mead Johnson]).

14. **Why can't I mix half juice and half rehydration solution to make it taste better?**
Juice and soda have high sugar contents, and a 50% mixture raises the sugar content above the amount that allows for maximum sodium/glucose transport across the cell membrane in the gastrointestinal tract. Use flavored solutions or add only a small amount (1:8 solution) to the rehydration solution.

15. **When should oral rehydration not be used?**
   - Severe dehydration
   - Inability to tolerate oral fluids because of vomiting
   - Altered mental status with risk of aspiration
   - Ileus
   - Short gut or carbohydrate malabsorption, which limit absorption

Batra B, Stanton B: Oral rehydration therapy, 2006. Available at www.uptodate.com.

16. **What concerns should I have about a child with hypertonic dehydration?**

    The deficit in children with hypertonic dehydration may be underestimated because they appear less dry since their intravascular space is maintained longer. Additionally, rapid rehydration can cause cerebral edema, hemorrhage, or thrombosis. Hyperglycemia or hypocalcemia may also occur.

17. **How do I treat hyponatremia?**

    Treat the patient, not the laboratory value. Treat children with seizures, severe lethargy, hypoventilation, coma, or shock immediately. For children with dehydration and low serum sodium, a fluid bolus of 20–40 mL/kg NS quickly corrects symptomatic hyponatremia. For water-intoxicated children or those with syndrome of inappropriate antidiuretic hormone secretion—-in whom sodium, not fluid, is needed—give 2–4 mL/kg of 3% saline to stop seizures, followed by 6–12 mL/kg of 3% saline over the next 2–4 hours.

18. **How do I treat hypoglycemia?**

    A 0.5-gm/kg bolus is adequate to treat most cases of hypoglycemia. This can be given as 5 mL/kg of D10 or 2 mL/kg of D25. D50 is not used in children.

19. **How and when do I treat metabolic acidosis?**

    Give sodium bicarbonate to children with a pH < 7.1 who are critically ill or are unable to compensate. Most children with dehydration whose serum bicarbonate level is > 8 correct their metabolic acidosis with fluid resuscitation and do not require bicarbonate. Bicarbonate should be given only for metabolic acidosis, not respiratory acidosis. Children with respiratory insufficiency should not receive bicarbonate. Also, bicarbonate should be given slowly because it does not cross the blood–brain barrier. However, its byproduct, carbon dioxide, does cross this barrier and may cause cerebral acidosis. Usually 1–2 mEq/kg is given over a minimum of 30–60 minutes. Administration of bicarbonate is the only treatment factor found to be associated with development of cerebral edema in patients with diabetic ketoacidosis.

    Glaser N, Barnett P, McCaslin I, et al, for the Pediatric Emergency Medicine Collaborative Research Committee of the American Academy of Pediatrics: Risk factors for cerebral edema in children with diabetic ketoacidosis. N Engl J Med 344:264–269, 2001.

20. **How do I treat hypercalcemia?**

    Give furosemide, 1–2 mg/kg, and address the etiology.

21. **How do I treat hyperkalemia?**

    The type and speed of treatment depend on the potassium levels and electrocardiogram changes. Potassium may be forced out of the cell by acidosis. Treatment of the acidosis causes potassium to return to the cell and out of the serum (Table 34-2).

KEY POINTS: ACIDOSIS/HYPERKALEMIA ✔

1. Beware of bicarbonate—especially in the treatment of diabetic ketoacidosis—because it has been associated with cerebral edema.

2. Treat hyperkalemia on the basis of the electrocardiogram, clinical picture, and etiology, not just the serum value.

TABLE 34-2. TREATMENT OF HYPERKALEMIA		
Potassium Level (mEq/dL)	ECG Finding	Treatment
<7.0	Peaked t waves only, or normal	Remove K source, treat acidosis, Kayexalate (1g/kg orally or rectally) every 4–6 hr
7.0	Widespread ECG changes without arrhythmia	Glucose (0.5 g/kg or 5 mL/kg of D10 over 30–60 minutes) *and* insulin (0.1 U/kg over 30–60 minutes) *plus* bicarbonate (2 mEq/kg over 30–60 minutes)
8.0	Arrhythmia	10% calcium gluconate (0.5 mL/kg over 2–5 minutes with ECG monitoring, discontinue if heart rate <100 beats per minute) *plus* glucose *and* insulin, bicarbonate as above

ECG = electrocardiogram.

22. **How do I treat hypocalcemia?**
First, check the ionized calcium and confirm the diagnosis. If the patient is symptomatic, treat with 2–4 mg/kg of elemental calcium over 5 minutes with electrocardiographic monitoring. Calcium gluconate, 10% solution, can be given via peripheral IV route (0.5 mL/kg).

Cronan KM, Kost SI: Renal and electrolyte emergencies. In Fleisher GR, Ludwig S, Henretig FM (eds): Textbook of Pediatric Emergency Medicine, 5th ed. Philadelphia, Lippincott Williams & Wilkins, 2006, pp 873–919.

GASTROINTESTINAL EMERGENCIES

Susan Fuchs, MD

1. **What is the most common cause of vomiting in older children?**
   Acute gastroenteritis. Although usually associated with diarrhea, vomiting can occur alone in the early stages of gastroenteritis. The most common infectious viral etiology is rotavirus. *Salmonella, Shigella, Yersinia, Campylobacter* spp. and *Escherichia coli* can also cause bacterial gastroenteritis with vomiting.

   Stevens MW, Henretig FM: Vomiting. In Fleisher GR, Ludwig S, Henretig FM (eds): Textbook of Pediatric Emergency Medicine, 5th ed. Philadelphia, Lippincott Williams & Wilkins, 2006, pp 681–689.

2. **What are other medical causes of vomiting in children?**
   Metabolic disorders, such as galactosemia, fructose intolerance, or amino acid or organic acid defects (phenylketonuria, urea cycle defects) usually present in infancy. Along with vomiting, symptoms such as lethargy, seizures, or coma may occur. Diabetes mellitus can cause vomiting because of ketoacidosis or slowed gastric motility (gastroparesis may occur after 10 years of diabetes mellitus). Other causes include milk/soy protein allergies, pancreatitis, urinary tract infection, neurologic disorders associated with increased intracranial pressure (tumor, hydrocephalus), migraines, pregnancy, and psychological causes (rumination, bulimia).

   Stevens MW, Henretig FM: Vomiting. In Fleisher GR, Ludwig S, Henretig FM (eds): Textbook of Pediatric Emergency Medicine, 5th ed. Philadelphia, Lippincott Williams & Wilkins, 2006, pp 681–689.

3. **What are the most common anatomic regions to find a coin that has not passed?**
   In the esophagus, the cricopharyngeus/thoracic inlet (proximal third) is the most common place, followed by the level of the aortic arch (middle third), then the gastroesophageal junction/sphincter (lower third). Other areas of the gastrointestinal (GI) tract include the stomach, pylorus, ligament of Treitz, and ileocecal valve. Objects larger than 2 cm in diameter or longer than 5 cm are more likely to get "caught" at the pylorus.

   Karaman A, Cavusoglu YH, Karaman I, et al: Magill forceps technique for removal of safety pins in upper esophagus: A preliminary report. Int J Pediatr Otorhinolaryngol 68:1189–1191, 2004.

4. **What is the best way to remove an esophageal coin?**
   This is a highly controversial topic. One study demonstrated that when the foreign body is lodged for less than 24 hours, no respiratory symptoms are present, and the child has no prior esophageal disease or surgery, 28% pass spontaneously, including 22–33% of those in the upper esophagus and midesophagus. In such cases, observation for 12–24 hours with repeat radiography may be appropriate.

   There are several methods of coin removal in infants and children with no respiratory symptoms and no history of esophageal disease. Some advocate the use of Foley catheter extraction under fluoroscopic guidance for coins that have been lodged less than 24 hours, while others extend this time to 3 days. Others use esophageal bougienage for coins lodged in the distal esophagus less than 24 hours. Laryngoscopy with Magill forceps removal, esophagoscopy, or endoscopy under general anesthesia are also options. In the presence of respiratory symptoms, a history of esophageal disease, esophageal edema, or focal narrowing of the adjacent trachea (seen on the lateral neck radiograph), the best way to remove the foreign body is under direct vision via esophagoscopy or endoscopy. The choice of method is often based upon the expertise and availability of the specialists (radiology, otolaryngology, surgery, or gastroenterology) at a particular hospital.

Harned RK, Strain JD, Hay TC, et al: Esophageal foreign bodies: Safety and efficacy of Foley catheter extraction of coins. AJR 168:443–446, 1997.

Karaman A, Cavusoglu YH, Karaman I, et al: Magill forceps technique for removal of safety pins in upper esophagus: A preliminary report. Int J Pediatr Otorhinolaryngol 68:1189–1191, 2004.

Macpherson RI, Hill JG, Othersen HB, et al: Esophageal foreign bodies in children: Diagnosis, treatment and complications. AJR 166:919–924, 1996.

Schunk JE, Harrison M, Corneli HM, et al: Fluoroscopic Foley catheter removal of esophageal foreign bodies in children: Experience with 415 episodes. Pediatrics 94:709–714, 1994.

Soprano JV, Fleisher GR, Mandl KD: The spontaneous passage of esophageal coins in children. Arch Pediatr Adolesc Med 153:1073–1076, 1999.

5. **What is the "big deal" about button batteries?**
Although they are small (watch or hearing aid batteries), the risk is corrosion of the ingested battery. If the battery remains in the esophagus, there is fear of tissue damage, with resultant erosions, tracheoesophageal fistulas, and strictures. When a child swallows a button battery, obtain a radiograph to determine the battery's location. If it remains in the esophagus, it should be removed under direct visualization (not a Foley catheter) to assess for any damage to the esophageal mucosa. The proposed mechanisms of injury include electrolyte leakage, alkali production, mercury toxicity, and pressure necrosis.
Fun fact: Many batteries are made of mercuric oxide. There is little risk of mercury poisoning, however, because mercuric oxide is poorly absorbed from the GI tract.

Lin VYW, Daniel SJ, Papsin BC: Button batteries in the ear, nose and upper aerodigestive tract. Int J Pediatr Otorhinolaryngol 68:473–479, 2004.

6. **How should a caustic ingestion be managed?**
First, ensure that there is a patent airway. Next, determine what was ingested. This may require calling the poison control center (1-800-222-1222) or going to a computer-based system that determines treatment, signs/symptoms, and toxicity in the emergency department. The child may have symptoms such as drooling, mouth pain, pain on swallowing, chest pain, or cough. Examine the mouth for mucosal and oral burns. Alkali ingestions (lye, drain cleaners) are more damaging to the oropharynx and esophagus than are acid burns because they cause deeper injury. In addition, after an alkali burn, esophageal burns can occur without an oral burn. The amount of caustic ingested does not correlate with the degree of burns, or the symptoms. Induced vomiting is contraindicated in these children because of the risk of injury and aspiration. After a thorough examination, if any burns are seen, or if the child ingested alkali, the child should undergo endoscopy under general anesthesia. If there are no burns and no symptoms, and if a weak or very dilute formulation of an acid was ingested, observation is indicated.

Erickson TB: Toxicology: Ingestions and smoke inhalation. In Gausche-Hill M, Fuchs S, Yamamoto L (eds): APLS: The Pediatric Emergency Medicine Resource, 4th ed. Sudbury, MA, Jones & Bartlett Publishers, 2004, pp 244–245.

7. **Distinguish among hematemesis, hematochezia, and melena.**
   - Hematemesis is the vomiting of bright red or denatured blood ("coffee-ground" appearance). The source of the blood is proximal to the ligament of Treitz.
   - Hematochezia is bright red blood or maroon-colored stools per rectum and implies a lower GI source (colon).
   - Melena is the rectal passage of black tarry stools (black from the bacterial breakdown of blood); the source is proximal to the ileocecal valve.

Squires RH: Gastrointestinal bleeding. In Altschuler SM, Liacouras CA (eds): Clinical Pediatric Gastroenterology. Philadelphia, Churchill Livingstone, 1998, pp 31–42.

8. **Distinguish between upper GI and lower GI bleeding in terms of site of bleeding.**
   - Upper GI bleeding occurs when the site of bleeding is proximal to the ligament of Treitz or the second portion of the duodenum.
   - Lower GI bleeding implies a site distal to the ligament of Treitz, or those structures supplied by mesenteric vessels.

   Squires RH: Gastrointestinal bleeding. In Altschuler SM, Liacouras CA (eds): Clinical Pediatric Gastroenterology. Philadelphia, Churchill Livingstone, 1998, pp 31–42.

9. **What are some of the common tests used to determine the presence of blood? What causes them to be falsely positive or falsely negative?**
   The Hematest is a qualitative stool test that uses orthotolidine (a leukodye). False-positive results occur when the patient has ingested red meats, iron preparations, or plant peroxidases (found in horseradish, turnips, tomatoes, and fresh red cherries). False-negative results occur in the presence of ascorbic acid (vitamin C). The Hemoccult test is a qualitative stool test that uses guaiac (also a leukodye). False-positive results occur with red meats, broccoli, grapes, cauliflower, iron preparations, plant peroxidases, and cimetidine. False-negative results occur with hard stool, penicillamine, antacids, and ascorbic acid. The HemoQuant test is the only quantitative test (2 mg hemoglobin/gm stool) and uses a fluorescent antibody to porphyrin. It is falsely positive with red meat. Gastroccult tests check gastric fluids for blood.

   Cadranel S, Scaillon M: Approach to gastrointestinal bleeding. In Guandalini S (ed): Textbook of Pediatric Gastroenterology and Nutrition. London, Taylor & Francis, 2004, pp 639–654.
   Squires RH: Gastrointestinal bleeding. In Altschuler SM, Liacouras CA (eds): Clinical Pediatric Gastroenterology. Philadelphia, Churchill Livingstone, 1998, pp 31–42.

10. **What ingested foods can cause red stools?**
    Fruit punch, Kool-Aid beverage (especially cherry or strawberry), red beets, tomatoes, and gelatin. Note that commercial dyes can also be found in breakfast cereals.

    Cadranel S, Scaillon M: Approach to gastrointestinal bleeding. In Guandalini S (ed): Textbook of Pediatric Gastroenterology and Nutrition. London, Taylor & Francis, 2004, pp 639–654.
    Markel H, Oski JA, Oski FA, McMillan JA: The Portable Pediatrician. Philadelphia, Hanley & Belfus, 1992.

11. **What foods or items can cause black stools?**
    Bismuth (Pepto-Bismol), iron preparations, charcoal, licorice, beets, spinach, blueberries, grape juice, dark chocolate, and swallowed blood.

    Cadranel S, Scaillon M: Approach to gastrointestinal bleeding. In Guandalini S (ed): Textbook of Pediatric Gastroenterology and Nutrition. London, Taylor & Francis, 2004, pp 639–654.

12. **What is the APT-Downey test? How is it used?**
    This test is for fetal red cells and is used when an infant spits up blood. If the infant is breast-feeding, it is often unclear if the blood is from the baby's GI tract or maternal milk. Adult hemoglobin, eluted from erythrocytes, is denatured to alkaline globin hematin in an alkaline solution (sodium hydroxide), resulting in a yellow-brown color. Fetal hemoglobin resists the effect of alkali and stays pink. However, if the blood you use for the test is coffee-ground color (not red), it will be read falsely as adult blood.

    Cadranel S, Scaillon M: Approach to gastrointestinal bleeding. In Guandalini S (ed): Textbook of Pediatric Gastroenterology and Nutrition. London, Taylor & Francis, 2004, pp 639–654.

13. **What is another test that can help localize the source of GI bleeding?**
    The blood urea nitrogen (BUN)–to–creatinine ratio can help. A BUN–creatinine ratio > 30 indicates upper GI bleeding. In a study done at the Children's Hospital of Los Angeles, the specificity was 100% (although the sensitivity was 39%). The BUN level is thought to rise after upper GI bleeding as a result of increased hepatic catabolism of the absorbed amino acid load

from the intraluminal blood. Therefore, the bleeding must occur proximal to the ligament of Treitz. A BUN–creatinine ratio of 30 can occur with upper or lower GI bleeding.

Markel H, Oski JA, Oski FA, McMillan JA: The Portable Pediatrician. Philadelphia, Hanley & Belfus, 1992.

14. **What are some common causes of upper GI bleeding in infants and children?**
   - **Neonates:** Swallowed maternal blood, esophagitis, coagulopathy, sepsis, gastritis (stress ulcer)
   - **Infants (age 1–12 months):** Gastritis, esophagitis, Mallory-Weiss tear, duplication
   - **Children (age 1–12 years):** Epistaxis, esophagitis, gastritis, ulcers, Mallory-Weiss tear, esophageal varices, toxic ingestion
   - **Adolescents:** Ulcers, esophagitis, varices, gastritis, Mallory-Weiss tear, toxic ingestion

Squires RH: Gastrointestinal bleeding. In Altschuler SM, Liacouras CA (eds): Clinical Pediatric Gastroenterology. Philadelphia, Churchill Livingstone, 1998, pp 31–42.

Stevens MW, Henretig FM: Vomiting. In Fleisher GR, Ludwig S, Henretig FM (eds): Textbook of Pediatric Emergency Medicine, 5th ed. Philadelphia, Lippincott Williams & Wilkins, 2006, pp 681–689.

15. **What are some common causes of lower GI bleeding in infants and children?**
   - **Neonates:** Swallowed maternal blood, anorectal lesions, milk allergy, necrotizing enterocolitis, midgut volvulus, Hirschsprung's disease
   - **Infants (age 1–12 months):** Anal fissure, midgut volvulus, intussusception, Meckel's diverticulum, infectious diarrhea, milk allergy
   - **Children (age 1–12 years):** Anal fissures, polyps, Meckel's diverticulum, intussusception, infectious diarrhea, inflammatory bowel disease, duplications, hemangiomas, Henoch-Schönlein purpura, hemolytic uremic syndrome
   - **Adolescents:** Inflammatory bowel disease (ulcerative colitis, Crohn's disease), polyps, hemorrhoids, anal fissure, infectious diarrhea

Squires RH: Gastrointestinal bleeding. In Altschuler SM, Liacouras CA (eds): Clinical Pediatric Gastroenterology. Philadelphia, Churchill Livingstone, 1998, pp 31–42.

Stevens MW, Henretig FM: Vomiting. In Fleisher GR, Ludwig S, Henretig FM (eds): Textbook of Pediatric Emergency Medicine, 5th ed. Philadelphia, Lippincott Williams & Wilkins, 2006, pp 681–689.

16. **Distinguish between malrotation and volvulus.**
   Malrotation is the incomplete or reverse rotation of the embryonic midgut about the superior mesenteric artery. The small bowel then hangs on a mesenteric stalk. Volvulus occurs when the midgut twists around the stalk, resulting in small bowel obstruction and vascular compromise due to compression of the mesenteric vessels. Midgut volvulus occurs in 70% of infants with malrotation.

Okada PJ, Hicks BA: Nontraumatic surgical emergencies. In Gausche-Hill M, Fuchs S, Yamamoto L (eds): APLS: The Pediatric Emergency Medicine Resource, 4th ed. Sudbury, MA, Jones and Bartlett Publishers, 2004, pp 367–371.

17. **What are the clinical features of malrotation with volvulus?**
   An infant with malrotation and volvulus is usually less than 1 month of age. Symptoms include bilious vomiting, irritability, and abdominal pain. When volvulus is present, there are bloody or heme-positive stools. The infant can rapidly progress to a shocklike state. The physical examination reveals abdominal distention with dilated loops of bowel, lethargy, pallor, and possibly hypotension. Therapy includes fluid resuscitation, nasogastric tube, broad-spectrum antibiotics, and emergent surgery (Ladd's procedure).

Okada PJ, Hicks BA: Nontraumatic surgical emergencies. In Gausche-Hill M, Fuchs S, Yamamoto L (eds): APLS: The Pediatric Emergency Medicine Resource, 4th ed. Sudbury, MA, Jones and Bartlett Publishers, 2004, pp 367–371.

18. **What is the radiographic finding in an infant with malrotation and volvulus?**
The abdominal radiographs may be normal (50–60% of patients) or show duodenal obstruction (double bubble). The upper GI study shows a displaced duodenal–jejunal junction (both to the right of the spine), with the jejunum on the right side of the abdomen. There may be a corkscrew appearance of contrast. A lower GI study shows a displaced cecum, usually in the right upper quadrant, or an abnormally oriented superior mesenteric artery.

    Okada PJ, Hicks BA: Nontraumatic surgical emergencies. In Gausche-Hill M, Fuchs S, Yamamoto L (eds): APLS: The Pediatric Emergency Medicine Resource, 4th ed. Sudbury, MA, Jones and Bartlett Publishers, 2004, pp 367–371.

KEY POINTS: ETIOLOGY OF VOMITING ✔️

1. The most common cause of vomiting in older children is acute gastroenteritis.

2. Vomiting can occur from extra-GI problems, such as infections (meningitis, urinary tract infections), metabolic (inborn errors of metabolism, diabetic ketoacidosis), drugs/toxins (iron, lead), and pregnancy.

3. An infant under 1 month of age (outside of the nursery) with bilious vomiting and abdominal pain and distention has malrotation (with or without volvulus) until proven otherwise.

19. **Is a "currant jelly" stool classic for intussusception?**
Up to 75% of children with intussusception never have visible blood in the stool (although the stool is guaiac-positive). A currant jelly stool is a late finding because it implies that bowel necrosis has occurred. Intussusception generally occurs in children under 2 years of age, with a peak age range of 5–9 months. Classic symptoms occur in 10% of cases and include the sudden onset of severe, intermittent, crampy abdominal pain, with crying and drawing up of legs in episodes every 15 minutes. This is followed by vomiting and the passage of a "currant jelly" stool. There is also a "neurologic presentation," which consists of lethargy followed by brief periods of irritability. Abdominal radiographs (Fig. 35-1) may show a soft tissue mass, a nascence of cecal gas and stool, a target sign, a meniscus or crescent sign, a paucity of bowel gas, or a bowel obstruction. Definitive diagnosis and treatment in >75% of cases are made by barium or air contrast enema (hydrostatic reduction). The most common location for the intussusception is ileocolic. Lead point is usually not present in younger children but is somewhat common in older children (e.g., Meckel's diverticulum, duplication, vasculitis due to Henoch-Schönlein purpura).

    Okada PJ, Hicks BA: Nontraumatic surgical emergencies. In Gausche-Hill M, Fuchs S, Yamamoto L (eds): APLS: The Pediatric Emergency Medicine Resource, 4th ed. Sudbury, MA, Jones & Bartlett Publishers, 2004, pp 376–381.

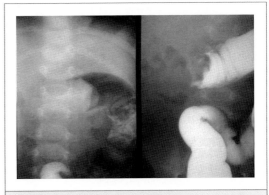

Figure 35-1. Radiograph of intussusception.

20. **What is a Meckel's diverticulum?**

Meckel's diverticulum is a remnant of the vitellointestinal or omphalomesenteric duct that may result in painless rectal bleeding. It is present in 2% of the population, is 2 inches long (or less), and is found within 2 feet of the ileocecal valve. It contains ectopic gastric mucosa in 60–90% of patients and in almost all of those who have painless rectal bleeding. (The gastric mucosa can result in an ulcer, which bleeds.) Diagnosis is by a Meckel's scan (technetium 99m pertechnetate scan). Gastric mucosa concentrates the technetium 99. An intestinal duplication may also contain gastric mucosa and can cause GI bleeding or symptoms of obstruction or intussusception. A duplication occurs most commonly in the ileocecal region, but also is found in the distal esophagus, stomach, and duodenum.

Azizkhan RG: Meckel's diverticulum. In Guandalini S (ed): Textbook of Pediatric Gastroenterology and Nutrition. London, Taylor & Francis, 2004, pp 729–738.

21. **A child who has had surgical correction for Hirschsprung's disease presents with fever, abdominal distention, and diarrhea. What is your concern?**

This child probably has Hirschsprung's enterocolitis and requires IV fluids, nasogastric drainage, broad-spectrum antibiotics, and decompression of the rectum or colon by rectal stimulation or irrigation. Enterocolitis is the most common cause of death in children with Hirschsprung's disease. Other complications include persistent obstructive symptoms and fecal incontinence.

Dasgupta R, Langer JC: Hirschsprung disease. Curr Prob Surgery 41: 949–988, 2004.

22. **True or false: Pain is worse after meals in younger children with ulcers.**

False. In most young children with ulcers, pain is not related to meals. In some older children and adolescents, pain may be exacerbated by acidic foods or spicy meals, as in adults. Symptoms in neonates include vomiting; infants may feed poorly or vomit; toddlers may have poorly localized abdominal pain or vomiting; adolescents may have epigastric pain. All age groups can have melena or upper GI bleeding.

Stevens MW, Henretig FM: Vomiting. In Fleisher GR, Ludwig S, Henretig FM (eds): Textbook of Pediatric Emergency Medicine, 5th ed. Philadelphia, Lippincott Williams & Wilkins, 2006, pp 681–689.

23. **What is the relationship between *Helicobacter pylori* and gastritis/peptic ulcers in children?**

Helicobacter pylori is a gram-negative, spiral-shaped bacterium present in over 50% of the population that causes gastritis and peptic ulcers. Although seroprevalence in the United States is 10%, the risk is higher for those who live with an infected family member, those in crowded living conditions, those who attend day care, those who have poor hygiene, American-born children of immigrant parents, and internationally adopted children. *H. pylori* colonizes and persists only in the gastric mucosa and causes gastritis and primarily duodenal ulcers. *H. pylori* infection has been associated with gastric adenocarcinoma and lymphoma, decades after infection.

Czinn SJ: *Helicobacter pylori* infection: Detection, investigation, and management. J Pediatr 146:S21–S26, 2005.

Gold BD, Colletti RB, Abbott M, et al: *Helicobacter pylori* infection in children: Recommendations for diagnosis and treatment. J Pediatr Gastroenterol Nutrition 31:490–497, 2000.

24. **What are some therapies for *H. pylori* infection in children?**

Eradication therapy is recommended for children with a definitive peptic ulcer and *H. pylori* on histology. Triple therapy is recommended and includes the following first-line therapies in a twice-daily fashion for 7–14 days:

- Amoxicillin, 50 mg/kg/d (up to 1 gm twice daily)
- Clarithromycin, 15 mg/kg/d (up to 500 mg twice daily)

- Proton-pump inhibitor (e.g., omeprazole), 1 mg/kg/d (up to 20 mg twice daily)
One can substitute metronidazole, 20 mg/kg/d (up to 500 mg twice daily), for clarithromycin, or use clarithromycin, metronidazole, and omeprazole.

Czinn SJ: *Helicobacter pylori* infection: Detection, investigation, and management. J Pediatr 146:S21–S26, 2005.

Gold BD, Colletti RB, Abbott M, et al: *Helicobacter pylori* infection in children: Recommendations for diagnosis and treatment. J Pediatr Gastroenterol Nutrition 31:490–497, 2000.

KEY POINTS: GASTRITIS/PEPTIC ULCERS AND *HELICOBACTER PYLORI* ✓

1. *H. pylori* is associated with gastric and duodenal ulcers in children.

2. Endoscopy with biopsy is the preferred method for diagnosis. The serologic tests are not reliable in children. The urea breath tests are reliable in older children, but have not been studied adequately in children under 2 years.

3. *H. pylori* is an infrequent cause of recurrent abdominal pain in children.

4. Treatment is indicated in symptomatic patients with proven *H. pylori* infection.

25. **Describe some of the anatomic and histologic differences between ulcerative colitis and Crohn's disease.**
    - **Ulcerative colitis:** Inflammation of the mucosa and submucosa limited to the colon and rectum, continuous involvement in these regions. There are various degrees of ulceration, hemorrhage, edema, and pseudopolyps.
    - **Crohn's disease:** Can involve any portion of the alimentary tract, including the upper GI tract (30–40% of cases), small bowel (90%), and distal ileum (70%). There is transmural inflammation, with discrete lesions ("skip lesions"). Because of the full-thickness involvement, there can be focal ulcerations, fistulae, strictures, adhesions, and a cobblestone appearance.

Brown JB, Li BUK: Inflammatory bowel disease. In Green TP, Franklin WH, Tanz RR (eds). Pediatrics: Just the Facts. New York, McGraw-Hill, 2005, pp 316–319.

Mamula P, Markowitz JE, Baldassano RN: Inflammatory bowel disease in early childhood and adolescence: Special considerations. Gastroenterol Clin North Am 32:967–995, 2003.

26. **What are some of the extraintestinal features of ulcerative colitis and Crohn's disease?**
    Since both can present with bloody diarrhea, abdominal pain, weight loss, and fever, extraintestinal manifestations may help determine which is more likely prior to endoscopy.
    - **Ulcerative colitis:** Growth failure, arthropathy/arthritis, pyoderma gangrenosum
    - **Crohn's disease:** Growth failure, delayed puberty, perianal disease, stomatitis, erythema nodosum, arthritis, clubbing, uveitis, nephrolithiasis

Brown JB, Li BUK: Inflammatory bowel disease. In Green TP, Franklin WH, Tanz RR (eds). Pediatrics: Just the Facts. New York, McGraw-Hill, 2005, pp 316–319.

Mamula P, Markowitz JE, Baldassano RN: Inflammatory bowel disease in early childhood and adolescence: Special considerations. Gastroenterol Clin North Am 32:967–995, 2003.

27. **What is a food allergy?**
This is an abnormal reaction after the ingestion of food. It can be non–immune-mediated (lactose intolerance, infectious [*Salmonella*], toxic [*Clostridium botulinum*]) or immune-mediated, including IgE-mediated (immediate hypersensitivity), non–IgE-mediated (food protein–induced enterocolitis, celiac disease), or mixed IgE and T cell (eosinophilic esophagitis).

Shah U, Walker WA: Food allergy. In Lifschitz CH (ed): Pediatric Gastroenterology and Nutrition in Clinical Practice. New York, Marcel Dekker, 2002, pp 601–613.
Spergel JM, Pawlowski NA: Food allergy: Mechanism, diagnosis and management in childhood. Pediatr Clin North Am 49:73–96, 2002.

28. **What are some of the food allergy disorders of infancy and their treatment?**
Food protein–induced enterocolitis syndrome occurs in the first few months of life and involves allergy mainly to milk protein and soy. The infant presents with vomiting, diarrhea, and irritability and can present in shock. Food protein–induced enteropathy presents in infancy with diarrhea and poor weight gain. Vomiting and malabsorption also occur. Milk sensitivity is the usual culprit, but soy, egg, wheat, and other food can cause this. Biopsy of the small intestine shows villous atrophy with cellular infiltration. These symptoms also improve when the agent is removed, but these reactions often resolve by 1 year of age.

In both of these cases, whole cow milk should be substituted with casein hydrolysate formulas (Nutramigen, Pregestimil, Alimentum). Even whey hydrolysate or soy protein formulas are not appropriate, as some children have allergies to these as well. An amino acid–based formula (Neocate, Vivonex) can also be used.

Shah U, Walker WA: Food allergy. In Lifschitz CH (ed): Pediatric Gastroenterology and Nutrition in Clinical Practice. New York, Marcel Dekker, 2002, pp 601–613.
Spergel JM, Pawlowski NA: Food allergy: Mechanism, diagnosis and management in childhood. Pediatr Clin North Am 49:73–96, 2002.

29. **What is celiac disease?**
This is a specific food protein–induced enteropathy due to gluten, a protein found in grains. The specific proteins are gliadin in wheat, secalines in rye, and hordeins in barley. Some patients may also have problems with oats. It is an HLA-associated condition. Presenting symptoms include weight loss/failure to thrive, chronic diarrhea, steatorrhea, and abdominal distention. Treatment is avoidance of these grains.

Shah U, Walker WA: Food allergy. In Lifschitz CH (ed): Pediatric Gastroenterology and Nutrition in Clinical Practice. New York, Marcel Dekker, 2002, pp 601–613.
Shamir R: Advances in celiac disease. Gastroenterol Clin North Am 32:931–947, 2003.
Spergel JM, Pawlowski NA: Food allergy: Mechanism, diagnosis and management in childhood. Pediatr Clin North Am 49:73–96, 2002.

30. **List some of the malignant abdominal masses in children.**
Wilms' tumor, neuroblastoma, hepatoblastoma, hepatocarcinoma, pelvic sarcoma, lymphoma, teratomas, and ovarian tumors.

Rheingold SR, Lange B: Oncologic emergencies. In Fleisher GR, Ludwig S, Henretig FM (eds): Textbook of Pediatric Emergency Medicine, 5th ed. Philadelphia, Lippincott Williams & Wilkins, 2006, pp 1239–1274.

31. **What is the classic triad of findings associated with hemolytic uremic syndrome?**
Acute hemolytic anemia, thrombocytopenia, and renal injury (oliguria, abnormal urinalysis, increasing BUN and creatinine levels). Although usually associated with bloody diarrhea, there are actually two phenotypes of hemolytic uremic syndrome (HUS). One is diarrhea-associated

(D+ HUS or typical HUS), the other nondiarrheal (D−, or atypical HUS). D+ HUS is usually caused by *Shiga* toxins elaborated by *E. coli* O157:H7 or *Shigella dysenteriae* type 1.

Cronan K, Kost S: Renal and electrolyte abnormalities. In Fleisher GR, Ludwig S, Henretig FM (eds): Textbook of Pediatric Emergency Medicine, 5th ed. Philadelphia, Lippincott Williams & Wilkins, 2006, pp 873–919.

Wong CS, Jelacic S, Habeeb RL, et al: The risk of hemolytic-uremic syndrome after antibiotic treatment of *Escherichia coli* O157:H7 infections. N Engl J Med 342:1930–1936, 2000.

32. **A child has diarrhea as a result of *E. coli* O157:H7. Should he receive antibiotics?**
    No, because there is an increased risk (adjusted relative risk, 17.2) of that child developing HUS. This is true for sulfa-containing drugs as well as β-lactams.

    Wong CS, Jelacic S, Habeeb RL, et al: The risk of hemolytic-uremic syndrome after antibiotic treatment of *Escherichia coli* O157:H7 infections. N Engl J Med 342:1930–1936, 2000.

33. **What laboratory tests should you order for a child you think has pancreatitis?**
    Serum amylase levels become elevated within 2–12 hours of symptoms of acute pancreatitis, peak at 12–72 hours, and often return to normal in 3–5 days. Since amylase is produced in the salivary glands and ovaries, an isolated serum amylase level does not necessarily reflect pancreatic origin. Serum lipase increases 4–8 hours after the onset of symptoms, peaks at 24 hours, and remains elevated for 8–14 days. A serum lipase level three times normal has better diagnostic accuracy for pancreatitis than serum amylase.

    Azzam R, Li BUK: Pancreatic disorders. In Green TP, Franklin WH, Tanz RR (eds). Pediatrics: Just the Facts. New York, McGraw-Hill, 2005, pp 325–327.

    Pietzak MM: Acute and chronic pancreatitis. In Guandalini S (ed): Textbook of Pediatric Gastroenterology and Nutrition. London, Taylor & Francis, 2004, pp 303–318.

34. **What causes pancreatitis in children?**
    Acute pancreatitis in children is due to one of several causes:
    - Anatomic/structural abnormalities (choledochal cysts, biliary stone, tumors)
    - Drugs and toxins (acetaminophen overdose, antibiotics, anticonvulsants, antihypertensives, anti-inflammatories, neoplastic agents)
    - Infections (*E. coli*, *Ascaris lumbricoides*, varicella, mumps, influenza B, HIV)
    - Trauma (disruption of pancreatic ducts, compression injury)
    - Familial/hereditary (cystic fibrosis)
    - Metabolic (hyperlipidemia, hyperparathyroidism, malnutrition)
    - Idiopathic

    Pietzak MM: Acute and chronic pancreatitis. In Guandalini S (ed): Textbook of Pediatric Gastroenterology and Nutrition. London, Taylor & Francis, 2004, pp 303–318.

35. **What is cyclic vomiting syndrome?**
    This is a syndrome of vomiting in a cyclic pattern that is severe, recurring, and stereotypical. There is a high intensity of vomiting (6–12 times an hour) that occurs 1–2 times a month and lasts approximately 24 hours. The child is well between episodes. It is often precipitated by psychological stress, infection, exhaustion, a menstrual period, or certain foods (cheese, chocolate, caffeine, monosodium glutamate), and there is usually a strong family history of migraine headaches. Treatment includes IV fluids with 10% dextrose in 0.2 normal saline (D10.2NS), 10 mL/kg bolus, then give at 1.5 times maintenance, ondansetron and lorazepam (or chlorpromazine and diphenhydramine).

    Sunku B, Li BUK: Cyclic vomiting syndrome. In Guandalini S (ed): Textbook of Pediatric Gastroenterology and Nutrition. London, Taylor & Francis, 2004, pp 289–302.

    Li BUK, Misiewicz L: Cyclic vomiting syndrome: A brain-gut disorder. Gastroenterol Clin North Am 32:997–1019, 2003.

36. **What are the criteria necessary to make the diagnosis of cyclic vomiting syndrome?**
    - Three or more episodes of vomiting within the last year
    - No symptoms between episodes of vomiting
    - Acute onset of vomiting with each episode, with each one lasting no more than 1 week
    - No identifiable organic cause of the vomiting

    Li BU: New hope for children with cyclic vomiting syndrome. Contemp Pediatr 19:121, 2002.

37. **What is the typical history of the GI symptoms associated with Henoch-Schönlein purpura?**
    GI symptoms normally include nausea, vomiting, and abdominal pain and can occasionally result in intussusception, GI hemorrhage, and, rarely, bowel necrosis. The GI symptoms usually develop within 8 days of the rash. However, it has been noted that GI symptoms, including abdominal pain, precede the rash in about 15–35% of cases, making the diagnosis of the condition more challenging.

    Chang WL, Yang YH, Lin YT, Chiang BL: Gastrointestinal manifestations in Henoch-Schönlein purpura: A review of 261 patients. Acta Paediatr 93:1427–1431, 2004.

38. **What causes the abdominal pain in Henoch-Schönlein purpura?**
    The pain is thought to be caused by submucosal hemorrhage as well as edema. Endoscopy may reveal purpura in the stomach, duodenum, terminal ileum, and colon.

39. **What is the suggested imaging study in suspected intussusception associated with Henoch-Schönlein purpura?**
    Abdominal ultrasonography is recommended as opposed to air or barium contrast enema (typically ordered when intussusception is suspected in patients without Henoch-Schönlein purpura). Contrast enemas cannot make the diagnosis of ileoileal intussusception, which is typically seen in patients with Henoch-Schönlein purpura–related intussusception.

CHAPTER 36

GYNECOLOGIC EMERGENCIES

Kate M. Cronan, MD, FAAP

1. **What are the best ways to perform a genital examination in a prepubertal girl?**
   The external genitalia should be examined with the child lying supine in a "frog-leg" position, either on the examining table or on the parent's lap. Use gentle lateral traction on the labia majora to obtain an adequate view of the introitus. To visualize the vaginal vault, examine the child in the "knee-chest" position. Ask the child to get up on her hands and knees ("like you are going to crawl"), and to rest her head on her folded arms. The labia and buttocks can be separated while the child relaxes her abdominal muscles. An otoscope *without* speculum can be used as a light source. If discharge or bleeding is noted, return the child to the supine position to take samples/cultures. If there is vaginal bleeding from an injury, it may be necessary to perform a speculum examination under sedation.

   Paradise J: Vaginal bleeding. In Fleisher G, Ludwig S, Henretig FM (eds). The Textbook of Pediatric Emergency Medicine, 5th ed. Philadelphia, Lippincott Williams & Wilkins, 2006, pp 669–670.

2. **A mother brings her 2-year-old daughter to the emergency department (ED) because she has noticed that her "vagina seems to be closing up." What could this be caused by?**
   Labial adhesions are a benign condition occurring in 3–7% of girls between the ages of 3 months and 5 years. The medial epithelial surfaces of the labia minora gradually adhere to one another, and the fusion proceeds anteriorly. Physical examination using labial traction reveals a flat area of adherent tissue, with a characteristic vertical raphe obscuring the introitus. A small opening remains through which urine may pass. Therapy consists of twice-daily applications of estrogen cream at the point of midline fusion. Continue treatment until the lesions resolve. Once the adhesions have separated, zinc oxide or petroleum jelly should be applied for an additional 2 weeks to prevent readherence. Medical therapy may rarely fail when the adhesions are thick (3–4 mm in width) with no evidence of a thin raphe.

   Do not confuse labial adhesions with congenital abnormalities of the genitalia, such as ambiguous genitalia or imperforate hymen.

   Bacon JL: Prepubertal labial adhesions: Evaluation of a referral population. Am J Obstet Gynecol 187: 327–331, 2002.

3. **A healthy 14-year-old girl presents with symptoms of urgency, frequency, and dysuria, as well as intermittent lower-abdominal pain. Her urinalysis is normal. Although her sexual development has been normal, she has never menstruated. What might be the problem?**
   A thorough physical examination, including a genital examination, will reveal the source of her distress. This patient probably has a congenital obstruction of the vagina, either an imperforate hymen or vaginal atresia. If this condition is not noticed during infancy, a young adolescent girl can present as above, with large quantities of menstrual blood accumulated behind the hymen. The collection of blood is termed *hematocolpos*. Examination of the abdomen may reveal a mass, which might initially be confused with a tumor or even pregnancy. Examination of the genitalia shows a bulging, membranous covering over the introitus, often appearing bluish from the blood behind. Treatment is surgical.

4. **How does hydrocolpos differ from hematocolpos?**

   Vaginal obstruction during infancy leads to vaginal distention that is due to a buildup of mucous. This is called **hydrocolpos** or **mucocolpos**. Infants present with an abdominal mass, trouble with urinating, and a bulging membrane at the introitus. When the amount of mucous secretion is large, the uterus also becomes distended and results in **hydrometrocolpos**. If vaginal obstruction is not recognized until menarchal age, menstrual blood accumulates and distends the vagina, producing **hematocolpos**. In late puberty the child may present with amenorrhea. Eventually urinary symptoms may develop as the collection of blood increases in size. A lower-abdominal mass is often palpable.

5. **How does perineal trauma in young girls occur?**

   Most perineal trauma in young girls results from a "straddle injury," wherein the girl falls on a narrow object (e.g., bicycle crossbar, jungle gym, chair arm, fence). The most common injuries are vulvar hematomas and superficial lacerations. Most of these may be treated conservatively with sitz baths several times a day. Ensuring that the patient can void in the ED is crucial.

6. **How should urinary retention after a straddle injury be managed?**

   In most cases urinary retention is mild and brief, and it occurs because of the discomfort of the urine passing over the injured perineum. Girls may be more comfortable urinating while sitting in a tub of warm water.

7. **What concerns must you have regarding more complicated perineal trauma?**

   With a very forceful straddle injury, deep lacerations may occur in the vagina, and may extend into the rectum or urethra. Some hematomas may expand rapidly and become massive, requiring evacuation. These injuries must be explored thoroughly, either with effective sedation or under general anesthesia in the operating room. Consultation should be initiated with colleagues from pediatric gynecology or pediatric urology as appropriate for surgical repair. Concerns are similar for penetrating trauma to the perineum by a foreign object.

8. **What are the causes of vaginal bleeding before menarche?**

   In the prepubertal child, "vaginal bleeding" may originate in the vagina, the vulva, or both. Causes of apparent vaginal bleeding can be divided into nonhormonal and hormonal:
   - **Nonhormonal** causes include trauma, tumor, urethral prolapse, infectious vaginitis, intravaginal foreign body, and genital warts.
   - **Hormonal** causes include neonatal bleeding, exogenous estrogen, and precocious puberty.

9. **A 3-year-old African-American girl presents to the ED with vaginal bleeding and a donut-shaped mass of purplish tissue protruding from her vagina. Her mother is concerned that she might have been abused. What's your diagnosis?**

   Although sexual assault must always be in the differential diagnosis of genital trauma, the soft donut-shaped mass in this child is most likely *not* protruding from the vagina but rather is a urethral prolapse (Fig. 36-1). It is the most common cause of apparent vaginal bleeding in childhood, with the bleeding resulting from ischemia of the protruding urethral mucosa. For reasons that remain obscure, 95% of cases

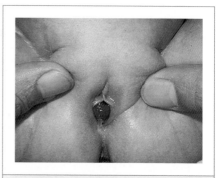

Figure 36-1. Urethral prolapse.

reported in the literature are in African-American girls. If the segment of prolapsed urethra is not necrotic, warm compresses or sitz baths in combination with 2 weeks of topical estrogen may be effective. Dark red necrotic mucosa requires surgical reduction of the prolapse within several days.

10. **A mother brings in her 6-year-old daughter and tells you that the girl seems to be urinating more frequently than usual and says that it hurts when she urinates. You are sure she has a urinary tract infection, and you confidently send a sample to the lab. The urinalysis is normal. What could be causing her dysuria and frequency?**
Symptoms of vulvovaginitis can include urinary frequency and dysuria. The most frequent reason for vulvovaginitis is simple irritation, either as the result of poor hygiene or cleansing products, such as bubble bath, shampoo, powders, soaps, and some feminine hygiene products. Infectious etiologies include *Shigella* spp., group A streptococci, *Neisseria gonorrhoeae*, and *Candida* spp. Pinworm infections, although rectal in origin, may lead to such intense itching and vigorous scratching that the patient presents with perineal excoriations and bleeding.
    Treatment is frequent sitz baths. If the vulva is irritated, the patient may be more comfortable voiding while sitting in a tub of warm water. If symptoms of nonspecific vulvovaginitis persist for 2–3 weeks, consider a 10-day course of oral antibiotics (e.g., amoxicillin). When a specific microbial etiology has been identified in a prepubertal child (such as gonorrhea or chlamydia, coliform bacteria, group A streptococci, *Candida albicans*, *Trichomonas* spp., or *Gardnerella* spp.), give appropriate antimicrobial treatment and alert child protective services.

11. **What is the most common cause of vaginal discharge in young girls?**
Foul-smelling discharge most commonly signals a retained foreign body in the vagina. The most common foreign body is toilet paper, which may be contaminated with feces. To assess for a foreign body, first place the patient in the knee-chest position to examine the vaginal area. Attach a 60-mL syringe filled with warmed saline to an 8-Fr feeding tube. Place the patient in the supine position and separate the labia majora. Viscous lidocaine may be applied prior to the insertion of the catheter. Then place the tube past the hymenal orifice and irrigate with saline.

   Giardino A, Christian C: Vaginal foreign body removal. In Henretig F, King C (eds): The Textbook of Pediatric Emergency Procedures, 5th ed. Philadelphia, Lippincott Williams & Wilkins, Philadelphia, 2005, pp 971–974.

12. **What causes vaginal bleeding after menarche?**
Vaginal bleeding in the adolescent patient can result from hormonal contraception, endometritis, dysfunctional uterine bleeding, bleeding diathesis, or complications of pregnancy (spontaneous abortion, ectopic pregnancy, placenta previa, placental abruption).

13. **What is the first test to send on *any* adolescent patient with abnormal vaginal bleeding?**
Qualitative urine pregnancy test. An ectopic pregnancy can rapidly progress into a life-threatening emergency. In many instances, the urine sample can be obtained even before the physical examination is begun.

14. **A 13-year-old female patient arrives in your ED with abnormal vaginal bleeding. Her menarche was around age 12. Her menstrual periods generally occur 24–32 days apart, but it has been only 18 days since the start of her last period. Should you be concerned?**
Probably not. During the first 2 years following menarche, it is not uncommon to have irregularities in both duration of menses and number of days between cycles. Note that 95% of adolescents' periods last 2–8 days. Ten or more days of bleeding should be considered

abnormal. Most cycles start 21 days or more from the first day of the last period. While occasional intervals of less than 21 days are normal for young teens, several short cycles in a row are abnormal. Although any amount of bleeding may be more than young teenagers would like, it is uncommon for adolescents to soak more than 6–8 pads or tampons per day.

15. **What are the most common organisms causing sexually transmitted disease (STD) in the adolescent population?**

    C. trachomatis and *N. gonorrhoeae* infections are the most commonly reported STDs among adolescent patients. In fact, reported rates of chlamydial and gonorrheal infections are highest among females age 15–19 years. Human papillomavirus is probably the most common viral STD among teens, with herpes simplex virus type 2 also frequent. Neither are reportable diseases, so exact prevalence rates are not known. HIV infection is increasing among adolescents, while rates of both primary and secondary syphilis have steadily declined in all age groups since peaking in 1990.

    Centers for Disease Control and Prevention: Sexually transmitted diseases treatment guidelines. MMWR Morb Mortal Wkly Rep 55:1–94, 2006.

16. **Pelvic inflammatory disease (PID) can be caused by a number of different microorganisms. What are they?**

    C. trachomatis, *N. gonorrhoeae*, or both can be identified in nearly 50% of cases of PID, with almost all first episodes of PID in adolescents attributable to these organisms. Evidence from laparoscopically obtained cultures demonstrates that upper tract infection can be polymicrobial, involving both aerobic and anaerobic organisms. Isolates have included genital mycoplasmas, such as *Mycoplasma hominis* and *Ureaplasma urealyticum*, aerobic and anaerobic streptococci, *Gardnerella vaginalis*, *Haemophilus influenzae*, and enteric organisms such as *Escherichia coli* and *Bacteroides* spp.

17. **What distinguishes PID from uncomplicated cervicitis?**

    Cervicitis is an inflammation of the cervix characterized by a mucopurulent vaginal discharge; cervical inflammation with friability, edema, and ectopy; and presence of white blood cells in the cervical os. Symptoms may include vaginal discharge, dysuria, dyspareunia, and postcoital bleeding. Unlike with PID, systemic signs of infection are *not* characteristic of cervicitis, nor is cervical motion tenderness or adnexal tenderness evident on examination. Cervicitis can be caused by a variety of organisms, including *Chlamydia trachomatis*, *N. gonorrhoeae*, *Trichomonas vaginalis*, *Candida albicans*, and herpes simplex virus. Cervicitis can also be noninfectious, resulting from a foreign body or chemical irritation. In contrast to PID, in which there should be a low threshold for starting empiric antibiotics, treatment for uncomplicated cervicitis can be deferred until a specific microbial etiology is identified.

18. **How is PID diagnosed?**

    Acute PID is often difficult to diagnose because of the nonspecific nature of symptoms and the broad differential diagnosis of abdominal pain in an adolescent female. Diagnosis is made through a combination of historical and clinical findings. Laboratory and radiologic studies may be helpful. In evaluating an adolescent female with abdominal pain, the patient should be interviewed and examined in private (without the parent in the room). A thorough gynecologic and sexual history should be taken, including menstrual history, number of sexual partners, contraceptive practices, and history of previous STDs. Physical examination should focus on the many possible causes of abdominal pain, including pregnancy, complications of prior abdominal surgery, and pneumonia. Careful examination of the abdomen and a thorough pelvic examination (both speculum and bimanual examination, checking for cervical motion tenderness, adnexal masses, or tenderness) should be performed, and culture or DNA probe samples should be taken for chlamydia and gonorrhea.

19. **When should you treat for PID?**
    In the ED, physicians should have a low threshold for initiating empiric antibiotic treatment for any adolescent female patient with a history or physical examination suggestive of PID. Only minimal laboratory evaluation (testing for gonorrhea and chlamydia) need be performed. This approach minimizes the chance of missing PID in a patient presenting with only mild symptoms. If the patient presents with a severe clinical picture or is pregnant, undertake more extensive evaluation (laboratory and ultrasonography) to rule out other diagnoses. If no other definitive diagnosis is reached (e.g., appendicitis, urinary tract infection, pneumonia), start treatment.

20. **What are the indicators for treating sexual partners?**
    Identification and treatment of sexual partners are key in limiting the spread of STD. Any sexual partners within the past 3 months should be thoroughly evaluated and tested for gonorrhea and chlamydia, whether or not they are symptomatic. In general, empiric treatment is appropriate for all sexual contacts of a patient with PID.

21. **Do all adolescents with PID need to be hospitalized for treatment?**
    No. The Centers for Disease Control and Prevention recommends hospitalization when "surgical emergencies such as appendicitis cannot be excluded; the patient is pregnant; the patient does not respond clinically to oral antimicrobial therapy; the patient is unable to follow or tolerate an outpatient oral regimen; the patient has severe illness, nausea and vomiting, or high fever; or the patient has a tubo-ovarian abscess." There is no evidence that adolescents benefit from hospitalization for treatment of PID. Nonetheless, many practitioners believe that hospitalization is appropriate for adolescents, especially when adherence to treatment is in question. Hospitalization also affords an opportunity for education regarding "safe sex" practices.

    Centers for Disease Control and Prevention: Sexually transmitted diseases treatment guidelines 2006. MMWR Morb Mortal Wkly Rep 55:1–94, 2006.

KEY POINTS: INDICATIONS FOR ADMISSION OF PATIENTS WITH PID ✓

1. Pregnancy
2. Surgical emergency that cannot be ruled out
3. No response to oral antimicrobials
4. Nonadherent patient
5. Evidence of severe illness
6. Tubo-ovarian abscess
7. Immunodeficiency

22. **What are the long-term complications of PID?**
    Long-term complications may occur in as many as 25% of females who have had PID. These include tubo-ovarian abscesses, Fitz-Hugh-Curtis syndrome, a sixfold to tenfold increased risk of ectopic pregnancy, infertility as a result of scarring (with the risk of infertility increasing with the number of episodes of PID), dyspareunia, and chronic and recurrent pelvic pain.

23. **Why are adolescent patients at such high risk for STD?**
Adolescents have some of the highest rates of STD. Many factors put adolescents at increased risk, including a high frequency of risky sexual behaviors and basic physiologic differences. Teenagers who are beginning to experiment with sexual behaviors often have multiple sexual partners and change partners frequently, with each new partner constituting a potential exposure to STD. Adolescents generally use contraceptives inconsistently, particularly barrier methods such as condoms, which prevent the passage of infectious organisms. Human papilloma virus infects actively dividing cells, and both *Chlamydia trachomatis* and *N. gonorrhoeae* adhere more easily to columnar epithelial cells. Finally, adolescents lack immunity to STDs.

24. **What are the most typical presenting features of ovarian torsion, and which patients are most likely to have this condition?**
- Stabbing abdominal pain
- Nausea and vomiting
- Pain radiating to the back or groin
- Sudden onset of sharp pain
A history of recent vigorous activity may be the precipitating event. Ovarian torsion is most frequently seen in postmenarchal females because it occurs more often when an ovarian cyst is present. However, ovarian torsion can occur in premenarchal females with normal ovaries.

Growdon WB, Laufer MR: Ovarian torsion, 2006. Available at www.uptodate.com.

25. **How is the clinical diagnosis of ovarian torsion made?**
In a female patient with symptoms of severe lower abdominal pain and nausea or vomiting, the differential diagnosis includes ectopic pregnancy, appendicitis, ovarian torsion, PID, tubo-ovarian abscess, endometriosis, and hemorrhagic cyst. Two-dimensional ultrasonography with Doppler and three-dimensional ultrasonography are the most effective modalities used to diagnose ovarian torsion. These studies demonstrate limited or absent blood flow in the ovary, which is suggestive of torsion. Open laparotomy provides definitive diagnosis.

26. **A 15-year-old female presents to the ED with left-lower abdominal pain. She has had some nausea but no vomiting or fever. On examination there is mild tenderness in the left-lower quadrant. Ultrasonography of the pelvis is negative. What is the likely diagnosis?**
Menarchal females who are ovulatory may have midcycle pain suggesting *mittelschmerz,* which means "middle pain." Mittelschmerz is attributable to follicular enlargement prior to ovulation. It can also be caused by bleeding associated with follicular rupture. The pain is usually mild and unilateral. It lasts from a few hours to several days.

27. **What are the risk factors for ectopic pregnancy?**
Risk factors include tubal abnormalities, history of assisted reproduction, use of an intrauterine device, prior upper gynecologic tract infection, and use of progestin-only contraceptives.

Mollen C, Pletcher J, Lavelle J: Adolescent emergencies. In Fisher G, Ludwig S, Henretig FM (eds): The Textbook of Pediatric Emergency Medicine, 5th ed. Philadelphia, Lippincott Williams & Wilkins, 2006, pp 1842–1843.

28. **What is the clinical profile of a ruptured ectopic pregnancy, and what is the most crucial therapy?**
Patients with ruptured ectopic pregnancy generally have a history of intermittent pelvic pain in association with abnormal vaginal bleeding. Shock (compensated or uncompensated) may be evident on physical examination. Abdominal examination reveals tenderness, and an adnexal mass may or may not be palpated after rupture. Surgical assessment must be immediate.

Imperative components of treatment are ongoing cardiovascular monitoring, fluid resuscitation, and transfusion of packed red blood cells as needed.

Mollen C, Pletcher J, Lavelle J: Adolescent emergencies. In Fisher G, Ludwig S, Henretig FM (eds): The Textbook of Pediatric Emergency Medicine, 5th ed. Philadelphia, Lippincott Williams & Wilkins, 2006, pp 1842–1843.

29. **What is the most common presenting sign of early pregnancy in adolescents?**
A missed or abnormal period is the most common sign of pregnancy in teens. However, the menstrual history is often unreliable in adolescents because of anovulatory cycles. Therefore, other symptoms should raise a red flag. These include fatigue, weight gain, nausea, morning sickness, and nonspecific gastrointestinal or genitourinary symptoms. Less common symptoms consist of vaginal bleeding or discharge, hyperemesis, and headache.

30. **What is the preferred oral regimen for emergency contraception?**
Levonorgestrel, 0.75 mg every 12 hours, is preferred over estrogen-progestin regimens because it has fewer side effects and greater efficacy. Nausea and vomiting are less common in patients treated with this medication. The treatment should begin as soon after unprotected intercourse as possible, preferably within 72 hours of intercourse. Other options include a combination of levonorgestrel and ethinyl estradiol and insertion of a copper intrauterine device. The duration of effectiveness of emergency contraception medications is not known. Medical contraindications include allergy, vaginal bleeding that has not been diagnosed, and pregnancy.

Zieman M: Emergency contraception. Available at www.uptodate.com.

31. **What is the leading cause of teenage short-term recurring school absenteeism in the United States?**
Primary dysmenorrhea. The prevalence of dysmenorrhea is highest in adolescent females, and severe dysmenorrhea occurs in approximately 15% of adolescents. The etiology of dysmenorrhea is thought to be secretion of prostaglandins in the menstrual fluid, leading to uterine contractions and subsequent pain. Vasopressin may also be involved. It increases uterine contractility, leading to vasoconstriction. Nonsteroidal anti-inflammatory drugs remain the most effective initial therapy for dysmenorrhea. They inhibit prostaglandin synthesis and are thought to decrease menstrual flow volume.

French L: Dysmenorrhea. Am Fam Physician 71:285–291, 2005.

CHAPTER 37

HEMATOLOGIC AND ONCOLOGIC EMERGENCIES

Paul Ishimine, MD, and Jenny Kim, MD

HEMATOLOGIC EMERGENCIES

1. **How should one approach the evaluation of a child presenting with anemia to the emergency department (ED)?**
Anemia is caused by problems of red cell destruction, red cell or hemoglobin production, or blood loss. After patient stabilization, the following features can help determine the underlying cause:
   - **Historical features:** Rapidity of onset, hemorrhage, diet, history of easy bruising or bleeding, family history of blood disorders
   - **Physical examination findings:** Jaundice, splenomegaly, enlarged lymph nodes, bruising/bleeding, occult blood on rectal examination
   - **Laboratory studies:** Complete blood count with manual differential, mean corpuscular volume (MCV), peripheral smear, reticulocyte count, Coombs test

   Cohen AR: Pallor. In Fleisher GR, Ludwig S, Henretig FM (eds): Textbook of Pediatric Emergency Medicine, 5th ed. Philadelphia, Lippincott Williams & Wilkins, 2006, pp 535–543.

2. **What is the underlying pathophysiology of sickle cell disease (SCD)?**
SCD is due to an inherited hemoglobinopathy in which a single mutation causes an amino acid substitution in the β-globin chain. This results in abnormally shaped red blood cells (RBCs) that are prone to aggregation and vascular injury, resulting in vaso-occlusion and resultant complications, such as splenic infarction (resulting in increased susceptibility to infection), stroke, and pain from ischemia. There are many genotypes of sickle cell disease, including SCD-SS, -SC, -Sβ^+ thalassemia, and -Sβ^0 thalassemia. Patients with SCD-SS and SCD-Sβ^0 thalassemia usually have a more severe clinical course.

3. **What are the life-threatening complications of SCD?**
   - Sepsis
   - Stroke
   - Splenic sequestration crisis
   - Acute chest syndrome
   - Aplastic crisis

   National Institutes of Health/National Heart, Lung, and Blood Institute Division of Blood Diseases and Resources: The Management of Sickle Cell Disease, 4th ed. Bethesda, MD, National Institutes of Health, 2002, NIH publication no. 02–2117, 2002, pp 1–188.

4. **Why is a patient with SCD immunocompromised?**
Splenic microinfarctions due to sickling of red cells cause altered splenic function. As a result, patients with SCD are prone to infection with encapsulated organisms, such as *Streptococcus pneumoniae*.

5. **What causes painful crisis in patients with SCD?**
Vaso-occlusive crises are due to localized sickling and vascular occlusion. This can occur in any organ, but most frequently affects bone and viscera. Most older children report long bone,

back, and abdominal pain. Precipitating events may include infection, dehydration, fever, or exposure to cold.

6. **How should painful crisis be treated?**
   Assess the severity of pain and associated organ systems. IV hydration, usually at 1.5 times the maintenance rate, and narcotic administration are frequently required. Administration of oxygen is often recommended. It is important to inquire about pain medications given at home, and if these were ineffective to administer an appropriate dose of a more potent analgesic medication. Morphine is often used at an IV dose of 0.1 or 0.2 mg/kg/dose every 1–4 hours.

7. **What is dactylitis?**
   Dactylitis, or "hand-foot syndrome," results from vaso-occlusion of the nutrient arteries that supply the metacarpal and metatarsal bones, causing bone marrow infarction in patients with SCD. This is a form of vaso-occlusive crisis most common in young infants (mostly under age 2 years) and results in pain and swelling of the hands and feet, irritability, and refusal to walk. It is usually bilateral, distinguishing it from cellulitis.

8. **Define acute chest syndrome and its causes and treatment.**
   Acute chest syndrome is a serious complication of SCD and can be life threatening. The syndrome is defined as a new pulmonary infiltrate and chest pain, hypoxia, fever, tachypnea, wheezing, or cough. Both infectious (e.g., chlamydia, mycoplasma, viruses, bacteria) and noninfectious (e.g., fat embolism, pulmonary infarction) causes have been described. Supportive care measures include analgesia, cautious hydration, oxygen, antibiotics, bronchodilators, and blood transfusions.

   Vichinsky EP, Neumayr LD, Earles AN, et al: Causes and outcomes of the acute chest syndrome in sickle cell disease. N Engl J Med 342:1855–1865, 2000.

9. **What is splenic sequestration crisis?**
   Splenic sequestration crisis is a life-threatening complication of SCD that occurs when a large portion of a patient's blood volume becomes acutely trapped in the spleen. This leads to massive splenomegaly, acute anemia, and hypovolemic shock. Treatment is supportive and includes hospitalization, fluid resuscitation, and blood transfusion. Splenic sequestration is seen in young children, typically between 3 months and 5 years of age.

KEY POINTS: LIFE-THREATENING COMPLICATIONS OF SICKLE CELL DISEASE ✔

1. Sepsis

2. Stroke

3. Splenic sequestration crisis

4. Acute chest syndrome

5. Aplastic crisis

10. **Which virus frequently leads to aplastic crisis in children with SCD?**
    Parvovirus B19. This causes brief suppression of erythropoiesis, which is not tolerated in patients with SCD who are already anemic, and patients may present with fatigue, shortness of

breath, and severe anemia with reticulocytopenia. Treatment is supportive, and RBC transfusions are often necessary.

11. **Are aplastic crises due to parvovirus B19 seen only in patients with SCD?**
No. Parvovirus B19 can also cause aplastic crises in patients with other chronic hemolytic diseases, such as thalassemia or hereditary spherocytosis. These patients have shortened RBC survival and frequently cannot tolerate even a brief suppression of erythropoiesis.

12. **How should patients with SCD and fever be treated in the ED?**
Because these children are at high risk for serious bacterial infections, febrile children with SCD need rapid treatment with parenteral antibiotics after appropriate cultures are obtained. The greatest risk of serious bacterial infection is between the ages of 6 months and 3 years, when protective antibodies are not adequate and splenic function is greatly diminished. After administration of IV antibiotics, the conventional approach has been to admit these patients to the hospital. Currently, some hematologists advocate cautious outpatient management of selected well-appearing febrile patients.

13. **What are considered to be low-risk criteria for outpatient management of febrile patients with SCD?**
   - Well appearance
   - No focal findings
   - Temperature $< 40°$ C
   - White blood cell count > 5000 but $< 30,000$ cells/mm^3
   - No pulmonary infiltrates
   - Baseline hemoglobin, white blood cell, and platelet counts

   Wilimas JA, Flynn PM, Harris S, et al: A randomized study of outpatient treatment with ceftriaxone for selected febrile children with sickle cell disease. N Engl J Med 329:472–476, 1993.

14. **If a patient with SCD meets the above criteria, what is the recommended treatment plan?**
These patients should receive an initial dose of parenteral ceftriaxone in the ED. Further treatment may consist of oral amoxicillin. Close follow-up must be arranged if febrile patients with SCD are discharged, including telephone follow-up or scheduling of a revisit within the next 24 hours.

   Wilimas JA, Flynn PM, Harris S, et al: A randomized study of outpatient treatment with ceftriaxone for selected febrile children with sickle cell disease. N Engl J Med 329:472–476, 1993.

15. **An ill-appearing 6-year-old girl presents with weakness for 2 days. On examination she has jaundice and pale conjunctivae but no bruising or petechiae. Her hemoglobin level is 4 g/dL, but her white blood cell and platelet counts are normal. Her reticulocyte count is 20%. She has unconjugated hyperbilirubinemia, and she has dark-brown urine (which is dipstick-positive for blood but has no RBCs on microscopic examination). This presentation suggests what broad category of anemia?**
Hemolytic anemia. Hemolytic disease may be seen in children with red cell membrane defects, such as hereditary spherocytosis or liver disease. Enzyme defects, such as glucose-6-phosphate dehydrogenase deficiency, predispose the patient to hemolysis following an oxidant exposure. Autoimmune hemolysis occurs when antibodies directed against red cells cause hemolysis. This may be triggered by drugs, infections, autoimmune diseases, or maternal–fetal transfer, or it may be idiopathic. Nonimmune acquired hemolysis may be caused by drugs, infections, or chemicals that cause direct red cell injury. Patients with

hemoglobinopathies, such as SCD and thalassemias, can have periods of increased hemolysis and worsening anemia. Finally, mechanical causes of red cell fragmentation, such as hemolytic uremic syndrome, may also cause hemolysis.

16. **What are the typical laboratory findings in iron-deficiency anemia?**
    - Low hemoglobin and hematocrit
    - Low MCV and RBC
    - High RBC distribution width
    - Low serum iron and ferritin
    - Increased transferrin
    - Increased free erythrocyte protoporphyrin
    - Microcytosis, hypochromia, poikilocytosis, and anisocytosis on smear
    - Elevated platelet count

17. **Why is excessive cow's milk consumption associated with iron-deficiency anemia in young children?**
    Overconsumption of cow's milk decreases the toddler's appetite for other foods, and cow's milk does not contain adequate iron for nutrition. There may also be a concomitant cow's milk enteropathy, causing microscopic intestinal blood loss.

18. **Describe appetite abnormalities associated with iron-deficiency anemia.**
    - **Pica** refers to an appetite for unusual substances not regarded as food, such as clay, paper, or dirt.
    - **Pagophagia**, or pica for ice, is thought to be a specific finding in iron-deficiency anemia. Patients are treated with iron.

    Osman YM, Wali YA, Osman OM: Craving for ice and iron-deficiency anemia: A case series from Oman. Pediatr Hematol Oncol 22:12, 2005.

19. **What is transient erythroblastopenia (TEC) of childhood? How does it present?**
    TEC is an idiopathic disorder of acquired RBC aplasia characterized by a gradual onset of pallor. The median age at the time of diagnosis is 23 months, and there is often a history of a preceding viral illness. Except for pallor, the patient's physical examination is otherwise normal, with the absence of bruising, fever, lymphadenopathy, and hepatosplenomegaly. The CBC in a patient with TEC shows an isolated normochromic normocytic anemia with reticulocytopenia. TEC can be confused with leukemia, and bone marrow biopsy may be needed to exclude this diagnosis in a patient suspected of having TEC.

20. **What are the causes of methemoglobinemia?**
    Methemoglobinemia may occur after exposure to oxidizing drugs (e.g., benzocaine, sulfonamide antibiotics), well water that contains nitrites, mothballs, and aniline dyes. Acute gastroenteritis can lead to methemoglobinemia in infants. The heme iron is converted from a ferrous to a ferric state, resulting in hemoglobin with impaired oxygen binding and manifests as cyanosis. Congenital methemoglobinemia is a rare cause of cyanosis in the newborn.

21. **How do patients with idiopathic (or immune) thrombocytopenic purpura (ITP) typically present?**
    ITP most commonly presents in children ages 1–4 years with the acute onset of bruising and petechiae. There is often a history of a preceding viral illness. Children with ITP generally do not appear ill, and frank bleeding is surprisingly less common than would be expected in patients with thrombocytopenia.

22. **What is the most serious complication of ITP?**
The most serious concern in young children with ITP is intracranial hemorrhage. The risk of intracranial hemorrhage is highest in the first week after diagnosis and when the platelet count is less than 20,000 cells/mm^3. Intracranial hemorrhage is seen more frequently in patients who present with mucosal bleeding.

23. **How is ITP treated?**
The treatment of ITP is controversial. Options include close observation only, IV γ-globulin (which is thought to block the uptake of antibody-coated platelets by the spleen), antibodies directed against the D-antigen of RBCs (only effective in Rh-positive patients), steroids, or splenectomy. Some physicians feel that not all patients with ITP need treatment, given the generally benign course and significant costs and side effects of treatment.

Tarantion MD, Buchanan GR: The pros and cons of drug therapy for immune thrombocytopenic purpura in children. Hematol Oncol Clin North Am 18:1301–1314, 2004.

24. **Name the three most common bleeding disorders and the deficient factors associated with each.**
The most common inherited bleeding disorders are:
- Hemophilia A (factor VIII deficiency)
- Hemophilia B (factor IX deficiency)
- Von Willebrand disease (von Willebrand factor)

25. **What are the typical findings of an acute hemolytic transfusion reaction?**
- Fever and chills
- Apprehension
- Chest tightness
- Abdominal or flank pain
- Hypotension

26. **How is a suspected hemolytic transfusion reaction initially treated?**
- Stop the transfusion immediately.
- Give saline at twice the maintenance rate.
- Confirm that the blood was intended for this patient.
- Examine the urine for hemoglobin.
- Send a tube of blood from the unit of transfused blood to the blood bank for confirmation of initial compatibility.

Cohen A, Manno C: Hematologic emergencies. In Fleisher G, Ludwig S, Henretig FM (eds): The Textbook of Pediatric Emergency Medicine, 5th ed. Philadelphia, Lippincott Williams & Wilkins, 2006, p 948.

ONCOLOGIC EMERGENICIES

27. **What are the most common childhood malignancies?**
- Leukemia is the most common childhood malignancy, and acute lymphoblastic leukemia (ALL) is the most common type of childhood leukemia.
- The most common solid organ tumors are brain tumors, and most of these tumors are infratentorial. Medulloblastomas and cerebellar astrocytomas are the most common central nervous system tumors in children.

National Cancer Institute. Available at www.cancer.gov/.

28. **Why are children with malignancies at risk for sepsis?**
Several factors contribute to the risk of severe infections and sepsis in pediatric oncology patients:

- Most importantly, there can be replacement of the bone marrow by malignant cells and direct suppression of granulocyte production by chemotherapeutic agents, resulting in neutropenia.
- Other mechanisms of defense against infection, including mechanical barriers (e.g., intact mucous membranes and skin), cell-mediated and humoral immunity, and splenic function, are frequently impaired in patients with cancer.
- Indwelling central venous catheters, ventriculoperitoneal shunts, and other implanted devices may become sites of infection.

29. **How should febrile children with cancer be managed?**
Febrile children with cancer must be approached carefully. The most important component in the evaluation of a febrile oncologic patient is the patient's overall appearance. Any ill-appearing child needs broad-spectrum antibiotic coverage and admission to the hospital. If a febrile child is neutropenic (absolute neutrophil count < 500 cells/mm^3) or if his or her absolute neutrophil count is < 1000 cells/mm^3 and expected to drop further, broad-spectrum antibiotic therapy should be administered after blood and other appropriate cultures are obtained. These patients are also admitted to the hospital. Well-appearing febrile patients who are not neutropenic may be treated more selectively. The treatment and disposition of all febrile children with cancer should be discussed with the child's oncologist.

Rheingold SR, Lange BJ: Oncologic emergencies. In Pizzo PA, Poplack DG (eds): Pediatric Oncology, 4th ed. Philadelphia, JB Lippincott, 2002, pp 1177–1203.

30. **An ill-appearing 6-year-old boy with acute myelogenous leukemia presents with fever and right-lower-quadrant abdominal pain. In addition to the usual causes of fever and right-lower-quadrant pain, what other entity needs to be considered in a neutropenic patient?**
Typhlitis, a necrotizing colitis and inflammation of the cecum, can be seen in neutropenic patients. The etiology is multifactorial and includes infection and mucosal injury from chemotherapy or radiation therapy. Typhlitis usually presents with fever, abdominal pain, and bloody diarrhea. The diagnosis is best made by computed tomography, and treatment includes gut rest, antibiotic therapy and, rarely, surgery. The mortality rate with typhlitis is very high.

31. **A teenager with a diffuse headache is found to have a white blood cell count of 200,000 cells/mm^3. What treatment should be initiated in the ED while awaiting confirmatory studies?**
This child has hyperleukocytosis, which is very suggestive of leukemia. This degree of white blood cell elevation leads to increased blood viscosity, which, in turn, predisposes a patient to thrombosis, leading to neurologic, pulmonary, and hemorrhagic symptoms. These patients are also at high risk for tumor lysis syndrome. Treatment includes hydration and alkalinization; more refractory cases are treated with leukapheresis. Platelet transfusions should be given if the platelet count is $< 20,000$ cells/mm^3 to reduce the risk of central nervous system hemorrhage. RBC transfusions should be given judiciously because they can increase blood viscosity.

32. **What comprises the differential diagnosis of an anterior mediastinal mass in a child?**
    1. The "Terrible Ts":
       - T-cell lymphoma/leukemia
       - Thymoma
       - Thyroid carcinoma
       - Teratoma/germ cell tumors
    2. Hodgkin's disease

3. Non-Hodgkin's lymphoma
4. Neuroblastoma
5. Cystic hygroma
6. Congenital diaphragmatic hernia

33. **What are some of the risks associated with an anterior mediastinal mass?**
Anterior mediastinal masses are associated with superior mediastinal syndrome in 12% of patients at the time of presentation. This is defined as compression of the superior vena cava (SVC syndrome) and trachea.

34. **What are the presenting symptoms of anterior mediastinal mass?**
These symptoms may include stridor, cough, dyspnea, hemoptysis, and orthopnea.

35. **How should a patient with an anterior mediastinal mass be studied?**
The initial diagnostic test should be a chest radiograph, with posteroanterior and lateral views. Perform chest computed tomography to investigate tracheal involvement. Finally, echocardiography and pulmonary function tests will further delineate circulatory and respiratory functional impairment.

KEY POINTS: METABOLIC DISTURBANCES SEEN IN ONCOLOGY PATIENTS ✓

1. **Hyperkalemia:** Seen with tumor lysis syndrome

2. **Hyperphosphatemia:** Seen with tumor lysis syndrome

3. **Hyperuricemia:** Seen with tumor lysis syndrome

4. **Hypercalcemia:** Seen in patients being treated with cis-retinoic acid or those with significant bony metastases

5. **Hypernatremia:** Seen in patients with diabetes insipidus, which can occur frequently in patients with central nervous system tumors or Langerhans cell histiocytosis

6. **Hyperglycemia:** Seen in patients on steroids or asparaginase

36. **What are the pitfalls of managing the ABCs of a patient with an anterior mediastinal mass?**
Endotracheal intubation may be difficult because of tracheal or bronchial compression. Cardiac output may be compromised by positive-pressure ventilation. Be particularly wary of the patient who has worsening respiratory difficulty when placed in the recumbent position, and avoid sedating patients and lying patients flat because doing so may result in cardiorespiratory arrest.

37. **A 4-year-old girl with lymphoma presents with shortness of breath. What are some possible causes of her symptoms?**
See Table 37-1.

TABLE 37-1. CAUSES OF SHORTNESS OF BREATH IN PATIENTS WITH CANCER
Superior vena cava (SVC) syndrome: Compression or thrombosis of the SVC can cause dyspnea, and may result in facial plethora, jugular venous distention, and headache
Superior mediastinal syndrome: Compression of the trachea by tumor; often used interchangeably with SVC syndrome
Pleural effusions
Pericardial effusion
Cardiomyopathy: Commonly associated with anthracycline chemotherapeutics
Dysrhythmias: Electrolyte disturbances
Pneumonia
Pulmonary embolism
Anemia

38. **Describe some of the symptoms and signs of neuroblastoma.**

Symptoms:
- Abdominal pain
- Bone pain
- Back pain
- Constipation
- Fever
- Weight loss

Signs:
- Abdominal mass
- Proptosis
- Horner's syndrome
- Raccoon eyes
- Hypertension

39. **An 8-year-old girl who has been reporting back pain intermittently for several months presents to the ED with a sudden inability to move her right leg. What does this presentation suggest, and what is the treatment?**
Spinal cord compression can present with back pain (typically worse when lying down), leg paresis or paralysis, and bowel and/or bladder incontinence or retention. Examination may reveal back tenderness, leg weakness, decreased rectal tone, and hyperreflexia or hyporeflexia. Plain radiography may reveal vertebral abnormalities, but the diagnostic study of choice is magnetic resonance imaging. Treatment should be initiated immediately to minimize permanent neurologic sequelae and may include a combination of chemotherapy, radiation therapy, and surgical decompression.

40. **What is tumor lysis syndrome (TLS)?**
TLS is a metabolic syndrome of hyperkalemia, hyperphosphatemia, and hyperuricemia resulting from release of intracellular contents from dying cells. This is seen most commonly in cancers with large tumor burdens and rapid cellular turnover, such as lymphomas and leukemias.

Although TLS usually occurs soon after initiation of chemotherapy, patients can present at the time of initial diagnosis with TLS, especially in patients who present with Burkitt's lymphoma. TLS can cause numerous complications, such as dysrhythmias and renal failure.

41. **How is TLS treated?**

Treatment of TLS consists of hydration and alkalinization of the urine. The recommendation is to start 5% dextrose in one-quarter normal saline with 50–100 mEq/L sodium bicarbonate at 2–4 times maintenance rates. Potassium should not be added to the IV fluids. Allopurinol or rasburicase is administered to reduce uric acid, and aluminum hydroxide or calcium carbonate is started for hyperphosphatemia. Hyperkalemia can be treated with a potassium-binding resin, calcium gluconate, sodium bicarbonate, or insulin with glucose, depending on the patient's clinical status. Hemodialysis may be used for uncontrolled TLS and renal failure.

42. **A 5-year-old girl with all presents with fever and hypotension. Antibiotics and IV fluid resuscitation are started immediately, but she has persistent hypotension. In addition to fluids and pressors, what other therapies should be considered?**

Consider adrenal suppression in patients with persistent hypotension who recently (in the past year) have been treated with steroids. These patients may need stress-dose hydrocortisone. If worsening hypotension is associated with flushing of the central line or infusion of IV antibiotics through the central line, be suspicious of central line infection.

ACKNOWLEDGMENT

The authors would like to thank Janet Friday, MD, for writing this chapter for the first edition of this book.

CHAPTER 38

INFECTIOUS DISEASE EMERGENCIES

*Robert P. Olympia, MD; Julie-Ann Crewalk, MD; Theoklis
Zaoutis, MD, MSCE; Joel D. Klein, MD, FAAP; and Stephen C. Eppes, MD*

FEVER

1. **A 10-day-old, full-term male infant presents to the emergency department (ED) with a 1-day history of being fussy but consolable, slightly decreased oral intake, and a temperature of 38.5° C rectally. What is the risk for serious bacterial illness?**

   A published study demonstrated that the incidence in infants with fever who are < 28 days old is approximately 13%. Among 372 such infants, the etiology of fever was determined to be a nonspecific viral syndrome (65%), serious bacterial infection (12%), aseptic meningitis (8.1%), otitis media (5.1%), bronchiolitis (5.1%), nonbacterial gastroenteritis (2.7%), and viral stomatitis (1.0%).

   Kadish H, Loveridge B, Tobey J, Bolte RG, Corneli HM: Applying outpatient protocols in febrile infants 1–28 days of age: Can the threshold be lowered?. Clin Pediatr 39:81–88, 2000.

   Teague JA, Harper MG, Bachur R, et al: Epidemiology of febrile infants 14–28 days of age. Pediatr Res 53:214A, 2003.

2. **Which bacterial agents are of most concern in an infant < 28 days old presenting to the ED with a fever?**

   Group B streptococci, gram-negative enteric organisms (*Escherichia coli*, *Enterococcus* spp.), *Listeria monocytogenes*, and, less commonly, *Streptococcus pneumoniae*, *Haemophilus influenzae*, *Staphylococcus aureus*, *Neisseria meningitidis*, and *Salmonella* spp.

3. **A 26-day-old infant presents to the ED with a 1-day history of fever up to 39° C rectally. What should your initial management include?**

   For initial management of a newborn infant < 28 days old presenting to the ED with a temperature of 38.0° C:

   - Perform a complete history (including prenatal history) and physical examination of the newborn.
   - Obtain laboratory studies, including a complete blood count (CBC) with differential and blood culture; urine obtained by catheterization or suprapubic aspiration for urinalysis, Gram stain, and culture; cerebrospinal fluid (CSF) for protein/glucose, cell count, Gram stain, and bacterial/viral cultures; chest radiograph if signs of respiratory distress (tachypnea, cyanosis, wheezing, retractions, grunting, nasal flaring, rales, rhonchi, or decreased breath sounds); and stool for heme testing and culture if bloody or watery stool is noted.
   - Admit patient to the hospital and administer parenteral antibiotics (ampicillin *plus* cefotaxime or gentamycin).
   - Consider IV acyclovir if neonatal herpes is suggested by history or physical examination.

4. **How is an infant < 28 days of age classified as low-risk?**

   Several screening tools (Boston and Philadelphia protocols for the outpatient management of infants with fever) have been applied to infants < 28 days old presenting with fever to predict which of these newborns are less likely to have a positive bacterial culture on initial evaluation. Several of these criteria are as follows: gestational age > 37 weeks, uncomplicated prenatal course, no history of hyperbilirubinemia, no focal bacterial infection on physical examination except otitis media, no previous use of antibiotics, nontoxic appearance, and normal laboratory values (white blood count [WBC], 5000–15,000 cells/mm^3, absolute band count < 1500 cells/mm^3, < 10 WBCs/high-power field on urinalysis, and < 5 WBCs/high-power field on stool sample). Negative predictive values determined on infants assigned to the low-risk category were 95.4–99.1%.

5. **A 6-week-old male infant presents to the ED with a temperature of 38.4° C. The infant appears nontoxic and is without an obvious source for the fever. How likely is this infant to have a bacterial infection?**
A normal physical examination does not correlate well with the presence of a bacterial infection in this age group. In a study evaluating 747 febrile infants age 1–2 months, two thirds of infants with a documented bacterial infection appeared well to the attending pediatric emergency physician. The incidence of serious bacterial infection in febrile infants 1–2 months of age is 7.3%.

Bachur RG, Harber MB: Predictive model for serious bacterial infections among infants younger than three months of age. Pediatrics 108:311–316, 2001.
Baker MD, Bell LM, Avner JR: Outpatient management without antibiotics of fever in selected infants. N Engl J Med 329:1437–1441, 1993.

6. **What is the cause of a temperature of 38.0° C in infants age 1–3 months who present to the ED?**
A published study of 422 such infants determined the following sources:
- Viral syndrome, 54.0%
- Nonbacterial gastroenteritis, 16.4%
- Aseptic meningitis, 11.8%
- Serious bacterial illness, 10.2% (growth of pathogen in cultures of blood, spinal fluid, urine, stool)
- Bronchiolitis, 4.7%
- Pneumonia, 1.9%
- Otitis media, 0.5%
- Varicella infection, 0.2%
- Conjunctivitis, 0.2%

Baker MD, Bell LM, Avner JR: The efficacy of routine outpatient management without antibiotics of fever in selected infants. Pediatrics 103:627–630, 1999.

7. **A 2-month-old presents with a temperature of 40.5° C and otherwise appears nontoxic. Do infants with hyperpyrexia have a higher risk of having a serious bacterial infection?**
A recently published retrospective study of infants younger than 3 months of age demonstrated that the prevalence of serious bacterial infection among febrile infants with temperatures > 40° C was 38% compared with 8.8% of those with temperature < 40° C.

Stanley R, Pagon Z, Bachur R: Hyperpyrexia among infants younger than 3 months. Pediatr Emerg Care 21:291–294, 2005.

8. **What is the most common cause of sepsis in newborns?**
Early-onset (birth to 7 days) group B streptococcal (GBS) infections, which may be secondary to maternal obstetric complications, prematurity, or lack of prophylactic antibiotics prior to delivery. Late-onset GBS infection (7 days to 3 months) is uncommonly associated with these factors (Table 38-1).

TABLE 38-1. EARLY-ONSET VERSUS LATE-ONSET GROUP B STREPTOCOCCAL INFECTIONS

Type of GBS	Usual Clinical Presentations	Comments
Early-onset GBS	Septicemia (25–40%)	5–20% mortality
	Meningitis (5–15%)	
	Respiratory illness (35–55%)	
Late-onset GBS	Meningitis (30–40%)	2–6% mortality
	Bacteremia without focus (40–50%)	
	Osteomyelitis/septic arthritis (5–10%)	

GBS = group B streptococcus.

9. **Does the immature neutrophil (band) count help in distinguishing bacterial infections from viral infections in infants age 3–36 months presenting to the ED with a temperature > 39.0° C?**

    In a prospective cohort study of 100 febrile children younger than 2 years old, the investigators concluded that there was no difference in percentage band count, absolute band count, or band–neutrophil ratio between bacterial and viral infections. Furthermore, children with bacterial infections had a higher mean absolute neutrophil count than children with respiratory viral infections.

    Kuppermann N: Immature neutrophils in the blood smears of young febrile children. Arch Pediatr Adolesc Med 153:261–266, 1999.

10. **Has the introduction of the heptavalent pneumococcal conjugate vaccine (PCV7) affected the incidence of occult bacteremia?**

    A retrospective cohort study of febrile infants age 2 months to 36 months conducted from 2001 to 2003 demonstrated that three of 329 blood cultures yielded a pathogenic bacterium (0.91% [95% confidence interval, 0–2.4%]); all were *Streptococcus pneumoniae*. One patient had a nonvaccine serotype, one was unimmunized, and the third was infected with an unknown serotype.

    Stoll ML, Rubin LG: Incidence of occult bacteremia among highly febrile young children in the era of the pneumococcal conjugate vaccine. Arch Pediatr Adolesc Med 158:671–675, 2004.

11. **How helpful is C-reactive protein in detecting serious bacterial infection in febrile children?**

    In a prospective cohort study of febrile children (> 39° C) age 1–36 months with clinically undetectable source of fever, only C-reactive protein (CRP) remained a predictor of serious bacterial infection after multivariate logistic regression analysis compared with WBC count and absolute neutrophil count. Receiver-operating characteristic analysis demonstrated CRP to be superior to WBC count and absolute neutrophil count. A CRP cutoff point of 7 mg/dL maximized both sensitivity and specificity.

    Pulliam PN, Attia MW, Cronan KM: C-reactive protein in febrile children 1 to 36 months of age with clinically undetectable serious bacterial infection. Pediatrics 108:1275–1279, 2001.

12. Do prophylactic antibiotics have a role in children with presumed bacteremia?
Studies comparing one dose of intramuscular ceftriaxone versus oral amoxicillin have had varied results. One study found that the use of ceftriaxone correlated with less persistent fever as compared to amoxicillin, although the incidence of subsequent bacterial infections was equivalent in both groups. Another study using meta-analysis to evaluate the efficacy of oral antibiotics in children with pneumococcal bacteremia concluded that there is a decrease in the risk of serious bacterial infections, but insufficient evidence to prove that oral antibiotics prevent meningitis.

13. Are febrile infants with influenza at lower risk for a serious bacterial infection?
A recently published retrospective cross-sectional study of infants age 0–36 months presenting to the ED with fever demonstrated that febrile infants with influenza A had lower prevalence of bacteremia (0.6% vs. 4.2%), urinary tract infections (1.8% vs. 9.9%), consolidated pneumonia (25.4% vs. 41.9%), meningitis (0% vs. 2.2%), or any serious bacterial infection (9.8% vs. 28.2%) compared with infants without influenza A.

Smitherman HF, Caviness AC, Macias CG: Retrospective review of serious bacterial infections in infants who are 0 to 36 months of age and have influenza A infection. Pediatrics 115:710–718, 2005.

OPHTHALMIC INFECTIONS

14. Distinguish between the presentation of preseptal and orbital cellulitis in children.
See Table 38-2.

TABLE 38-2. PRESEPTAL VERSUS ORBITAL CELLULITIS IN CHILDREN		
Feature	Preseptal Cellulitis	Orbital Cellulitis
Location	Infection of the eyelids anterior to the orbital septum	Infectious process posterior to the orbital septum involving the tissues within the orbit (eye, fat, muscles, optic nerve)
Etiology	• Direct inoculation following trauma • Direct spread from adjacent structures (skin) • Secondary to bacterial spread from ethmoid sinuses	• Extension of bacterial infection from sinuses (75%) • Direct inoculation from penetrating trauma or surgery • Spread from adjacent structure (skin)
Clinical presentation		
Fever/malaise	+/−	Usually +
Orbital/eye pain	+/−	+
Conjunctival hyperemia or swelling	+	+
Upper-/lower-eyelid edema or erythema	+	+

Signs of external trauma (insect bite, etc.)	+	+
Fluctuance	+/−	+/−
Photophobia	−	+/−
Proptosis*	−	+
Orbital pain	−	+
Pain on eye movement	−	+
Normal movement of eye*	+	−
Visual loss or abnormal pupillary reactivity*	−	+ (if severe)
Signs of cavernous sinus thrombosis, meningitis, or intracranial abscess formation	−	+ (if severe)

+ indicates present, − indicates absent.
*The three most important features.

15. **How should a patient with suspected orbital cellulitis be managed?**
Almost 75% of the cases of orbital cellulitis result from an extension of a sinus infection (most often the ethmoid sinus). *Streptococcus pneumoniae* and *H. influenzae* are the usual infectious agents. Acute diagnostic work-up and management may include:
- WBC count (often reveals leukocytosis with predominance of bands)
- Blood cultures obtained before antibiotics
- Orbital computed tomography (CT) with thin and coronal cuts, including frontal lobes
- Lumbar puncture if meningeal signs are present (only after negative findings on CT of the head for signs of increased intracranial pressure)
- Admission to the hospital for IV antibiotics (IV ceftriaxone or cefotaxime)
- Consultation with ophthalmology, otorhinolaryngology, or infectious diseases, as necessary

16. **What are the indications for hospital admission of infants and children who present with preseptal cellulitis?**
- Age < 1 year
- Moderate to severe preseptal cellulitis
- Inability to rule out orbital cellulitis
- Anorexia or inability to tolerate oral medication
- Irritability and other signs of meningitis
- Presence of a subcutaneous abscess

17. **For children discharged from the ED with the diagnosis of preseptal cellulitis, which antibiotics are best?**
Amoxicillin/clavulanate potassium (or clindamycin if methicillin-resistant *Staphylococcus aureus* is a concern) may be used if the preseptal cellulitis is secondary to trauma, specifically a bite (human or animal). If you suspect preseptal cellulitis secondary to an extension from an adjacent structure (conjunctivitis or skin dermatitis), treat the original infection with the appropriate antibiotic (cloxacillin or penicillin).

18. **What is ophthalmia neonatorum?**
Ophthalmia neonatorum, also known as **neonatal conjunctivitis**, is defined as conjunctival inflammation during the first month of life. Infants typically present with eyelid edema, conjunctival hyperemia, and ocular discharge. Maternal history may reveal exposure to sexually transmitted diseases (STDs) or previous genital infections. Birth history may reveal premature rupture of membranes in infants born via cesarean section, or vaginal discharge with a vaginal delivery. Infectious causes for ophthalmia neonatorum include *Chlamydia trachomatis*, *N. gonorrhoeae*, and, less frequently, *Staphylococcus aureus*, *Streptococcus pneumoniae*, *Haemophilus* species, enterococci, and viral agents (herpes simplex virus [HSV], adenovirus, Coxsackie virus, cytomegalovirus, and echovirus).
    Time of onset and type of eye discharge may help with the diagnosis, but Gram stain, culture on chocolate or Thayer-Martin agar (*N. gonorrhoeae*), chlamydial culture, direct immunofluorescent monoclonal antibody testing for chlamydia, and HSV immunochemical testing should be ordered on every infant with these symptoms.

19. **Distinguish between conjunctivitis caused by *C. trachomatis* and *N. gonorrhoeae*.**
See Table 38-3.

TABLE 38-3. CHLAMYDIA TRACHOMATIS VS. NEISSERIA GONORRHOEAE CONJUNCTIVITIS

Features	Chlamydia trachomatis	Neisseria gonorrhoeae
Presentation	First 3 weeks of life	24–48 hours after birth
Distinctive clinical features	Initially serous then mucopurulent discharge Unilateral or bilateral	Acute onset of purulent conjunctival discharge, marked eyelid edema, and chemosis Septicemia, meningitis, or arthritis
Potential complications	Self-limited Rarely conjunctival or corneal-scarring Potential development of upper and lower respiratory tract infections	Potential corneal ulceration and perforation
Treatment	Oral erythromycin estolate syrup for 2 weeks *plus* *topical erythromycin four times a day*	Parenteral ceftriaxone or cefotaxime, penicillin G, penicillin G topical

20. **A 5-year-old girl presents to the ED with "burning and itchy" eyes. She describes a sensation of "chalk in her eyes," with some blurry vision. On physical examination, she has bilateral conjunctival hyperemia, chemosis, and ocular discharge, and has preauricular lymph nodes bilaterally. What is the differential diagnosis?**
The presence of preauricular lymph nodes and conjunctivitis is associated with conjunctivitis caused by *N. gonorrhoeae* and adenoviral keratoconjunctivitis. Adenoviral keratoconjunctivitis is often associated with fever, other upper respiratory symptoms, or vomiting and diarrhea.

21. **What is the treatment for adenoviral keratoconjunctivitis?**
Treatment includes cold compresses and acetaminophen to help with ocular discomfort, gentle removal of conjunctival membranes with a cotton swab, and possibly topical corticosteroids for severe conjunctival inflammation. Ophthalmologic consultation is strongly recommended before using steroids. Prevention of transmission includes frequent hand washing and the recommendation to keep the child out of day care or school until complete resolution of the conjunctival hyperemia.

NECK INFECTIONS

22. **What organisms are associated with deep neck infections (peritonsillar abscess, retropharyngeal abscess, and lateral pharyngeal abscess) in children?**
Aerobic (*Streptococcus pyogenes, Staphylococcus aureus,* and *H. influenzae*) and anaerobic (*Prevotella, Fusobacterium, and Peptostreptococcus* spp.) organisms are typically associated with deep neck infections in children. Almost 66% of deep neck abscesses contain β-lactamase–producing organisms.

23. **Distinguish the features of deep neck infections in children.**
See Table 38-4.

TABLE 38-4.	FEATURES OF DEEP NECK INFECTIONS IN CHILDREN		
Deep Neck Infection	Age Associated	Historical/Clinical Features	Management
Peritonsillar abscess	Adolescents and young adults	Difficulty swallowing or speaking, throat pain radiating to the ear, foul breath, swelling of one tonsil with lateral displacement of the uvula, trismus, drooling	Hospitalization, possible surgical drainage, IV antibiotics, tonsillectomy
Retropharyngeal abscess	<4 years	High fever, difficulty swallowing, drooling, dysphagia, dyspnea, hyperextension of the neck, unilateral posterior pharyngeal fullness	Hospitalization, lateral neck x-ray (retropharyngeal space >½ diameter of adjacent vertebral body), possible surgical drainage, IV antibiotics
Lateral pharyngeal abscess	Older children, adolescents, and young adults	Ill-appearing, high fever, odynophagia, dysphagia, dyspnea; if anterior compartment (swelling of parotid region, trismus); if posterior compartment (minimal pain or trismus)	Hospitalization, possible surgical drainage, IV antibiotics

24. **Which IV antibiotics are appropriate for retropharyngeal abscess?**

As with other pediatric deep neck infections, the antibiotics expected to be efficacious include cefoxitin, clindamycin, imipenem or meropenem, and combination penicillin and β-lactamase inhibitors (ticarcillin-clavulanate).

25. **Do all children with retropharyngeal abscess require surgical treatment?**

Recent evidence suggests that the majority of patients with retropharyngeal abscess can be treated successfully with IV antibiotics. Surgical incision and drainage should be used in cases that do not respond to antibiotic therapy or in cases of persistent large abscesses.

Craig FW, Shunk JE: Retropharyngeal abscesses in children: Clinical presentation, utility of imaging, and current management. Pediatrics 111:1394–1398, 2003.

EAR, NOSE, AND THROAT INFECTIONS

26. **A 3-year-old boy with a history of mild to moderate eczema presents to the ED with ear pain and drainage. On physical examination, his tympanic membrane appears normal, although swelling of the ear canal makes it difficult to view the entire tympanic membrane. There is pain on movement of the tragus. There is no lateral displacement of the ear and no signs of mastoiditis. What is the likely diagnosis?**

The clinical findings are consistent with *otitis externa*. Otitis externa is associated with *Pseudomonas* spp. in > 50% of patients; *Escherichia*, *Proteus*, *Enterobacter*, and *Klebsiella* spp. affect the other half. There is an increased incidence of otitis externa in children with eczema and other dermatologic disorders, as well as in children with a history of swimming, extensive cleaning of the ear, hearing aid use, immunocompromised state, and histiocytosis X.

27. **How should otitis externa be managed?**

Management of otitis externa includes the following: (1) gentle irrigation and suction of debris with hypertonic saline, 2% acetic acid, or alcohol with acetic acid; (2) topical antibiotics, such as neomycin-polymyxin B-hydrocortisone mixture or fluoroquinolone (using a wick in cases of severe canal edema); and (3) culturing the exudate in severe or unresponsive cases.

28. **What is the best treatment for a young child with a runny nose, sore throat, cough, and fever?**

The "common cold" or rhinosinusitis is caused by viruses, primarily rhinoviruses and coronaviruses. Rhinovirus has been associated with wheezing in the asthmatic child. Coronavirus causes most of the colds in young children. Antibiotics should not be used to treat the common cold because of their lack of efficacy and, more importantly, to prevent the further emergence of resistant bacteria. Over-the-counter cold remedies, such as antihistamines and decongestants, have not shown significant benefit, and in younger children may have significant side effects such as somnolence or hyperactivity. Nasal saline drops can be safely used for nasal congestion, although aggressive suctioning should be avoided.

29. **List the three major causes of exudative pharyngitis in children.**

Exudate refers to white or gray debris on the tonsils or pharynx. Causes include:
- Group A β-hemolytic streptococcus (GABHS)
- Adenoviruses
- Epstein-Barr virus

In developing countries, *Corynebacterium diphtheriae* should be included in this list. In sexually active adolescents or abused children, *Neisseria gonorrhoeae* should be considered. More recently, *Arcanobacterium haemolyticum* has been shown to cause an exudative pharyngitis, especially in adolescents.

30. **A 7-year-old has fever, sore throat, tender anterior cervical lymph nodes, and lack of significant upper respiratory tract symptoms. Are these clinical features suggestive of GABHS pharyngitis?**

Unfortunately, there are no clinical findings that are specific or sensitive for streptococcal pharyngitis. The absence of symptoms of upper respiratory tract infection and the presence of tender cervical nodes and a scarlatiniform rash are suggestive of the diagnosis. Some children may present with headache, abdominal pain, or nausea and vomiting. Exudative pharyngitis in children younger than 3 years of age does not tend to be streptococcal. Viral causes, such as adenovirus, predominate, especially in younger children. The diagnosis of GABHS infection is best made through culture or rapid streptococcal antigen tests.

Gerber MA: Diagnosis and treatment of pharyngitis in children. Pediatr Clin North Am 52:729–747, 2005.

31. **What is the drug of choice for the treatment of streptococcal pharyngitis?**

Amoxicillin or penicillin for a full 10 days to prevent rheumatic fever is the oral drug of choice. Erythromycin can be used in the penicillin-allergic patient. A single dose of intramuscular penicillin G benzathine may be indicated in specific cases in which nonadherence is a concern.

Gerber MA: Diagnosis and treatment of pharyngitis in children. Pediatr Clin North Am 52:729–747, 2005.

32. **How is the diagnosis of otitis media made?**

Otitis media is diagnosed as an acute otitis media or otitis media with effusion. See Table 38-5.

TABLE 38-5. DIAGNOSIS OF OTITIS MEDIA			
Diagnosis	**TM Abnormalities**	**Symptoms**	**Treatment**
Acute otitis media	Abnormal color: white, yellow Dullness Decreased or absent mobility Inflammation Full or bulging TM Redness	Pain, fever, anorexia, vomiting	Antibiotics
Otitis media with effusion	Air fluid levels and/or bubbles Translucent TM Retracted TM improved with insufflation No acute inflammation	Irritability, fever	No antibiotics

TM = tympanic membrane.
Adapted from Pelton SI: Otitis media: Re-evaluation of diagnosis and treatment in the era of antimicrobial resistance, pneumococcal conjugate vaccine, and evolving morbidity. Pediatr Clin North Am 52:711–728, 2005.

33. **Which pathogens are implicated in acute otitis media?**

- *Streptococcus pneumoniae* (35%)
- *Haemophilus influenzae*, nontypeable (25%)
- *Moraxella catarrhalis*

- **Viruses:** Adenoviruses, coxsackie virus, measles virus, parainfluenza virus, rhinoviruses, respiratory syncytial virus
- **Others:** Anaerobes; *Chlamydia*, *Mycoplasma*, and *Staphylococcus* spp., *Mycobacterium tuberculosis* agent

Pelton SI: Otitis media: Re-evaluation of diagnosis and treatment in the era of antimicrobial resistance, pneumococcal conjugate vaccine, and evolving morbidity. Pediatr Clin North Am 52:711–728, 2005.

34. **What is the drug of choice for treatment of acute otitis media?**
Amoxicillin remains the drug of choice. High-dose amoxicillin (80–90 mg/kg) divided twice daily for 10 days is the best for the treatment of drug-resistant strep pneumococci, which causes 35% of cases and is less likely to resolve without treatment. Acute otitis media caused by *H. influenzae* and *M. catarrhalis* is more likely to resolve spontaneously. Recurrent acute otitis media may require the use of other antibiotics to address the problem of β-lactamase–producing bacteria or highly resistant *Streptococcus pneumoniae*. Shorter courses of treatment may be considered in nontoxic children older than 2 years.

35. **What is the mechanism of pneumococcal resistance?**
Pneumococcal resistance is mediated by alterations in the penicillin-binding proteins. Resistance of *H. influenzae* and *M. catarrhalis* is mediated by a β-lactamase. This difference has important therapeutic implications, since β-lactamase–stable agents, such as amoxicillin-clavulanate, are more effective against *H. influenzae* and *M. catarrhalis*, but do not provide any advantage over amoxicillin in treating penicillin-resistant pneumococci.

36. **Which antibiotics are considered second-line agents for the treatment of acute otitis media?**
Amoxicillin-clavulanic acid, newer macrolides such as azithromycin, or cephalosporins such as cefdinir are suitable alternative agents if amoxicillin has failed. Intramuscular ceftriaxone, a broad-spectrum, third-generation cephalosporin, should be reserved for children who are vomiting and cannot tolerate oral medication, or for those with possible concomitant occult bacteremia.

37. **List the risk factors for infection with drug-resistant pneumococci.**
- Age under 2 years
- Antibiotic nonadherence
- Recent antibiotic use
- Winter months
- Day care attendance

38. **You decide to intubate the trachea of a young patient who presents with severe respiratory distress and stridor. On endotracheal intubation, purulent tracheal secretions are seen. What is the likely diagnosis?**
Bacterial tracheitis, also called pseudomembranous tracheitis. This infection requires immediate attention and treatment. Copious amounts of secretions can obstruct the trachea or a major bronchus. This condition may resemble croup, which may be a predisposing risk factor. Because of inspiratory and expiratory wheezing, foreign-body aspiration may also be part of the differential diagnosis. The most common organisms recovered from infected patients are *Staphylococcus aureus*, *H. influenzae*, *Streptococcus pyogenes*, *Streptococcus pneumoniae*, and *M. catarrhalis*. Antimicrobial selection should be based on these pathogens, and cefuroxime or a combination of oxacillin plus a third-generation cephalosporin is a reasonable choice.

39. **What are the common causes of stomatitis? How can they be distinguished?**
Inflammation of the oral mucous membrane (stomatitis) is a common finding in children, usually presenting with ulcers or vesicles ("canker sores"). The differential diagnosis is based on the location of the lesions and clinical picture:
- **Buccal stomatitis** may be due to infectious agents, Behçet's syndrome, or trauma.
- **Gingivitis** may be due to herpes simplex virus (HSV) or enteroviruses (coxsackie virus: hand-foot-mouth disease).
- **Gingivostomatitis** may be due to an infectious agent: (HSV, *Candida albicans*) or Stevens-Johnson syndrome.
- **Glossitis** may be due to group A streptococci or HSV.

Recurrent lesions may be due to abnormalities in the immune system, such as in cyclic neutropenia or chemotherapy-induced neutropenia and chronic granulomatous disease. In association with recurrent fever, stomatitis may be due to **PFAPA** (**p**eriodic **f**ever, **a**denitis, **p**haryngitis, and **a**phthous stomatitis).

Fisher RG, Boyce TG: Moffet's Pediatric Infectious Diseases: A Problem-Oriented Approach. 4th ed. Philadelphia, Lippincott Williams & Wilkins, 2005, pp 62–67.

40. **What are the clinical manifestations and management of a child with suspected acute mastoiditis?**
Mastoiditis is an infection of the mastoid bones or air spaces that surround them. The mastoid air cells transmit to the middle ear, and their mucous membrane is in contact with the middle ear. It is a severe but rare complication of otitis media. It manifests as fever, ear pain, erythema, and retroauricular swelling resulting in a downward and outward deviation of the auricle. Computed tomography (CT) may be helpful when intracranial complications of mastoiditis are suspected. Children with mastoiditis should be admitted to the hospital and treated with IV antibiotics and myringotomy with tympanostomy tube placement.

41. **What are the typical organisms causing sinusitis?**
The typical organisms associated with acute sinusitis include:
- *Streptococcus pneumoniae*
- Nontypeable *H. influenzae*
- *M. catarrhalis*

42. **What criteria define sinusitis?**
- **Acute bacterial sinusitis** is an infection of the paranasal sinuses lasting less than 30 days that presents with either persistent or severe symptoms.
- **Persistent symptoms** are those that last longer than 10–14, but less than 30, days and include nasal or postnasal discharge (of any quality), daytime cough (which may be worse at night), or both.
- **Severe symptoms** include a temperature of at least 102°F and purulent nasal discharge present concurrently for at least 3–4 consecutive days in a child who seems ill.

American Academy of Pediatrics: Clinical practice guideline: Management of sinusitis. Pediatrics 108: 798–808, 2001.

43. **What is the differential diagnosis of acute bacterial sinusitis?**
- Mucopurulent rhinitis
- Allergic rhinitis
- Pharyngitis
- Nasal foreign body
- Adenoiditis
- Poor dental hygiene

44. **When is imaging necessary in the diagnosis of acute bacterial sinusitis?**
    The American Academy of Pediatrics recommends that for children < 6 years of age who have persistent respiratory symptoms that have not improved for > 10 but < 30 days, the diagnosis of acute bacterial sinusitis can be made on clinical criteria without radiographs. For children > 6 years of age with persistent symptoms and for all children with severe symptoms, radiography may be indicated. CT and plain radiographic findings in children with acute sinusitis include:
    - Diffuse opacification
    - Mucosal thickening of at least 4 mm
    - Presence of air-fluid levels
      In children < 6 years old with persistent upper respiratory tract symptoms, 88% have abnormal sinus radiographs. Therefore, in uncomplicated cases of sinusitis in children < 6 years, radiographs are not necessary.

    American Academy of Pediatrics: Clinical practice guideline: Management of sinusitis. Pediatrics 108:798, 2001.

    Wald ER: Clinical features, diagnosis, and evaluation of acute bacterial sinusitis in children, 2006: www.uptodate.com

45. **When is CT useful in the diagnosis of sinusitis?**
    CT (Fig. 38-1) is helpful in children with complications of acute bacterial sinus infection or those with very persistent or recurrent infections that do not respond to medical management.

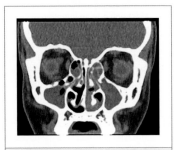

Figure 38-1. Computed tomographic scan of sinusitis.

46. **Describe the treatment of acute bacterial sinusitis.**
    1. For uncomplicated acute bacterial sinusitis of mild to moderate severity:
       - Amoxicillin (45–90 mg/kg/d twice daily)
       - *Or* amoxicillin-clavulanate (45–90 mg/kg/d in two divided doses)
    2. For children with acute bacterial sinusitis of at least moderate severity or who have received an antibiotic in the past 90 days or who attend day care:
       - Amoxicillin-clavulanate (80–90 mg/kg/d in two divided doses)
       - *Or* cefdinir (14 mg/kg/d in one or two doses)
       - *Or* cefuroxime (30 mg/kg/d)
       - *Or* cefpodoxime (10 mg/kg/d once daily)
    3. **Children with vomiting** can be treated with one dose of IV ceftriaxone followed by oral antibiotics after vomiting has subsided.

    Wald ER: Microbiology and treatment of acute bacterial sinusitis, 2006: www.uptodate.com

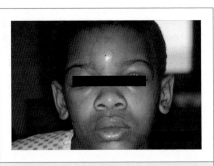

Figure 38-2. Pott's puffy tumor.

47. **What is Pott's puffy tumor?**
    Pott's puffy tumor (Fig. 38-2) was first described by Sir Percivall Pott in 1760, and appears as a soft, fluctuant, painful forehead or scalp swelling usually associated with frontal

sinusitis. Patients tend to be febrile and appear toxic. It is usually seen in children after 8 years of age when the frontal sinuses begin to develop. It represents osteomyelitis of the frontal bone with subsequent subperiosteal elevation. CT is essential for diagnosis and to evaluate other possible areas of spread. Successful treatment usually involves both antibiotics and surgical drainage.

CARDIAC INFECTIONS

48. **Which infectious organisms are associated with the three primary cardiac infections?**
See Table 38-6.

TABLE 38-6. INFECTIOUS ORGANISMS ASSOCIATED WITH THE THREE PRIMARY CARDIAC INFECTIONS			
Infection	Bacterial	Viral	Others
Myocarditis	*Borrelia Burgdorferi* *Neisseria meningitidis*	Enteroviruses Adenovirus Influenza	
Endocarditis	*Streptococcus viridans* Enterococci *Staphylococcal aureus* Coagulase-negative staphylococci Gram-negative bacilli		
Pericarditis	*S. aureus* *N. meningitides* *Streptococcus pneumoniae*	Enteroviruses	*Mycobacterium tuberculosis* *Mycoplasma pneumoniae*

49. **What are some of the signs and symptoms of myocarditis in infants and children?**
Children presenting to the ED with myocarditis may initially report a nonspecific, flulike illness or gastroenteritis. Within 1–4 weeks, fever, malaise, dyspnea, tachypnea, chest pain, pallor, or cool, poorly perfused distal extremities may develop. Infants may present with feeding difficulties, listlessness, cardiac signs, or respiratory distress. The cardiac examination may reveal sinus tachycardia at rest, muffled and distant heart sounds, lateral displacement of the point of maximal impulse, and a gallop rhythm suggestive of congestive heart failure. Other findings on physical examination associated with heart failure include jugular venous distention, weak pulses, cyanosis, poor perfusion, or hepatosplenomegaly.

50. **What diagnostic test results in the ED support the suspicion of myocarditis?**
   - Chest radiography can demonstrate cardiomegaly, interstitial pulmonary edema, or an engorged pulmonary venous pattern.
   - Electrocardiography may demonstrate mild to moderate PR interval prolongation, generalized low-voltage QRS complexes, ST-segment elevation or depression, decreased precordial voltages, high-grade atrioventricular block, and complex ventricular arrhythmias.

- Echocardiography typically demonstrates global cardiac chamber enlargement with poorly contracting ventricles or atrioventricular valve regurgitation.
- WBC count, erythrocyte sedimentation rate, and creatine kinase–MB fraction may be abnormal but are nonspecific.

51. **What is the acute management of myocarditis in infants and children?**
    - Admission to the hospital (intensive care unit for infants and children with heart failure or arrhythmias) for serial echocardiography, electrocardiography, and monitoring
    - Diuretics or inotropic agents for heart failure
    - Specific antibiotics if a bacterial etiology is considered
    - Debated: corticosteroid and immunosuppressive agent use

52. **What are the common symptoms, signs, and laboratory findings in infants and children with infective endocarditis?**
    See Table 38-7.

TABLE 38-7. SYMPTOMS, SIGNS, AND LABORATORY FINDINGS IN INFECTIVE ENDOCARDITIS		
Symptoms	Signs	Laboratory Findings
Fever	Fever	Positive blood culture (75–100%)
Malaise	Petechiae	Elevated erythrocyte sedimentation rate (75–100%)
Anorexia/weight loss	Splenomegaly	Anemia (75–90%)
Arthralgias	New or changed murmur	
Less frequent		
Gastrointestinal symptoms	Embolic phenomenon	Hematuria (25–50%)
Neurologic deficits	Heart failure	Positive rheumatoid factor (25–50%)
Aseptic meningitis		Low complement level (5–40%)
Chest pain		

53. **Differentiate among Osler nodes, Janeway lesions, and Roth spots.**
    - **Osler nodes** are painful, red, nodular lesions seen most frequently on the pulp areas of the distal digits.
    - **Janeway lesions** are small, erythematous, nontender areas typically on the palms and soles.
    - **Roth spots** are retinal hemorrhages with central clearing.

    Although commonly seen in adults, these findings are rare in infants and children with infective endocarditis. Other embolic phenomena associated with endocarditis include splinter hemorrhages and conjunctival hemorrhages.

54. **How do you make the diagnosis of infective endocarditis?**
    For a *definitive diagnosis* of infective endocarditis, you must have evidence, either based on surgery or autopsy histology or positive bacteriology, of valvular vegetations or peripheral embolus. *Probable diagnosis* is based on (1) persistently positive blood culture *plus* either a new or changing cardiac murmur or predisposing heart disease *plus* vascular phenomenon

(petechiae, splinter hemorrhages, conjunctival hemorrhages, Roth spots, Osler nodes, Janeway lesions, aseptic meningitis, glomerulonephritis, pulmonary emboli, or coronary or peripheral emboli), or (2) negative or intermittently positive blood cultures *plus* all three of the following: fever, new or changing cardiac murmur, and vascular phenomenon as defined above.

55. **What antibiotics are recommended for the presumptive diagnosis of infective endocarditis?**
Vancomycin plus gentamicin is recommended for nosocomial infections associated with a vascular cannula or "early" prosthetic valve endocarditis (< 60 days after surgery), and a penicillinase-resistant penicillin plus gentamicin for a natural valve or "late" prosthetic valve endocarditis (> 60 days after surgery).

56. **What are the clinical manifestations and diagnostic findings associated with pericarditis?**
Clinical Manifestations:
- Precordial chest pain
- Irritability
- Grunting expiratory sounds
- Fever
- Exercise intolerance
- Muffled heart sounds
- Pericardial friction rub during deep inspiration with the patient kneeling or in the knee-chest position
- If tamponade: tachycardia, peripheral vasoconstriction, decreased arterial pulse pressure, or pulsus paradoxus

Diagnostic Findings:
- Pericardial fluid analysis suggestive of infection
- Increased size of cardiac shadow in the absence of pulmonary congestion on chest radiography ("water bottle heart")
- Electrocardiography: ST-segment elevations without reciprocal ST-segment depression, except in leads V1 and aVR; flattening or inversion of T waves (late), low-voltage QRS waves
- Echocardiography: presence of pericardial fluid
- Microbiological evaluation of the pericardial fluid by pericardiocentesis
- Viral cultures, serologic tests, and molecular genetic techniques

57. **What is the antimicrobial agent of choice for the presumptive diagnosis of bacterial pericarditis?**
Until pericardial cultures return, initial antibiotics should include oxacillin *or* nafcillin or vancomycin plus cefotaxime or ceftriaxone.

URINARY TRACT INFECTIONS

58. **How common are urinary tract infections in infants and children?**
Among infants and young children (males < 1 year and females < 2 years) who present to the ED with a temperature of 38.5° C without a source, approximately 3.3% have a urinary tract infection (UTI). The highest prevalence occurs in white females with temperature > 39.0° C without a potential source of fever on examination (30.6%).

Shaw KN, Gorelick M, McGowan KL, Yakscoe NM, Schwartz JS: Prevalence of urinary tract infections in febrile young children in the emergency department. Pediatrics 102:e16, 1998.

59. **What are the signs and symptoms of UTIs in infants and children?**
See Table 38-8. Approximately 50% of *adolescents* who present to the ED with dysuria, increased frequency, and urgency on urination have a UTI. Only 10% of *children* who present with these symptoms have a UTI; their symptoms may instead be due to bubble bath irritation, vaginitis, pinworms, or sexual abuse.

TABLE 38-8. SIGNS AND SYMPTOMS OF URINARY TRACT INFECTIONS ACCORDING TO AGE		
Newborns	**Infants and Toddlers**	**School-Age Children**
Fever	Fever	Fever
Hypothermia	Failure to thrive	Vomiting
Vomiting	Vomiting	Diarrhea
Failure to thrive	Diarrhea	Strong-smelling urine
Sepsis	Strong-smelling urine	Abdominal pain
Jaundice	Irritability	Dysuria
Irritability		Frequency
		Urgency
		Enuresis

60. **What is the definition of pyuria?**
Pyuria is the presence of 5 WBCs/high-power field (uncentrifuged) or 10 WBCs/mm^3 (centrifuged) specimens. Although pyuria can be an indication of a UTI, it also is seen with chemical irritation, fever, viral infection, appendicitis, glomerulonephritis, Kawasaki disease, and renal tuberculosis.

61. **What screening tests are most useful to rule out a UTI?**
Several rapid screening tests are used frequently in the ED to evaluate for a UTI in an infant or child presenting with a fever without a source. They include a dipstick biochemical analysis of urine for nitrites or leukocyte esterase and a microscopic analysis of urine for WBCs or bacteria. A meta-analysis examining screening tests for UTIs concluded that both Gram stain on an uncentrifuged urine specimen and dipstick analysis of an uncentrifuged urine specimen for nitrite and leukocyte esterase performed similarly, and these tests were superior to microscopic analysis for pyuria.

Gorelick MH: Screening tests for urinary tract infection in children: A meta-analysis. Pediatrics 104:e54, 1999.

62. **Should all infants age 2–24 months with a fever be evaluated for a UTI?**
In females, features increasing the likelihood of UTI include temperature of 39.0° C, fever for 2 or more days, white race, age < 1 year, and absence of another potential source of fever. In males, clinical features predictive of a UTI include age < 6 months, being uncircumcised, and absence

of another potential source for the fever. Consider screening tests and urine cultures in all infants and children with these risk factors.

63. **Can a urine specimen collected with a bag be used to diagnose a UTI in an infant < 2 years old?**
No. The false-positive rate of a positive urine culture obtained by the bag method is approximately 85%, although a negative result from bagged urine rules out a UTI. If a UTI is considered in an infant < 2 years of age, then transurethral catheterization of the urinary bladder (sensitivity of 95% and specificity of 99%) or suprapubic aspiration should be implemented. In older, toilet-trained children, the midstream clean-catch method is preferred (contamination rates of 0–29%).

64. **What treatment options are available for infants and children with simple cystitis?**
Outpatient therapy may be considered in infants who are well hydrated and nontoxic appearing, those who can tolerate oral medication, those without underlying urologic abnormalities, and those with reliable parents and social situations. When empiric therapy is chosen, the antibiotic should be based on patterns of antibiotic sensitivity in your community. A 5- to 7-day course of oral antibiotics is recommended. Cefixime or cefdinir is the first-line choice. There are increasing rates of resistance of *E. coli* to amoxicillin, trimethoprim, and first-generation cephalosporins are adequate for simple cystitis.

Ladhani S, Gransden W: Increasing antibiotic resistance among urinary tract isolates. Arch Dis Child 88:444–445, 2003.

65. **Which young children with UTIs need to be admitted to the hospital?**
Most pediatric and emergency medicine textbooks recommend treating febrile children with UTIs and those with acute pyelonephritis, regardless of age, with IV antibiotics. Recent literature concludes that if an infant or child suspected of having acute pyelonephritis is nontoxic and well hydrated, with a reliable social situation, then he or she may be treated with oral antibiotics. A multicenter, randomized clinical trial evaluated children age 1–24 months presenting with temperature > 38.3°C and either pyuria or bacteriuria. Some children received either oral cefixime for 14 days (double dose on day 1) or IV cefotaxime for 3 days followed by oral cefixime for 11 days. Both groups responded equally.

Hoberman A: Oral versus intravenous therapy for urinary tract infections in young febrile children. Pediatrics 104:79–86, 1999.

GYNECOLOGIC INFECTIONS

66. **What are the most likely etiologic agents for pelvic inflammatory disease (PID)?**
The etiologic agents causing PID include *N. gonorrhoeae* (25–50%), *C. trachomatis* (25–43%), and anaerobes (*Peptococcus, Peptostreptococcus, Bacteroides* spp.; 25–84%), although most cases of PID are of polymicrobial etiology.

67. **What is the etiology of vaginitis in postpubertal girls? What characteristics distinguish the infections?**
Patients with vaginitis typically present with a history of dysuria, vaginal discharge, burning, or vulvar lesions. Physical examination reveals vulvar irritation and vaginal discharge. The infectious etiologies in postpubertal girls include bacterial vaginosis (40–50%), vulvovaginal candidiasis (20–25%), and *Trichomonas vaginitis* (15–20%) (Table 38-9).

TABLE 38-9. FEATURES OF VAGINITIS IN POSTPUBERTAL GIRLS

Feature	Bacterial Vaginosis	Vulvovaginal Candidiasis	Trichomonas
Clinical presentation	Gray-white homogenous vaginal discharge with fish odor without signs of erythema or infection	Intense burning, pruritus, erythema of vulva with milky white discharge, cottage cheese–appearing, dysuria and dyspareunia	Vaginal pruritus; malodorous, green-gray or cream-colored discharge that is bubbly or frothy; cervix with strawberry appearance
Diagnosis	Clue cells on wet prep, pH >4.5, positive result on whiff test and routine culture	Wet prep with potassium hydroxide revealing budding yeast with pseudohyphae, vaginal culture, pH normal	Culture, wet prep revealing organism, polymerase chain reaction on urine sample
Treatment	Metronidazole × 7 days Clindamycin vaginal cream × 7 days Metronidazole gel × 5 days	Monistat (cream or suppository) Gyne-Lotrimin (cream or vaginal tablet) Nystatin vaginal tablet × 14 days Fluconazole orally × 1 dose	Metronidazole orally × 1 dose or for 7 days

68. **What is the differential diagnosis for genital ulcers? How do you distinguish between each disease process?**
See Table 38-10.

TABLE 38-10. DIFFERENTIAL DIAGNOSIS FOR GENITAL ULCERS

Disease	Clinical Presentation	Diagnosis	Treatment
Herpes genitalis	Single or multiple vesicles on the genitalia that rupture to form shallow ulcers; very painful and resolve without scarring	Tzanck smear: multinucleated giant cells, HSV viral culture, DFA, or PCR	No cure; symptomatic treatment (acyclovir, valacyclovir, famciclovir)
Syphilis	Chancre at site of the incubation (painless papule eroding to an indurated ulcer) with lymphadenopathy; heals in 4–6 weeks	Dark field examination of chancre, serologic tests (VDRL, RPR)	Benzathine penicillin IM × 1 dose (doxycycline or tetracycline × 14 days if penicillin allergic)
Lymphogranuloma venereum	Lesion (papule, ulcer, herpetiform, or urethritis/cervicitis), painful regional unilateral inguinal or	Clinical presentation, culture of *Chlamydia* of node, or complement fixation	Doxycycline, tetracycline, or erythromycin for 21 days

	femoral adenopathy with constitutional symptoms or systemic complications		
Chancroid	Usually single, superficial, painful ulcer surrounded by an erythematous halo; bleeds easily with purulent exudate; unilateral adenopathy	Clinical appearance, smears from ulcer or aspiration from infected lymph nodes, or culture positive for *Haemophilus ducreyi*	Azithromycin orally × 1 dose *or* IM ceftriaxone × 1 dose

DFA = direct fluorescent antibody, IM = intramuscular, HSV = herpes simplex virus, PCR = polymerase chain reaction, RPR = rapid plasmin reagin, VDRL = Venereal Disease Research Laboratory.

CELLULITIS

69. **What organisms most commonly cause cellulitis?**
    Cellulitis, which is an infection of the dermis and subcutaneous fat, is caused most often by *Staphylococcus aureus* and β-hemolytic streptococci in children.

70. **Are cultures helpful in diagnosing cellulitis?**
    In a published study, blood cultures were positive in only 2% of children with cellulitis. Furthermore, cultures of fluid aspirated from the point of maximum inflammation along with blood cultures are positive in only 25% of children with cellulitis.
    Sadow KB: Blood cultures in the evaluation of children with cellulitis. Pediatrics 101:e4, 1998.

71. **When is parenteral treatment recommended for cellulitis?**
    Criteria for parenteral antibiotics include signs of systemic toxicity, rapidly progressing involvement, lymphangitis, involvement of face or neck, and absence of improvement following 48 hours of outpatient management. A penicillinase-resistant penicillin or a first-generation cephalosporin may be used for empiric outpatient therapy. Consider clindamycin or trimethoprim-sulfamethoxazole for suspected methicillin-resistant *Staphylococcus aureus* (MRSA) infection.

72. **A 9-year-old child presents to the ED with a chief complaint of right foot pain. Four days ago he stepped on a nail that went through his sneaker into his sole. He presents with no history of fever, but with erythema and warmth of the sole of his foot and point tenderness at the proximal end of his fifth metatarsal. What diagnosis do you suspect?**
    This scenario is classic for a *Pseudomonas aeruginosa* infection (most likely osteochondritis) in a child who has a history of stepping on a nail through a sweaty sneaker. This child should be admitted for IV antibiotics following a workup for osteomyelitis (i.e., magnetic resonance imaging or nuclear bone scanning, CBC with differential, erythrocyte sedimentation rate/CRP, blood culture). Consult orthopedic surgery for probable surgical debridement.

73. **What is the differential diagnosis of perianal dermatitis/cellulitis?**
    Streptococcal infections (GBS in infants, group A β-hemolytic streptococci [GABHS] in older children), inflammatory bowel disease, sexual abuse, pinworms, diaper dermatitis, psoriasis, and seborrheic dermatitis.

74. **Match the superficial bacterial skin infection with its classical presentation and treatment.**

   1. May begin following minor trauma or an insect bite; initially vesiculopapular with surrounding erythema and later developing a thick, adherent crust that, when removed, reveals a punched out, painful ulcerative lesion. Treatment includes cleansing, and topical and systemic antibiotics covering streptococci and *Staphylococcus aureus*. Typically seen in immunocompromised patients.

   2. Results from local injury to the nail fold seen in children who suck their fingers or bite their nails; lateral nail fold becomes warm, erythematous, edematous, and painful. Treatment includes warm compresses and, for deep infections, incision and drainage and antibiotics covering mixed oral flora.

   3. Either isolated nodular subcutaneous abscesses or multiple abscesses separated by connective tissue septae clinically presenting as painful red papules or boils in a nontoxic-appearing child. Treatment includes local care, incision and drainage, and systemic antibiotics for larger lesions.

   4. Superficial infection of the skin caused by either *Staphylococcus aureus* or GABHS appearing as mildly painful lesions with an erythematous base and honey-crusted exudates in a nontoxic child; absence of constitutional symptoms and presence of regional adenopathy. Treatment includes topical mupirocin or systemic antibiotics (widespread lesions, lesions near the mouth, evidence of deeper infection, constitutional symptoms).

   5. Clearly demarcated, raised, and advancing red border extending from the site of inoculation with lymphangitic streaks extending from the involved area; shiny and warm to touch; presence of systemic signs and high fever. Treatment with IV antibiotics until patient is afebrile and lesion begins to regress, then oral antibiotics.

   6. Small, red pustules at the site of hair follicles. Treatment includes local care and topical antibiotics.

   A. Impetigo
   B. Ecthyma
   C. Erysipelas
   D. Paronychia
   E. Folliculitis
   F. Furuncles/ carbuncles

   Answers: 1, B; 2, D; 3, F; 4, A; 5, C; 6, E

75. **A 4-year-old presents with a boggy, purulent, eczematoid mass measuring 5 × 5 cm on his right temporal scalp area. He also has alopecia and a right-sided, posterior chain cervical adenopathy. What is the likely diagnosis?**
   This presentation is consistent with a kerion, which is a cell-mediated response to tinea capitis often confused with a bacterial skin infection. Therapy includes a minimum of 4 weeks of oral antifungal therapy (griseofulvin or ketoconazole). Systemic antibiotics are not indicated.

76. **What findings may be associated with an invasive skin or soft tissue infection?**
   - Necrosis of skin or soft tissue
   - Crepitance on physical examination
   - Nonadherence of skin and subcutaneous tissue to underlying fascia on exploration
   - Abnormal skin color other than erythema (such as bronzed, cyanotic, violaceous)
   - Severe systemic toxicity, anxiety, or confusion
   - Pain on palpation out of proportion to physical findings
   - Tachycardia out of proportion to fever (suggestive of clostridial infection)
   - Hypocalcemia (calcium deposition in necrotic subcutaneous fat)
   - Gas present on radiograph
   - Failure to respond to medical management
   - Bullae with thin, brown discharge with "sweet but foul" odor (clostridial infection), or "dishwater" fluid (anaerobic fluid)

LYMPH NODES

77. **What characteristics of lymph nodes distinguish infectious from noninfectious causes?**

Soft, nontender, small (usually < 2 cm), and discrete nodes either found in a specific region or generalized may be associated with hyperplasia secondary to a viral infection. These nodes typically lack signs of edema, erythema, or abscess formation. **Acute bacterial lymphadenitis** is associated with soft, unilateral, fixed, and large (usually > 2 cm) nodes with surrounding erythema or swelling. These usually are tender and warm, and poorly defined. When acute bacterial lymphadenitis progresses to chronic infections, the nodes become larger, less erythematous, and more fluctuant, and adhere to overlying skin.

Lymph nodes associated with malignancy are firm, discrete, freely movable, nontender, rubbery in texture, and lacking in signs of inflammation. They increase in size and, over time, become matted with adjacent lymph nodes.

78. **Lymphadenopathy isolated to a particular region may indicate a specific infection. List some of these associations**

See Table 38-11.

TABLE 38-11. REGIONAL LYMPHADENOPATHY AND ASSOCIATED INFECTIOUS ETIOLOGY

Region	Infectious Etiology	
	Common	Less Common
Occipital	Impetigo Tinea capitis Seborrhea	Toxoplasmosis Rubella
Preauricular	Pediculosis Chlamydial conjunctivitis Adenoviral conjunctivitis	Tularemia Herpes simplex Parinaud's syndrome
Cervical	Viral upper respiratory tract infection Bacterial infection of head/neck Primary bacterial adenitis Epstein-Barr virus/cytomegalovirus Cat scratch disease Atypical mycobacterium *Mycobacterium tuberculosis*	Kawasaki disease Toxoplasmosis Anaerobic infection Tularemia Histoplasmosis Leptospirosis Brucellosis
Axillary	Local pyogenic infection Cat scratch disease	Toxoplasmosis
Epitrochlear	Local infection Chronically inflamed hand	Secondary syphilis Tularemia
Inguinal	Lower-extremity infection Genital herpes Primary syphilis	Chancroid Lymphogranuloma venereum
Iliac	Lower-extremity infection Abdominal infection Urinary tract infection	
Popliteal	Severe local pyogenic infection	

79. **How does a child with cat scratch disease typically present?**

    Typically there is a history of a scratch by a kitten on an extremity or the face, followed by the appearance (3–10 days after the inoculation) of a macule, papule, or vesicle, which may last several days to weeks. Single lymph nodes occur 1–2 weeks after the scratch in approximately 50% of children; several lymph nodes appear in the same region in 20%. Other clinical manifestations of cat scratch disease include fever, malaise/fatigue, headaches, splenomegaly, anorexia/emesis/weight loss, sore throat, exanthems, conjunctivitis, and parotid swelling. Lymphadenopathy associated with cat scratch disease is self-limited, although recent studies demonstrate the efficacy of azithromycin in decreasing the duration of local and systemic symptoms.

    Spach DH, Myers SA, Kaplan SL: Cat scratch disease, 2006: www.uptodate.com

80. **What are *atypical* clinical manifestations seen in cat scratch disease (5–20% of all presentations)?**

    - Parinaud oculoglandular syndrome (conjunctival granuloma and preauricular adenopathy)
    - Thrombocytopenic purpura
    - Osteitis resembling bacterial osteomyelitis
    - Central nervous system (CNS) manifestations (encephalopathy, encephalitis, radiculitis, polyneuritis, myelitis, neuroretinitis)
    - In immunocompromised children, bacteremia, bacillary angiomatosis, and bacillary peliosis

81. **What is appropriate treatment for a nontoxic-appearing child who presents with lymphadenitis?**

    For a child with a nonfluctuant node consistent with an acute bacterial infection, or a staphylococcal or streptococcal infection, a β-lactamase–resistant penicillin (e.g., dicloxacillin) or a cephalosporin (e.g., cephalexin) for 2 weeks is appropriate treatment. For a penicillin-allergic child, clindamycin or erythromycin may be used. In those patients who are toxic-appearing or unresponsive to oral antibiotics, or in young infants, IV antibiotics (e.g., nafcillin, cefazolin, or clindamycin) are effective. Percutaneous aspiration or incision and drainage may be necessary for fluctuant nodes.

SEPSIS

82. **Distinguish among bacteremia, systemic inflammation response syndrome (SIRS), sepsis, severe sepsis, and septic shock.**

    Bacteremia: The presence of bacteria in the blood

    SIRS: A clinical syndrome in response to a variety of insults (e.g., infection, trauma, acute respiratory distress syndrome, neoplasms, pancreatitis, burns) manifested by at least two of the following conditions:

    - Temperature $> 38.0°$ C or $< 36.0°$ C
    - Tachycardia (heart rate > 160 beats per minute in infants, > 150 beats per minute in children)
    - Tachypnea (respiratory rate > 60 breaths per minute in infants, > 50 breaths per minute in children)
    - WBC count $> 12,000$ cells/mm^3 or $> 10\%$ immature forms

    Sepsis: The systemic response to infections manifested by two or more of the criteria for SIRS

    Severe sepsis: Sepsis associated with hypotension (systolic blood pressure < 65 mmHg in infants, < 75 mmHg in children, and < 90 mmHg in adolescents, or reduction > 40 mmHg from baseline), hypoperfusion (lactic acidosis, oliguria, hypoxemia, or acute change in mental status), or organ dysfunction

    Septic shock: Sepsis with hypotension, despite adequate fluid resuscitation, with the presence of perfusion abnormalities, which may include lactic acidosis, oliguria, or acute change in mental status.

83. What are the common signs/symptoms and laboratory values associated with septic shock in infants and children?

Infants:

Signs/Symptoms	Laboratory Results
Hyperthermia or hypothermia	Lactic acidosis
Tachycardia	Leukocytosis or leukopenia
Tachypnea	Increased bands, myelocytes, promyelocytes

Children:

Signs/Symptoms	Laboratory Results
Hypotension	High or low serum glucose level
Delayed capillary refill	Hypocalcemia
Weak peripheral pulses	Hypoalbuminemia
Cool extremities	Positive blood, urine, CSF cultures
Irritability	Abnormal coagulation factors/disseminated intravascular coagulation
Lethargy	Thrombocytopenia
Confusion	Abnormal renal function
Oliguria	
Petechiae or purpura	

84. What are the antibiotic choices for empirical therapy in infants and children presenting in septic shock?
See Table 38-12.

TABLE 38-12. EMPIRICAL THERAPY FOR SEPTIC SHOCK ACCORDING TO AGE		
Age/ Condition	Bacterial Etiology	Antibiotic Choice for Empirical Therapy
Neonate	GBS	Ampicillin plus aminoglycoside or cefotaxime; if nosocomial, then add vancomycin
	Gram-negative bacilli	Cefotaxime or ceftriaxone plus vancomycin (if you suspect gram-positive infection)
Child	S. pneumoniae, N. meningitidis, S. aureus, GAS	If nosocomial, vancomycin plus antibioticagainst gram-negative bacteria (ceftazidime, cefepime).
	Invasive GAS (e.g., postvaricella)	Aminoglycoside, carbapenem, or extendedspectrum penicillin with β-lactamase inhibitor Penicillin and clindamycin

GAS = group A streptococci, GAB = group B streptococci.

FEVER AND RASH

85. **What is the differential diagnosis of fever and petechiae?**

    Children and infants who present to the ED with fever and petechiae require immediate attention because there are life-threatening causes that may progress rapidly to death. The differential diagnosis of common infectious causes includes both treatable and nontreatable organisms:

Treatable	Nontreatable
N. meningitidis (meningococcemia)	Adenovirus
N. gonorrhoeae (gonococcemia)	Rubeola (atypical measles)
Pseudomonas aeruginosa	Enterovirus
Streptococcus pyogenes	Epstein-Barr virus
Rickettsia prowazekii (epidemic typhus)	
Rickettsia rickettsii (Rocky Mountain spotted fever)	
Staphylococcus aureus (endocarditis)	

86. **When is fever associated with a petechial rash less concerning?**

    A child with fever and petechiae is less likely to have serious bacterial illness if he or she appears well and has one isolated petechial lesion, petechiae only above the nipple line, a mechanical cause of the petechiae (coughing, emesis, screaming or crying, blood pressure cuff or tourniquet), or normal WBC count. Most can be safely discharged from the ED.

    Mandl KD: Incidence of bacteremia in infants and children with fever and petechiae. J Pediatr 131: 398–404, 1997.

87. **What factors predict poor prognosis in infants and children with meningococcemia?**
    - Absence of CSF pleocytosis
    - Rapidly evolving hemorrhagic skin lesions
    - Shock
    - Hyperpyrexia
    - Leukopenia
    - Thrombocytopenia
    - Low plasma levels of fibrinogen
    - Disseminated intravascular coagulation
    - Metabolic acidosis
    - Rapid clinical deterioration
    - Low serum CRP level
    - Low absolute neutrophil count
    - Low serum potassium level

88. **What is acute arthritis and dermatitis syndrome?**

    Also known as disseminated gonococcal infection, acute arthritis and dermatitis syndrome occurs in approximately 1–3% of persons with untreated mucosal gonorrhea. Clinical findings include dermatitis (tender necrotic pustule with an erythematous base located distally on an upper extremity), migratory polyarthralgias or tenosynovitis affecting smaller joints, and arthritis (pyogenic monoarticular or polyarticular with effusion, especially of knee, ankle, or wrist). Gonococcal bacteremia may also be seen.

89. **List clinical criteria that define toxic shock syndrome.**
    The diagnosis is made by the presence of three major criteria and at least three minor criteria, with negative blood, throat, and CSF cultures (except for *Staphylococcus aureus*) and no rise in titers to Rocky Mountain spotted fever (RMSF), leptospirosis, and rubeola antigens.

    Major Criteria:
    - Temperature > 38.9°C
    - Hypotension (shock or orthostatic)
    - Macular erythroderma—late desquamation within 1–2 weeks of the illness (especially of palms and soles)

    Minor Criteria:
    - Mucous membrane inflammation (conjunctival or pharyngeal)
    - Gastrointestinal (vomiting, diarrhea)
    - Musculoskeletal (myalgia or elevation of creatine phosphokinase)
    - Central nervous (alteration of consciousness)
    - Hepatic (elevated bilirubin, aminotransferase levels)
    - Renal (elevated blood urea nitrogen level, > 5 WBCs/high-power field on urinalysis)
    - Decreased platelet count (< 100,000/mm^3)

90. **Distinguish between staphylococcal and streptococcal toxic shock syndrome.**
    See Table 38-13.

TABLE 38-13.	STAPHYLOCOCCAL VS. STREPTOCOCCAL TOXIC SHOCK SYNDROME	
Feature	Staphylococcal Toxic Shock Syndrome	Streptococcal Toxic Shock Syndrome
General presentation	Acute onset of severe symptoms (vomiting/diarrhea)	Gradual onset of mild symptoms (malaise/myalgia)
Fever	High; abrupt onset	Gradual onset (if fever present)
Rash	Erythroderma	Scarlatina
Shock	Responds to aggressive intravascular volume expansion	Unpredictable response to intravascular volume expansion
Source of infection	Menstrual related, sinusitis, surgical wound	Cellulitis, necrotizing myositis, fasciitis, pneumonitis
Response to antibiotics	Beneficial for treatment of acute infection and recurrence; β-lactamase–resistant penicillins or cephalosporins	More difficult in treating acute infection; clindamycin more superior than β-lactam agents
Complications	Infrequent coagulopathies, complicated hospitalizations, gangrene	Common coagulopathies, complicated hospitalization, gangrene
Mortality rate	10%	30–50%

91. **Which two infectious agents are most commonly associated with erythema multiforme minor and major (Stevens-Johnson syndrome), respectively?**
    Erythema multiforme minor is most commonly associated with HSV, and Stevens-Johnson syndrome is most commonly associated with *Mycoplasma pneumoniae*.

92. **What is staphylococcal scalded skin syndrome?**

Staphylococcal scalded skin syndrome is a dermatosis caused by an epidermolytic toxin produced by certain strains of staphylococci. It generally affects children < 5 years old, and classically presents with fever, irritability, and tender erythematous skin. The skin begins to exfoliate, with crusting and exudation around the mouth, eyes, and paranasal areas, within 2–3 days of the initial rash. The presence of the **Nikolsky sign** (wrinkling of the upper layer of the epidermis and removal of the layer by light stroking, like the peeling of wet tissue paper) may be present. A skin biopsy from the blister base can distinguish staphylococcal scalded skin syndrome from toxic epidermal necrolysis. The mortality rate is < 4%. Hospitalization is often required for skin care, fluid management, and IV antibiotics.

93. **What are the typical cutaneous findings associated with scarlet fever?**

These follow a 2- to 5-day incubation period and accompany the abrupt onset of fever, headache, vomiting, malaise, abdominal pain, and sore throat:

- Erythematous oral mucous membranes with scattered palatal petechiae
- White or red strawberry tongue
- Circumoral pallor
- Erythematous, punctate rash with sandpaper-like texture; first appears on upper trunk, and then becomes more generalized over 3–4 days (more intense in skin folds of axillae, antecubital, popliteal, and inguinal regions, and sites of pressure such as buttocks and small of back)
- Pastia's lines (transverse areas of hyperpigmentation with petechial character in antecubital fossa, axilla, and inguinal regions)
- Scaly exfoliation on the hands, palms, knees, feet, and perineum within 4–5 days of beginning of sandpaper rash

94. **Match the following ED scenarios with the appropriate management.**

Management Options

A. A 10-month-old, ill-appearing infant has a history of multiple episodes of vomiting, lethargy, and rapidly spreading rash consistent with petechiae and purpura. The infant is resuscitated immediately (oxygen applied by face mask; IV access obtained; blood, urine, and lumbar puncture performed and laboratory tests ordered; antibiotics given). What antibiotic prophylaxis is needed for the ED staff?

B. An 18-year-old man is escorted to the ED from prison with a chief complaint of "coughing up blood." He has had a chronic cough for approximately 6 months and has lost 10 pounds over the last year. What should the ED staff do to protect themselves from possibly being exposed to this disease?

1. The scenario is most consistent with tuberculosis. Airborne precautions should be taken, which include a private room with negative air-pressure ventilation and properly fitted or sealing respiratory masks to be worn by all health care providers in contact with the patient.

2. The scenario is most consistent with meningococcemia. Droplet precautions should be taken, which include the use of a respiratory mask if within 3 feet of the child. Chemoprophylaxis is strongly recommended if mouth-to-mouth resuscitation is provided or there is unprotected contact during endotracheal intubation. Options for chemoprophylaxis include oral rifampin for 2–4 days, intramuscular ceftriaxone for one dose, or oral ciprofloxacin for one dose (the latter is not recommended for use in children < 18 years old).

C. A 16-year-old boy with a medical history of mental retardation and cerebral palsy who lives in a long-term care facility has extensive infected decubitus ulcers on his buttocks and lower extremities. What should the ED staff do to protect themselves from being exposed to this disease?

3. The scenario is most consistent with possible MRSA. Contact precautions should be used, including a private room, gloves at all times, hand washing with an antimicrobial agent after glove removal, and gown use at all times.

Answers: A, 2; B, 1; C, 3.

95. **What is PANDAS?**
This is a condition that has been described as **p**ediatric **a**utoimmune **n**europsychiatric **d**isorders **a**ssociated with **s**treptococcal infections. The association between group A streptococci and PANDAS is not proven.

American Academy of Pediatrics: Group A streptococcal infections. In: Pickering, LK (ed): Red Book: 2006 Report of the Committee on Infectious Diseases, 27th ed. Elk Grove Village, IL, American Academy of Pediatrics, 2006, p 611.

CNS INFECTIONS

96. **What are the most common etiologic agents of bacterial meningitis?**
   - **0 to 4 weeks:** Group B streptococci, *Escherichia coli*, *Klebsiella pneumoniae*, *Salmonella* spp., other gram-negative bacilli, *Listeria monocytogenes*, enterococci
   - **4 weeks to 3 months:** Group B streptococci, *Streptococcus pneumoniae*, *N. meningitides*, *Escherichia coli*, *Haemophilus influenzae*, *Listeria monocytogenes*
   - **3 months to 18 years:** *Streptococcus pneumoniae*, *N. meningitides*, *Haemophilus influenzae*

   Wubbel L, McCracken GH: Management of bacterial meningitis: 1998. Pediatr Rev 19:78–84, 1998.

97. **You are evaluating a 12-month-old infant for possible meningitis. He comes from a community that does not believe in immunization for religious reasons. Given the history, of the three possible pathogens, which should you be most concerned about?**
Haemophilus influenzae type B (Hib). The epidemiology and microbiology of childhood meningitis have changed dramatically since the introduction of the Hib conjugate vaccines. Prior to the vaccine, Hib caused the majority of cases of bacterial meningitis in children. Peak incidence of meningitis was between 6 and 18 months. It is no longer a significant pathogen in countries where Hib vaccination is used because of the vaccine's ability to decrease pharyngeal colonization. Since 1988, when the Hib vaccine was introduced, we now see < 1/100,000 cases of meningitis caused by Hib in children younger than 5 years old. Hib disease is currently seen in the United States in closed communities that do not believe in immunizations, or in very young infants who have not completed their vaccination series.

   Wubbel L, McCracken GH: Management of bacterial meningitis: 1998. Pediatr Rev 19:78–84, 1998.

98. **Which antibiotics should be used to treat neonatal meningitis (age 0–3 months)?**
Ampicillin and cefotaxime. Ampicillin and gentamicin are commonly used for the treatment of neonatal sepsis, but if the CSF findings are consistent with meningitis, consider a third-generation cephalosporin in addition to ampicillin because of its superior CNS penetration.

99. **Why is ampicillin used to treat meningitis in the 0- to 3-month-old infant?**
It is used to provide adequate antimicrobial coverage for *Listeria monocytogenes*. Frequently, an aminoglycoside, such as gentamicin, is added to improve the effectiveness of the ampicillin. Penicillin-allergic patients may be treated with trimethoprim-sulfamethoxazole.

100. **What empirical antibiotic therapy should be initiated for the treatment of bacterial meningitis outside the neonatal period ($>$ 3 mo)?**
Administer vancomycin and ceftriaxone to all infants with definite or presumed bacterial meningitis. Vancomycin is recommended for all CNS infections that may involve pneumococcus as a pathogen because of pneumococcal resistance to penicillin and other β-lactam antibiotics. For the child with hypersensitivity to β-lactam antibiotics, consider the combination of rifampin plus vancomycin. Vancomycin should not be given alone.

American Academy of Pediatrics: Pneumococcal infections. In Pickering LK (ed): Red Book: 2006 Report of the Committee on Infectious Diseases, 27th ed. Elk Grove Village, IL, American Academy of Pediatrics, 2006, pp 529–530.

101. **Should corticosteroids be administered as adjunctive therapy in the treatment of bacterial meningitis?**
Corticosteroids have been shown to reduce hearing loss and neurologic sequelae in children with Hib meningitis. The effectiveness of corticosteroids in disease caused by *Streptococcus pneumoniae* and *N. meningitidis* is less clear, although retrospective studies have shown significant reductions in hearing loss among those treated with dexamethasone with antibiotics versus antibiotics alone. There is evidence that dexamethasone reduces the incidence of neurologic complications in adults with *Streptococcus pneumoniae* meningitis. Current recommendations suggest that dexamethasone be considered for children with pneumococcal meningitis. If used, dexamethasone should be given before or at the time of antibiotic administration.

van de Beek D, de Gans J, McIntyre P, Prasad K: Corticosteroids in acute bacterial meningitis. Cochrane Database Syst Rev 2003; CD004305

102. **What is aseptic meningitis?**
This term has become synonymous with viral meningitis but in fact describes meningitis caused by viruses, fungi, or certain bacteria that cannot be seen on Gram stain. It also applies to meningitis caused by drugs (nonsteroidal anti-inflammatory drugs), systemic illness, neoplasms, or parameningeal conditions. This term does not imply an aseptic course of illness or an aseptic-appearing child. A more accurate term would be *Gram stain–negative meningitis*.

103. **How can viral meningitis be distinguished from bacterial meningitis?**
It is often difficult to distinguish these two clinical entities. Both can present with fever, headache, stiff neck, vomiting, and photophobia. Young infants may show nonspecific signs such as irritability, poor oral intake, and somnolence. The typical CSF findings can sometimes be used to distinguish viral from bacterial meningitis, although considerable overlap can exist (Table 38-14).

TABLE 38-14.   TYPICAL CEREBROSPINAL FLUID FINDINGS IN VIRAL AND BACTERIAL MENINGITIS

CSF Variable	Bacterial	Viral
WBC count (cells/mm^3)	$>$1000	$<$ 500
Neutrophils (%)	$>$50	$<$50
Glucose level (mg/dL)	$<$20	$>$30
Protein level (mg/dL)	$>$100	50–100

CSF = cerebrospinal fluid, WBC = white blood cell.

104. **On a hot summer day, a 5-year-old boy presents with fever, headache, and photophobia. You suspect meningitis and perform a lumbar puncture. The CSF evaluation reveals a WBC count of 400 cells/mL with a polymorphonuclear cell predominance, normal glucose, normal protein, and negative Gram stain. What is the most likely diagnosis?**

Enteroviral meningitis is the most likely diagnosis. Nonpolio enteroviruses are the leading cause of viral meningitis, accounting for 80–90% of all cases from which an etiologic agent is identified. This group includes group A and B coxsackie viruses, echoviruses, and enteroviruses (types 68–71 and 73). They are called *summer viruses* because resulting infections occur during the warmer months. The CSF examination in this patient is typical of enterovirus infection. The predominance of neutrophils is often seen *early* in the course of the disease. The presence of other identifiable enteroviral syndromes in the community, such as herpangina and hand-foot-mouth disease, can be useful in diagnosis because outbreaks tend to be epidemic and seasonal. The availability of reliable enteroviral polymerase chain reaction in CSF makes it easier to distinguish these two entities.

Zaoutis TE, Klein JD: Enterovirus infections. Pediatr Rev 19:183–191, 1998.

105. **A 2-week-old infant presents with fever and focal seizures. What therapy should be instituted immediately?**

Ampicillin, cefotaxime, and acyclovir should be started as soon as possible. This child's presentation, especially the seizures, is consistent with HSV encephalitis. Typically, fever, lethargy, and seizures occur at 2–3 weeks of age. Skin lesions are present in about 50% of patients, and in most will appear late in the illness if at all. CSF examination usually reveals fewer than 100 WBCs, but may have an increased number of red blood cells. CSF cultures are usually negative for HSV. HSV DNA in the CSF can best be detected using polymerase chain reaction. Neonatal infections are serious, with high mortality and morbidity rates even with prompt treatment. About one third of neonatal HSV infections involve the CNS, and while most patients survive, there is a high incidence of neurologic impairment. This patient should begin receiving empirical therapy for both bacterial and HSV infection.

Kohl S: Herpes simplex infections in newborn infants. Semin Pediatr Infect Dis 10:154–160, 1999.

106. **A 10-year-old boy has a fever and is suddenly acting strangely, with combative behavior and garbled speech. What is the differential diagnosis for this presentation?**

Fever in combination with a change in mental status suggests a diagnosis of encephalitis. Increased intracranial pressure without signs of meningitis can also be seen. Infectious causes of encephalitis are predominately viral in origin. Epidemic acute encephalomyelitis is usually due to arboviruses (*ar*thropod *bor*ne viruses) such as West Nile and LaCrosse viruses. Sporadic acute encephalitis can be due to many viruses such as enteroviruses, HSV, varicella, cytomegalovirus, and Epstein-Barr virus. Bacterial causes are less common, but in a child with exposure to cats (especially kittens), consider infection with *Bartonella henselae* (cat scratch disease). Other infectious diseases that cause encephalitis include RMSF, Lyme disease, and *Mycoplasma pneumoniae* infection. Acute disseminated encephalomyelitis (ADEM), also known as a postinfectious encephalomyelitis, is a rare monophasic inflammatory disorder of the CNS that can also present in this manner. ADEM has a propensity to occur after minor upper respiratory tract infections. CSF, by definition, reveals no bacterial or viral etiology. The existence of bilateral optic neuritis and transverse myelitis, however, is consistent with the diagnosis of ADEM.

Russell CD: Acute disseminated encephalomyelitis. Semin Pediatr Infect Dis 14:90–95, 2003.

107. **A 12-year-old boy with a 2-week history of sinusitis presents with persistent fever, headache, and altered mental status. What serious complication of sinusitis should be considered?**

Brain abscess is an uncommon but serious complication of frontal sinusitis. It is seen in older children and teenagers because of the late development of the frontal sinuses. Maintain a high index of suspicion when patients with sinusitis present with persistent symptoms and neurologic findings. Other potential complications include epidural abscess or meningitis.

Wald ER: Clinical features, evaluation and diagnosis of acute bacterial sinusitis in children, 2006: www.uptodate.com

108. **An 8-year-old boy has fever and back pain. What is your approach to diagnosis and management?**

Back pain is an unusual reason for children to be seen in the ED. Frequently, back pain in children indicates significant disease. The differential diagnosis includes infectious, neoplastic, and rheumatologic disorders. The major infections producing back pain in children include discitis, vertebral osteomyelitis, spinal epidural abscess, and sacroiliac joint infection (Table 38-15).

TABLE 38–15.	DISTINGUISHING BETWEEN INFECTIOUS CAUSES OF BACK PAIN			
Variable	Discitis Osteomyelitis	Vertebral	Spinal Epidural Abscess	Sacroiliac Joint Infection
Age (y)	<5	≥8	>8	Any
Symptoms	Gradual	Gradual onset	Severe	Gradual
	Increased with activity	Constant, dull	Constant	Sciatica
			Radiation to legs	Buttock pain
Fever	Low	High	High	High
Examination	Locally tender	Locally tender	Locally tender	
	↓ Lumbar lordosis	↓ Spinal mobility	↓ Spinal mobility	
	↓ Spinal mobility		↓ DTRs	
	Refusal to walk		↓ Strength	

DTRs = deep tendon reflexes.

TICK-BORNE DISEASE

109. **What is the appropriate treatment for a child who presents with erythema migrans?**

Erythema migrans is the characteristic rash of Lyme disease, seen in approximately 70% of patients. It begins as a red papule or macule that rapidly expands to become a round or oval lesion at least 5 cm in diameter, with an erythematous periphery and central clearing. The treatment of choice is doxycycline, for children 8 years old or older. Amoxicillin is recommended for younger children (because of possible tetracycline toxicity). Treatment for 2–3 weeks is recommended. Cefuroxime axetil is an approved alternate therapy.

110. **What is the recommended treatment for Lyme disease in children?**
See Table 38-16.

TABLE 38-16. TREATMENT OF LYME DISEASE BY STAGE

Disease Stage	Clinical Manifestations	Drug
Early localized	Erythema migrans, malaise, myalgia	Doxycycline (amoxicillin*), 14–21 days
Early disseminated	Multiple erythema migrans rashes	Doxycycline (amoxicillin), 21 days
	Facial palsy	Doxycycline (amoxicillin), 21–28 days
	Arthritis	Doxycycline (amoxicillin), 28 days
Late disseminated	Persistent arthritis, carditis	IV ceftriaxone, 14–21 days
	Meningitis or encephalitis	IV ceftriaxone, 30–60 days

*$\geq$8 years old, treat with doxycycline; <8 years old, treat with amoxicillin.
Penicillin-allergic patients can be treated with cefuroxime axetil and erythromycin.
Adapted from American Academy of Pediatrics: Lyme disease. In: Pickering LK (ed): Red Book:
2006 Report of the Committee on Infectious Diseases, 27th ed. Elk Grove Village, IL, American Academy
of Pediatrics, 2006, pp 428–432.

111. **A child presents with bilateral facial palsy. What disease entities would you consider?**
In areas that are endemic for Lyme disease in the United States (Northeast, upper Midwest, and Pacific Northwest), Lyme disease should always be suspected. It is one of the few diseases that can produce bilateral facial palsy. Other causes of facial palsy, usually unilateral, include mastoiditis, Guillain-Barré syndrome, herpesvirus infection, and tumors.

112. **A 16-year-old otherwise healthy girl presents with a syncopal episode. electrocardiography reveals complete heart block. What is the differential diagnosis?**
- Lyme carditis
- Systemic lupus erythematosus
- Enteroviral myocarditis
- Digoxin toxicity

113. **What is the time course of clinical manifestations of Lyme disease?**
See Table 38-17.

114. **Describe the distribution of the rash in RMSF.**
RMSF is a small vessel vasculitis caused by *Rickettsia rickettsii*. The rash usually occurs before the sixth day of the febrile illness (temperature, 38.5° C) as a blanching maculopapular rash on the ankles and wrists. It spreads centripetally to the trunk but spares the face. In most patients, the rash involves the palms and soles and eventually becomes petechial or purpuric.

KEY POINTS: POSSIBLE PRESENTATIONS OF LYME DISEASE IN CHILDREN ✓

1. Rash
2. Arthritis
3. Heart block
4. Meningeal signs
5. Facial palsies

TABLE 38-17.	TIME COURSE OF CLINICAL MANIFESTATIONS OF LYME DISEASE	
Stage	**Clinical Manifestations**	**Time after Exposure**
Early localized	Single EM lesion, myalgia, headache, arthralgia, fever, fatigue	3–32 days
Early disseminated	Single or multiple EM lesions, arthralgia, neck pain and/or stiffness, cranial neuritis (facial nerve palsy), meningitis, radiculoneuritis	3–10 weeks
Late disseminated	Arthritis, carditis, encephalomyelitis	2–12 months

EM = erythema migrans.

Other clinical features of RMSF include headache, myalgia, conjunctival hyperemia, and photophobia. Approximately 20% of cases never develop a rash.

American Academy of Pediatrics: Rocky Mountain spotted fever. In Pickering LK (ed): Red Book: 2006 Report of the Committee on Infectious Diseases. 27th ed. Elk Grove Village, IL, American Academy of Pediatrics, 2006, pp 570–572.

115. What electrolyte abnormality is commonly associated with RMSF?
Hyponatremia (sodium level < 130 mEq/L) is seen in about 25% of affected patients. Other laboratory abnormalities commonly include thrombocytopenia, anemia, and a variable WBC count with a left shift.

116. In which Rocky Mountain state is RMSF most commonly seen?
None. "Rocky Mountain" is a misnomer. Most cases of RMSF occur in the South Atlantic, South Central, and the Southeastern United States.

117. What laboratory abnormalities are found in ehrlichiosis?
- Leukopenia
- Hepatitis (elevated aminotransferase levels)
- CSF pleocytosis (with predominance of lymphocytes)

- Anemia
- Thrombocytopenia
- Hyponatremia

GASTROINTESTINAL INFECTIONS

118. **When a child is found to have bloody diarrhea, which infectious agents are most likely responsible?**
The most common agents are *Salmonella, Shigella,* and *Campylobacter* spp.; shiga toxin producing *E. coli* (*E. coli* O157:H7); and *Yersinia* spp. Other infectious agents, including *Vibrio parahaemolyticus, Aeromonas* spp., and acute amebiasis, should be considered.

119. **Which bacterial stool pathogens require antimicrobial treatment?**
- ***Shigella:*** Most infections are self-limiting; however, antibiotics can reduce the length of symptoms. Antibiotics are therefore recommended for severe disease with dehydration, or in immunocompromised individuals.
- ***Salmonella:*** Treatment does not shorten the duration of the symptoms and may actually prolong the carrier state. However, bacteremia is common in infants younger than 3 months of age, in patients with sickle cell disease, and in other immunocompromised individuals. Therefore, treatment should be considered if bacteremia is suspected in this population.
- ***E. coli* O157:H7:** No treatment because there is no proven benefit. A meta-analysis failed to confirm an increased risk of hemolytic uremic syndrome in patients treated with antibiotics.

American Academy of Pediatrics: *Escherichia coli* diarrhea. In Pickering LK (ed): Red Book: 2006 Report of the Committee on Infectious Diseases, 27th ed. Elk Grove Village, IL, American Academy of Pediatrics, 2006, pp 291–295.

120. **A 2-year-old presents with vomiting, profuse diarrhea, and new-onset seizures. What could be responsible for this clinical picture?**
Shigella infections are associated with CNS symptoms, including seizures and toxic encephalopathy (Ekiri syndrome). Severe diarrhea regardless of the etiology, however, may cause electrolyte abnormalities that result in seizures.

Fisher RG, Boyce TG: Moffet's Pediatric Infectious Diseases: A Problem-Oriented Approach, 4th ed. Philadelphia, Lippincott Williams & Wilkins, 2005, p 551.

121. **Should antimotility agents be used to manage gastroenteritis in children?**
No. The medications have limited benefit and have a high rate of side effects. Products with opiate derivatives are actually contraindicated. Nonnarcotic antimotility agents may be used in afebrile patients with nonbloody diarrhea.

122. **Which organisms cause food-borne illnesses? How can you distinguish them?**
See Table 38-18.

123. **A 3-month-old infant presents with a 3-day history of constipation, progressively poor feeding, and lethargy. On physical examination you notice a quiet, inactive child who is otherwise alert with good perfusion. The neurologic examination reveals a weak cry, poor suck, and hypotonia. What is the likely diagnosis?**
Infant botulism. Infants with botulism may appear to be septic, but usually are afebrile and have stable vital signs. Botulism occurs after ingestion of airborne spores from soil or dust. The ingested spores produce toxin in the intestine of the infant. Peak incidence is infants 6 weeks to 6 months of age. Breast-feeding is a significant risk factor. The ingestion of honey or corn syrup is often implicated, but not proven to be a risk factor. A history of soil

TABLE 38-18. ONSET, SYMPTOMS, AND ETIOLOGY OF FOOD-BORNE ILLNESS

Time of Onset	Main Symptoms	Organism or Toxin
Upper GI Tract		
1–6 hours	Nausea, vomiting, usually afebrile	*Staphylococcus aureus*
1–6 hours	Nausea, vomiting, afebrile	*Bacillus cereus* (emetic form)
Lower GI Tract		
8–16 hours	Diarrhea, afebrile	*Bacillus cereus* (diarrheal form)
6–24 hours	Foul-smelling diarrhea, cramps, afebrile	*Clostridium perfringens*
16–48 hours	Abdominal cramps, diarrhea, fever	*Vibrio cholerae*, Norwalk virus, *Escherichia coli* O157:H7, *Cryptosporidium* spp.
16–72 hours	Bloody diarrhea, fever, abdominal cramps	*Salmonella, Shigella*, and *Campylobacter* spp., *E. coli*
16–72 hours	Bloody diarrhea, fever, pseudoappendicitis, pharyngitis	*Yersinia enterocolitica*
1–6 weeks	Mucoid diarrhea (fatty stools), abdominal pain, weight loss	*Giardia lamblia*
Neurologic Infection		
12–36 hours	Vertigo, diplopia, areflexia, weakness, difficulty breathing and swallowing, constipation	*Clostridium botulinum*
Generalized Infection		
14 days	All of the above symptoms, plus vomiting, rose spots, constipation, abdominal pain, fever, chills, malaise, swollen lymph nodes	*Salmonella typhi*

Adapted from American Academy of Pediatrics: Appendix VI: Clinical syndromes associated with food borne diseases. In Pickering LK (ed): Red Book: 2006 Report of the Committee on Infectious Diseases, 27th ed. Elk Grove Village, IL, American Academy of Pediatrics, 2006, pp 858–860.

disruption, which occurs near construction sites, has been a common epidemiologic finding in reported cases. Infants should be hospitalized and observed for progressive weakness and respiratory failure. Botulism immune globulin intravenous is an antitoxin that, when given early, has been found to decrease duration of illness and hospital stay.

American Academy of Pediatrics: Clostridial infections. In Pickering LK (ed): Red Book: 2006 Report of the Committee on Infectious Diseases, 27th ed. Elk Grove Village, IL, American Academy of Pediatrics, 2006, pp 257–260.

124. Why is the diagnosis of *Clostridium difficile* colitis difficult in infants?
Almost 50% of infants (< 2 years) can have asymptomatic colonization, so toxin production is present without symptoms. Immature enterocytes with decreased amount of toxin-binding

capacity and maternal antibodies have been postulated as mechanisms for disease protection in infants. Disease is sometimes seen in infants younger than 3 months of age.

American Academy of Pediatrics: Clostridial infections. In Pickering LK (ed): Red Book: 2003 Report of the Committee on Infectious Diseases, 27th ed. Elk Grove Village, IL, American Academy of Pediatrics, 2006, pp 261–263.

125. **A 5-year-old who resides in a group home is transported to the ED because he looks "yellow." What are the diagnostic considerations?**
Hepatitis A virus (HAV) is highly contagious and spreads among children with poor hygiene or those in close quarters. Outbreaks at child care facilities usually represent an extension of a community outbreak. HAV infection is abrupt in onset and self-limiting, consisting of fever, anorexia, nausea, and headache. Jaundice is uncommon in young children compared with older children and adults, in whom jaundice can occur in 70% of cases. Liver failure in HAV is not common. The differential diagnosis should include hepatitis B or C (obtain a good history for associated risk factors: maternal history, blood transfusions, sexual contact), Epstein-Barr virus, adenoviruses, enteroviruses, varicella zoster, and HIV.

KEY POINTS: BLOODY DIARRHEA ✔

1. Send stool cultures for *Salmonella, Shigella, Yersinia,* and *Campylobacter* spp., and *E. coli* testing.

2. Initiate antimicrobial treatment for *Salmonella* and *Shigella* infections if the patient is clinically unstable, severely dehydrated, immunocompromised, or < 3 months of age.

3. Consider other noninfectious causes (e.g., inflammatory bowel disease).

BITES

126. **Which animals should be considered at high risk for transmission of rabies? How is rabies managed?**
Bats, foxes, and raccoons should be considered rabid. Between 1990 and 2001, 74% of human deaths from rabies have been associated with bats. Cats and dogs also carry rabies. Rabies in small rodents (squirrels, hamsters, rats, and mice) is uncommon. If bitten, patients should receive postexposure prophylaxis, including both passive and active therapy. Rabies immune globulin can be used for passive immunization. An exposed individual will need five total doses of active immunization with an approved rabies vaccine. Domestic animals, such as dogs, can be observed for 10 days after a bite for observation, since canine rabies in the United States is rare.

American Academy of Pediatrics: Rabies. In Pickering LK (ed): Red Book: 2006 Report of the Committee on Infectious Diseases, 27th ed. Elk Grove Village, IL, American Academy of Pediatrics, 2006, pp 552–558.

127. **Should a child who has been in proximity to bats (e.g., in the same room during sleep), but without known physical contact, receive prophylaxis?**
Yes. Cases of rabies have been reported in the absence of known contact with a rabid animal. Insignificant physical contact or airborne transmission of the virus may be responsible.

American Academy of Pediatrics: Rabies. In Pickering LK (ed): Red Book: 2006 Report of the Committee on Infectious Diseases, 27th ed. Elk Grove Village, IL, American Academy of Pediatrics, 2006, pp 552–558.

128. **True or false: Cat bites have a greater chance of becoming infected than dog bites.**
True. Wounds from cat bites are more than twice as likely to become infected, in part because of the deep puncture wound they cause. Rate of infection from cat bites can be more than 50% in some cases. *Pasteurella multicoda* is the most common organism seen in cat bite infections; it is seen in 25% of dog bites.

129. **When should antibiotics be prescribed for animal bites?**
Antibiotic use is recommended for all deep puncture wounds (e.g., cat bites), moderate and severe wounds (with edema or crush injury), bites involving certain areas of the body (face, hand/foot, genitals), and bites in the immunocompromised or asplenic patients. Recommended oral antibiotics include amoxicillin-clavulanate or amoxicillin. Intravenous antibiotics include ampicillin-sulbactam. Include coverage for *Staphylococcus aureus* and anaerobes as well as *Pasteurella multocida*.

RESPIRATORY ILLNESSES

130. **An afebrile 2-month-old presents with tachypnea and cough. What are the causes of pneumonia in this age group?**
Respiratory viruses account for up to 90% of pneumonias in the 1- to 3-month-old age group. Pneumonitis without fever in this age group may represent an infection with *Chlamydia trachomatis* or *Bordetella pertussis*. *C. trachomatis* is perinatally acquired and peaks at 4–11 weeks of age. Infants usually present with nasal discharge and a staccato cough, and have a history of conjunctivitis (50%). The chest radiograph reveals interstitial infiltrates and hyperinflation. *B. pertussis* in this age group presents with paroxysms of cough, often followed by vomiting, and a recent history of upper respiratory tract symptoms.

131. **Describe the acute management of bronchiolitis due to respiratory syncytial virus.**
   - Supportive treatment (mist treatments, suction, oxygen if needed)
   - Ensure hydration (IV fluid if dehydrated)
   - Chest radiographs to determine severity
   - Trial of bronchodilator (albuterol nebulized treatment), although various studies have demonstrated variable response
   - Racemic epinephrine for moderate to severe cases of bronchiolitis (has been shown to decrease respiratory distress [i.e., respiratory rate, oxygen saturation, and clinical scores])
   - Dexamethasone is not indicated in respiratory syncytial virus bronchiolitis, although several studies using nebulized budesonide demonstrate variable results

132. **What is the treatment of choice for presumed *C. trachomatis* infection (either conjunctivitis or pneumonia)?**
Oral erythromycin, clarithromycin, or azithromycin. Treatment for chlamydial pneumonia or conjunctivitis should be systemic. Chlamydial conjunctivitis alone is treated systemically to prevent the pneumonitis. Caution should be exercised with use of macrolides in infants younger than 6 weeks of age since they have been associated with hypertrophic pyloric stenosis.

American Academy of Pediatrics: Chlamydial infections. In Pickering LK (ed): Red Book: 2006 Report of the Committee on Infectious Diseases, 27th ed. Elk Grove Village, IL, American Academy of Pediatrics, 2006, pp 252–256.

133. **Describe the characteristics of pertussis in infancy.**
Most pertussis cases occur in infants younger than 6 months of age. This population does not often have the classic "whoops" with cough. Apnea can be a common presenting

symptom. Fever is absent or low grade. Adolescents and adults in the household are a major reservoir for transmission of pertussis because of their waxing vaccine-induced immunity. Pertussis should be considered in any infant with cough longer than 10–14 days. Pertussis in infants has a high mortality and morbidity. Complications in infants with pertussis include pneumonia, seizures, encephalopathy, and death.

134. **What is the drug of choice for the treatment of pertussis?**
Oral erythromycin estolate for 14 days is preferred. After the cough is present, however, antibiotics have no effect on the illness and are used more for prevention of spread to others. Oral azithromycin for 5 days has also been shown to be effective and is associated with better adherence.

135. **What are the most common types of pneumonia in a 2-year-old?**
Respiratory viruses are the most common causes of pneumonia in toddlers. Causes include:
- Respiratory syncytial virus
- Influenza
- Parainfluenza
- Adenovirus

Viral pneumonia is usually gradual in onset and preceded by upper respiratory tract symptoms; examination reveals diffuse auscultatory findings. Most of these children appear ill but not toxic.

Hendricskon KJ: Viral pneumonia in children. Semin Pediatr Infect Dis 3:217–233, 1998.

136. **When should you consider admitting an older child with pneumonia?**
- Hypoxia
- Toxic appearance
- Failed outpatient treatment
- Respiratory distress
- Questionable adherence
- Inability to maintain oral intake

137. **What clinical clues suggest typical bacterial pneumonia?**
Bacterial pneumonia is usually characterized by abrupt onset of high fever, respiratory distress (tachypnea, shortness of breath, hypoxia), and sometimes vomiting. Physical examination may reveal rales or decreased breath sounds. Chest radiograph may show lobar or segmental dense infiltrates associated with pleural effusion. A WBC count > 15,000 cells/mm^3 or elevated CRP level may indicate a bacterial process.

Lichenstein R, Suggs A, Campbell J: Pediatric pneumonia. Emerg Med Clin North Am 21:437–451, 2003.

138. **What are the typical bacterial causes of pneumonia in children outside the neonatal period?**
Streptococcus pneumoniae accounts for most bacterial pneumonias in children. Other uncommon causes include group A streptococci and *Staphylococcus aureus*. All these pathogens may cause severe, life-threatening pneumonias often associated with pneumatoceles.

139. **A 10-year-old presents with nonproductive cough, low-grade fever, and malaise. On physical examination, the patient appears well, has minimal respiratory distress, and has bilateral lower lung field crackles. What is the most frequent cause of pneumonia in this age group?**
This is a classic presentation of a child with atypical pneumonia caused by *Mycoplasma pneumoniae* or *C. pneumoniae*. *M. pneumoniae* is a common cause of pneumonia in older

children and young adults. It accounts for about 40% of community-acquired pneumonias in certain populations. Bilateral diffuse infiltrates are the most common radiographic findings, which are frequently out of proportion to clinical findings. Extrapulmonary manifestations, including a maculopapular rash (10%), CNS disease, hemolytic anemia, arthritis, and hepatitis, are occasionally seen in atypical pneumonia syndromes caused by *M. pneumoniae*.

Katz B, Waites K: Emerging intracellular bacterial infections. Clin Lab Med 24:627–649, 2004.

KEY POINTS: COMMON ETIOLOGIC AGENTS OF PNEUMONIA IN CHILDREN ✓

1. **Neonate:** Group B streptococci, *E. coli,* and other gram-negative bacilli, *Listeria monocytogenes, Ureaplasma urealyticum* (premature)

2. **Infant (< 3 months):** Respiratory syncytial virus, influenza, parainfluenza, adenovirus, *Chlamydia trachomatis*

3. **Infant to toddler (< 5 years):** Respiratory viruses, *Streptococcus pneumoniae, Mycoplasma pneumoniae*

4. **School age to adolescence:** *M. pneumoniae, C. pneumoniae, S. pneumoniae,* respiratory viruses

140. **What test can be used to assist in the diagnosis of *M. pneumoniae* infection?**
Cold agglutinins are IgM antibodies that agglutinate human red blood cells and are found in approximately 50% of patients with acute mycoplasma infection, and in some viral infections as well (adenovirus, Epstein-Barr virus, and measles virus). Although available, cold agglutinins have a poor specificity profile. Serology is not very useful in the ED management of these patients. If available, culture may be used for diagnosis as well.

141. **Which antimicrobials can be used for outpatient treatment of community-acquired pneumonia?**
The treatment of community-acquired pneumonia (CAP) is based on the most likely etiologic agents. When typical bacterial pneumonia is suspected, treatment should include adequate coverage against penicillin-resistant *Streptococcus pneumoniae*. Among available oral antibiotics, amoxicillin at high dose (80–100 mg/kg) provides the best coverage against resistant *Streptococcus pneumoniae*. Two recent studies comparing erythromycin, azithromycin, and amoxicillin-clavulanate showed comparable efficacy for the treatment of CAP. In the older child, treatment options should include coverage against atypical organisms such as *M. pneumoniae* and *C. pneumoniae* with erythromycin-azithromycin (< 8 years of age); tetracycline-doxycycline is an option in children > 8 years of age.

KEY POINTS: COMMUNITY-ACQUIRED PNEUMONIA ✓

1. In younger children, consider viruses and coverage for *Streptococcus pneumoniae*.

2. In older school-aged children, consider treatment to cover *Mycoplasma pneumoniae*.

ORTHOPEDIC INFECTIONS

142. **What are the most common sites for septic arthritis?**
The lower-extremity joints, such as the hip, knee, and ankle (less common), are
common sites for septic arthritis. Primary pyogenic arthritis is uncommon in
the post–*H. influenzae* era. Always suspect associated osteomyelitis when the
joint "looks septic."

143. **A 2-year-old presents with a limp. A radiograph of the suspected limb
is negative. Does a negative radiograph eliminate the possibility of
osteomyelitis?**
No. In the first 2 weeks of osteomyelitis, plain radiographs are not sensitive for the
detection of osteomyelitis (bony changes may not be evident yet). The gold standard
for diagnosis is magnetic resonance imaging or radionuclide bone scanning.

   Frank G, Mahoney HM, Eppes SC: Musculoskeletal infections in children. Pediatr Clin North
   Am 52:1083–1106, 2005.

144. **What is the classically described position that the leg is held in by a
child with septic arthritis of the hip?**
The leg is externally rotated and abducted.

145. **What are the most common bones affected in osteomyelitis?**
The long bones of the leg—femur and tibia—are most affected. In neonates and
infants, osteomyelitis may affect any bone, including the humerus, hips, mandible, or
calcaneus.

146. **Aspiration of the hip joint in a 2-year-old febrile child with a limp reveals
a WBC count of 60,000 cells/mm^3 with a neutrophil predominance. What
diagnosis is likely?**
Septic arthritis is most likely. However, Table 38-19 can aid in diagnosis based on the
WBC count and differential but demonstrates considerable overlap. Epidemiology,
presence of fever, and detailed history may help.

   Frank G, Mahoney HM, Eppes SC: Musculoskeletal infections in children. Pediatr Clin North
   Am 52:1083–1106, 2005.

TABLE 38-19. DIFFERENTIAL DIAGNOSIS OF SEPTIC ARTHRITIS BASED ON WHITE BLOOD CELL COUNT AND NEUTROPHILS		
Diagnosis	White Blood Cells (cells/mm^3)	Neutrophils (%)
Normal	<200	10–20
Traumatic effusion	<2000	10–30
Rheumatologic	10,000–50,000	50–80
Septic arthritis	>50,000	≥80
Lyme disease	15–125,000	>50

147. **Match the disease with the appropriate management plan.**

1. Osteomyelitis	**A.** No antibiotics needed. Anti-inflammatory medications may
2. Septic arthritis of hip	be needed.
3. Toxic synovitis	**B.** Admission to hospital. No IV antibiotics until patient is
	evaluated by orthopedic surgery and cultures of bone have
	been obtained.
	C. Emergency, requiring surgical drainage and IV antibiotics.

Answers: 1, B; 2, C; 3, A

148. **What are the most common organisms found in bone and joint infections?**
See Table 38-20.

TABLE 38-20. ORGANISMS MOST COMMONLY FOUND IN BONE AND JOINT INFECTIONS*

Age	Septic Arthritis	Osteomyelitis
Neonate	*Staphylococcus aureus*	*S. aureus*
	Group B streptococci	Group B streptococci
	Gram-negative bacilli	Gram-negative bacilli
Toddler	*S. aureus*	*S. aureus*
	Group A streptococci	Group A streptococci
	Streptococcus pneumoniae	*Kingella kingae*
	Kingella kingae	
School-age	*S. aureus*	*S. aureus*
	Group A streptococci	Group A streptococci

*In sexually active adolescents, also consider *Neisseria gonorrhoeae*. *Salmonella* sp. is a common cause of osteomyelitis in children with sickle cell disease.
Adapted from Frank G, Mahoney HM, Eppes SC: Musculoskeletal infections in children. Pediatr Clin North Am 52:1083–1106, 2005; and Gutierrez K: Bone and joint infections in children. Pediatr Clin North Am 52:779–794, 2005.

149. **What is pyomyositis?**
Pyomyositis is an infection of skeletal muscle that may be associated with antecedent trauma. The etiology is often *Staphylococcus aureus* or GABHS in immunocompetent children, but gram-negative organisms may also be involved in infections seen in immunocompromised children. Fever, myalgias, muscle tenderness to palpation, or swelling of the involved muscle may be seen. Magnetic resonance imaging is extremely helpful in making the diagnosis. Treatment includes surgical drainage if abscesses are involved and IV antibiotics.

VIRAL ILLNESSES/EXANTHEMS

150. **What is the classic description of roseola (primary human herpesvirus-6 infection)?**
High fever (temperature > 39.5° C) for 3–7 days, nonspecific signs (e.g., irritability, decreased feeding, or toxic appearance), and a diffuse maculopapular rash soon after defervescence

(about day 4–6 of illness) lasting hours to days. This classic presentation is seen in only 20% of patients. Human herpesvirus 6 infection accounts for approximately 20% of acute febrile illness visits for children 6–8 months of age. Seizures may occur in about 10% patients during the febrile period. A bulging anterior fontanel occurs occasionally.

151. **A medical student reports to you that a 3-year-old, febrile child appears to have been slapped on both cheeks by someone. What infectious disease are you considering?**
Erythema infectiosum is the most common manifestation of parvovirus B19 infection. This infection is associated with a rash, characterized by intense erythema of the cheeks (slapped-cheek appearance) with circumoral pallor. On the trunk and extremities, the rash is maculopapular with a lacelike or reticular appearance.

152. **A 15-year-old with fever, exudative pharyngitis, lymphadenopathy, and splenomegaly presents to the ED. You suspect infectious mononucleosis. What laboratory tests should be obtained to aid in diagnosis?**
A CBC and heterophil antibody (IgM) test should be done. The WBC count can vary, but sometimes anemia, leukopenia, and thrombocytopenia can be seen. An increase in the number of atypical lymphocytes (10%) is a characteristic finding. The heterophil antibody test (Monospot) is specific for Epstein-Barr virus. In adolescents, the heterophil response occurs more reliably after the first week of illness. Its sensitivity is poor in young children (< 4 years of age). The younger child is more likely to be asymptomatic or have a nonspecific infection.

153. **What should you recommend to a patient with infectious mononucleosis upon discharge from the ED?**
The patient should avoid contact sports until examined by a physician and until the spleen is no longer palpable to avoid traumatic rupture of the spleen, which can be life-threatening.

154. **Should patients with infectious mononucleosis be treated with corticosteroids?**
Steroids are indicated for significant tonsillar inflammation with impending airway obstruction, hemophagocytic syndrome, massive splenomegaly, hemolytic anemia, and carditis.

American Academy of Pediatrics: Epstein Barr viral infections. In: Pickering LK (ed): Red Book: 2006 Report of the Committee on Infectious Diseases, 27th ed. Elk Grove Village, IL, American Academy of Pediatrics, 2006, pp 286–290.

155. **Match the disease with the clinical description.**

1. Varicella (chicken pox)
2. Measles
3. Rubella

A. Fever, cough, coryza, and conjunctivitis. Confluent maculopapular rash beginning on upper part of body; can involve palms and soles.

B. Fever; coalescent, pink, maculopapular rash that begins on face and extends downwards; tender postauricular, suboccipital, and posterior cervical lymph nodes. Prodromal symptoms of cough, malaise, and conjunctivitis are uncommon.

C. Prodrome of fever, papules, vesicles, and umbilicated and scabbed lesions. Hallmark is lesions present in different stages at the same time. Lesions develop in crops. Initial lesion typically in scalp and lesions can involve oral mucosa.

Answers: 1, C; 2, A; 3, B.

156. **How long is the child with chicken pox contagious?**
The period of communicability begins 1–2 days prior to the outbreak of lesions and lasts until all lesions are crusted over.

157. **A child with varicella presents with chicken pox, high fever, and toxic appearance. What should you suspect?**
Examine the child closely for evidence of secondary bacterial infection with *Staphylococcus aureus* and *Streptococcus pyogenes* (group A). Secondary bacterial infection is the most common cause of morbidity in children with varicella infection. Clinical features include high fever, toxic appearance, and a varicella lesion that has become erythematous, warm, and painful. Superinfection with group A streptococci can progress to soft tissue necrosis, necrotizing fasciitis, and sepsis.

158. **A 1-year-old infant has fever and rash 10 days after the annual visit to the pediatrician. What important history should be obtained regarding the recent visit to the pediatrician?**
Immunization history. Determine if the measles, mumps, and rubella vaccine was administered. Fever with body temperature as high as 39°C develops in 5–15% of children 7–12 days after vaccination. The fever typically lasts 1–2 days, and approximately 5% of patients develop a rash. Varicella vaccination may also be given at 1 year of age. Within 1 month of vaccination, 5–10% of children develop a mild maculopapular or varicelliform rash. The rash is limited to only a few lesions that can be at the injection site or elsewhere.

159. **A 4-year-old boy presents with a chief complaint of body temperature of 40°C for 7 days. On physical examination, you notice bilateral conjunctivitis, a strawberry red tongue, anterior cervical lymphadenopathy, and diffuse erythema of the perineal area. What is your diagnosis?**
Kawasaki disease. This is a multisystem vasculitis with a peak incidence in childhood; 80% of cases occur in children < 4 years old.

KAWASAKI DISEASE

160. **What are the diagnostic criteria for Kawasaki disease?**
   1. Fever for at least 5 days
   2. Presence of four of the following:
      - Swelling and erythema of hands and feet
      - Cervical lymphadenopathy
      - Bilateral, nonpurulent conjunctival injection
      - Mucous membrane changes
      - Diffuse polymorphous rash

   Newburger JW: Diagnosis, treatment and long-term management of Kawasaki disease: A statement for health professionals from the committee on rheumatic fever, endocarditis, and Kawasaki disease. Council on Cardiovascular Disease in the Young; American Heart Association. Pediatrics 114:1708–1733, 2004.

161. **What is the differential diagnosis of Kawasaki disease?**
   - Measles
   - Scarlet fever
   - Toxic shock syndrome
   - Juvenile rheumatoid arthritis
   - Viral syndromes (adenovirus, Epstein-Barr virus, enteroviruses)
   - RMSF
   - Leptospirosis
   - Mercury poisoning
   - Drug reactions

   Dedeoglu F, Sundei RP: Vasculitis in children. Pediatr Clin North Am 52:547–575, 2005.

162. **What laboratory findings support the diagnosis of Kawasaki disease?**
    - WBC count increased with left shift ($>$ 20,000 cells/mm^3 in 50% of patients, $>$ 30,000 cells/mm^3 in 15% of patients)
    - Increased erythrocyte sedimentation rate
    - Platelets increased during second week of illness
    - Sterile pyuria
    - Mild elevation of aminotransferase levels
    - Mild anemia
    - Hypoalbuminemia
    - Low phosphorus level

163. **What is the management of a patient with suspected Kawasaki disease?**
    Management includes admission to the hospital for treatment with high-dose aspirin and IV immunoglobulin within 10 days of fever onset. All patients should have echocardiography performed as part of the initial hospital evaluation and then a repeat test 6–8 weeks after onset. Treatment within the first 10 days of the illness has been shown to substantially decrease the risk of coronary artery disease (a known complication of Kawasaki disease) from 20% to $<$ 5%.

    Newburger JW: Diagnosis, treatment and long-term management of Kawasaki disease: A statement for health professionals from the committee on rheumatic fever, endocarditis, and Kawasaki disease. Council on Cardiovascular Disease in the Young; American Heart Association. Pediatrics 114:1708–1733, 2004.

BIOTERRORISM INFECTIONS

164. **What are some agents of bioterrorism?**
    Agents are broken down into categories A, B, and C. Category A agents provide the greatest risk. They can be easily transmitted from person to person and tend to have the highest mortality rates. Category B agents have lower mortality rates and are not as easily spread as category A agents. Category C agents can be engineered to be biological weapons of mass destruction with the potential for high morbidity and high mortality rates.
    - **Category A agents:** Anthrax, smallpox, plague, tularemia, hemorrhagic fever viruses, botulinum toxin
    - **Category B agents:** *Coxiella burnetii* (Q fever), *Brucella* species, *Burkholderia mallei*, alphaviruses (Venezuelan, eastern, and western equine encephalomyelitis), *Salmonella* species, *Shigella dysenteriae*, *E. coli* O157:H7, *Vibrio cholerae, Cryptosporidium parvum*
    - **Category C agents:** Hantavirus, tick-borne hemorrhagic fever viruses, yellow fever, and *Mycobacterium tuberculosis* (multidrug-resistant).

    Shannon M: Management of infectious agents of bioterrorism. Clin Pediatr Emerg Med 5:63–71, 2004.

165. **Match the bioterrorist disease with the organism and symptoms.**

    A. Anthrax
    B. Tularemia
    C. Plague
    D. Smallpox

    1. Gram-negative rod resulting in pneumonia-like illness with fever, cough, dyspnea, large lymph node (bubo), and hemoptysis 2–4 days after exposure. Chest radiograph reveals bilateral infiltrates or lobar consolidation.
    2. Spore forming gram-positive bacillus resulting in a flulike illness: fever, chills, malaise, nonproductive cough, absence of rhinorrhea. Chest radiograph reveals widened mediastinum.
    3. Gram-negative coccobacillus resulting in possible skin ulceration, pharyngitis, conjunctival injection, lymphadenitis, fever, pneumonia. Chest radiograph reveals hilar adenopathy.

4. Member of the Poxviridae family and resulting in low-grade fever, vesicular centrifugal rash 14 days after exposure. Lesions are umbilicated and in the same stage of development.

Answers: A, 2; B, 3; C,1; D, 4.

Shannon M: Management of infectious agents of bioterrorism. Clin Pediatr Emerg Med 5:63–71, 2004.

METHICILLIN-RESISTANT *STAPHYLOCOCCUS AUREUS* INFECTIONS

166. **What are some epidemiologic concerns regarding community-acquired MRSA?**
Community-acquired MRSA infections have increased dramatically in the last 3–4 years. They may include furunculoses, carbuncles, and invasive staphylococcal infections. There are apparent differences between racial groups, with African-American children having two to four times the frequency of these types of infections. Community-acquired MRSA infection may be seen in multiple family members, day care attendees, and athletes.

Kaplan SL: Implications of methicillin-resistant *Staphylococcus aureus* as a community-acquired pathogen in pediatric patients. Infect Dis Clin North Am 19:747–757, 2005.

167. **What antimicrobials would you use to treat community-acquired MRSA?**
When considering community-acquired MRSA as a source of infection, antibiotics such as β-lactams, oxacillin, or cefazolin should not be used. Clindamycin and trimethoprim-sulfamethoxazole can be considered. However, in parts of the United States where community-acquired MRSA with resistance to clindamycin is greater than 10%, alternative therapies such as vancomycin and linezolid should be used.

Lowy FD, Kaplan SL: Treatment of methicillin-resistant *Staphylococcus aureus* in children, 2006: www.uptodate.com

168. **What is the relevance of the D-test?**
The D-test is a disk diffusion test to evaluate isolates of community-acquired MRSA, which may have macrolide inducible resistance to clindamycin. It looks for the presence of macrolide lincosamide streptogramin B (MLS$_B$) resistance coded for by ermA and ermC. In the laboratory, an erythromycin disk is placed 15–26 mm away from the clindamycin disk. An observed "D" shape indicates an induced resistance to clindamycin.

UNUSUAL INFECTIONS

169. **What is SARS and how can it be diagnosed?**
SARS stands for "severe acute respiratory syndrome." It is a severe lower respiratory tract infection caused by a coronavirus also called SARS-associated coronavirus (SARS-CoV). Symptoms are often nonspecific, including fever, dyspnea, and extreme hypoxia in adults. Children appear to have a less severe course and outcome. Children younger than age 12 years present with fever, rhinorrhea, cough, and lymphopenia. Children older than 12 years of age present with malaise, chills, rigors, and higher fevers. A good history is crucial in the diagnosis of SARS, including a recent travel history to China, Hong Kong, or Taiwan, contact with someone from that region or recent travel to, or occupation in a high-risk environment (hospital, laboratory). Diagnosis can be made by culture of respiratory secretions or by using reverse-transcriptase polymerase chain reaction. Serum can be tested for coronavirus serologies.

Williams JV: The clinical presentation and outcomes comes of children infected with newly identified respiratory tract viruses. Infect Dis Clin North Am 19:569–584, 2005.
Centers for Disease Control and Prevention: www.cdc.gov.

170. **What do pigs and birds have in common with the flu?**
The influenza A (H5N1) virus is a virus that occurs mainly in birds. During late 2003–2004, outbreaks occurred among poultry in Asia. In 1997, the first cause of spread from bird to human was seen in Hong Kong, with more cases seen with the outbreaks during 2003–2004. It is also possible for strains that have passed through an intermediate host, most often the pig, to infect a human. H5N1 virus spread from person to person is rare.

Williams JV: The clinical presentation and outcomes of children infected with newly identified respiratory tract viruses. Infect Dis Clin North Am 19:569–584, 2005.
Centers for Disease Control and Prevention: www.cdc.gov

171. **What is the treatment for H5N1 virus? Is there a vaccine to protect humans?**
H5N1 has been shown to be resistant to amantadine and rimantadine, two antiviral medications we use now for influenza. Both oseltamavir and zanamavir may be active against H5N1, but more studies need to be done. To date, there is no human vaccine for the H5N1 virus.

Centers for Disease Control and Prevention: www.cdc.gov

172. **What are the distinguishing features of malaria?**
Malaria is characterized by paroxysms of fever, chills, and rigors occurring at certain time intervals depending on the species. Infection with *Plasmodium falciparum* carries a high morbidity and mortality (secondary to cerebral malaria in addition to renal and respiratory failure).

BIBLIOGRAPHY

1. Fleisher GR: Infectious disease emergencies. In Fleisher GR, Ludwig S, Henretig FM (eds): Textbook of Pediatric Emergency Medicine, 5th ed. Baltimore, Lipppincott, Willliams & Wilkins, 2006, pp 783–853.
2. Long SS, Pickering LK, Prober CG (eds): Principles and Practice of Pediatric Infectious Diseases, 2nd ed. New York, Churchill Livingstone, 2003.

CHAPTER 39

POISONINGS

Kevin C. Osterhoudt, MD, MSCE, and James F. Wiley II, MD, MPH

EPIDEMIOLOGY

1. **How many poisonings occur in the united states each year? How many exposures involve children < 6 years?**
   Over 2 million calls are made to regional poison control centers annually. Of these, 50–60% involve toxic exposures in children younger than 6 years of age. Not all poisonings are reported to poison control centers. Estimates suggest that 4 million people are poisoned in the United States each year.

   Watson WA, Litovitz TL, Rodgers Jr GC, et al: 2004 annual report of the American Association of Poison Control Centers toxic exposure surveillance system. Am J Emerg Med 23:589–666, 2005.

2. **How often can poisoning be managed at home with the assistance of a regional poison control center?**
   Of all poison calls to a regional center, 80–90% are typically handled safely via phone advice and home observation.

   Watson WA, Litovitz TL, Rodgers Jr GC, et al: 2004 annual report of the American Association of Poison Control Centers toxic exposure surveillance system. Am J Emerg Med 23:589–666, 2005.

3. **When was the first poison control center established and why?**
   Dr. Edward Press in Chicago established the first center in 1953 in response to an American Academy of Pediatrics study published in 1952, which found that 50% of all childhood injuries were due to potentially poisonous ingestions.

   Press E, Mellins RB: A poisoning control program. Am J Public Health 44:1515–1525, 1954.

4. **What is the poison prevention packaging act?**
   Passed in 1970, this act mandated safety packaging for pharmaceuticals. It followed other important landmark legislation, including the Federal Hazardous Substances Labeling Act of 1960, which promoted product labeling, and the Child Protection Act of 1966, which required appropriate labeling of pesticides and other previously unlabeled hazardous substances.

5. **What was the impact of the poison prevention packaging act?**
   Frequency of poisoning and death due to poisoning in children decreased significantly in 1969, one year prior to the passage of the act. This effect was due to voluntary initiation of safety packaging (childproof caps) by manufacturers in anticipation of the law.

   Arena J: The pediatrician's role in the poison control movement and poison prevention. Am J Dis Child 137:870–873, 1983.

6. **What are the most common poisons to which young children are exposed?**
   In 2004, the top 10 exposures in young children, from most frequent to least frequent, were cosmetics, cleaning substances, topicals, foreign bodies (e.g., coins, button batteries), cough and cold preparations, plants, pesticides, vitamins, and antihistamines.

Watson WA, Litovitz TL, Rodgers GC Jr, et al: 2004 annual report of the American Association of Poison Control Centers toxic exposure surveillance system. Am J Emerg Med 23:589–666, 2005.

7. **Who is more likely to ingest a poison: A 2-year-old boy or a 2-year-old girl?**
The boy is more likely to ingest a poison.

8. **Who is more likely to ingest a poison: A 15-year-old boy or a 15-year-old girl?**
The girl is more likely to ingest a poison and usually does so intentionally.

9. **What is the typical setting for a pediatric poisoning incident?**
The child is usually younger than 6 years of age and is at home. The poison is typically readily available to the child. Prescription medicines that children ingest frequently belong to a grandparent or older nonparent relative. In most cases, only one poison is ingested. Social history often discloses a recent stress in the household, such as a recent move, new baby, marital discord, visiting relatives, or distracting event (holiday, wedding).

Henretig FM: Special considerations in the poisoned pediatric patient. Emerg Med Clin North Am 12: 549–567, 1994.

10. **What is the most common cause of death due to poisoning?**
Carbon monoxide inhalation is widely felt to be the most common cause of death due to poisoning because this gas can be implicated in the numerous fire deaths that occur annually, in addition to the intentional and unintentional deaths reported to the American Association of Poison Control Centers.

Homer CD, Engelhart DA, Lavins ES, et al: Carbon monoxide-related deaths in a metropolitan county in the USA: An 11-year study. Forens Sci Int 149:159–165, 2005.

11. **What are the most dangerous substances, according to reports to the American Association of Poison Control Centers?**
Investigators have devised the **hazard factor**, which calculates the sum of the number of deaths and major effects (patients requiring antidotes or life-saving supportive measures after exposure) for each substance divided by the total number of exposures. This number is then normalized by using a constant reflecting the overall rate of major effects and deaths for data reported between 1985 and 1989 (six major effects or deaths per 10,000 exposures). A factor of 1 suggests that the poison is no worse than the average poison on the database. A factor of 50 implies that the poison is 50 times more likely to cause major effects or death after exposure than the average poison. On the basis of this analysis, the following substances are particularly hazardous:

Substance	Hazard Factor
Rattlesnake envenomation	245
Methadone	75
Chloral hydrate	66
Cyclic antidepressant	57
Strychnine	50
Selenious acid (gun bluing)	48
Acid drain cleaner (toilet bowel cleaner)	47
Carbamazepine	33
Chloroquine (antimalarial)	32
Carbon monoxide	31
Paraquat	24

Litovitz TL, Manoguerra A: Comparison of pediatric poisoning hazards: an analysis of 3.8 million exposure incidents. A report from the American Association of Poison Control Centers. Pediatrics 89:999–1006, 1992.

12. **Which medicinals are potentially life-threatening or fatal to a 10-kg toddler following ingestion of a single dose?**
    Benzocaine, camphor, chloroquine, clonidine, cyclic antidepressants, diphenoxylate/atropine (Lomotil), lindane, methadone (and other opioids), methyl salicylate (oil of wintergreen), oral hypoglycemics, quinidine, propranolol, theophylline, thioridazine, and verapamil.

    Osterhoudt KC: The toxic toddler: Drugs that can kill in small doses. Contemp Pediatr 17:73–88, 2000.

KEY POINTS: POISONING EPIDEMIOLOGY ✔

1. More than half of all poisoning exposures are reported among children younger than age 6 years.

2. Natural exploratory behaviors of young children put them at risk for poisoning.

3. Drug abuse, experimental risk taking, and depression put adolescents at risk for poisoning.

4. Poisoning can be prevented.

INITIAL MANAGEMENT

13. **Which three antidotal drugs should be immediately considered in the resuscitation of the comatose child?**
    Two are often not thought of as drugs per se, but they are essential substrates for brain function: oxygen and glucose. Administration of the opioid antagonist naloxone may also be warranted.

14. **What is a "toxidrome"?**
    The word *toxidrome* can be thought of as a combination of the words "toxic" and "syndrome." Toxidromes are groupings of physical signs that may help to suggest the drug class responsible for a poisoning. These signs should be noted in the examination of every potentially poisoned patient: mental status, vital signs, pupil size and reactivity, skin color and moisture, and bowel sounds.

    Osterhoudt KC: No sympathy for a boy with obtundation. Pediatr Emerg Care 20:403–406, 2004.

15. **Describe the most common toxidromes.**
    See Table 39-1.

16. **How can the anticholinergic toxidrome be differentiated from the sympathomimetic toxidrome?**
    Anticholinergic agents and sympathomimetic agents may both produce altered mental status, tachycardia, hypertension, hyperthermia, and mydriatic pupils, so distinguishing between these drugs is not easy. Look to the skin, the bowels, and the eyes for help. Anticholinergic poisoning is likely to produce flushed skin that is surprisingly dry to the touch, diminished or absent bowel sounds, and less reactive pupils. Many people remember the characteristics of

TABLE 39–1. COMMON TOXIDROMES

Variable	Sympathomimetics	Anticholinergics	Organophosphates	Opiates/Clonidine	Barbiturates/ Sedative-Hypnotics	Salicylates
Mental status	A, D, P, S	C, D, P, S	C, D, F	C	C	C, S
Heart rate	↑	↑	↓ (↑)	↑	–	– (↑)
Blood pressure	↑	↑	– (↑)	↓	↓	–
Temperature	↑	↑	–	↓	↓	↑
Respirations	–	–	↑	↓	↓	↑
Pupil size	↑ (reactive)	↑ (sluggish)	↓	↓↓	–	–
Bowel sounds	–	↓	↑	↓	–	–
Skin	Sweaty	Flushed/dry	Sweaty	–	Bullae (IV use)	Sweaty

A = agitation, C = somnolence/coma, D = delirium, F = fasciculations, P = psychosis, S = seizure.

the anticholinergic toxidrome with the mnemonic: "Mad as a hatter, blind as a bat (pupils do not accommodate well), red as a beet, dry as a bone, and hot as Hades."

17. **What would be the significance of a bitter almond smell to your morning coffee?**
Consider the possibility of cyanide in the coffee.

18. **What other toxicants are associated with characteristic odors?**

Odor	Agent
Acetone	Acetone, isopropyl alcohol, phenol
Almonds	Cyanide
Garlic	Arsenic, thallium, organophosphates, selenious acid
Pears	Chloral hydrate, paraldehyde
Rotten eggs	Hydrogen sulfide
Wintergreen	Methyl salicylate

19. **List the most commonly considered methods of gastrointestinal decontamination of the poisoned patient.**
   - **Gastric emptying:** Induced emesis, gastric lavage
   - **Prevention of drug absorption:** Activated charcoal
   - **Catharsis:** Simple cathartics, whole-bowel irrigation

20. **Elaborate the indications for ipecac-induced emesis.**
Induced emesis has little role in the emergency department setting. Indeed, its use as out-of-hospital first aid is now discouraged by the American Academy of Pediatrics.

   American Academy of Pediatrics Committee on Injury, Violence, and Poison Prevention: Poison treatment in the home. Pediatrics 112:1182–1185, 2003.

21. **What is the proper technique for gastric lavage?**
Consider the need for airway protection with endotracheal intubation. Place the patient in left lateral decubitus position with the head slightly lower than feet if tolerated. Use a large-bore orogastric tube (24 Fr in toddlers and up to 36 Fr in adolescents). Lavage with saline aliquots until the effluent is clear of toxic materials.

22. **Under what circumstances is gastric lavage indicated?**
Gastric lavage, once the stalwart of emergency department management of poisonings, is falling from favor after recent investigation has questioned its efficacy. It may still have a role in the management of *life-threatening overdoses presenting within the first hour*. Gastric lavage may be considered more strongly for poisoning scenarios that lack dependable antidotes.

23. **What is the gastrointestinal decontamination technique of choice for most poisonings?**
In most cases, gastric emptying can be omitted in preference to administration of activated charcoal.

   Osterhoudt KC, Durbin D, Alpern ER, et al: Activated charcoal administration in a pediatric emergency department. Pediatr Emerg Care 20:493–498, 2004.

24. **What is activated charcoal?**

Most would recognize charcoal as the byproduct of the pyrolysis of wood or other organic materials. "Activation" of charcoal refers to a process of further oxidizing the charcoal, either chemically or at high temperatures, to increase its surface area and adsorptive capacity.

25. **List common drugs and toxicants that are poorly adsorbed by activated charcoal.**

- **Ineffective:** Alcohols, iron, lithium
- **Poorly effective:** Hydrocarbons, metals

26. **What is whole-bowel irrigation?**

Whole-bowel irrigation uses nonabsorbable polyethylene glycol solution (well-known as a surgical bowel prep) to wash intestinal contents through before absorption can take place. Typical administration is 500 mL/hour in a toddler and to 2 L/hour in an adolescent, continued until the rectal effluent is clear and clinical signs of continued drug absorption have subsided.

27. **List the possible indications for whole-bowel irrigation.**

Although not yet proven to improve patient outcomes, use of whole-bowel irrigation has been advocated for the following situations:

- Body packers/stuffers
- Ingestion of metals, lithium
- Ingestion of sustained-release preparations
- Ingestion of pharmaceutical patches
- Massive overdoses
- Concretions of pills

28. **What is a body packer or a body stuffer?**

Body packers are smugglers who attempt to evade customs officials by swallowing packages (typically tied condoms) of drugs. Body stuffers are drug sellers or users who hurriedly ingest illicit substances to hide evidence from authorities. Because of the planning involved, packers are less likely to become toxic than stuffers; however, packers typically ingest more dangerous quantities of drug.

Traub SJ, Hoffman RS, Nelson LS: Body packing: The internal concealment of illicit drugs. N Engl J Med 349:2519–2526, 2003.

29. **How often do poisoned patients require special therapy, such as antidote administration, elimination enhancement, or extracorporeal elimination?**

Antidotes and elimination enhancement, such as urinary alkalinization or multiple-dose activated charcoal, are performed in about 1% of all reported poisonings. Extracorporeal elimination (hemodialysis or hemoperfusion) is needed in less than 0.1%.

Watson WA, Litovitz TL, Rodgers GC, et al: 2004 annual report of the American Association of Poison Control Centers toxic exposure surveillance system. Am J Emerg Med 23:589–666, 2005.

30. **What are the characteristics of the ideal toxic agent that would be amenable to multiple-dose activated charcoal?**

The ideal toxicant has a small volume of distribution (< 1 L/kg), has low protein binding, binds to activated charcoal, and either has an enterohepatic circulation of an active metabolite in the bowel or undergoes enteroenteric dialysis with evidence of excretion of agent from the microvillous blood circulation into the gut, where it is bound by the charcoal. Multiple-dose activated charcoal may also be of benefit after ingestion of sustained-release compounds or after a toxic gastric concretion has formed.

31. **Multiple doses of activated charcoal are believed to enhance clearance of what poison(s)?**
Good evidence exists to support the use of multiple-dose activated charcoal to treat certain cases of poisoning from carbamazepine, dapsone, phenobarbital, quinine, and theophylline. Elimination of amitriptyline, dextropropoxyphene, digoxin, disopyramide, nadolol, phenylbutazone, phenytoin, piroxicam, and sotalol increases with multiple-dose activated charcoal; however, improved outcomes for ingestion of these poisons with respect to morbidity and mortality have not been shown in controlled trials.

American Academy of Clinical Toxicology, European Association of Poisons Centers and Clinical Toxicologists. Position statement and practice guideline on the use of multi-dose activated charcoal in the treatment of acute poisoning. Clin Toxicol 37:731–751, 1999.

32. **What is extracorporeal removal?**
Extracorporeal removal refers to elimination of a poison from the blood after removing the blood or a portion of the blood from the body. The forms of extracorporeal elimination include hemodialysis, charcoal hemoperfusion, arteriovenous hemofiltration, venovenous hemofiltration, exchange transfusion, and plasmapheresis. Of these, hemodialysis is used most commonly.

33. **What factors predict adequate removal of a poison by hemodialysis?**
The substance should have the following characteristics: small volume of distribution, little protein binding, water solubility, low molecular weight, low endogenous clearance, and single-compartment kinetics.

34. **For which toxic agents is hemodialysis most commonly considered?**
- Ethylene glycol
- Lithium
- Methanol
- Salicylate
- Theophylline

Dargan PI, Jones AL: Acute poisoning: Understanding 90% of cases in a nutshell. Postgrad Med J 81: 204–216, 2005.

35. **When should hemodialysis be used?**
The decision to perform hemodialysis should be based on physical findings as well as drug levels. Always repeat an elevated level and check units of measurement before instituting hemodialysis.

36. **What is the rationale behind urinary alkalinization?**
Urinary alkalinization refers to the administration of sodium bicarbonate to raise the urine pH to 8.0. This procedure converts renally excreted toxins, which are weak acids to their ionized form within the proximal renal tubules, and thereby prevents reabsorption in the distal tubules (ion trapping). This technique is most useful for enhancing the excretion of salicylates and phenobarbital (but not other barbiturates). Urinary alkalinization is also useful to protect the kidney during rhabdomyolysis.

Proudfoot AT, Krenzelok EP, Vale JA: Position paper on urine alkalinization. J Toxicol Clin Toxicol 42:1–26, 2004.

37. **What are the pitfalls of urinary alkalinization?**
Urine alkalinization is inhibited by the presence of hypokalemia. Urinary alkalinization has been associated with pulmonary and cerebral edema, and fluid administration must be monitored

carefully. Electrolyte and acid-base disturbances can result from sodium bicarbonate administration and merit frequent monitoring.

Proudfoot AT, Krenzelok EP, Vale JA: Position paper on urine alkalinization. J Toxicol Clin Toxicol 42:1–26, 2004.

38. **List some drugs that may lead to a delayed expression of clinical toxicity.**
   - Acetaminophen
   - Monoamine oxidase inhibitors
   - Oral hypoglycemic agents
   - Sustained-release drug formulations
   - Thyroid hormones
   - Warfarin

KEY POINTS: INITIAL POISONING MANAGEMENT ✔

1. Toxidrome analysis is more clinically useful than toxicology urine analysis.

2. In most cases, gastrointestinal decontamination with activated charcoal is preferred to gastric emptying measures.

PHARMACEUTICALS

39. **Describe the pathophysiology of acetaminophen poisoning.**
   Acetaminophen is the drug most commonly administered to children. Toxicity may occur after acute overdose of 150–200 mg/kg or after repeated supratherapeutic ingestions. Overdose of acetaminophen saturates typical hepatic metabolism pathways, and expends glutathione, resulting in the production of an intermediate metabolite, N-acetyl-p-benzoquinoneimine via cytochrome oxidase (P450) metabolism. This metabolite binds to hepatocytes and causes centrilobular liver necrosis.

40. **What are the three stages of acetaminophen overdose poisoning?**
   - **Stage I** (1/2–24 hours after ingestion): Often asymptomatic; occasionally nausea, vomiting, diaphoresis, and pallor are seen.
   - **Stage II** (24–48 hours after ingestion): Nausea, vomiting, right-upper-quadrant abdominal pain, elevation of hepatic aminotransferase levels.
   - **Stage III** (72–96 hours after ingestion): Fulminant hepatic failure with jaundice, thrombocytopenia, prolonged prothrombin time, and hepatic encephalopathy. Renal failure and cardiomyopathy may occur. If the patient survives, complete resolution of liver abnormalities is possible.

41. **How is acetaminophen intoxication diagnosed?**
   The potential for acetaminophen poisoning must be thoughtfully considered since most patients are initially asymptomatic. The serum acetaminophen level should be measured in all patients with intentional drug overdose. Frequently, acetaminophen is overlooked as a coingestant with cough/cold preparations and combination analgesics such as Darvocet (propoxyphene and acetaminophen) and Percocet (oxycodone and acetaminophen). An acetaminophen level at 4–24 hours after ingestion can predict the potential for toxicity and determine the need for antidote administration based on the Rumack-Matthew nomogram.

42. **What is the antidote for acetaminophen overdose? How does it work?**

    N-acetyl cysteine (NAC) replenishes, and substitutes for, depleted glutathione stores in the liver and detoxifies the toxic metabolite. NAC also seems to alleviate existing hepatotoxicity through antioxidant and procirculatory properties.

43. **When is NAC given after acute acetaminophen overdose?**

    All patients with acute overdose whose acetaminophen levels fall within the potential toxicity area on the Rumack-Matthews nomogram merit administration of NAC. This therapy is most effective when initiated within 8 hours of ingestion, though it may provide benefit even if given later.

44. **How is NAC administered?**

    Historically, within the United States, the inhalational form of NAC had been given enterally with a loading dose of 140 mg/kg, followed by 17 doses of 70 mg/kg given every 4 hours. Recently, an IV form of NAC has been approved; it is given as a continuous infusion over 21 hours. The IV route may be preferred in a pregnant patient to ensure adequate NAC delivery to the fetus via the placenta and in patients who present late with acetaminophen toxicity to augment the potential antioxidant effect.

45. **Does IV NAC have any particular risks?**

    The IV administration of NAC may cause a life-threatening anaphylactoid reaction, which most commonly occurs during the first, higher-dose infusion. Patients with asthma may be at highest risk.

46. **Can the oral NAC regimen be shortened?**

    Some poison centers will recommend "short-course" NAC therapy for patients who have received at least 24 hours of the antidote and have no evidence of liver toxicity by enzyme studies. Such a practice, if proven efficacious, may lead to favor of oral NAC over IV NAC in risk-benefit analysis.

    Marzullo L: Update of N-acetylcysteine treatment for acute acetaminophen toxicity in children. Curr Opin Pediatr 17:239–245, 2005.

    Rowken AK, Norvell J, Eldridge DL, Kirk MA: Updates on acetaminophen toxicity. Med Clin North Am 89:1145–1159, 2005.

47. **Detail the pathophysiology of salicylate overdose.**

    Salicylate overdose commonly causes gastritis and vomiting. Salicylates uncouple oxidative phosphorylation from the production of energy in the form of adenosine triphosphate. Metabolic consequences include hyperthermia, metabolic acidosis, increased glucose utilization, fatty acid catabolism, and increased free water loss. Salicylates also directly stimulate the medullary respiratory center, causing hyperpnea with respiratory alkalosis; impede platelet aggregation; and cause direct renal and hepatic impairment. Seizures and coma denote severe toxicity. Noncardiogenic pulmonary edema complicates treatment in severely affected patients.

48. **Describe the treatment for acute salicylate poisoning.**

    Activated charcoal may be considered early after overdose. Intravascular volume should be restored. Urinary alkalinization is appropriate for patients with symptoms and a peak salicylate level of > 35 mg/dL (350 mg/L). Mild alkalemia will reduce salicylate access to the brain. Patients with unremitting metabolic acidosis, pulmonary edema, severe renal impairment, coma or seizures, liver impairment, and salicylate level > 70 mg/dL meet criteria to receive hemodialysis.

    Dargan P, Wallace CI, Jones AL: An evidence based flowchart to guide the management of acute salicylate (aspirin) overdose. Emerg Med J 19:206–209, 2002.

49. **What hazard is associated with endotracheal intubation of salicylate-poisoned patients?**
    Salicylate-poisoned patients typically have profound respiratory alkalosis. This process is abruptly reversed by paralytic and sedative medications, and resulting acidemia may increase salicylate entry to the brain.

50. **How does iron produce toxicity?**
    Iron acts as a gastrointestinal mucosal irritant and as an inhibitor of oxidative phosphorylation in the mitochondria. The body has no mode of excretion of excess iron.

51. **How much iron is toxic?**
    Expected toxicity can be estimated by the amount of elemental iron ingested (Table 39-2).

TABLE 39-2. EXPECTED TOXICITY OF ELEMENTAL IRON	
Dose Ingested (mg/kg Elemental Iron)	Toxicity
20–60	Mild gastrointestinal symptoms
60–100	Moderate toxicity
100–200	Serious toxicity
>200	Possibly lethal

52. **How much elemental iron is present in commonly available preparations?**

Product	Elemental Iron
Ferrous sulfate, 325 mg	65 mg (20% of tablet strength)
Ferrous gluconate, 325 mg	40 mg (12% of tablet strength)
Ferrous fumarate, 325 mg	105 mg (32% of tablet strength)
Feosol elixir (sulfate)	44 mg/5 mL
Children's chewable vitamins	4–18 mg
Infant liquid vitamins	10 mg/mL

53. **Has the epidemiology of childhood iron poisoning changed?**
    For more than a decade, iron poisoning was the leading cause of pediatric overdose death from pharmaceutical products, but this pattern abated with changes in iron formulations and packaging.

    Tenenbein M: Unit-dose packaging of iron supplements and reduction of iron poisoning in young children. Arch Pediatr Adolesc Med 159:557–560, 2005.

54. **What are the clinical manifestations of iron poisoning?**
    Gastrointestinal irritation leads to vomiting, diarrhea, abdominal pain, melena, and hematemesis. Coma and shock are the hallmarks of severe poisoning. Multiorgan system failure may ensue. Patients recovering from severe iron poisoning may develop gastric scarring with pyloric obstruction 4–6 weeks later.

55. **What laboratory studies are helpful in the management of iron poisoning?**
    An abdominal radiograph can confirm iron ingestion and give an impression of the amount of unabsorbed iron. However, a negative radiograph does not rule out iron ingestion, particularly more than 2 hours after ingestion since dissolved or absorbed iron is *not* radio-opaque. A serum iron level 4–6 hours after ingestion confirms and helps categorize iron poisoning:

Serum Iron Level (μg/dL)	Toxicity
<350	Minimal
350–500	Mild
>500	Serious

    The presence of metabolic acidosis may be the most telling indicator of cellular dysfunction from iron poisoning.

56. **What special decontamination issues arise with iron poisoning?**
    Activated charcoal does *not* bind iron. Gastric emptying via large-bore lavage may be warranted after massive ingestion with evidence of retained gastric iron tablets. Gastric concretions of iron tablets frequently occur and sometimes require endoscopy or gastrotomy for removal and to prevent perforation. Whole-bowel irrigation has been recommended for iron poisoning.

    Tenenbein M: Whole bowel irrigation in iron poisoning. J Pediatr 111:142–145, 1987.

57. **What is the antidote for iron poisoning?**
    Deferoxamine is an iron chelator. The dose is 5–15 mg/kg/h, up to 6 gm/day intravenously. As use of deferoxamine has been associated with pulmonary fibrosis and the acute respiratory distress syndrome, children given deferoxamine infusion for longer than 24 hours should have the infusion stopped for 6 hours per each 24-hour period.

    Yatscoff RW, Wayne EA, Tenenbein M: An objective criterion for the cessation of deferoxamine therapy in the acutely iron poisoned patient. J Toxicol Clin Toxicol 29:1–10, 1991.

58. **List the major toxicities of cyclic antidepressants.**
    - Sodium-channel blockade in the cardiac conduction system (dysrhythmia)
    - Seizures
    - α_1-adrenergic blockade (hypotension)
    - Inhibition of norepinephrine reuptake
    - Anticholinergic toxicity

59. **What electrocardiographic findings correlate with potential toxicity from cyclic antidepressants?**
    - QRS > 0.1 second
    - Corrected QT interval prolonged for age
    - R height > 3 mm in aVR

    Boehnert MT, Lovejoy FH: Value of the QRS duration versus the serum drug level in predicting seizures and ventricular arrhythmias after an acute overdose of tricyclic antidepressants. N Engl J Med 313:474–479, 1985.
    Liebelt E, Ulrich A, Francis PD, Woolf A: Serial electrocardiogram changes in acute tricyclic antidepressant overdoses. Crit Care Med 25:1721–1726, 1997.
    Neimann JT, Bessen HA, Rothstein RJ, Laks MM: Electrocardiographic criteria for tricyclic antidepressant cardiotoxicity. Am J Cardiol 57:1154–1159, 1986.

60. **Why is sodium bicarbonate helpful for drug-induced ventricular dysrhythmias associated with a prolonged QRS interval?**
Many agents that cause ventricular tachycardia in overdose block fast sodium channels, which are essential to proper myocardial conduction. Sodium bicarbonate competitively inhibits this blockade by increasing available serum sodium. In addition, the modest serum alkalinization appears to promote, in a synergistic fashion, improved conduction that clinically appears as narrowing of the QRS interval and cessation of ventricular tachycardia.

Liebelt E: Targeted management strategies for cardiovascular toxicity from tricyclic antidepressant overdose: The pivotal role for alkalinization and sodium loading. Pediatr Emerg Care 14:293–298, 1998.

61. **What are some special considerations for drug-induced bradydysrhythmias?**
Bradydysrhythmias commonly follow ingestion of β-blockers, calcium-channel blockers, and digitalis-containing compounds. These rhythm disturbances may not be amenable to standard therapy with atropine, epinephrine, and pacing.

62. **Name antidotes that may be useful for specific causes of drug-induced bradydysrhythmias.**

Overdose	Antidote
β-blocker	Glucagon
Calcium-channel blocker	Calcium, insulin/glucose
Digoxin	Digoxin-specific F_{ab} fragments (Digibind, Digifab)

Kenny J: Treating overdose with calcium channel blockers. BMJ 308:992–993, 1994.
Weinstein RS: Recognition and management of poisoning with beta-adrenergic blocking agents. Ann Emerg Med 13:1123–1131, 1984.
Woolf AD, Wenger T, Smith TW, et al: The use of digoxin-specific F_{ab} fragments for severe digitalis intoxication in children. N Engl J Med 326:1739–1744, 1992.

63. **What signs and symptoms are expected after isolated benzodiazepine overdose in children?**
Benzodiazepines usually do not cause severe symptoms when ingested alone. They typically cause sedation, ataxia, and, in rare cases, respiratory depression. Ataxia without lethargy may occur in up to 30% of children after benzodiazepine ingestion. Apnea, deep coma, or cardiovascular instability suggests co-ingestion of another agent (e.g., ethanol, barbiturates, other sedative-hypnotics). Benzodiazepines have frequently been implicated in child abuse by poisoning. Typically, the situation involves an elderly caretaker sedating a normally active toddler.

Wiley C, Wiley JF: Pediatric benzodiazepine ingestion resulting in hospitalization. J Toxicol Clin Toxicol 36:227–231, 1998.

64. **What is flumazenil?**
Flumazenil is a specific benzodiazepine receptor antagonist that reverses benzodiazepine-induced central nervous system depression.

65. **List problems associated with flumazenil administration after drug overdose.**
- May precipitate benzodiazepine withdrawal
- May precipitate seizures and their complications
- Has short duration of action compared with duration of benzodiazepine toxicity

Perry HE, Shannon MW: Diagnosis and management of opioid- and benzodiazepine-induced comatose overdose in children. Curr Opin Pediatr 8:243–247, 1996.

66. **How are poison-induced seizures treated?**
Benzodiazepines and barbiturates are the treatments of choice. Seizures may recur and be difficult to treat. The cardiovascular effects of IV phenytoin may complicate cyclic antidepressant overdose. Pyridoxine is a specific antidote for seizures caused by isoniazid overdose. Drug-induced status epilepticus requires advanced modalities, such as pentobarbital coma or general anesthesia, more frequently than does status epilepticus complicating other types of seizure disorders.

> Wills B, Erickson T: Drug- and toxin-associated seizures. Med Clin North Am 89:1297–1321, 2005.

KEY POINTS: PHARMACEUTICALS ✔

1. Dangerous acetaminophen poisoning may be asymptomatic initially but can be predicted with serum levels.

2. Prevention of acidemia, maintenance of intravascular volume, and urinary alkalinization are key goals in the treatment of moderate aspirin poisoning.

3. Prevention strategies are important in reducing the pediatric mortality of iron products.

4. Sodium bicarbonate therapy may be beneficial for toxic cardiac syndromes manifested by wide QRS tachycardia.

DRUGS OF ABUSE

67. **How do opiates cause toxicity?**
Opiates bind specific opiate receptors in the brain (μ, κ, σ, δ), causing global depression of the central and autonomic nervous systems. Meperidine (Demerol) and propoxyphene with acetaminophen (Darvocet) also have active metabolites that can cause seizures and cardiac dysrhythmias.

68. **What is the mnemonic for the opiate toxidrome?**
FAME: **F**laccid coma, **A**pnea, **M**iosis, and **E**xtraocular paralysis.

69. **Which opioids may require high doses of naloxone to reverse toxicity?**
Doses up to 10 mg of naloxone may be required to completely reverse the following opioids: methadone, LAAM (levo-α-acetyl-methadol), propoxyphene, dextromethorphan, pentazocine, and fentanyl and its derivatives. Also, anyone habituated to opioids that primarily bind μ receptors and are shorter acting (e.g., heroin, morphine) may need only small doses of naloxone to reverse respiratory depression. A dose of 1–2 mg of naloxone may induce opiate withdrawal in these patients.

70. **What common pediatric drug toxicity closely mimics opiate intoxication but does not reliably respond to naloxone?**
The α_2-adrenergic agonist clonidine acts centrally to reduce sympathetic outflow, and its toxidrome may mimic opiate poisoning. Naloxone reverses coma and respiratory depression in 10–15% or less of severely poisoned patients and cannot be considered a consistent antidote for clonidine poisoning. A trial of naloxone is reasonable in severely poisoned children.

Yohimbine has been proposed as a specific α_2 antagonist but is available only in oral form and may cause clonidine withdrawal in patients receiving clonidine therapeutically.

Wiley JF: Clonidine poisoning: Is there any effective therapy? Clin Ped Emerg Med 1:207–212, 2000.

71. **Describe the typical findings after clonidine ingestion.**
As little as 0.1 mg (one tablet) of clonidine has been associated with miosis, coma, apnea, bradycardia, and hypotension. Transient hypertension may also occur. More rare findings include modest hypothermia and pallor.

72. **Are there any other distinguishing features between clonidine poisoning and opiate poisoning?**
Children with clonidine poisoning often have transient arousal and improvement in respiratory and hemodynamic instability with stimulation. Patients comatose from opiate poisoning are usually not arousable despite painful stimulation.

73. **Hallucinations or psychosis may be prominent from which drugs of abuse?**
- Anticholinergics (antihistamines, Jimson weed)
- Dissociatives (phencyclidine, ketamine, dextromethorphan)
- Hallucinogens (lysergic acid diethylamide, psilocybin, mescaline)
- Sympathomimetics (amphetamines, cocaine, ecstasy)
- Withdrawal from ethanol or sedative-hypnotics

74. **Why should neuroleptics, such as haloperidol, be used cautiously in the treatment of drug-induced psychoses?**
These agents may lower the seizure threshold of the overdose patient, may add to the cardiovascular toxicity of some drugs, and may limit the patient's ability to dissipate heat.

75. **What adverse effects are associated with cocaine intoxication?**
Cocaine abusers seek a pleasurable "rush" of euphoria and increased energy. However, intoxicating doses may produce agitation, tachycardia, hypertension, hyperthermia, mydriasis, and tremor. Altered judgment may lead to an increased incidence of accidents and interpersonal violence, and abusers may neglect societal obligations while engaging in high-risk behaviors. Seizures, intracranial hemorrhage, myocardial ischemia, rhabdomyolysis, pneumothorax, psychosis, and death may occur from cocaine abuse.

76. **What is the treatment for the tachycardia, hypertension, and hyperpyrexia associated with cocaine overdose?**
High doses of benzodiazepines are the most effective and safest pharmacotherapy for cocaine intoxication. Extreme hyperthermia may also warrant aggressive environmental cooling methods. Rhabdomyolysis should be treated with mechanical ventilation, paralysis, and bicarbonate infusion to reduce the chance of renal failure. Sympatholytics should be reserved for the most extreme cases. β-adrenergic antagonist therapy may lead to detrimental unopposed α-adrenergic toxicity. Persistent hypertensive crisis may respond well to nitroprusside infusion or phentolamine.

77. **Name seven hyperthermic syndromes in toxicology.**
1. Sympathomimetic poisoning
2. Anticholinergic poisoning
3. Neuroleptic malignant syndrome
4. Malignant hyperthermia
5. Serotonin syndrome
6. Uncoupling of oxidative phosphorylation
7. Acute withdrawal syndrome

78. **Describe the serotonin syndrome.**
The serotonin syndrome is characterized by autonomic hyperactivity, increased neuromuscular tone (especially prominent in the lower extremities), hyperreflexia, and central nervous system depression after exposure to a drug or drugs with proserotonergic properties.

   Boyer EW, Shannon M: The serotonin syndrome. N Engl J Med 352:1112–1120, 2005.

79. **Name some of the methods by which inhalants are abused.**
   - *Sniffing* describes direct inhalation of vapors from an open container.
   - *Huffing* implies inhaling from a cloth soaked with the volatile substance.
   - *Bagging* involves holding a volatile-containing bag over the nose.

80. **Describe the most widely proposed mechanism for "sudden sniffing death."**
Inhaled hydrocarbons are believed to potentiate the cardiovascular effects of catecholamines. Ventricular dysrhythmia may occur, especially if an inhalant abuser becomes surprised (perhaps by parents or police) or agitated.

81. **What modification to advanced cardiac life support protocol might be beneficial in the treatment of tachydysrhythmia after inhalant abuse?**
Theoretical and anecdotal evidence suggests that β-adrenergic antagonists may help reverse these catecholamine-driven cardiac disturbances. Epinephrine may be relatively contraindicated in this scenario.

   Albertson TE, Dawson A, de Latorre F, et al: TOX-ACLS: Toxicologic-oriented advanced cardiac life support. Ann Emerg Med 37:S78–S90, 2001.

82. **γ hydroxybutyrate and γ butyrolactone are drugs that have received considerable attention recently. What are they?**
Both γ hydroxybutyrate (GHB) and γ butyrolactone (GBL) are central nervous system depressants similar to GABA (γ aminobutyrate). They produce mild euphoria in low doses but can produce rapid onset of coma in larger doses. They have been promoted as aids to sleeping or bodybuilding, and more recently have become popular as drugs of abuse. These tasteless, colorless chemicals are easily manufactured at home and have become notorious for alleged use as "date rape drugs." Treatment is supportive.

KEY POINTS: DRUGS OF ABUSE ✓

1. Naloxone dosing in patients overdosed on heroin requires careful consideration of habituation to avoid precipitation of withdrawal.

2. Overdoses with long-acting or synthetic opioids often require increased doses of naloxone to achieve adequate reversal of respiratory depression.

3. Benzodiazepines are the most appropriate initial treatment for agitation caused by sympathomimetic and hallucinogenic drugs of abuse.

4. Malignant hyperthermia from overdoses of cocaine, amphetamines, or serotonergic drugs requires rapid treatment, including cooling measures, benzodiazepine administration, and mechanical ventilation with paralysis and bicarbonate infusion in the setting of rhabdomyolysis.

5. γ hydroxybutyrate and γ butyrolactone (GBL) are popular club drugs that are easily manufactured at home and are widely promoted on the Internet.

ENVIRONMENTAL POISONS AND VENOMS

83. **What is the differential diagnosis for an increased anion gap metabolic acidosis?**
One can make mountains out of the mnemonic **MUDPILES:**
- **M** = **M**ethanol, metformin
- **U** = **U**remia
- **D** = **D**iabetic, alcoholic, or starvation ketoacidosis
- **P** = **P**araldehyde (and other aldehydes)
- **I** = **I**ron, isoniazid, inborn errors of metabolism
- **L** = **L**actic acidosis
- **E** = **E**thylene glycol
- **S** = **S**alicylates

    Louie JP, Peterson J: Pick your poison: Not a basic case. Pediatr Emerg Care 22:461–463, 2006.

84. **What is the differential diagnosis for lactic acidosis?**
Lactic acidosis may be caused by sepsis, shock, seizures, anoxia, ischemia, or trauma. Toxic causes include poisoning from carbon monoxide, cyanide, sodium azide, hydrogen sulfide, ibuprofen, adrenergic agents, isoniazid, and others.

85. **How is the osmolar gap calculated?**
- Osmolar gap = measured osmolality − calculated osmolarity
- Calculated osmolarity = 2 ([sodium] mEq/L) + ([blood urea nitrogen] mg/dL)/2.8 + ([glucose] mg/dL)/18

86. **What is a "normal" osmolar gap?**
−7 to 10 mOsm

87. **List the potential causes of a large osmolar gap.**

Acetone	Mannitol
Ethanol	Methanol
Glycols	Renal failure
Isopropanol	Severe ketoacidemia
Magnesium	Severe lactic acidemia

88. **How do toxic alcohols produce an increased osmolar gap?**
Once absorbed into the bloodstream, alcohols are osmotically active. This principle explains why people have to urinate so frequently at Happy Hour. It is also the principle behind administering mannitol to head-injured patients.

89. **How can the osmolar gap be used to estimate the levels of toxic alcohols?**
This calculation is based upon the molecular weight of the alcohols:
- **Methanol:** molecular weight = 32 mg/mmol; conversion factor = 3.2
- **Ethanol:** molecular weight = 46 mg/mmol; conversion factor = 4.6
- **Ethylene glycol:** molecular weight = 62 mg/mmol; conversion factor = 6.2
Alcohol level (mg/dL) = [osmolar gap] × [conversion factor]

90. **How does ethanol intoxication lead to life-threatening hypoglycemia in young children?**
Ethanol is metabolized by the enzymes alcohol dehydrogenase and acetaldehyde dehydrogenase. This process involves the production of NADH (nicotinamide-adenine

dinucleotide). An increased ratio of NADH to NAD inhibits gluconeogenesis, and may lead to hypoglycemia in patients with insufficient stores of glycogen.

Hoffman RS, Goldfrank LR: Ethanol-associated metabolic disorders. Emerg Med Clin North Am 7:943–961, 1989.

91. **How fast does an inebriated 14-year-old metabolize an ethanol level of 150 mg/dL to zero?**

Ethanol is metabolized at a constant rate according to zero order kinetics. The typical decrease is 15 mg/dL/h in the noninduced (nonalcoholic) patient. Therefore, the level should be zero in 10 hours.

Gershman H, Steper J: Rate of clearance of ethanol from the blood of intoxicated patients in the emergency department. J Emerg Med 9:307–311, 1991.

92. **How do some toxic alcohols lead to metabolic acidosis?**

Early after methanol or ethylene glycol ingestion, there will be increased serum osmolality but little acidosis. The body subsequently metabolizes methanol to formic acid, and ethylene glycol to glycolic and oxalic acids. The osmolar gap may drop while the anion gap increases. Isopropyl alcohol is somewhat distinctive as it is metabolized to acetone and typically does not lead to profound acidosis.

93. **True or false: Ethylene glycol in the urine fluoresces when examined with a Wood's lamp.**

False, but not entirely. The most common source of ethylene glycol exposure is automobile antifreeze. Some manufacturers put fluorescein in the antifreeze solution to allow detection of radiator leaks. Lack of fluorescent urine does not rule out ethylene glycol poisoning.

Casavant MJ, Shah MN, Battels R: Does fluorescent urine indicate antifreeze ingestion by children? Pediatrics 107:113–114, 2001.

94. **What is the physiologic basis for the treatment of methanol or ethylene glycol poisoning?**

Formic acid is toxic to the retina, and glycolic and oxalic acids are toxic to the kidneys. The treatment goal is to prevent metabolism to these toxic metabolites. Alcohol dehydrogenase is the enzyme responsible for this biotransformation, and inhibition of this enzyme will be protective.

95. **What agents can be used to inhibit alcohol dehydrogenase in the setting of methanol or ethylene glycol poisoning?**

- Fomepizole
- Ethanol

Barceloux DG, Krenzelok EP, Olson K, et al: American Academy of Clinical Toxicology practice guidelines on the treatment of ethylene glycol poisoning. J Toxicol Clin Toxicol 37:537–560, 1999.

96. **Do any vitamins or nutritional supplements have a role in the treatment of methanol or ethylene glycol poisoning?**

Folic acid may promote the metabolic degradation of formic acid. Pyridoxine and thiamine may speed transformation of glycolic acids to nontoxic metabolites.

97. **When should an ingested button battery be emergently removed?**

Disc batteries may contain potentially toxic components, such as mercury or lithium, but are most dangerous as mucosal corrosives. Disc batteries lodged in the nares, ear canal, or esophagus should be removed immediately. Once in the stomach they will almost always pass uneventfully.

98. **List some of the dangerous caustic agents frequently found in U.S. households.**
Many cleaning products, especially phosphate dishwashing detergents, are mildly corrosive. Hair-relaxing products typically have basic pH. Oven cleaners, toilet bowl cleaners, and drain products often contain hydrochloric acid or sodium hydroxide.

99. **What characteristics of a caustic agent are most predictive of injury?**
    - pH
    - Concentration
    - Volume ingested
    - Viscosity of product
    - Manner of exposure
    - Duration of exposure

    Therefore, thick hair-relaxer creams licked by an explorative child rarely lead to severe esophageal injury, but suicidal ingestions of liquid acids can be expected to lead to significant morbidity.

    Friedman EM, Lovejoy FH Jr: The emergency management of caustic ingestions. Emerg Med Clin North Am 2:77–86, 1984.

100. **What are the complications of ingestion of caustic agents?**

    Acute:
    - Upper airway obstruction
    - Aspiration pneumonitis
    - Gastrointestinal bleeding and/or perforation
    - Systemic acidosis and/or disseminated intravascular coagulation
    - Sepsis

    Chronic:
    - Esophageal stricture
    - Impaired gastric function/pyloric obstruction

101. **Which patients should be examined endoscopically after caustic ingestion?**
    - Ingestion involving a concentrated, strong acid or base
    - Suicidal ingestions
    - Large-volume ingestions
    - Patients with vomiting, or two or more signs or symptoms of injury

    Note: The absence of oral burns is not a sensitive sign for excluding esophageal injury.

102. **Give the advantages and disadvantages for using corticosteroids to palliate caustic esophageal burns.**

    Advantages:
    - Anti-inflammatory
    - May decrease tissue scarring and stricture

    Disadvantages:
    - May increase perforation risk
    - May increase infection risk
    - May mask signs of infection or perforation

103. **When should steroids be used to palliate caustic esophageal burns?**
Esophageal burns should be graded at endoscopy. First-degree burns do not lead to stricture formation, so steroids are not warranted. Third-degree burns will probably lead to stricture regardless of treatment, and the benefit is not likely worth the risk. Controversy surrounds the value of using steroids together with antibiotics to treat circumferential second-degree burns of the esophagus. Many clinicians believe that corticosteroids may modestly reduce stricture formation in this situation. Note that a less controversial indication for steroid therapy is the palliation of glottic edema and airway obstruction.

104. **What are the indications for surgical exploration after caustic ingestion?**
- Evidence of perforation
- Abdominal tenderness after acid ingestion
- Inability to evaluate injuries endoscopically
- Significant central nervous system depression
- Progressive metabolic acidosis
- Hypotension with tachycardia

105. **What is the major long-term concern for patients recovered from caustic burns of the esophagus?**
These patients are at a 1000-fold increased risk for esophageal carcinoma. The mean latency period is over 40 years.

Appelqvist SM: Lye corrosion carcinoma of the esophagus: A review of 63 cases. Cancer 45:2655–2658, 1980.

106. **Which characteristics of certain hydrocarbon products make them prone to aspiration?**
- Low viscosity
- Low surface tension
- High volatility

107. **Describe the time course of aspiration injury after hydrocarbon ingestion.**
Children may cough, gag, or sputter at the time of ingestion. A gradual evolution of radiographic findings occurs, but most children who will develop pneumonitis will have visible abnormality by 6 hours. More than 98% of children who will develop clinical pneumonitis will do so by 24 hours.

108. **Do any hydrocarbons have serious systemic toxicity?**
Central nervous system depression, seizures, hepatotoxicity, nephrotoxicity, and bone marrow toxicity are among the injuries that can occur after specific hydrocarbon ingestions. The hydrocarbons most noted for systemic toxicity can be remembered with this **CHAMP**ion of mnemonics:
- **C** = **C**amphor
- **H** = **H**alogenated hydrocarbons (e.g., carbon tetrachloride, trichloroethane)
- **A** = **A**romatic hydrocarbons (e.g., Benzene, toluene)
- **M** = **M**etal-containing hydrocarbons
- **P** = **P**esticide-containing hydrocarbons

109. Which features in the evaluation of an encephalopathic child suggest acute lead encephalopathy?

History:
- Prodrome of listlessness, anorexia, vomiting, clumsiness, seizures
- History of pica or plumbism
- Source of exposure to lead

Studies:
- Microcytic anemia
- Basophilic stippling of erythrocytes
- Radiopaque flecks on abdominal radiograph
- Radiographic "lead lines" at bony metaphyses
- Increased cerebrospinal fluid opening pressure or radiographic cerebral edema

110. List the clinical manifestations of organophosphate or carbamate insecticide poisoning.
These insecticides are examples of "cholinergic" poisoning.
1. **Muscarinic effects** (pre- and postganglionic parasympathomimetic)
   - "**SLUDGE**" = **s**alivation, **l**acrimation, **u**rination, **d**efecation, **g**astric cramping, **e**mesis
   - Bronchorrhea, bronchoconstriction
   - Bradycardia
   - Miotic pupils
2. **Nicotinic effect** (preganglionic sympathomimetic)
   - Tachycardia (often prominent early after exposure in children)
3. **Nicotinic effects** (neuromuscular endplate)
   - Muscle fasciculations
   - Muscle weakness
4. **Central nervous system effects**
   - Depressed consciousness
   - Seizures

111. What antidotes are used to treat organophosphate poisoning?
Atropine may be needed in large doses to reverse muscarinic toxicity. Pralidoxime regenerates active acetylcholinesterase, the enzymatic site of action of organophosphate insecticides.

112. What is the appropriate response to an exploratory anticoagulant rodenticide ingestion by a toddler?
Suicidal ingestions of anticoagulant rodenticides have led to catastrophic consequences. Single exploratory ingestions by curious children have not been reported to produce dangerous bleeding diatheses. Some poison centers recommend decontamination with activated charcoal at the time of the event, and evaluation of a prothrombin time 2 to 3 days afterward. Other poison centers recommend no treatment other than expectant observation at home.

113. How should coagulopathy from the warfarin-like rodenticides be treated?
These rodenticides inhibit hepatic production of the vitamin K–dependent coagulation factors II, VII, IX, and X. Acute bleeding can be palliated with transfusion of fresh-frozen plasma. Administration of vitamin K_1 will restore production of clotting factors with a lag time of approximately 6 hours. Prophylactic use of vitamin K_1 often complicates evaluation of

the anticoagulant-poisoned patient. As the "superwarfarins" have a very long duration of effect, any patient treated with vitamin K_1 warrants monitoring for at least 5 days after the last dose.

114. Describe the typical symptoms of carbon monoxide poisoning.
Typical symptoms are nonspecific and include malaise, nausea, lightheadedness, and headache, leading many children to be misdiagnosed with a viral illness. More severe poisoning may manifest as confusion, coma, syncope, seizure, or death. Survivors of acute intoxication are at risk of delayed neurologic sequelae, including cognitive deficits, personality changes, and movement disorders.

115. Which member of the family is most likely to suffer the most from equivalent carbon monoxide (CO) exposure?
Infants and small children have higher oxygen consumption and a higher basal metabolic rate than adults. Therefore, they may be most susceptible to the effects of CO. This is the basic concept behind the "canary in a coal mine."

116. Describe the pathophysiology of toxicity from CO exposure.
1. CO displaces oxygen from the hemoglobin molecule, leading to decreased oxygen-carrying capacity. CO has an affinity for hemoglobin approximately 250 times that for O_2.
2. Allosteric inhibition of oxygen release to tissues occurs (displacement of the oxyhemoglobin dissociation curve to the left).
3. Cellular oxidative metabolism is reduced through inhibition of cytochrome oxidase enzyme systems.
4. Oxidative injury to the brain endothelium begins a cascade of leukocyte activation, lipid peroxidation, and impaired cerebral metabolism.

Martin JD, Osterhoudt KC, Thom SR: Recognition and management of carbon monoxide intoxication in children. Clin Pediatr Emerg Med 1:244–250, 2000.

117. How long does it take the body to eliminate carboxyhemoglobin?
Carboxyhemoglobin elimination depends on inspired oxygen concentration.
- **Room air:** 4–6 hours
- **100% O_2:** 40–90 minutes
- **Hyperbaric O_2 (3 atm):** 15–30 minutes

118. When is hyperbaric oxygen therapy indicated for CO intoxication?
Oxygen, in the highest concentration possible, should be administered to all symptomatic patients until CO levels are below 5% and symptoms subside. Hyperbaric oxygen therapy may prevent oxidative cerebral vasculitis, and prevent delayed neurologic injury. Proposed criteria for considering hyperbaric oxygen include syncope, confusion, central nervous system depression, or very high carboxyhemoglobin levels.

Weaver LK, Hopkins RO, Chan KJ: Hyperbaric oxygen for acute carbon monoxide poisoning. N Engl J Med 347:1057–1067, 2002.

119. Describe the characteristic brain abnormalities after significant CO poisoning on magnetic resonance imaging of the brain.
Approximately half of patients with neurologic dysfunction will have bilateral lucencies in the basal ganglia. They are most prominent in the globus pallidus, an area of high metabolic demand. Less frequently, subcortical white matter lesions may also be noted.

120. **Cyanosis, unreponsive to supplemental oxygen therapy and in the face of a normal partial pressure of oxygen in arterial blood, is characteristic of what physiologic abnormality?**
Poor response to oxygen makes a pulmonary disorder unlikely. Normal partial pressure of oxygen rules out intracardiac shunting. This is the characteristic clinical scenario of an abnormal hemoglobin, most commonly methemoglobinemia.

121. **What is methemoglobin?**
Hemoglobin is a heme (iron-containing) protein. Methemoglobin exists when the iron moiety is ferric (3^+) rather than ferrous (2^+). Methemoglobin is incapable of transporting oxygen.

122. **Provide the differential diagnosis for methemoglobinemia.**

   Congenital
   - Hemoglobin M
   - NADH (reduced form of nicotinamide adenine dinucleotide)–dependent methemoglobin reductase deficiency
   - Cytochrome b0005 deficiency

   Acquired
   - Transient, illness-associated methemoglobinemia of infancy
   - Toxicant-induced

123. **Describe the transient, illness-associated methemoglobinemia of infancy.**
Young infants have been found to be cyanotic with methemoglobinemia in conjunction with a number of illnesses, including diarrheal dehydration, metabolic acidosis, urinary tract infection, and others. Babies are uniquely susceptible to oxidant stress, and this condition should be considered in the evaluation of septic-appearing infants.

124. **What are some of the more common toxicants associated with the production of excessive methemoglobin?**
Many chemicals and pharmaceuticals can produce methemoglobinemia in susceptible people. Among the most commonly noted exposures are benzocaine, dapsone, environmental (i.e., well water) nitrates, nitrites (i.e., amyl nitrite), and phenazopyridine.

125. **What is the appropriate therapy for methemoglobinemia?**
Provide supplemental oxygen. Eliminate or treat the oxidative stress responsible for methemoglobin formation. Antidotal therapy with methylene blue (1–2 mg/kg of a 1% solution) is indicated in the presence of tissue hypoxia. Methylene blue is unlikely to be effective, and may worsen illness, when administered to patients with severe forms of glucose-6-phosphate dehydrogenase deficiency.

   Wright RO, Lewander WJ, Woolf AD: Methemoglobinemia: Etiology, pharmacology, and clinical management. Ann Emerg Med 34:646–656, 1999.

126. **What are the clinical classifications syndromes for toxic mushrooms syndromes, typical clinical findings, and poisoning treatment syndromes?**
See Table 39-3.

TABLE 39-3. DESCRIPTION OF TOXIC MUSHROOM SYNDROMES

Class	Onset of Action (h)	Toxicity/Symptoms	Treatment
I. Cyclopeptides (e.g., *Amanita virosa, Amanita phalloides,* and *Galerina marginata*)	6–10 (late)	6–12 h: GI symptoms 12–24 h: transient improvement 1–6 days: hepatic and renal failure Mortality: 10–50%	Multiple-dose activated charcoal Supportive care for hypovolemia, liver and renal failure Transplantation Unproven therapies: High-dose penicillin, silibinin, cimetidine, thioctic acid
II. Monomethylhydrazine-containing (e.g., *Gyromitra esculenta*)	6–10 (late)	GI symptoms, seizures, hepatorenal failure	Pyridoxine, 25 mg/kg, for seizures
III. Muscarinic (e.g., *Clitocybe dealbata*)	0.5–2 (early)	Salivation, lacrimation, vomiting, diarrhea, bronchospasm	Atropine, 0.02 mg/kg
IV. Coprine-containing (e.g., *Coprinus atramentarius*)	0.5–2 (early) after co-ingestion of ethanol	Disulfiram-like effect with ethanol: flushing, tachycardia, vomiting	Supportive, abstinence from ethanol
V. Ibotenic acid-containing (e.g., *Amanita muscaria*)	0.5–2 (early)	Early stimulation, delirium, seizures, followed by somnolence	Benzodiazepines for delirium or seizures

VI.	Psilocybin-containing (e.g., *Psilocybe cubensis*, "little brown mushrooms," "lawn mower mushrooms")	0.5–1 (early)	Hallucinations, LSD-like effects	Benzodiazepines for agitation
VII.	Gastrointestinal (e.g., *Chlorophyllum molybdites*)	0.5–3 (early)	GI symptoms	IV fluids as needed for losses
VIII.	Orellanine-, orelline-containing, (e.g., *Cortinarius orellanus*)	24 or longer (up to 2 weeks)	Acute renal tubular necrosis	Fluids, electrolytes Hemodialysis for renal failure
IX.	*Amanita smithiana*	0.5–12	GI symptoms, renal failure	Hemodialysis
X.	*Tricholoma equestre*	24–72	Fatigue, muscle weakness, diaphoresis, myocarditis	None

GI = gastrointestinal. LSD= lysergic acid diethylamide.
Adapted from Goldfrank LR: Mushrooms. In Goldfrank LR, Flomenbaum NE, Lewin NA, Howland MA, Hoffman RS, Nelson LS (eds): Goldfrank's Toxicologic Emergencies, 7th ed. New York, McGraw-Hill, 2002, pp 1115–1128.

127. **What are the most common toxic plant poisonings?**
Of the 20 most common plant exposures, the most commonly encountered toxic plants are:
- The Arum family (*Dieffenbachia*, *Philodendron*), which may cause severe pharyngeal edema and possible airway obstruction through the elaboration of calcium oxalate crystals and proteolytic enzymes and direct mucosal irritation
- The *Taxus* species (yew), which cause gastrointestinal irritation, cardiac dysrhythmias, coma, and seizures if large amounts of leaves or seeds are ingested
- Solanum family (Jerusalem cherry, black nightshade, climbing nightshade), which cause gastrointestinal effects, lethargy, or delirium
- *Rhododendron* and *Azalea* spp., which cause gastrointestinal effects, bradycardia, lethargy, and paresthesias through elaboration of grayanotoxins

128. **What other plants have potential for severe toxicity? Describe the treatment.**
See Table 39-4.

TABLE 39-4. CATEGORIES OF TOXIC PLANTS

Symptom Class	Plants	Potential Treatment
GI irritants	Pokeweed Horse chestnut English ivy	Supportive care
Toxalbumin	Castor bean Rosary pea Autumn crocus (colchicine-containing)	Multisystem organ failure Supportive care
Digitalis-like toxin	Foxglove Oleander Lily of the valley	Digoxin F_{ab} fragments
Other cardiac effects	Mistletoe Monkshood False hellebore Mountain laurel	Supportive care, standard treatment for dysrhythmias
Nicotinic effects	Wild tobacco Tobacco Poison hemlock	Atropine, supportive care for weakness, paralysis
Anticholinergic effects	Jimsonweed Angel's trumpet Matrimony vine Henbane Belladonna	Physostigmine for seizures, malignant hyperthermia Benzodiazepines for delirium
Seizures	Water hemlock	Anticonvulsants
Hallucinations	Morning glory Nutmeg Peyote	Sedation

Cyanogenic	Chokecherry	Cyanide antidote
	Cherry (pit)	(rarely needed)
	Plum (pit)	
	Peach (pit)	
	Apple (seeds)	
	Pear (seeds)	
	Cassava	
	Elderberry	
	(leaves and shoots)	
	Black locust	

129. What venomous snakes are indigenous to the United States?

The Crotalinae family includes rattlesnakes, copperheads, and water moccasins. The Elapidae family includes the coral snakes.

130. What are the clinical differences between bites from rattlesnakes and bites from coral snakes?

Rattlesnakes, copperheads, and water moccasins are long-fanged "pit vipers" whose bites produce significant local inflammation and may lead to shock, thrombocytopenia, and coagulopathy. The venom of coral snakes is less irritating locally and more typically produces neuromuscular paralysis. Of note, envenomation from the Mojave rattlesnake may more closely mimic that of coral snakes.

131. When should a bystander use his or her mouth to suck the venom out of a bite site?

Never! This is more likely to infect the wound than it is to reduce toxicity. The Sawyer extractor, a commercial suction device, is also of little value.

Bush S: Snakebite suction devices don't remove venom: They just suck. Ann Emerg Med 43:187–188, 2004.

132. What are the most important principles of first aid for a North American snakebite victim?

Remove the victim from the snake and, if possible, wash the wound with soap and water. Keep the victim calm. Activate emergency medical systems to transport the victim to a hospital as soon as possible. Remove any potentially constricting apparel. Immobilize a bitten extremity near the level of the heart. Tourniquets are more likely to increase injury to an extremity and are not routinely advised. Ice is not advised.

133. What are the indications for administration of antivenin to a patient following Crotaline envenomation?

Antivenin should be administered to most patients with progressive local injury, cardiovascular compromise, or coagulopathy.

Gold BS, Barish RA, Dart RC: North American snake envenomation: Diagnosis, treatment, and management. Emerg Med Clin North Am 22:423–443, 2004.

134. **Name the two antivenin products available for treatment of North American pit viper envenomation.**
    - Antivenin (Crotalidae) polyvalent (equine origin)
    - Crotalidae polyvalent immune Fab (ovine)

135. **What are the side effects of equine- or ovine-derived antivenin administration?**
    Anaphylaxis is a potentially life-threatening complication of antivenin administration. Serum sickness is a common delayed side effect. These adverse events are less frequent with the purified F_{ab} antivenin.

136. **Compare the toxic manifestations of bites from black widow spiders *(Latrodectus)* to those of brown recluse spiders *(Loxosceles).***
    The venom of black widow spiders leads to increased stimulation of the motor endplate. Restlessness, tachycardia, hypertension, muscular fasciculations, and muscle cramping are common signs and symptoms. In severe cases, black widow bites can mimic a surgical abdomen. In contrast, brown recluse venom is predominantly digestive in nature. Local inflammation may progress to tissue necrosis at the bite site. Systemic toxicity is possible but uncommon.

KEY POINTS: ENVIRONMENTAL POISONS AND VENOMS ✓

1. Fomepizole is an antidote that inhibits alcohol dehydrogenase to provide protection in methanol and ethylene glycol poisoning.

2. After carbon monoxide poisoning, hyperbaric oxygen is most beneficial in its ability to halt an inflammatory cascade in the brain.

3. The low surface tension and viscosity of hydrocarbons create great risk for pulmonary injury after ingestion.

4. Snake antivenin purified to F_{ab} fragments poses less risk of anaphylaxis and serum sickness than whole immunoglobulin products.

BIBLIOGRAPHY

1. Flomenbaum NE, Goldfrank LR, Hoffman RS, et al (eds): Goldfrank's Toxicologic Emergencies, 8th ed. New York, McGraw-Hill, 2006.
2. Osterhoudt KC, Burns Ewald M, Shannon M, Henretig FM: Toxicologic emergencies. In Fleisher G, Ludwig S, Henretig F (eds): Textbook of Pediatric Emergency Medicine, 5th ed. Philadelphia, Lippincott Williams & Wilkins, 2006, pp 951–1031.
3. Osterhoudt KC, Perrone J, De Roos F, et al (eds): Toxicology Pearls. Philadelphia, Elsevier Mosby, 2004.
4. Shannon MW: Ingestion of toxic substances by children. N Engl J Med 342:186–191, 2000.

CHAPTER 40

PSYCHIATRIC EMERGENCIES

Philip V. Scribano, DO, MSCE

1. **What constitutes a psychiatric emergency?**
Most practically defined, this is a potentially preventable or treatable condition that threatens:
   - The patient's own bodily integrity by suicide, self-mutilation, or drug ingestion
   - Someone else's bodily integrity by assault or homicide
   - The patient's own psychological and functional integrity (i.e., ability to perceive reality, feel appropriately, make judgments, remember)
   - The psychological and functional integrity of the family unit.

2. **What is the epidemiology of psychiatric illness in children?**
   - Between 6 and 9 million children and adolescents have serious emotional disturbances, and this accounts for 9–13% of all children in the United States.
   - In addition, only an estimated 20% of children in the United States with some form of mental health problem severe enough to require treatment are actually identified as such, and are receiving mental health services.
   - Emergency department (ED) visits for psychiatric conditions accounts for 1.6% of all ED visits and 3.2% of visits requiring an inpatient admission.

   Sills MR, Bland SD: Summary statistics for pediatric psychiatric visits to US emergency departments, 1993–1999. Pediatrics 110:e40, 2002.

3. **Which is the most common psychiatric emergency in children?**
Pediatric psychiatric visits to emergency departments in the United States reveal unspecified neurotic disorders (13%), depressive disorders (13%), and anxiety states (11%) as the three most common principal diagnoses; whereas the most common *Diagnosis and Statistical Manual of Mental Disorders*, 4th edition, axis I disorders are substance abuse (24%), anxiety disorders (17%), and attention deficit and disruptive disorders (11%).

   Sills MR, Bland SD: Summary statistics for pediatric psychiatric visits to US emergency departments, 1993–1999. Pediatrics 110:e40, 2002.

KEY POINTS: EPIDEMIOLOGY OF PSYCHIATRIC EMERGENCIES ✓

1. Up to 6–9 million children suffer from serious emotional disturbances, accounting for 9–13% of all children in the United States.
2. Psychiatric conditions account for under 2% of all emergency department visits but for over 3% of emergency department visits requiring inpatient hospitalization.
3. Suicide is the leading cause of death from a psychiatric cause and the third leading cause of death overall in older adolescents.

4. **What is the leading cause of death due to psychiatric emergencies?**
Suicide is the leading cause of adolescent death due to psychiatric illness and is the third leading cause of death behind accidents and homicides overall in older adolescents.

Sills MR, Bland SD: Summary statistics for pediatric psychiatric visits to US emergency departments, 1993–1999. Pediatrics 110:e40, 2002.

EVALUATION

5. **What are the ABCs of the mental status examination in the ED?**
A = **A**ppearance/affect: dress/grooming; abnormal movements; eye contact; facial expression; affect (depressed, blunted, flat, anxious, constricted, hostile, euphoric)
B = **B**ehavior: attitude (cooperative, manipulative, guarded, suspicious, angry, violent, withdrawn)
C = **C**ognition:
- Thought content—delusions, suicidal or homicidal; paranoia; somatic preoccupation; depression, obsessions, fears, phobias; belief of special powers; thought control; depersonalization; feelings of helplessness or hopelessness; guilt
- Thought process—rate, organization, goal directedness, tangential, flight of ideas
- Level of consciousness—orientation, attention, concentration, abstraction

6. **How should the initial approach be conducted in evaluating a child with a possible psychiatric emergency?**
First, perform an acute medical evaluation, assessing the airway, breathing, circulation, vital signs, and central nervous system (CNS) function, including pupillary response. An assessment for possible toxic ingestions should include a history of all possible medications in the home or accessible to the child, obtained by asking the caregiver and the child, and an identification of possible toxidromes. Obtain a history of potential traumatic injury. Evaluate past medical history that might indicate an organic basis for the acute emergency. Consider laboratory aids, such as electrolytes, glucose, osmolality, blood gas, toxicologic screen, electrocardiography, and cranial computed tomography. Obtain a urine pregnancy test in all adolescent females.

7. **List some of the medical considerations of acute psychosis.**
- **Trauma:** Intracranial hemorrhage
- **Drug intoxication:** Ethanol, barbiturates, cocaine, opiates, amphetamines, hallucinogens, marijuana, phencyclidine, anticholinergic medications (antihistamines, tricyclics), heavy metals, corticosteroids, neuroleptic medications
- **CNS lesions/infections:** Tumor, hemorrhage, temporal lobe epilepsy, abscess/meningitis/encephalitis, HIV
- **Cerebral hypoxia:** Carbon monoxide poisoning, cardiopulmonary failure
- **Metabolic/endocrinologic:** Hypoglycemia, hypocalcemia, hyperthyroidism or hypothyroidism, adrenal insufficiency, uremia, liver failure, diabetes mellitus, porphyria, Wilson's disease
- **Collagen vascular diseases:** Lupus
- **Miscellaneous causes:** Malaria, typhoid fever, Wilson's disease, Epstein-Barr virus infection

8. **How should the psychiatric evaluation be incorporated into the ED management of a child with a psychiatric emergency?**
Once the child has been medically evaluated and organic causes of the mental disturbance have been ruled out, the psychiatric assessment may proceed. The appropriate interview setting is crucial to effectively assess the child's and family's crisis. A private room away from the

noisy distractions of the main ED setting is optimal. An effort to establish rapport is necessary to engage the child and family to discuss the issues as well as to develop trust. Avoid confrontation and escalation of the crisis, and attempt to de-escalate the arousal of any potentially violent patient. Use psychiatric emergency services and/or social services for the risk assessment of the crisis event.

RESTRAINTS

9. **What are the indications for the use of physical restraint or seclusion in the ED setting?**
   When attempts to provide verbal restraint have been unsuccessful, the following are indications for escalating to physical restraint:
   - To prevent imminent harm to the patient or other persons when other means of control are not effective or appropriate
   - To prevent serious disruption of the treatment plan or significant damage to the physical environment
   - To decrease the stimulation a patient receives (i.e., for those with PCP [phencyclidine] or ethanol intoxications)
   - When the patient is feeling out of control and requests it

   Joint Commission on Accreditation of Healthcare Organizations. 2005 Restraint and Seclusion. Available at www.jointcommission.org/AccreditationPrograms/BehavioralHealthCare/Standards/FAQs/ Provision+of+Care+Treatment+and+Services/Restraint+and+Seclusion/Restraint_Seclusion.htm

10. **Describe the proper procedure in the use of physical restraint.**
    - Explain to the patient why physical restraint is necessary.
    - Enlist at least five caretakers, one for each limb and one for the head. Avoid pressure on the patient's throat or chest and keep hands away from the patient's mouth.
    - Closely supervise (1:1) the patient in physical restraints; assess restraints at least every 30 minutes and document findings.
    - Avoid placement of the restrained child in the prone position (this could interfere with ventilation).
    - Remove restraints only with adequate staff present, and when the patient has regained control (either on his or her own volition, or with the use of chemical restraint).

KEY POINTS: PROPER ADMINISTRATION OF PHYSICAL RESTRAINTS ✓

1. Explain to the patient why physical restraint is necessary.

2. Have at least five caretakers.

3. Avoid pressure on the patient's throat or chest.

4. Avoid placement of the restrained child in a prone position.

5. Provide close supervision (1:1) while the patient is in physical restraints.

6. Assess restraints at least every 30 minutes and document assessment.

7. Remove restraints only with adequate staff present, and when the patient has regained control.

11. **What are the drugs of choice to use as a restraint of a child?**
See Table 40-1.

TABLE 40-1. DRUGS OF CHOICE TO USE AS A RESTRAINT IN CHILDREN		
Drug	**Dose**	**Comment**
Benzodiazepines		
Diazepam (Valium)	0.1 mg/kg PO or IM/IV	Dose range, 2–10 mg
Lorazepam (Ativan)	0.05 mg/kg PO or IM/IV	Dose range, 1–2 mg with titrated dose every 30 minutes
High-potency neuroleptics*		
Haloperidol (Haldol)	0.05 mg/kg PO or IM/IV	Dose range, 2–5 mg
Droperidol (Inapsine)[†]	0.05 mg/kg IM/IV	Dose range, 2.5–5 mg
(0.1–0.15 mg/kg maximum dose) (has shorter half-life [2–4 hours] than haloperidol)		
Low-potency neuroleptics		
Chlorpromazine (Thorazine)	0.5–1 mg/kg PO or IM/IV	Usually 200 mg/d
Thioridazine (Mellaril)	0.5–3 mg/kg PO	May cause hypotension
Antihistamines		
Diphenhydramine (Benadryl)	1–2 mg/kg PO or IM/IV	Usually 12.5–75 mg

IM = intramuscularly, IV = intravenously, PO = orally.
*Children have a slightly higher risk of dystonia compared to adults. Although very rare, neuroleptic malignant syndrome can occur with these medications.
†Droperidol has come under increased scrutiny since the U.S. Food and Drug Administration has issued a "black box" warning because of concerns of a weak association with QT prolongation and torsades de pointes. The extensive experience and safety of this agent in rapid sedation of severely agitated and violent patients leave a quandary with the use of this drug.
Notes: For substance-induced psychosis due to hallucinogens (such as PCP), benzodiazepines given at 30- to 60-minute intervals appear to be more effective than the neuroleptic medications. For substance-induced psychosis due to stimulant intoxication (such as with cocaine or amphetamine), droperidol may be the optimal choice because of its shorter half-life. Some authors advocate concomitant use of antihistamine with neuroleptics to decrease the likelihood of dystonia.
Adapted from Shale JH, Shale CM, Mastin WD: A review of the safety and efficacy of droperidol for the rapid sedation of severely agitated and violent patients. J Clin Psychiatry 64:500–505, 2003.

DRUG-INDUCED PSYCHIATRIC EMERGENCIES

12. **What is neuroleptic malignant syndrome? How is it treated?**
Neuroleptic malignant syndrome (NMS) is an acute, life-threatening reaction to dopamine receptor–blocking agents (typical and atypical antipsychotics) that presents with fever, axial muscular rigidity, autonomic instability/shock, and altered consciousness. An elevated creatine kinase and leukocytosis are common. Treatment is supportive with IV fluids, antipyretics, and stopping the neuroleptic medication. Bromocriptine and dantrolene are specific medications

to treat NMS. The differential diagnosis of hyperthermia includes malignant hyperthermia, anticholinergic poisoning, serotonin syndrome, and reactions to sympathomimetics. The presence of rigidity and elevated creatine kinase levels are distinguishing features of NMS that are rare in serotonin syndrome.

13. **What is serotonin syndrome? How is it treated?**
Given the rise in use of selective serotonin reuptake inhibitors (SSRIs) as well as increased abuse of amphetamines such as ecstasy (MDMA), serotonin syndrome has become more common. The following clinical features must be present: use of SSRI, agitation, stupor, myoclonus, hyperreflexia, diaphoresis, shivering, tremor, diarrhea, incoordination, and fever. Treatment is supportive, with discontinuation of the offending agent.

Rodnitzky RL: Drug-induced movement disorders in children. Semin Pediatr Neurol 10:80–87, 2003.

LEGAL ISSUES

14. **What is required for hospital admission of a minor with a psychiatric emergency?**
For both involuntary and voluntary, most states require parental consent for commitment of a child under the age of 14 years. In children older than age 12–16 years, many states require consent of the minor. A legal process is required if the child does not consent to voluntary commitment. Most states include some period of emergency involuntary admission, however, this varies greatly from state to state. Commonly, involuntary commitment requires physician (and/or designee) documentation of patient's danger to self or others and can be in effect for several days without a court order (depending on state statutes). In general, there are more inpatient psychiatric units that will accept patients under voluntary commitment than under involuntary commitment.

Fortunati FG, Zonana HV: Legal considerations in the child psychiatric emergency department. Child Adolesc Psychiatr Clin North Am 12:745–761, 2003.

DEPRESSION AND SUICIDAL IDEATION

15. **Identify risk factors for suicidal attempts in children and adolescents.**
- Male sex
- Age > 16 years
- Previous suicide attempt
- Substance abuse
- Poor social support
- Mood disorder
- Access to firearms or other lethal means

Recent psychosocial stressor, family history of mental illness, relationship with parents or guardians, history of physical or sexual abuse, and sexual orientation are additional factors to elicit to assess suicidal risk.

16. **How can a clinician assess the presence of depression and suicidal potential of the depressed patient?**
A modified **SAD PERSONS** Scale has been developed and used in the adult and adolescent populations (Table 40-2).

TABLE 40-2. MODIFIED SAD PERSONS SCALE		
Mnemonic	**Characteristic**	**Score**
Sex	Male	1
Age	<19 or >45 years	1
Depression/hopelessness	Admits to depression; poor concentration, appetite, or sleep	2
Prior attempts/psychiatric care	Prior inpatient or outpatient care	1
ETOH/drug use	Addiction or frequent use	1
Rational thinking lost	Psychosis	2
Single/separated/divorced		1
Organized/serious attempt	Life-threatening presentation, careful plan	2
No social supports	No family, friends, religious associations	1
Stated future intent	Determined to repeat, ambivalent	2

ETOH = ethanol.
A score > 6 suggests 1:1 observation and acute psychiatric evaluation; a score > 10 suggests psychiatric inpatient hospitalization.
Adapted from Hockberger RS, Rostein RJ: Assessment of suicide potential by nonpsychiatrists using the SAD PERSONS Score. J Emerg Med 6:99–107, 1988.

17. **What questions have been identifed as useful in screening for suicide risk?**
   The abbreviated (four-item) Suicide Ideation Questionnaire (SIQ) has high sensitivity (98%) and negative predictive value (97%) and can be used as a screening tool to detect suicidality in children and adolescents.
   1. Are you here because you tried to hurt yourself?
   2. In the past week, have you been having thoughts about killing yourself?
   3. Have you ever tried to hurt yourself in the past other than this time?
   4. Has something very stressful happened to you in the past few weeks?

   Horowitz, LM, Wang PS, Koocher GP, et al: Detecting suicide risk in a pediatric emergency department: Development of a brief screening tool. Pediatrics 107:1133–1137, 2001.

18. **What are some medical conditions associated with depression?**
   - **Neurologic:** Hydrocephalus, migraine, myasthenia gravis, seizure, tumor
   - **Endocrine:** Adrenal insufficiency, type 1 diabetes, hyperthyroidism or hypothyroidism, menses-related condition, postpartum status
   - **Metabolic:** Hypercalcemia or hypocalcemia, hyponatremia, uremia, porphyria, Wilson's disease
   - **Infectious/inflammatory:** HIV, influenza, Epstein-Barr virus, hepatitis, collagen vascular diseases
   - **Co-occurring illness:** Cancer, hypothyroidism, systemic lupus erythematosus, HIV, diabetes, epilepsy

   Guerrero APS: General medical conditions in child and adolescent patients who present with psychiatric symptoms. Child Adolesc Psychiatr Clin North Am 12:613–628, 2003.

19. **What are some medications associated with depression?**
   See Table 40-3.

TABLE 40-3. MEDICATIONS ASSOCIATED WITH DEPRESSION

Category	Specific Medications
Neuropsychiatric	Neuroleptics, barbiturates, benzodiazepines, carbamazepine, phenytoin, stimulants
Antimicrobial	Ampicillin, griseofulvin, metronidazole, trimethoprim
Anti-inflammatory/analgesic	Corticosteroids, opiates
Cardiovascular	Clonidine, propranolol
Miscellaneous	Chemotherapy, ethanol, caffeine, oral contraceptives

Adapted from Milner KK, Florence T, Glick RL: Mood and anxiety syndromes in emergency psychiatry. Psychiatr Clin North Am 22:755–777, 1999.

20. **Describe the specific ED management issues in the evaluation of a child with depression or suicidal ideation.**
First, assess the potential medical causes of the child's depression, with specific attention to evaluation of toxic ingestions. Maintain suicide precautions with 1:1 observation until the patient has been fully evaluated regarding this risk. Search the patient and his or her personal belongings for possible harmful objects.

21. **List essential criteria for outpatient disposition of the suicidal child/adolescent.**
    - No requirement of inpatient medical care, including intoxication or delirium
    - No prior history of suicidal attempt, psychiatric disorder, or substance abuse
    - No active suicidal ideation
    - Presence in home of supportive adult with good relationship to child/adolescent
    - Adult agreement to safety plan with close observation of patient until scheduled outpatient follow-up appointment
    - Adult agreement to remove or secure all lethal risks (firearms, medications, drugs, alcohol) in home
    - Adult and patient provided with indications to return to ED if condition deteriorates
    - Follow-up arranged for additional evaluation and treatment
    - Both patient and adult agreement with plan and recommendations

    Kennedy SP, Baraff LJ, Suddath RL, Asarnow JR: Emergency department management of suicidal adolescents. Ann Emerg Med 43:452–460, 2004.

KEY POINTS: CRITERIA FOR OUTPATIENT MANAGEMENT ✔ OF THE PATIENT WITH SUICIDAL IDEATION

1. No inpatient medical care is required.

2. No prior history of suicidal attempt, psychiatric disorder, or substance abuse .

3. No active suicidal ideation.

4. Presence in home of supportive adult who agrees with safety plan and agrees to remove or secure all lethal risks.

5. Follow-up information provided.

6. Agreement of both patient and adult with plan.

AGGRESSION

22. **How often do children with aggression and violence present to the ED?**
    Aggression or dangerous behavior is often the final common pathway from a variety of causes, such as psychosis, child maltreatment, mood disorders, and behavioral/cognitive deficiencies. Twenty-five percent of adolescent emergency psychiatric presentations are due to this phenomenon.

    Sills MR, Bland SD: Summary statistics for pediatric psychiatric visits to US emergency departments, 1993–1999. Pediatrics 110:e40, 2002.

23. **In assessing the child with aggression, what key information is necessary to accurately evaluate the cause of this behavior?**
    Providers must obtain a history of: the onset of the symptoms and their severity; use of weapons; injury to self or others, including animals; indications of intent to harm and lethality; presence of other related symptoms; response to limit setting; destruction of property, including history of firesetting; and the presence of precipitants versus impulsive acts.

24. **What approach is suggested to address the child with aggression?**
    Clinicians must avoid responding to the patient's aggression in a punitive manner. A respectful, nonjudgmental, and reassuring attitude fosters an internal rather than external effort in gaining control for the patient and can reduce the aggressive behavior.

25. **Is it possible to provide oral medications to an agitated/ aggressive child?**
    Most patients will cooperate with an oral dosing of a medication, despite the belief that they may be too agitated and uncooperative. Aggressive behavior frequently causes shame and embarrassment to the child. As such, actions that reflect a respectful, nonjudgmental and reassuring attitude, such as offering the patient the option of oral medication versus "a shot," can accomplish much in reducing the agitation and additionally avoid any potentially punitive medical provider response. Lastly, for some sedatives, oral administration can be as effective as intramuscular dosing to control agitation, and the onset of intramuscular dosing is not significantly more rapid to warrant its routine, first-line use.

    Yildiz A, Sachs GS, Turgay A: Pharmacological management of agitation in emergency settings. Emerg Med J 20:339–346, 2003.

EATING DISORDER

26. **What are the four diagnostic criteria for anorexia nervosa?**
    - Refusal to maintain weight within a normal range for height and age (more than 15% below ideal body weight)
    - Fear of weight gain
    - Severe body image disturbance in which body image is the predominant measure of self-worth with denial of the seriousness of the illness
    - In postmenarchal females, absence of the menstrual cycle, or amenorrhea (greater than three cycles).

    American Psychiatric Association: Diagnostic and Statistical Manual of Mental Disorders, 4th ed. Washington, DC, American Psychiatric Association, 1994.

27. **What are some of the medical complications of persistent purging or starvation seen in anorexia nervosa or bulimia?**
    - Osteopenia
    - Cardiac impairment, bradycardia
    - Cognitive changes
    - Psychological functioning difficulties
    - Nausea or bloating

- Amenorrhea
- Hypokalemia, hyponatremia, and metabolic alkalosis in patients who purge by vomiting, laxative abuse, or diuretic abuse
- Dental erosion and enlarged salivary glands in patients with bulimia
- Infertility

Miller KK, Grinspoon SK, Ciampa J, et al: Medical findings in outpatients with anorexia nervosa. Arch Intern Med 165:561–566, 2005.

28. **What is the initial medical evaluation for a patient with a suspected eating disorder?**
    - CBC, electrolytes, BUN, creatinine, Ca, Mg, PO_4, glucose
    - Uric acid, cholesterol, triglycerides, liver transaminases
    - Thyroid function tests, urine pregnancy test, urinalysis
    - EKG

CHAPTER 41

RESPIRATORY EMERGENCIES

Marc H. Gorelick, MD, MSCE, and Sabina B. Singh, MD, FAAP

ASTHMA

1. **What is the best clinical indicator of airway obstruction in children with asthma?**
   There is no single best indicator of obstruction. It is generally true that, in younger children, observation is often more revealing than auscultation; it is hard to listen for wheezes in a crying child. Signs of airway obstruction include:
   - Evidence of work of breathing (retractions, use of accessory muscles, nasal flaring, abdominal breathing)
   - Decreased breath sounds
   - Prolongation of the expiratory phase
   - Wheezing

2. **What is the pulmonary index?**
   The pulmonary index is one of many clinical scores used in the evaluation of acute asthma severity (Table 41-1). Although no single score has been shown to be superior, the pulmonary index has been used widely in asthma research. Also, there is not universal agreement on how to interpret the score. As a general guide, a score < 6 is considered mild, while a score > 10 is considered severe.

   Becker AB, Nelson NA, Simons FER: The pulmonary index: Assessment of a clinical score for asthma. Am J Dis Child 138:574–576, 1984.

	Respiratory Rate, by Age (breaths/min)				
Score	<6 y	≥6 y	Wheezing*	Inspiratory-to-Expiratory Ratio	Accessory Muscle Use
0	≤30	≤20	None	5:2	None
1	31–45	21–35	End expiration	5:3–5:4	+
2	46–60	36–50	Entire expiration	1:1	++
3	>60	>50	Inspiration and expiration	>1:1	+++

TABLE 41-1. PULMONARY INDEX

*If there is no wheezing because of minimal air entry, score = 3.

3. **Describe the role of measuring peak expiratory flow rate during acute asthma exacerbations in children.**

Clinical assessment, while helpful, may underestimate the degree of airway obstruction in a child with acute asthma. The most commonly used pulmonary function test in pediatric acute care is the pulmonary expiratory flow rate (PEFR), which is the maximal rate of airflow during forced exhalation after a maximal inhalation. It is easily measured using an inexpensive, handheld metering device. Children as young as 4 or 5 years old can be taught how to perform PEFR, although it is more difficult to learn in the setting of an acute exacerbation. Advantages of PEFR include ease of performance, low cost, and ability to track changes during therapy. However, PEFR is effort-dependent and cannot be performed by very young children. In addition, PEFR measures function in medium and large airways, while much of the pathology in asthma occurs in medium and small airways; thus, even PEFR can underestimate the severity of disease. Normal values depend on the age and height of the child (a table is usually included with the meter), as well as the severity of the underlying lung disease, so results should be expressed as a percentage of predicted value, or of the patient's usual best value if known. PEFR of at least 80% of predicted indicates **mild** disease, 50–80% of predicted is considered **moderate**, and less than 50% of predicted constitutes **severe** disease. Failure to achieve PEFR of at least 50% of predicted is one indication for hospital admission.

Gorelick MH, Stevens MW, Schultz TR, Scribano PV: Difficulty in obtaining peak expiratory flow measurements in children with acute asthma. Pediatr Emerg Care 20:22–26, 2004.

4. **How should pulse oximetry be interpreted in acute asthma?**

"Normal" values vary considerably between institutions and practitioners. An SaO_2 (saturation of O_2 measured by pulse oximetry) of 95% correlates with a PaO_2 of around 75, while an SaO_2 of 90% is close to a PaO_2 of 60, at the top of the steep portion of the oxygen desaturation curve. Most clinicians set a cut-off for normal somewhere in between. Remember that while a low saturation is worrisome, a normal oxygen saturation does *not* rule out severe disease.

Keahey L, Bulloch B, Becker AB, et al: Initial oxygen saturation as a predictor of admission in children presenting to the emergency department with acute asthma. Ann Emerg Med 40:300–307, 2002.

5. **Why does hypoxemia sometimes increase paradoxically after treatment with inhaled bronchodilators?**

Hypoxemia in asthma is due to ventilation–perfusion mismatch. The acute deleterious effects of bronchodilators on oxygenation are believed to be due to their effects on the circulation rather than on the airways. After treatment, particularly when administered with high concentrations of oxygen, there is improvement in local alveolar oxygenation. This, in turn, causes a reversal of hypoxia-induced pulmonary vasoconstriction, with the result that areas previously neither ventilated nor perfused are now perfused but not ventilated, increasing the mismatch.

6. **What is Poiseuille's law?**

$$\text{Airway resistance} = 8\ nl/r^4$$

where n = viscosity coefficient of the gas, l = length of the tube, and r = radius of the tube. Thus, resistance to airflow increases in inverse proportion to the fourth power of the radius of the air passages. The take-home message is that a little narrowing goes a long way toward blocking air flow.

7. **What are the indications for obtaining arterial blood gas (ABG) analysis in a patient with asthma?**

Since oxygenation can be measured noninvasively, ABG is useful primarily for monitoring carbon dioxide concentration and acid–base status. In deciding whether to obtain an ABG, it is worth considering that hypercarbia generally only develops when the PEFR is < 20–25% of predicted. Moreover, the decision to intubate a patient with asthma is rarely made on the basis of ABG results alone. Thus, ABG is usually reserved for the following patients:

- Those who present in extremis
- Those demonstrating signs of respiratory fatigue
- Those who fail to respond to aggressive traditional therapy in whom more invasive treatments (e.g., endotracheal intubation, intravenous beta-agonists) are being considered

8. **What is pulsus paradoxus?**

   Pulsus paradoxus is an exaggeration of the normal decrease in systolic blood pressure during inspiration. In acute asthma, it has been shown to correlate well with pulmonary function tests, and it can be useful in assessing asthma severity and response to treatment. A pulsus paradoxus < 10 is considered normal; 10–20 indicates moderate obstruction; and > 20 indicates severe obstruction.

   To measure pulsus paradoxus, inflate the cuff of a manual sphygmomanometer, then auscultate as pressure is gradually released. Initially, Korotkoff sounds are heard only during expiration and disappear with inspiration. The difference between the pressure at which the sounds are first heard and the pressure at which they cease to disappear with expiration is the pulsus paradoxus.

   Other conditions that may cause an elevated pulsus paradoxus include severe pneumonia, pericardial effusion, constrictive pericarditis, and conditions affecting myocardial compliance (e.g., amyloidosis, endomyocardial fibroelastosis).

9. **A 6-year-old with asthma is treated for acute wheezing in the ED with only partial relief and needs to be admitted to the hospital. Should a chest x-ray be obtained?**

   Chest radiography is of limited value in the evaluation of the patient with acute asthma. It may be useful in identifying those patients with airleak (i.e., pneumothorax or pneumomediastinum) or a concomitant pneumonia. However, routinely obtaining radiographs in all patients with acute asthma, or even all patients with exacerbation serious enough to require hospital admission, rarely leads to an unexpected finding that changes management. In patients with known asthma, chest radiographs should be limited to cases where there is clinical suspicion of a radiographic abnormality, such as persistent rales or asymmetry of breath sounds, high fever, crepitus in the neck, or very poor response to therapy or deterioration after initial therapy.

10. **What is the value of radiography in children with a first episode of wheezing?**

    Routine use of radiography in such children is of relatively low yield. However, most authorities recommend obtaining an x-ray in a child with a first episode of wheezing. A number of conditions other than reactive airways disease may present with wheezing, and these should be ruled out before a diagnosis of asthma is made (Table 41-2). Radiography is probably not necessary in children with clinical bronchiolitis of mild-to-moderate severity, or in older children with a family history of asthma who respond completely to inhaled bronchodilators; however, in most cases of first-time wheezing, a chest x-ray is prudent.

    Roback MG, Dreitlin DA: Chest radiograph in the evaluation of first time wheezing episodes: Review of current clinical practice and efficacy. Pediatr Emerg Care 14:181–184, 1998.

11. **What is the role of exhaled nitric oxide (NO) measurement in the assessment of asthma?**

    NO is generated from the action of nitric oxide synthase on L-arginine in the lung. NO synthase activity increases during the inflammatory process, producing increased concentrations of NO in exhaled air. Measurement of exhaled NO levels has been shown to be a sensitive, noninvasive means of measuring the degree of airway inflammation in adult and pediatric patients, and it correlates well with other markers of chronic asthma severity. Available data suggest, however, that exhaled NO levels correlate poorly with acute severity in ED patients.

Gill M, Walker S, Khan A, et al: Exhaled nitric oxide levels during acute asthma exacerbation. Acad Emerg Med 12:579–586, 2005.

TABLE 41-2. OTHER CAUSES OF WHEEZING

Inflammatory/Infectious	Intraluminal Obstruction	Extraluminal Obstruction
Bronchiolitis	Foreign body	Vascular ring
Aspiration (gastroesophageal reflux, tracheoesophageal fistula)	Tracheomalacia	Mediastinal mass
Bronchopulmonary dysplasia	Congestive heart failure	Cystic malformation of the lung
Cystic fibrosis	α_1-antitrypsin deficiency Cholinergic poisoning (e.g., organophosphate)	Congenital lobar emphysema

12. **What is the preferred initial treatment for children with acute asthma?**
Treatment is tailored to the severity of the exacerbation, but treatment with inhaled bronchodilators is the mainstay of initial therapy for all patients. Those with moderate to severe exacerbation (as determined by clinical status or PEFR) should receive 3–4 doses of an inhaled bronchodilator in the first hour of treatment until there is good response; those with more mild disease may require less aggressive treatment. In addition, systemic steroids should be given immediately in severely ill patients, to those who are symptomatic despite appropriate bronchodilator therapy at home, and to all patients who fail to show complete response to one or two inhalation treatments in the ED.

Expert Panel on Management of Asthma: Guidelines for the Diagnosis and Management of Asthma: Clinical Practice Guidelines. Available at: http://www.nhlbi.nih.gov/guidelines/asthma/asthgdln.htm

13. **Isn't nebulization a more effective means of delivering inhaled beta-agonists than a metered dose inhaler (MDI)?**
Several studies and meta-analyses have shown that nebulizer and MDI are clinically equivalent, provided that an appropriate dose is given and that a spacer device is used with the MDI. Standard doses of nebulized beta-agonist (0.15 mg/kg per dose, maximum 5 mg) are substantially higher than for MDI. However, the particles produced by the MDI deliver medication far more effectively to the lungs. Current recommendations of ED dosages of albuterol for acute asthma are for 2–4 puffs of albuterol for young children, 4–6 puffs for older children, and 4–8 puffs for adolescents and adults. Spacer devices (e.g., Aerochamber®) are available in a variety of sizes and configurations and can be used successfully even in young infants. In one sense the delivery systems are not equivalent: Studies have shown that use of MDI is less expensive and leads to shorter ED stays.

Cates CJ, Bara A, Crilly JA, Rowe BH. Holding chambers versus nebulisers for beta-agonist treatment of acute asthma. Cochrane Database of Systematic Reviews 2003, Issue 2. Available at: http://www.cochrane.org/cochrane/revabstr/AB000052.htm

14. **What are the adverse effects of albuterol?**
    - Tachycardia; tachyarrhythmias (rare)
    - Tremor
    - CNS stimulation, hyperactivity
    - Hypokalemia
    Note that even with high-dose therapy, while mild degrees of hypokalemia are common (one-third of children in one study), symptomatic hypokalemia requiring treatment is rare. Patients receiving high-dose continuous albuterol for more than 6–8 hours should have serum potassium monitored.

15. **What is levalbuterol?**
    Racemic (standard) albuterol is a mixture of two isomers. Levalbuterol (Xopenex) is the pure R-isomer, which is responsible for bronchodilation. Although some authors suggest that levalbuterol produces fewer side effects, particularly tachycardia and jitteriness, than albuterol, most of the clinical evidence supports the notion that equipotent doses of albuterol and levalbuterol have similar bronchodilator efficacy and side effect profiles for acute use. There is some evidence that the S-isomer may increase airway reactivity, suggesting that levalbuterol may be preferred for chronic use.

    Qureshi F, Zaritzky A, Welch C, et al: Clinical efficacy of racemic albuterol versus levalbuterol for the treatment of acute pediatric asthma. Ann Emerg Med 46:29–36, 2005.

16. **What is the mechanism of action of ipratropium?**
    Ipratropium bromide binds to cholinergic receptors, located primarily in the medium and large airways, leading to bronchodilation. Because vagally mediated bronchodilation is much less marked than that produced by adrenergic stimulation, ipratropium is a much less potent bronchodilator than albuterol and should not be used alone. However, the concomitant administration of both leads to a synergistic effect. Ipratropium is structurally related to atropine, but it is a quaternary compound, and therefore is poorly absorbed. Thus, systemic side effects are minimal.

17. **Which patients should receive ipratropium?**
    Ipratropium bromide binds to cholinergic receptors in the airways; concomitant administration with beta-agonists leads to a synergistic bronchodilator effect. Pediatric studies are fairly convincing that addition of ipratropium to albuterol leads to significant improvement in patients with severe asthma exacerbation. The benefit in those with more moderate disease is less clear. However, ipratropium has very little downside; costs and adverse effects are both minimal. It should be given to those patients with severe disease at presentation and those who fail or have failed to respond well to beta-agonists alone.

    Plotnick LH, Ducharme FM: Combined inhaled anticholinergics and beta2-agonists for initial treatment of acute asthma in children. Cochrane Database of Systematic Reviews 2000, Issue 3. Available at: http://www.cochrane.org/cochrane/revabstr/AB000060.htm

18. **What is the optimum dose of ipratropium?**
    This has not yet been well established. Young children (< 10 kg) should get 250 μg (one-half vial) per dose; larger children can get 500 μg per dose. While multiple doses have been shown to be better than a single dose, the optimum schedule is not known. Most authorities recommend adding ipratropium to two or three of the first three doses of albuterol given in the ED, then every 2–4 hours.

19. **When should steroids be administered?**
    The sooner, the better. Asthma is an inflammatory disease. Bronchodilators control only the symptoms, not the underlying pathology. Therefore, nearly all children with acute asthma should receive systemic corticosteroids, preferably at the start of their ED treatment. That said, there

is a trade-off in that too-frequent steroid administration may lead to problems. Patients with particularly mild disease, who require no or only a single treatment in the ED and have complete relief of symptoms with infrequent (no more than three to four times a day) treatments at home, may be managed without steroids.

20. **What are the actions of corticosteroids in acute asthma?**
Steroids have multiple actions, including:
- Inhibition of mediator release and synthesis
- Interference with mediator action
- Up-regulation of beta-adrenergic receptors

The last two help explain the observed onset of clinical effect within 2 hours of administration—during the time course of a typical ED visit. Peak effect of steroids requires interference with cellular synthetic pathways and occurs after 6–12 hours.

21. **When are IV steroids preferred over the oral route?**
Almost never. There are several pediatric studies, and more from the adult literature, showing oral and IV corticosteroids to be equally effective, even among severely ill patients. The IV route should be reserved for those unable to take oral medicine (persistent vomiting, severe respiratory distress) and perhaps those patients ill enough to be admitted to an intensive care unit.

Barnett PL, Caputo GL, Baskin M, Kuppermann N: Intravenous versus oral corticosteroids in the management of acute asthma in children. Ann Emerg Med 29:212–217, 1997.

22. **How can steroids be given to the child who is vomiting but does not require hospital admission?**
Although pediatric data are sparse, a short course of high-dose inhaled steroids may be a useful alternative in children with mild-to-moderate exacerbation. Another option is the intramuscular route using dexamethasone. Two studies in children support this; one used a dose of 0.3 mg/kg, and the other used 1.7 mg/kg.

Edmonds ML, Camargo CA Jr, Brenner BE, Rowe BH: Inhaled steroids for acute asthma following emergency department discharge. The Cochrane Database of Systematic Reviews 2000, Issue 3: http://www.cochrane.org/cochrane/revabstr/AB002316.htm

23. **What are the contraindications to systemic steroids?**
- **Absolute contraindications:** Active varicella or herpes infection
- **Relative contraindication:** Exposure to varicella in an unprotected child

Note that concomitant bacterial infection (e.g., otitis media, pneumonia) is *not* a contraindication to the use of steroids.

24. **Describe the role of magnesium sulfate in acute asthma.**
Magnesium sulfate produces bronchodilation via direct effect on smooth muscle because of calcium antagonism. It may provide added benefit when adrenergic and vagal receptors have been saturated. In children with severe exacerbations, the addition of magnesium sulfate to aggressive beta-agonist therapy and systemic steroids leads to greater clinical improvement and improved pulmonary function and SaO_2. The effectiveness in patients with less severe illness is equivocal.

Rowe BH, Bretzlaff JA, Bourdon C, et al: Magnesium sulfate for treating exacerbations of acute asthma in the emergency department. Cochrane Database of Systematic Reviews 2000, Issue 1. Available at: http://www.cochrane.org/cochrane/revabstr/AB001490.htm

25. **What is the dose of magnesium sulfate for asthma?**
50–100 mg/kg (maximum 2–2.5 g) administered intravenously over 20–30 minutes.

26. **What is heliox?**

Heliox is a mixture of helium and oxygen, usually in a ratio of 60–70% He:30–40% O_2. Because helium is a smaller molecule than either nitrogen (the major component of air) or oxygen, heliox is less viscous than air. According to Poiseuille's law, gas flow is inversely proportional to viscosity; thus, heliox may be better able to diffuse past constricted air passages than air mixtures or pure oxygen. The evidence for its effectiveness in status asthmaticus is mixed. Case series and uncontrolled trials have shown improvement among severely ill patients given heliox. However, controlled clinical trials have failed to show significant benefit in terms of pulmonary function or clinical score. Among the disadvantages are the relatively low oxygen concentration permitted and the need for a tight-fitting mask (which may limit compliance in younger children). It remains an investigational agent but may be considered in patients with severe illness that fails to respond to other treatment.

Rodrigo G, Pollack C, Rodrigo C, Rowe BH: Heliox for nonintubated acute asthma patients. Cochrane Database of Systematic Reviews 2003, Issue 2. Available at http://www.cochrane.org/cochrane/revabstr/AB002884.htm

27. **What are the indications for endotracheal intubation and mechanical ventilation in a patient with asthma?**
    - Failure of maximal pharmacologic therapy
    - Hypoxemia unrelieved by O_2 therapy
    - Hypercarbia with rising pCO_2
    - Deteriorating mental status
    - Respiratory fatigue
    - Respiratory arrest

28. **Which medications should be used during endotracheal intubation of an asthmatic patient?**

Rapid sequence induction, including sedation and neuromuscular blockade, should be used. Ketamine is a good choice as a sedating agent because of its intrinsic bronchodilating properties. However, because it also increases airway secretions, it should be used in combination with an anticholinergic agent such as atropine or glycopyrrolate. Some medications, including opiates (morphine, meperidine) and muscle relaxants (curare, atracurium), potentiate histamine release and may worsen bronchospasm.

29. **What are the two most common complications of mechanical ventilation?**
    - **Air leak**, including pneumomediastinum and pneumothorax, is common due to barotrauma.
    - **Hypotension** often occurs shortly after endotracheal intubation. It results from a combination of relative hypovolemia in severely ill patients and decreased venous return to the heart due to positive intrapleural pressure.

KEY POINTS: TREATMENT OF ACUTE ASTHMA ✔

1. Provide frequent (every 20 minutes) inhaled albuterol.
2. Provide early oral steroids (before or after first treatment).
3. Add ipratropium bromide to beta-agonists in case of incomplete response.
4. Monitor response to therapy with clinical assessment or peak expiratory flow.
5. Consider intravenous magnesium sulfate for severe or refractory cases.

BRONCHIOLITIS

30. **What is bronchiolitis?**
    Bronchiolitis is a viral infection of the upper and lower respiratory tract (medium and small airways). The peak incidence is in the winter. Children less than 2 years of age are most commonly affected. Respiratory syncytial virus accounts for approximately 80% of cases; parainfluenza, human metapneumovirus, adenovirus, influenza, and other respiratory viruses are less common causes.

31. **Is there a test for respiratory syncytial virus (RSV)? How good is it?**
    RSV can be identified in nasal secretions by viral culture. Rapid antigen testing is also widely available in many hospital laboratories. The sensitivity of the commercially available tests is generally in the range of 80–90%, and specificity is greater than 90%. However, the clinical utility of these tests is limited, since treatment is directed toward the clinical manifestations rather than the etiologic agent; treatment generally is the same regardless of the results of the test.

    Bordley WC, Viswanathan M, King VJ, et al: Diagnosis and testing in bronchiolitis: A systematic review. Arch Pediatr Adolesc Med 158:119–126, 2004.

32. **What are the clinical characteristics and natural history of bronchiolitis?**
    Bronchiolitis begins as an upper respiratory infection, with coryza and cough. (In older children and adults, as well as many infants, RSV infection remains confined to the upper respiratory tract.) Over a period of several days, the lower tract becomes involved, with the development of wheezing and rhonchi, as well as signs of respiratory distress. Typically, signs and symptoms peak in severity on the third to fifth day of illness and then begin to wane. The total duration of illness is generally 10 to 14 days, although some infants may have a prolonged course. In one study, 18% of children were still symptomatic at 3 weeks. Central apnea can occur in young infants, usually at the onset of illness, before respiratory signs manifest.

    Swingler GH, Hussey GD, Zwarenstein MZ: Duration of illness in ambulatory children diagnosed with bronchiolitis. Arch Pediatr Adolesc Med 154:997–1000, 2000.

33. **Who is at risk for severe disease?**
    Among the risk factors for severe illness are very young age, prematurity, underlying cardiac or pulmonary disease, and immunodeficiency. Most previously healthy infants have mild to moderate disease and do not require hospitalization. However, several clinical features are predictive of development of more serious illness (Table 41-3). A score of 3 or more has a sensitivity and specificity of approximately 80% for severe disease (defined as needing hospitalization).

    Shaw KN, Bell LM, Sherman NH: Outpatient assessment of infants with bronchiolitis. Am J Dis Child 145:151–155, 1991.

TABLE 41-3. BRONCHIOLITIS SEVERITY SCORE			
	Points per Item		
Variable	0	1	2
Current age (mo)	≥ 3	< 3	
Gestational age at birth (wk)	≥ 37	34–36	< 34
General appearance	Well	Ill	Toxic
Respiratory rate (breaths/min)	< 60	60–69	≥ 70
Pulse oximetry (%)	≥ 97	95–96	< 95
Atelectasis on chest radiography	Absent	Present	

34. **What is the role of albuterol in the management of bronchiolitis?**

    Because wheezing is a clinical hallmark of bronchiolitis, inhaled beta-agonists are often administered. However, multiple clinical trials, summarized in two meta-analyses, have shown mixed results. On average, the benefit of beta-agonists is small. It appears that a subset of infants responds well, while a larger group responds minimally or not at all. It is not currently possible to predict responsiveness; therefore, a trial of albuterol, either 0.25–0.5 ml of a 0.5% solution via nebulizer or 2 puffs from an MDI with spacer/mask is warranted. Those children who respond are candidates for further treatment. It is not necessary to continue treatment in the absence of clinical responsiveness. Oral albuterol has *not* been shown to be efficacious.

    King VJ, Viswanathan M, Bordley WC, et al: Pharmacologic treatment of bronchiolitis in infants and children: A systematic review. Arch Pediatr Adolesc Med 158:127–137, 2004.

35. **A 3-month-old child with bronchiolitis has moderate distress and a pulse oximetry of 93% in room air. She does not respond to inhaled albuterol. Is there any other effective treatment?**

    Although several studies have found a superior clinical benefit of **inhaled epinephrine** compared to albuterol, more recent literature has shown that epinephrine and albuterol are similarly effective. It is not customary to administer inhaled epinephrine on an outpatient basis; a trial of epinephrine may be considered in those patients with more severe illness who are likely to require hospitalization. The usual dose is 3 ml of a 1:1000 solution via nebulizer.

    Hartling L, Wiebe N, Russell K, et al: Epinephrine for bronchiolitis. Cochrane Database of Systematic Reviews 2004, Issue 1: http://www.cochrane.org/cochrane/revabstr/AB003123.htm

36. **Is there a role for corticosteroids in bronchiolitis?**

    Most studies to date have shown no benefit of corticosteroids, either systemic or inhaled, in the treatment of bronchiolitis. One study by Schuh et al (J Pediatr 140:27–32, 2002) found that a single dose of dexamethasone decreased hospital admission by more than 50%; this finding has not yet been confirmed in larger, multicenter studies. Steroids may be of benefit in selected children with wheezing suspected of having intrinsic reactive airways disease, such as those with a prior history of wheezing, or strong family or personal history of atopy and good response to inhaled beta-agonists.

    Patel H, Platt R, Lozano JM, Wang EEL: Glucocorticoids for acute viral bronchiolitis in infants and young children. Cochrane Database of Systematic Reviews 2004, Issue 3. Available at: http://www.cochrane.org/cochrane/revabstr/AB004878.htm

37. **What is ribavirin?**

    Ribavirin is an antiviral agent with activity against RSV. Although previously recommended for patients with or at risk for severe RSV infection, experts have recommended more recently that ribavirin not be used routinely, even in severe cases.

38. **What is palivizumab?**

    Palivizumab (Synagis) is a humanized mouse monoclonal antibody against RSV. Palivizumab prophylaxis has been shown to reduce the incidence and severity of RSV bronchiolitis in high-risk patients. It is administered as a monthly intramuscular injection.

KEY POINTS: MANAGEMENT OF BRONCHIOLITIS ✓

1. Care is mainly supportive.

2. Trial of inhaled beta-agonists may be useful, but most children do not respond.

3. Use of corticosteroids for bronchiolitis not supported by majority of evidence.

4. Typical course is progression of symptoms over first 3–5 days, resolution over 2–3 weeks.

CROUP

39. **What is croup? How is it diagnosed?**
Croup is a viral infection of the upper respiratory tract lasting 7–10 days. It is the most common cause of stridor in a febrile child. Parainfluenza virus can be recovered from the nasopharynx in over 90% of cases. The rest of the cases are caused by influenza, respiratory syncytial virus, measles, or adenovirus. It is most often seen in the fall months with a peak in October, and it typically affects children between the ages of 6 and 36 months.

Croup usually begins with a fever (temperature 38–39° C) and rhinorrhea. The cricoid cartilage causes the mucosal swelling to occur inwards, encroaching on the airway. A harsh, barky, "seal-like" cough begins within 12–48 hours. There may be associated tachypnea, stridor, and subcostal retractions in the more severe cases. The symptoms may be relieved by cool or humidified air and are exacerbated by crying.

40. **What is the differential diagnosis of croup?**
Conditions that may be mistaken for croup include bacterial tracheitis, retropharyngeal abscess, and epiglottitis (Table 41-4). The last is a much less common entity since 1990, with the introduction of the Hib vaccine. In a 6- to 24-month-old afebrile child, an index of suspicion should be kept for an aspirated foreign body. Often a clear history of choking is not obtained.

TABLE 41-4.   DIFFERENTIAL DIAGNOSIS OF CROUP

Variable	Croup	Epiglottitis	Retropharyngeal Abscess	Bacterial Tracheitis
Anatomic area affected	Subglottic	Supraglottic	Retropharynx	Trachea
Age	6–36 mo	Any	6 mo–4 y	Any
Onset	Hours	1–3 days	1–3 days	3–5 days
Toxicity	None	Marked	Marked	Marked
Drooling	No	Yes	Yes	No
Voice	Hoarse	Muffled	Muffled	Normal
Cough	Barky	None	None	Painful
Radiographic finding	"Steeple"	"Thumb"	Widened retropharynx	"Shaggy"

41. **When are diagnostic tests indicated (or of value) in croup?**
Croup is diagnosed on the basis of presenting signs and symptoms. Children with characteristic disease do not require further diagnostic testing. Anteroposterior and lateral radiographs of the neck may be indicated in children with atypical features (e.g., age less than 6 months, recurrent or prolonged croup, toxicity on exam). The typical radiographic findings are shown in Table 41-4.

42. **How do you assess the severity of croup?**
Several scoring systems have been devised to assess croup severity. The most commonly used is the modified Westley score (Table 41-5). A score of < 4 indicates mild disease, 4–6 indicates moderate disease, and a score of 7 indicates severe disease.

   Super DM, Cartelli NA, Brooks LJ, et al: A prospective randomized double-blind study to evaluate the effect of dexamethasone in acute larygotracheitis. J Pediatr 115:323–329, 1989.

43. **What are indications for admission?**
A child with a croup score = 7, significant respiratory compromise, dehydration, unreliable caretaker, or lack of adequate follow-up should be admitted to the hospital. For those severely ill patients not responding to therapy, an ABG may be helpful in deciding admission to the general ward versus the pediatric ICU.

TABLE 41-5. WESTLEY CROUP SCORE*				
Variable	0	1	2	3
Stridor	None	With stethoscope	At rest	
Retraction	None	Mild	Moderate	Severe
Air entry	Normal	Mild decrease	Marked decrease	

*Cyanosis = 4 points; altered mental status = 5 points.

44. **Is there any scientific evidence that humidified air is beneficial in the treatment of children with croup?**
No. In theory, the humidified air moistens secretions and soothes the inflammation of the mucosa. However, despite the ubiquitous recommendations for the use of "the steamy bathroom" and "misty ox," controlled trials have failed to demonstrate a clinical benefit.

   Nieto GM, Kentab O, Klassen TP, Osmond MH: A randomized controlled trial of mist in the acute treatment of moderate croup. Acad Emerg Med 9:873–879, 2002.
   Scolnik D, Coates AL, Stephens D, et al: Controlled delivery of high vs low humidity vs mist therapy for croup in emergency departments: A randomized controlled trial. JAMA 295:1274, 2006.

45. **Is there any scientific evidence that steroids are beneficial in the treatment of croup?**
Yes. Although many of the randomized trials involving the use of steroids in croup have involved relatively small numbers of patients, meta-analyses of these trials have shown significant decreases in clinical croup scores and decrease in risk of intubation in patients with croup who receive steroids. In addition, one study has also demonstrated that steroids reduce symptom

duration even in children with mild symptoms. In general, patients with more than minimal symptoms (e.g., a croup score = 1) should be treated with steroids.

Bjornson CL, Klassen TP, Williamson J, et al: A randomized trial of a single dose of oral dexamethasone for mild croup. N Engl J Med 351:1306, 2004.

Russell K, Wiebe N, Saenz A, et al: Glucocorticoids for croup. Cochrane Database of Systematic Reviews 2004, Issue 1. Available at: http://www.cochrane.org/cochrane/revabstr/AB001955.htm

46. **Which method of corticosteroid delivery is better: intramuscular, oral, or nebulized? What is the ideal dose?**

Both dexamethasone (given orally or intramuscularly) and the newer synthetic glucocorticoid budesonide (inhaled) have been shown to be effective in the treatment of croup, although recent studies have suggested that systemic dexamethasone is superior. Comparisons of oral and intramuscular dexamethasone have found similar rates of clinical improvement. The usual dose of dexamethasone for croup has traditionally been 0.6 mg/kg IM or PO, though doses of 0.15 and 0.3 mg/kg have been shown to be similarly effective.

47. **Is racemic epinephrine superior to "regular" L-epinephrine in the treatment of croup?**

Nebulized epinephrine has been shown to provide short-term benefit in the treatment of croup, presumably by reducing tracheal secretions and mucosal edema. Racemic epinephrine has been advocated traditionally, based on the belief that a mixture of D- and L- isomers would lead to less tachycardia. However, in a randomized trial directly comparing the two drugs, they were equivalent in terms of efficacy and side effects. A dose of 5 ml of L-epinephrine 1:1000 is equal to 0.5 ml of the racemic (2%) mixture.

Kunkel NC, Baker MD: Use of racemic epinephrine, dexamethasone, and mist in the outpatient management of croup. Pediatr Emerg Care 12:156–159, 1996.

48. **Do patients who receive nebulized epinephrine in the ED require admission to the hospital?**

Because of the "rebound phenomenon"—a tendency to return to the baseline clinical picture after the epinephrine wears off—administration of nebulized epinephrine to children with croup in the ED became a major reason for admission to the hospital in the 1980s and early 1990s. However, studies have demonstrated a lack of adverse outcome in children who are discharged after a period of observation (typically 2–4 hours) after epinephrine. To be safely discharged, it is recommended that the child remain clinically stable (no stridor at rest, normal air entry and oxygen saturation), and that the child receive a dose of dexamethasone prior to discharge.

PNEUMONIA

49. **How reliable are signs and symptoms in diagnosing pneumonia in young children?**

Infants and young children with pneumonia often have subtle and nonspecific pulmonary findings. The issue of "occult" pneumonia—pneumonia in the absence of any pulmonary findings—has been a controversial one. Several authors have found that the risk of pneumonia is very low in the absence of any findings, but they caution that tachypnea may be a sole finding. Tachypnea, in fact, has the greatest negative predictive value. A study of highly febrile children with leukocytosis (WBC > 20,000) found that 26% of such children in whom pneumonia was unsuspected clinically had infiltrates on chest x-ray. However, tachypnea in this study was evaluated qualitatively.

50. **What are the most common bacterial causes of pneumonia in children?**
See Table 41-6.

TABLE 41-6. MOST COMMON BACTERIAL CAUSES OF PNEUMONIA IN CHILDREN		
Neonate (0–2 mo)	**Infant (2 mo–3 y)**	**Preschool/School Age (>3 y)**
Group B streptococci	*Streptococcus pneumoniae*	*Mycoplasma pneumoniae*
Gram-negative bacilli	*Staphylococcus aureus*	*Streptococcus pneumoniae*
Staphylococcus aureus	*Haemophilus influenzae**	*Chlamydia pneumoniae*
Chlamydia trachomatis		
Streptococcus pneumoniae		
*In unimmunized populations.		

51. **What organisms are most commonly associated with pleural effusion?**
Pneumococci, *S. aureus*, and *M. tuberculosis* are the most common causes of effusion in
children with pneumonia.

CHAPTER 42

ACUTE CARE OF TECHNOLOGY-ASSISTED CHILDREN

Kate M. Cronan, MD, FAAP; Joel A. Fein, MD, MPH; and Jill C. Posner, MD

TRACHEOSTOMY

1. **What are the most common reasons for tracheostomy tube placement in a child?**
   In children, tracheostomies are indicated for respiratory insufficiency due to a variety of causes, most commonly bronchopulmonary dysplasia and airway anomalies (e.g., congenital anomalies and subglottic stenosis). Also relatively common indications are neuromuscular disorders or central disorders, such as a brain tumor or Chiari malformation. A child with a tracheostomy may or may not require additional ventilatory assistance.

   Hadfield PJ, Lloyd-Faulconbridge RV, Almeyda J, et al: The changing indications for paediatric tracheostomy. Int J Pediatr Otorhinolaryngol 67:7–10, 2003.
   Pilmer SL: Prolonged mechanical ventilation in children. Pediatr Clin North Am 41:473–512, 1994.
   Schreiner MS, Downes JJ, Kettrick RG, et al: Chronic respiratory failure in infants with prolonged ventilator dependency. JAMA 258:3398–3404, 1987.

2. **How do I determine the appropriate tracheostomy tube size?**
   A tracheostomy tube is sized by three dimensions: its inner diameter, its outer diameter, and its length. The size of the tube can be ascertained by checking the flanges of the tube where the inner diameter, and in many cases the outer diameter, are imprinted. Many caretakers of technology-assisted children become experts in their child's technology and are excellent resources for medical personnel. Often, children will travel with emergency boards or "go bags," which contain all the equipment necessary to change a tracheostomy tube, including a replacement tube. If a patient presents without a tube in place and no replacement tube on hand, a reasonable estimate would be to use the formula for endotracheal tube sizing (16 + age)/4 or 4 + age/4.

KEY POINTS: THREE DIMENSIONS OF A TRACHEOSTOMY TUBE ✔

1. ID (internal diameter)

2. OD (outer diameter)

3. L (length)

---

3. **What are the immediate management priorities for a child with a tracheostomy who presents in respiratory distress?**
   Assume this patient has an inadequate airway until proven otherwise. The tracheostomy tube may be obstructed or malpositioned. Assess airway patency and the adequacy of breathing through physical examination and the usual monitoring. Administer supplemental oxygen.

Suction the tracheal tube to evaluate patency and to clear secretions as this may be help to alleviate symptoms. Do not be falsely reassured by a tube entering into the stoma because it may actually descend into the soft tissues of the neck rather than into the trachea, especially if a prior tracheostomy tube change was attempted and unknowingly resulted in a false passage. An emergent tracheostomy tube change may be indicated if respiratory distress persists or the cannula clearly is dislodged.

4. **What are the most common causes of respiratory distress in a child who has a tracheostomy tube?**
   Mechanical failure (cannula obstruction or dislodgement), infectious causes (pneumonia, tracheitis, viral respiratory infections), asthma, or reactive airway disease.

5. **What are the causes of bleeding from the tracheostomy tube?**
   The most common cause of bleeding from the tracheostomy tube is drying and friability of the tracheal mucosa due to inadequate humidification. Anatomically, the tracheostomy tube inserts into the airway below the vocal cords. Therefore, inspired air bypasses the natural warming and humidification processes of the upper airway. Humidification is an important component of the ventilator circuit for patients with mechanical ventilation. For those patients who breathe independently from the ventilator, a heat-moisture exchanger device is inserted at the opening of the tube. This plastic device contains a hydrophilic substance that captures the patient's own heat and humidity on exhalation so that it can be inhaled on inspiration. Other causes of bleeding include granuloma formation, infection (i.e., tracheitis), and erosion of the tube tip into a blood vessel.

6. **How should I manage bleeding from the tracheostomy tube?**
   First, ensure the adequacy of the airway, breathing, and circulation. Suction frequently to avoid aspiration of blood. Minor bleeding usually indicates the need to increase inspired humidification. A larger amount of blood may indicate that the tip of the tube has eroded into a blood vessel. Treat this as a surgical emergency with immediate notification of surgical, anesthesia, and operating room personnel. Obtain IV access with two large-bore catheters and initiate resuscitation with isotonic fluids or blood products. Overinflating the tracheostomy tube may tamponade the bleeding vessel, thereby providing a temporizing measure. Importantly, leave the tracheostomy tube in place, as this may be the only way to ensure an airway.

7. **What can I do if I am unable to replace a dislodged tracheostomy tube?**
   When a tracheostomy tube becomes dislodged or decannulated, there is a tendency for the stoma to constrict, making it difficult to replace the tube. If stomal constriction prevents insertion of the replacement tube, several options are available: (1) insert a smaller tracheostomy tube; (2) insert a smaller endotracheal tube (being careful not to advance it into a mainstem bronchus), and then slowly dilate the stoma by inserting tubes of successively increasing size; (3) cover the stoma and use a bag-valve-mask device to ventilate by using traditional methods via the patient's upper airway; and (4) insert an oral tracheal tube. Oral intubation may be exceptionally difficult, especially if the original indication for tracheostomy was to overcome an airway anomaly. Therefore, use neuromuscular blocking agents with great caution and consider anesthesiology or otolaryngology assistance early.

Posner JC, Cronan K, Badaki O, Fein JA: Emergency care of the technology-assisted child. Clin Pediatr Emerg Med 7:38–51, 2006.

Posner JC: Acute care of the child with a tracheostomy. Pediatr Emerg Care 15:49–54, 1999.

ENTERAL FEEDING

8. **What are the indicators for placement of a gastrostomy tube in a child?**
   - Inability to feed orally (due to swallowing dysfunction, esophageal injury, neuromuscular disease)
   - Failure to thrive
   - Risk of aspiration from oral secretions

9. **What is the difference between a percutaneous endoscopic gastrostomy (PEG) tube and a surgically placed gastrostomy tube?**
   - A **PEG** procedure may be performed under sedation or general anesthesia. An endoscope is inserted into the esophagus and a light source indicates the appropriate location on the stomach wall. An incision is made on the external abdominal wall and the tube is placed via this aperture.
   - A **surgical or open gastrostomy tube** is placed via laparotomy under general anesthesia. A purse string suture is made in the stomach to secure the tube and the stomach is then sutured to the abdominal wall.

   Gauderer MW: Percutaneous endoscopic gastrostomy. A 10 year experience with 220 children. J Pediatr Surg 26:288–294, 1991.

10. **What are some of the complications of gastrostomy tubes in children?**
    - Dislodgement
    - Clogging
    - Leaking
    - Gastric outlet obstruction
    - Bleeding
    - Gastric ulceration
    - Worsened gastroesophageal reflux

    Kazi S, Gunasekaran TS, Berman JH, Kavin H, Kraut JR: Gastric mucosal injuries in children from inflatable low-profile gastrostomy tubes. J Pediatr Gastroenterol Nutr 24:75–79, 1997.
    Koulentaki M, Reynolds N, Steinke D, et al: Eight years' experience of gastrostomy tube management. Endoscopy 34:941–945, 2002.

11. **How is dislodgement of a gastrostomy tube managed in the emergency department (ED)?**
    The first step is to determine the age of the stoma. If the stoma is older than 8 weeks, the ED physician or nurse should take action. If the stoma is less than 8 weeks, obtain a surgical or gastroenterology consultation.

    As soon as possible, stent the stoma open with a temporizing device, such as a Foley catheter. This should be placed with lubricant; rarely, a mild sedative is required. When the stoma is located, place the appropriate-size replacement gastrostomy tube in the stoma after removing the Foley catheter. If the tube has been dislodged for an extended period of time (hours), smaller gastrostomy tubes may be initially required to dilate the stoma. Always check the balloon's function before replacing the tube. Fill the balloon and check the tube to ensure that it is snug.

KEY POINTS: STEPS TO REPLACE A DISLODGED GASTROSTOMY TUBE ✔

1. Determine the age of the stoma.

2. Stent the stoma open with a temporary device.

3. Check the balloon of the new gastrostomy tube.

4. Remove the temporary tube.

5. Place the new gastrostomy tube using lubricant.

6. Fill the balloon and check for adequate fit.

12. **What is the danger of inserting a tube into a stoma that has recently been placed?**
The stomach wall may not have adhered to the peritoneal lining and skin. The fistula tract can be disrupted and a false lumen into the peritoneum may be formed. Formula inserted through the tube can lead to chemical or bacterial peritonitis.

13. **What are some of the complications of replacing a gastrostomy tube?**
- Accidental insertion into the peritoneal cavity, which can occur in specific scenarios
- Lysis of adhesions of the stomach wall away from the abdominal wall, resulting in pneumoperitoneum
- If a false lumen is created, formula may be installed into the space, causing chemical peritonitis
- Inadequate advancement of the tip of the tube can result in the tube's staying in the fistula; the fistula can thus be disrupted when the balloon is dilated, and having the tip in the fistula can result in pain
- Bleeding at the site of insertion can occur from trauma during insertion

Graneto J: Gastrostomy tube replacement. In Henretig FM, King C (eds): Textbook of Pediatric Emergency Medicine Procedures. Baltimore, Williams & Wilkins, 1997, pp 915–920.

14. **Is it necessary to perform a dye study in order to verify gastrostomy tube location after replacement?**
Not usually. Aspiration of stomach contents after the gastrostomy tube is replaced confirms that the tube is in the stomach. Listening over the stomach for borborygmi when 15 mL of air is inserted into the tube's lumen is also confirmatory. If in doubt, radiographic studies may be indicated.

15. **What is the best treatment for a clogged gastrostomy tube?**
Warm water is the best irrigant and has been shown to be superior to vinegar, soda, and juices. Repeated gentle flushing is advised. Prevention includes regular flushing after feedings.

16. **What are some complications that can occur in relation to the stoma?**
- Peristomal infection
- Irritation
- Bleeding
- Stretching
- Granuloma formation

17. **How is a stomal granulation treated?**
Application of silver nitrate to the granuloma is most often successful.

CEREBROSPINAL FLUID SHUNTS

18. **Name the most common symptoms associated with cerebrospinal fluid (CSF) shunt obstruction**
Symptoms frequently include headache, vomiting, and some alteration of mental status, however subtle. Alteration in vital signs may reflect autonomic instability or brain herniation. Seizures are rarely the only manifestation of increased intracranial pressure, and more likely represent an underlying seizure disorder. When a CSF shunt is obstructed, parents often accurately state, "this is what my child looked like when she/he had the last shunt obstruction."

Browd SR, Ragel BT, Gottfried ON, Kestle JR: Failure of cerebrospinal fluid shunts: part I: Obstruction and mechanical failure. Pediatr Neurol 34(2):83–92, 2006.

KEY POINTS: SYMPTOMS OF VENTRICULOPERITONEAL ✔ SHUNT OBSTRUCTION

1. Headache

2. Vomiting

3. Change in mental status, may be subtle

4. Alteration of vital signs

---

19. **What is "pumping the shunt," and what does this tell me?**
Conventional wisdom, which need not always be conventional or wise, suggests that easy depression of a shunt reservoir bubble signifies that the distal end is patent, and rapid refilling of this bubble signifies that the proximal shunt is patent. In reality, the amount of useful information gleaned from this procedure is less than expected. One study found that an "abnormal finding" when pumping the shunt identified less than 40% of obstructed shunts, and that a finding of "normal function" on pumping the shunt would miss between 10% and 35% of shunt obstructions for various brands of shunts.

Piatt JH: Physical examination of patients with cerebrospinal fluid shunts: Is there useful information in pumping the shunt? Pediatrics 89, 470–473, 1992.
Woodward GA, Carey CM: Evaluation of ventricular shunt function. In King C and Henretig FM (eds), Textbook of Pediatric Emergency Procedures, 1st ed, Williams & Wilkins, Philadelphia, 1997.

20. **When should shunt infection be suspected? How can I differentiate CSF shunt infection from obstruction?**
Suspect shunt infection in any febrile child with a shunt. However, in one series, fever was present in fewer than half of the patients with shunt infection. Meningeal signs are also an insensitive indicator of infection. A history of surgical manipulation of the shunt in the prior 2 months should increase suspicion for infection; infections rarely occur more than 6 months after surgery. Gram-positive organisms, such as *Staphylococcus epidermidis* and *S. aureus*, acquired in the surgical suite cause most infections. Gram-negative organisms are uncommon but can originate from an abdominal source or, rarely, bacteremia.

Symptoms of CSF shunt infection overlap considerably with those of CSF shunt obstruction because the diagnoses often occur together. The higher viscosity of infected fluid may lead to a partial or complete obstruction of the small fenestrations on the shunt tubing.

Duhaime AC: Evaluation and management of shunt infections in children with hydrocephalus. Clin Ped 45(8):705–713, 2006.

Nelson JD: Cerebrospinal fluid shunt infections. Pediatr Infect Dis 3:30–32, 1984.

Odio C, McCracken GH Jr, Nelson JD: CSF shunt infections in pediatrics. A seven-year experience. Am J Dis Child 138:1103–1108, 1984.

Walters BC, Hoffman HJ, Hendrick EB, Humphreys RP: Cerebrospinal fluid shunt infection. Influences on initial management and subsequent outcome. J Neurosurg 60:1014–1021, 1984.

21. **What studies are helpful in diagnosing CSF shunt infections?**
Culture of an organism from the CSF is the most accurate method of diagnosing a shunt infection. Attention to the white blood cell count and Gram stain from the shunt fluid are helpful but not foolproof methods of determining if a shunt is infected. The Gram stain is positive in a little more than half of all shunt infections. CSF that is aspirated from an infected shunt usually reveals a moderate pleocytosis but can be misleadingly normal, as can the CSF glucose. Peripheral white blood cell counts and blood cultures are frequently normal in the presence of shunt infection.

Anderson EJ, Yogev R: A rational approach to the management of ventricular shunt infections. Pediatr Dis J 24(6):557–558, 2005.

22. **What techniques can an emergency medicine practitioner use to treat the critically ill patient with a CSF shunt obstruction?**
When a child with suspected CSF shunt obstruction is critically ill with signs of increased intracranial pressure, emergent action is required to reduce that pressure. Conventional therapies, such as hyperventilation and mannitol administration, may be used, but if possible the pressure should be relieved by accessing the shunt. If there is a distal obstruction or partial proximal obstruction, fluid can be withdrawn in a sterile fashion by using a 23-gauge butterfly needle and 20-mL syringe. This potentially lifesaving procedure is usually done by a neurosurgeon but should not be delayed if the patient's condition is deteriorating—the procedure is well described in pediatric emergency procedure textbooks.

Duhaime AC, Wiley JF II: Ventricular shunt and burr hole puncture. In King C, Henretig FM (eds): Textbook of Pediatric Emergency Procedures, 2nd ed. Lippincott Williams & Wilkins, Philadelphia, 2006.

IV. SURGICAL EMERGENCIES

DENTAL/PERIODONTAL EMERGENCIES

Susanne Kost, MD

1. **What is the typical age at which an infant acquires the full complement of primary teeth?**
   The second primary molars typically erupt at about 22 months of age; most children have the full complement of 20 primary teeth around their second birthday.

2. **Which are the first permanent teeth to erupt? Which teeth come next?**
   The first permanent teeth to erupt are usually the first permanent molars ("6-year" molars), followed by the mandibular central incisors, maxillary central incisors, lateral incisors, cuspids, and bicuspids. The mixed dentition phase concludes at about age 12 years with the eruption of the second permanent ("12-year") molars, but the adult complement of 32 teeth is not achieved until the eruption of the third molars ("wisdom" teeth) in late adolescence (Fig. 43-1).

3. **What are Epstein's pearls? How do they differ from Bohn's nodules and dental laminal cysts?**
   Cystic lesions in the oral cavity of newborns are quite common, occurring in 80% of normal newborns. They are generally small, and superficial, and are caused by entrapment of bits of embryologic tissue within dental epithelium.
   - **Epstein's pearls** are tiny, 1- to 2-mm keratin-filled cystic lesions located along the midpalatine raphe.
   - **Bohn's nodules** are small mucous gland cysts found on the alveolar ridges or posterior palate.
   - **Dental laminal cysts** are larger, more lucent, fluctuant cysts consisting of remnants of dental laminal epithelium. They are usually single lesions, and they are found only on the crest of the alveolar mucosa.

   Nelson LP, Shusterman S: Dental emergencies. In Fleisher GR, Ludwig S (eds): Pediatric Emergency Medicine, 4th ed. Philadelphia, Lippincott Williams & Wilkins, 2006.

4. **Does teething cause fever?**
   Teething has been blamed for a number of symptoms in infants throughout time, ranging from fever, congestion, diarrhea, and rashes to seizures and death. A recent prospective descriptive study of 425 tooth eruptions in 125 children looked at parental reports of 18 "teething symptoms" daily for 8 months. Symptoms that were statistically linked to the eruption of a tooth included mild temperature elevation (temperature $< 38.8°$ C), biting, drooling, facial rash, and decreased appetite for solids. Congestion, cough, vomiting, diarrhea, and temperature $> 38.8°$ C were not associated with teething.

   Macknin ML, Piedmonte M, Jacobs J, Skibinski C: Symptoms associated with infant teething: A prospective study. Pediatrics 105:747–752, 2000.

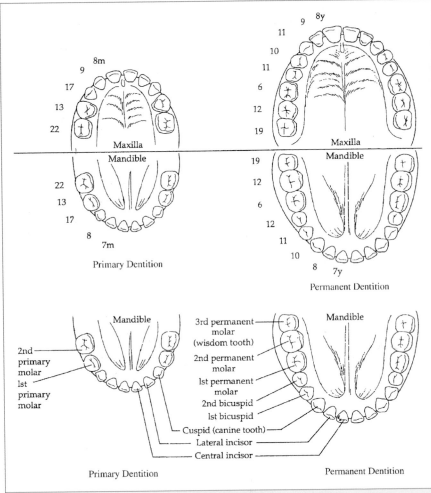

Figure 43-1. Primary and secondary tooth eruptions.(From Nazif MM, et al: Oral disorders. In Zitelli BJ, Davis HW [eds]: Atlas of Pediatric Physical Diagnosis, 2nd ed. New York, Harcourt, 1992, Fig. 20.9.)

KEY POINTS: CONDITIONS FOR WHICH TEETHING SHOULD NOT BE BLAMED ✓

1. Common viral symptoms of young children

2. Upper respiratory tract infections

3. Diarrhea

4. Significant fever

5. **An 8-year-old presents with a blue-black cystic lesion over an erupting tooth What is the cause?**
An eruption cyst is a nontender, fluid-filled cyst that sometimes forms over the crown of an erupting tooth. Occasionally, these cysts will fill with blood, creating the eruption hematoma described above. These cysts or hematomas are benign and self-limiting conditions that resolve when the tooth erupts.

6. **What are the three main "ingredients" in the development of dental caries?**
Dental caries is one of the most common disease processes in children, affecting about 5% of all children in the first few years of life, with much higher percentages in indigent children. The disease of dental caries is multifactorial in origin, requiring a susceptible host (genetic predisposition), a cariogenic diet (sticky sweets), and bacteria (most commonly *Streptococcus mutans*).

Tinanoff N, Kanellis MJ, Vargas CM: Current understanding of the epidemiology, mechanisms, and prevention of dental caries in preschool children. Pediatr Dent 24:543–551, 2002.

7. **Are dental caries contagious?**
In a sense, yes. *S. mutans* has been shown to be transmitted both vertically and horizontally and can colonize the mouths of infants even prior to the eruption of teeth. Thus, practices such as the "premoistening" of a pacifier with maternal saliva before insertion into the infant's mouth should be strongly discouraged.

Berkowitz RJ: Mutans streptococci: Acquisition and transmission. Pediatr Dent 28:106–109, 2006.

8. **Why is a dentoalveolar abscess more likely to "point" toward the buccal aspect of the gingiva than the lingual aspect?**
Dentoalveolar abscesses are a common cause of facial cellulitis based on the anatomy of the alveolar bone. The outer buccal aspect of the bone is much thinner than the inner lingual aspect; hence the path of least resistance for drainage is through the fascial planes of the cheek and face.

9. **What are the indications for hospital admission for a patient with a dental abscess?**
The majority of dental abscesses can be managed on an outpatient basis with oral antibiotics and close dental follow-up for drainage or extraction of the affected tooth. Facial cellulitis resulting from an abscessed tooth can be managed with outpatient antibiotics also, unless the orbit is involved or the amount of swelling and pain compromises the airway or the ability to take fluids. Children who are toxic-appearing, highly febrile, or lacking appropriate social support for follow-up should be admitted.

Nelson LP, Shusterman S: Dental emergencies. In Fleisher GR, Ludwig S (eds): Pediatric Emergency Medicine, 4th ed. Philadelphia, Lippincott Williams & Wilkins, 2006.

KEY POINTS: AREAS INTO WHICH UNTREATED DENTAL ABSCESSES CAN EXTEND ✔

1. Sinuses

2. Orbits

3. Brain

4. Airway

5. Mediastinum

10. **What are the most common complications of wisdom tooth extraction?**

Extraction of the third molars, or "wisdom teeth," is a common procedure in late adolescence and early adulthood. Complications resulting in a visit to the emergency department may include hemorrhage, infection, or alveolar osteitis ("dry socket"). The extraction site may normally ooze for 8–12 hours after the procedure; persistent oozing beyond 12 hours or frank bleeding at any point may require a coagulation profile. Most bleeding will be controlled with pressure, best achieved by biting on gauze sponges for 15–30 minutes. Moistened tea bags placed over the socket may facilitate clotting, based on the coagulating properties of tannic acid. If pressure fails to control the bleeding, the socket may be packed with Gelfoam or closed with sutures. Infection of the extraction socket is rare, but should be suspected in the presence of fever, swelling, or purulent exudate from the extraction site. Penicillin and pain control are the mainstays of treatment. Alveolar osteitis is a painful inflammatory process caused by disintegration of the clot in the tooth socket, typically occurring 3 days after extraction. Treatment consists of debridement and packing of the socket.

11. **What are the complications of oral piercings? Can they be life-threatening?**

Complications of oral (lip and tongue) piercing include:
- Pain and swelling
- Localized infection
- Gingival recession and chipping of teeth
- Poor cosmetic outcome (keloids, bifid tongue)
- Embedded jewelry

Potentially life-threatening complications include disseminated infection, such as mediastinitis and endocarditis, and hemorrhage, especially in patients with an underlying predisposition.

Larzo MR, Grimm Poe S: Adverse consequences of tattoos and body piercings. Pediatr Ann 35:187–192, 2006.

12. **What is meant by the term *geographic tongue*?**

Geographic tongue, or benign migratory glossitis, is a painless condition notable for erythematous "islands" of denuded papillae surrounded by elevated whitish borders (Fig. 43-2). The islands appear to migrate over the surface of the tongue over time, akin to the movement of continents on the globe. The etiology is unknown, with allergy, infection, and stress all implicated as potential contributors. It generally resolves without specific treatment over a period of weeks to months.

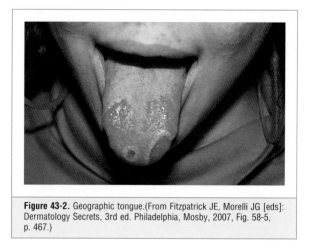

Figure 43-2. Geographic tongue.(From Fitzpatrick JE, Morelli JG [eds]: Dermatology Secrets, 3rd ed. Philadelphia, Mosby, 2007, Fig. 58-5, p. 467.)

13. **What is a ranula? How does it differ from a mucocoele?**

A ranula is a mucous retention cyst on the floor of the mouth, under the tongue (Fig. 43-3). A mucocele is a retention cyst located most commonly in the mucosa of the lower lip (Fig. 43-4). Both can range from several millimeters to a centimeter in diameter, are painless, and are felt to arise following trauma to the ducts of minor salivary glands. Treatment is surgical excision.

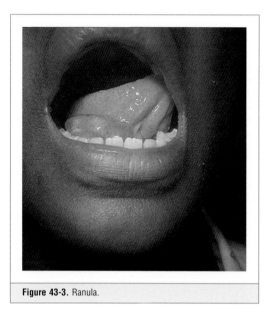

Figure 43-3. Ranula.

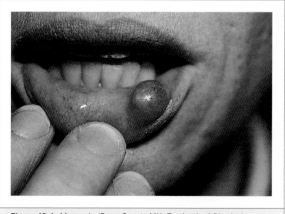

Figure 43-4. Mucocele.(From Swartz MH: Textbook of Physical Diagnosis: History and Examination, 4th ed. Philadelphia, Saunders, 2002, Fig. 11-13, p. 295.)

14. **What are the most common causes of stomatitis in young children?**
Viral infections most commonly cause stomatitis in young children (< 6 years old). Herpes simplex virus, usually type I, causes a syndrome of very painful vesicles and gingival inflammation, sometimes to the point of bleeding, in the anterior mouth and tongue. Herpes stomatitis is often associated with high fevers (temperature of 39–40° C), headache, and cervical adenopathy. Coxsackie viruses cause a more benign vesicular inflammation of the posterior pharynx. Also known as herpangina, this infection causes pain, low-grade fever, and drooling. An acral viral exanthem (hand, foot, and mouth disease) is seen with some strains of coxsackie virus. Both infections are most common in the toddler age group, and both are treated symptomatically with topical or systemic analgesics. There is some evidence that acyclovir given early in the course of herpetic stomatitis may alleviate the symptoms.

15. **Name three eponymous anaerobic infections associated with the mouth.**
    - **Vincent's disease**, also known as acute necrotizing ulcerative gingivostomatitis, or trench mouth, is a painful ulcerative gingivostomatitis caused by overgrowth of a spirochete, *Borrelia vincentii*. It is most common in adolescents. Treatment consists of vigorous oral hygiene, with the addition of penicillin in severe cases.
    - **Ludwig's angina** is a life-threatening cellulitis of the sublingual and submandibular spaces. Rapid spread of infection into the neck may result in airway obstruction.
    - **Lemierre syndrome**, or postanginal sepsis, involves infection of the lateral pharyngeal space with septic thrombophlebitis of the jugular vein, potentially leading to septic embolization to the lungs or brain. The most commonly associated organism is *Fusobacterium* sp.

    Fisher MC: Other anaerobic infections. In Behrmann RE, Kliegman RM, Jenson HB (eds): Nelson's Textbook of Pediatrics, 17th ed. Philadelphia, Saunders, 2004.

WEBSITE

American Academy of Pediatric Dentistry
www.aapd.org

GENERAL SURGERY EMERGENCIES

Kristine G. Williams, MD, MPH, and Dee Hodge III, MD

1. **What is the classic presenting history in a child with suspected appendicitis?**
   Usually the child presents with a history of diffuse abdominal pain, possibly associated with vomiting and a low-grade fever. Some may have a history of anorexia. Unlike in adults, it is often hard to obtain an accurate and consistent history. The presenting symptoms of appendicitis are similar to those of many other childhood diseases. Gastroenteritis, urinary tract infections, streptococcal pharyngitis, constipation, and pneumonia are just a few of the illnesses that appendicitis can mimic. Most children with appendicitis complain of pain in the right lower quadrant (RLQ) once peritoneal inflammation occurs.

   Bachur RG: Abdominal emergencies. In Fleisher GR, Ludwig S, Henretig FM (eds): Textbook of Pediatric Emergency Medicine, 5th ed. Philadelphia, Lippincott Williams & Wilkins, 2006, pp 1605–1630.
   eMedicine: General surgery articles: www.emedicine.com/ped/GENERAL_SURGERY.htm

2. **Where else might a child with appendicitis localize pain?**
   If the appendix is located in the lateral gutter, the child may exhibit tenderness in the lateral abdomen or flank. An appendix pointing toward the pelvis might cause pubic pain and diarrhea. A retrocecal appendix causes pain on deep palpation. This information is important, since not all children with appendicitis present with RLQ pain.

3. **Is diarrhea a presenting symptom of appendicitis?**
   Yes. Diarrhea may delay accurate diagnosis if the symptom is mistakenly associated with gastroenteritis rather than appendicitis. Children under 3 years old are the ones most likely to present with this symptom. A retrospective case series identified 63 children under the age of 3 who had an appendectomy for appendicitis at one of four teaching institutions. The mean age was 2.2 years. The mean delay from the onset of symptoms to presentation was 4.3 days, and 57% were misdiagnosed at initial presentation! Diarrhea was reported in one third of the patients. Although none of the children died, morbidity was increased: 84% had perforation or gangrene.

   Serious and life-threatening disease processes must be kept in mind when a young child presents with symptoms that may look like simple gastroenteritis.

   Horwitz JR, Gursoy M, Jaksic R, Lally KP: Importance of diarrhea as a presenting symptom of appendicitis in very young children. Am J Surg 173:80–82, 1997.

4. **Does a white blood cell (WBC) count of only 11.5 cells/mm³ rule out appendicitis?**
   A child with a nonperforated appendicitis usually has a WBC count of 11,000–15,000 cells/mm³ in the first 1–2 days of illness. A higher WBC count with a left shift may be found later in the course, as the appendix undergoes further degeneration, or if the appendix has ruptured. Although laboratory values may help to support your clinical diagnosis, they should not replace a good history and a careful physical examination.

5. **What laboratory findings *are* suggestive of appendicitis?**
   The two tests that should be done on all patients who are suspected of having appendicitis are a **complete blood count with differential** and a **urinalysis**. WBC counts appear to be highly associated with both uncomplicated acute and complicated acute appendicitis, and are a good

tool to aid in diagnosis. The urinalysis may show ketosis due to decreased oral intake. If the inflamed appendix lies near the bladder or ureter, sterile pyuria may be seen as well. However, a normal complete blood count or a normal urinalysis do not rule out appendicitis.

6. **Is C-reactive protein (CRP) helpful in diagnosing appendicitis?**
   Greatly elevated CRP levels (e.g., > 50 mg/L) have been found to be associated with *perforated* appendicitis. A patient with a normal WBC count AND a normal CRP level is unlikely to have appendicitis. Here is the evidence: Investigators have examined the use of CRP and WBC values to predict appendicitis at different stages. In one retrospective study, 100 adult and pediatric patients in each of the following categories had mean preoperative values calculated: uninflamed appendix, uncomplicated acute appendicitis, and complicated acute appendicitis. Although some of the patients with uninflamed appendices had increased WBC or CRP values, all patients with both values in the normal range had an uninflamed appendix. Those with uncomplicated acute appendicitis had either raised WBC counts and normal CRP levels, or elevated values of both. Most of those with complicated acute appendicitis had both values raised. A prospective study of pediatric patients with appendicitis showed a positive predictive value of 91% for perforation if the CRP level was > 50 mg/L. There was no difference in WBC counts among those with and without perforation.

   Chung JL, Kong MS, Lin SL, et al: Diagnostic value of C-reactive protein in children with perforated appendicitis. Eur J Pediatr 155:529–531, 1996.
   Gronoos JM, Gronoos P: Leukocyte count and C-reactive protein in the diagnosis of acute appendicitis. Br J Surg 86:501–504, 1999.

7. **Is a plain x-ray useful in diagnosing appendicitis?**
   Plain radiography is not very helpful. It usually reveals nonspecific findings for appendicitis, unless a calcified appendicolith is present (< 10% of patients). The presence of air–fluid levels in the RLQ suggests a localized ileus. Although this finding may heighten one's suspicion for appendicitis, beware! The same findings are also present in gastroenteritis. Plain films may reveal an alternate diagnosis, such as pneumonia.

   Heller RM, Hernanz-Schulman M: Applications of new imaging modalities to the evaluation of common pediatric conditions. J Pediatr 135:632–639, 1999.

8. **Is ultrasonography useful in evaluating for appendicitis?**
   Ultrasonography has a reported sensitivity of approximately 80% and a reported specificity of approximately 93% for the diagnosis of appendicitis. It is quick and does not involve large doses of radiation. It can identify ovarian pathology, such as ovarian cysts or torsion. However, there are limitations to this technology:
   - It requires an experienced technician.
   - It is difficult to scan overweight children.
   - It is uncomfortable for the patient because of a need for graded compression of overlying bowel.
   - It can be extremely difficult to perform on a crying or uncooperative child.
   - The appendix can be located anywhere in the abdomen, making visualization difficult at times. If visualized, the inflammation may be localized to a small segment that cannot be seen.
   Thus, a positive result is highly suggestive, but a negative result should be followed with repeated physical examination and reassessment of your level of suspicion for the diagnosis. If the appendix cannot be visualized, appendicitis is not ruled out.

9. **What is the value of computed tomography (CT) in diagnosing appendicitis?**
   CT is a valuable modality for appendicitis. It has a sensitivity of about 95% and a specificity of about 93% for the diagnosis of appendicitis. Of course, there are drawbacks to CT as well. The need for contrast material, exposure to radiation, higher cost, and a longer preparatory period

prior to the study are a few of them. Although some patients with a suspected inflamed appendix may not need imaging, the most sensitive imaging modality is abdominal CT.

Sivit CJ, Applegate KE, Stallion A, et al: Imaging evaluation of suspected appendicitis in a pediatric population: Effectiveness of sonography versus CT. AJR 175:977–980, 2000.

10. **What is focused CT of the abdomen?**
Focused CT of the lower abdomen, beginning at the lower end of the third lumbar vertebral body and extending to the pubic ramus, may effectively diagnose appendicitis. It offers a lower dose of radiation and is therefore a good option in the diagnosis of appendicitis.

Fefferman NR, Roche KJ, Pinkney LP, et al: Suspected appendicitis in children: Focused CT technique for evaluation. Radiology 220:691–695, 2001.

11. **Why does the pain of appendicitis typically start centrally (periumbilically) and then localize to the right lower quadrant?**
The initial pain of appendicitis is visceral: a dull, aching pain localized to the mid- or lower abdomen. **Visceral** or **splanchnic pain** originates in those abdominal organs, such as the appendix, that have visceral peritoneum. Increased hollow viscous wall tension and ischemia cause impulses to be sent from the organ to the spinal cord. In the case of the appendix, visceral afferent autonomic nerves enter the spinal cord at T8–T10. These segments supply the periumbilical area, which explains the initial, poorly localized pain associated with appendicitis.

As the appendix becomes more inflamed, it causes inflammation of the serosa and parietal peritoneum. The inflammation triggers local somatic pain fibers. **Somatic pain** is mediated by afferent nerve fibers in segmental spinal nerves. Thus, the pain is sharper and more localized, usually to the RLQ.

12. **Describe the pathophysiologic mechanism that leads to appendicitis.**
The appendix contains increasing amounts of lymphatic tissue as a child ages. Acute appendicitis occurs when the lumen of the appendix becomes obstructed. Sources of obstruction include fecaliths, lymphatic hypertrophy, worms, vegetable matter, and tumors. The appendix continues to secrete mucosal fluid, leading to distention of the viscus. Intraluminal bacterial overgrowth develops.

KEY POINTS: COMMON FINDINGS IN ACUTE APPENDICITIS ✔

1. Diffuse or periumbilical abdominal pain
2. Low-grade fever
3. Vomiting or diarrhea
4. Anorexia

13. **Which of these patients with appendicitis is most likely to present with a perforation? Why?**
A. A 2-year-old boy with pain for a few days
B. A 12-year-old girl with severe pain for 24 hours
C. An 8-year-old boy with a temperature of 40° C
D. A 16-year-old with a WBC count of 18,000 cells/mm³

Although any one of the patients could present with a perforated appendix, the 2-year-old with pain for 2 days is statistically most likely to have perforation at presentation. The rates of perforation are higher in younger children because of the following several factors: (1) the appendix is more thin walled, predisposing them to early perforation; (2) younger children are less able to communicate clearly, resulting in prolonged symptoms before diagnosis; and (3) the level of suspicion for appendicitis is often lower in younger age groups, leading to a delay in diagnosis.

14. **Why does perforated appendicitis progress to peritonitis more quickly in infants and children than in adults?**
The omentum is not as well developed in infants and children as it is in adults. Since the omentum is primarily responsible for walling off the infection in a perforated appendicitis, its insufficiency contributes to the development of peritonitis. This complication of perforated appendicitis may play a role in the increased mortality in young children with appendicitis.

15. **What conditions must be considered in a teenage girl with symptoms of appendicitis?**
Gynecologic conditions and emergencies should be a part of the differential diagnosis of any teenage girl with RLQ pain. In particular, ovarian cysts, corpus luteal cysts, mittelschmerz, tubal pregnancy, ovarian torsion, tubo ovarian abscess, and salpingitis can all present similarly to appendicitis.

16. **What is the most common cause of acute pancreatitis in children?**
Abdominal trauma.

17. **What are the radiographic findings in a child with acute mechanical bowel obstruction?**
Multiple, dilated loops of bowel and an air-fluid level visible in the upright or lateral decubitus views on plain films are common.

18. **What is the most common cause of acute intestinal obstruction in a child 3–12 months of age?**
Intussusception. This occurs when a proximal segment of bowel telescopes into a distal segment. It is commonly ileocolic, but small bowel may also telescope into itself.

19. **Define *lead point*.**
The lead point is the area that is thought to initiate the intussusceptum. The causes of lead points differ by age. In infants, lead points are often hypertrophied Peyer's patches. In older children, there are many possibilities for focal lead points, including intestinal polyps, Meckel's diverticulum, or a tumor.

Bachur RG: Abdominal emergencies. In Fleisher GR, Ludwig S, Henretig FM (eds): Textbook of Pediatric Emergency Medicine, 5th ed. Philadelphia, Lippincott Williams & Wilkins, 2006, pp 1605–1630.

20. **What causes intussusception?**
There is no definitive cause, though there is an association between intussusception and a history of a preceding viral illness, diarrhea, or, perhaps, Henoch-Schönlein purpura. The association between the rotavirus vaccine and increased frequency of intussusception led to the recall of the original rotavirus vaccine.

Centers for Disease Control and Prevention: Intussusception among recipients of rotavirus vaccine— United States 1998–1999. MMWR Morb Mortal Wkly Rep 282:520–521, 1999.

21. **How does the child with intussusception present?**
There may be several different presentations. The classic history is that the patient has crampy abdominal pain. Since this is a disease that mostly occurs in preverbal children, the parent may

give the history that the child acts normally or is only slightly irritable, but has episodic bouts of severe abdominal pain characterized by drawing his knees to his chest, lying still, or screaming inconsolably. Some children may present with profound lethargy. Vomiting may become bilious as the small bowel becomes completely obstructed. On physical examination, the child's abdomen may be normal or may be distended because of the partial or complete obstruction of the bowel. A sausage-like mass may be palpable in the right side of the abdomen.

eMedicine: General surgery articles: www.emedicine.com/ped/GENERAL_SURGERY.htm

22. **What is the origin of pain in intussusception?**
Intussusception is the result of invagination of a portion of proximal intestine into distal intestine. The intussuscepted mass can obstruct the intestinal lumen. Abdominal pain is due to distention and peristaltic rushes against the mass.

23. **What is "currant jelly" stool?**
Currant jelly is made from a small, round, acid berry that may be black or red. This term is used to describe the reddish, heme-positive stool of mixed mucous and blood associated with late stages of intussusception. It occurs when the edematous bowel causes compression of the mesenteric veins. It indicates mucosal damage and is present in only about one-third of patients. Intussusception cannot be ruled out in the absence of currant jelly stool.

24. **How do you diagnose intussusception?**
Aside from a good history and physical examination, **air contrast enema** is the best diagnostic test. However, you may choose to start with an **obstruction series**, which may demonstrate small bowel obstruction and free peritoneal air. Some authors suggest **ultrasonography** as a second step, since it can unequivocally identify intussusception and may help to identify the leading edge of the intussusceptum, the presence of a lead point, and the presence of blood flow within the intussusceptum. Whether or not you choose to begin with an obstructive series or ultrasonography, if the suspicion of intussusception remains, then contrast enema is the next step. Air contrast enema is preferred in many pediatric institutions, though some still use barium. Note that it is wise to inform your surgical colleagues of the case prior to the contrast enema because of the risk of perforation during the study.

Hadidi AT, El Shal N: Childhood intussusception: A comparative study of nonsurgical management. J Pediatr Surg 34:304–307, 1999.

25. **What are the only absolute contraindications to enema in the diagnosis of intussusception?**
The presence of free air or signs of peritoneal irritation are the only absolute contraindications.

KEY POINTS: CLASSIC FINDINGS IN INTUSSUSCEPTION ✓

1. Intense, intermittent abdominal pain

2. Currant jelly stool

3. Irritability

4. Vomiting

5. Lethargy

26. **How do you treat intussusception?**
This is a trick question because the diagnostic test (enema) is usually therapeutic as well. Intussusception can be reduced by air enema in the majority of cases. If the child is toxic, however, he or she may require surgical intervention. Recurrence rates are 5–8%, regardless of the means of reduction. Admit the patient to the hospital after the intussusception is reduced.

27. **Why are inguinal hernias usually repaired when detected in young infants?**
There is a high risk of intestinal incarceration in male infants and adnexal entrapment in female infants. Hernias that reduce spontaneously are generally repaired electively soon after detection. Those that require sedation or manual reduction are usually repaired 24–48 hours after reduction.

28. **Is an incarcerated hernia more common in girls or boys?**
Contrary to what you might think, it is more common in girls and usually involves the ovary rather than the intestine.

29. **What is the difference between an incarcerated and a strangulated hernia?**
Incarceration means that the intestine or ovary is nonreducible, but not necessarily gangrenous. However, if the hernia is not reduced, it can become strangulated. Once the hernia is strangulated, venous and lymphatic obstruction occur, leading to occlusion of arterial supply. This sets the stage for necrosis and possible perforation.

30. **On examination of a 3-month-old child brought in for a minor complaint, you notice a large umbilical hernia. The mother asks you what she should do about it. What do you tell her?**
Umbilical hernias are common in infants and young children, especially African Americans. Incarceration of an umbilical hernia is rare. Your best advice is to reassure the parent that most of these reduce spontaneously. If there is a *large* ring that has not diminished by age 2, or if an incarceration has occurred, the defect should be closed operatively. Otherwise, the hernia can be closed electively at age 5 or 6.

   Bachur RG: Abdominal emergencies. In Fleisher GR, Ludwig S, Henretig FM (eds): Textbook of Pediatric Emergency Medicine, 5th ed. Philadelphia, Lippincott Williams & Wilkins, 2006, pp 1605–1630.

KEY POINTS: WHICH TEST IS BEST? ✔

1. Appendicitis = CT

2. Pyloric stenosis = ultrasonography

3. Intussusception = air contrast enema

4. Malrotation = upper gastrointestinal series

31. **A 10-month-old, previously well child presents to the emergency department (ED) with acute onset of abdominal pain associated with bilious vomiting. The child is afebrile and ill-appearing and has a slightly distended abdomen that is diffusely tender. The rectal examination reveals blood on the examiner's finger. On routine abdominal radiography, the emergency physician notes air–fluid levels and a few dilated loops of bowel. The upright film shows a "double-bubble" sign. An upper gastrointestinal study reveals absence of the ligament of Treitz. What should the physician do next?**
The physician should call a surgeon and reserve the operating room as soon as possible. The "double-bubble" sign on the upright abdominal radiograph represents partial obstruction of the

duodenum causing distention of the stomach and the first part of the duodenum. The absence of the ligament of Treitz on the upper gastrointestinal study almost clinches the diagnosis (malrotation of the bowel with volvulus), especially if it is associated with finding the duodenum to the right of the spine and a coiled appearance of the jejunum in the RUQ. *This is a true surgical emergency.*

32. **What is the most common surgically correctable cause of vomiting in infants?**
Pyloric stenosis. This is estimated to occur in about 1 in 400 births.

33. **What is pyloric stenosis? How does it present?**
Pyloric stenosis is a narrowing of the outflow tract of the stomach due to hypertrophy of the pyloric musculature. Pyloric stenosis is often found among first-born males, and males predominate by a factor of 4 to 5. There may be a family history for this condition. The infants are usually clinically normal at birth. In the typical history, the infant does well for the first few weeks of life, usually regaining birth weight. At about the third week of life, the infant starts to vomit, usually at the end of feedings. The vomiting eventually becomes projectile. It is typically nonbilious, though blood may be seen because of associated gastritis or esophagitis. Most patients present between 2–6 weeks of age. The infant is often described as hungry all the time, eating even after vomiting, because the infant cannot achieve adequate nutrition. In time, the infant may become profoundly dehydrated and emaciated.

> Dinkevich E, Ozuah PO: Pyloric stenosis. Pediatr Rev 21:249–250, 2000.
> Hernanz-Schulman M: Infantile hypertrophic pyloric stenosis. Radiology 227:319–331, 2003.

34. **How do you examine an infant with suspected pyloric stenosis?**
Examine the infant on his or her back, preferably on the parent's lap, and while he or she is quiet. Hold the infant's legs and flex them to 90 degrees at the hips to help relax the abdominal musculature. A bit of sugar or juice on a pacifier may help to relax the child. Begin the examination from below the liver, palpating in a rocking motion. A firm, ballotable mass may be felt in the region of the pylorus. This is the classic physical finding of pyloric stenosis—**the "olive."** If you cannot palpate an olive and still have a high suspicion for pyloric stenosis, ultrasonography is the test of choice.

> Hernanz-Schulman M: Infantile hypertrophic pyloric stenosis. Radiology 227:319–331, 2003.

35. **Where is the "olive" usually found?**
Usually it is found to the right, just below the xiphoid.

36. **What ultrasonography findings are associated with pyloric stenosis?**
Ultrasonography allows visualization of the hypertrophied pylorus muscle. If the pyloric canal lengthening is > 16 mm and the wall thickness is > 4 mm, suspect pyloric stenosis. Ultrasonography is quickly becoming the favored radiologic test for diagnosing pyloric stenosis because that it involves no radiation and no need to introduce barium into the gastrointestinal tract of a potential surgical candidate who is at high risk for aspiration.

> Hernanz-Schulman M: Infantile hypertrophic pyloric stenosis. Radiology 227:319–331, 2003.

37. **What is the classic laboratory finding in a child with pyloric stenosis?**
The classic finding is hypochloremic, hypokalemic metabolic alkalosis. Serum bicarbonate levels may be as high as 65–75 mEq/L. Acidosis usually signifies a more dangerous metabolic state due to extreme dehydration.

38. **How does the metabolic derangement occur?**
The metabolic alkalosis is due to loss of acid and retention of bicarbonate. Several mechanisms play a part in achieving this. Frequent vomiting leads to depletion of potassium chloride and

hydrogen chloride. Additionally, as intravascular volume decreases with prolonged vomiting and dehydration, the concentration of bicarbonate in the plasma increases, resulting in a contraction alkalosis. As plasma potassium levels fall because of gastric losses, potassium moves out of the cells to restore extracellular concentrations. Hydrogen ions then move into cells to maintain electroneutrality. The net result is metabolic alkalosis. Although the serum potassium level may be normal or low, total-body potassium is often depleted.

However, this is only part of the picture. The kidneys also play a role in the development of metabolic alkalosis. To maximize intravascular volume in the face of ongoing gastric losses, the kidneys reabsorb bicarbonate in the distal tubules despite alkalosis. If excess bicarbonate is excreted in the urine, it obligates sodium loss (think electroneutrality, again). Remember that water follows sodium, which would result in further volume loss. A lot of chloride has been lost through vomiting. Decreased delivery of chloride to the macula densa of the kidneys results in renin release and secondary hyperaldosteronism, leading to increased distal hydrogen secretion and the paradoxical finding of aciduria in the presence of a metabolic alkalosis. Finally, in response to the total-body depletion of potassium, the distal tubules reabsorb potassium in exchange for hydrogen, leading to further acid loss.

Dinkevich E, Ozuah PO: Pyloric stenosis. Pediatr Rev 21:249–250, 2000.

KEY POINTS: FINDINGS THAT REQUIRE IMMEDIATE SURGICAL CONSULTATION ✔

1. Strangulated hernia on physical examination

2. Distended abdomen and "double-bubble" sign on upright abdominal radiograph

3. Bilious emesis, especially in the first few months of life

4. Absence of the ligament of Treitz on upper gastrointestinal study

5. Ultrasonography findings consistent with ovarian torsion

39. **How is pyloric stenosis treated?**
    Initially, the infant's fluid and electrolyte status must be corrected with IV fluids. Once the infant is euvolemic and the electrolytes have returned to normal, a surgeon should perform a **pyloromyotomy**.

    Bachur RG: Abdominal emergencies. In Fleisher GR, Ludwig S, Henretig FM (eds): Textbook of Pediatric Emergency Medicine, 5th ed. Philadelphia, Lippincott Williams & Wilkins, 2006, pp 1605–1630.

40. **What are the most common surgically correctable causes of vomiting in the following infant age groups: First week of life? First month of life? Beyond the neonatal period?**
    - **In the first week of life**, consider anatomic malformations. Esophageal atresia, duodenal or jejunal atresia, duodenal stenosis, midgut malrotation, ileal atresia, and meconium ileus are the most common causes.
    - **In the first month of life**, consider pyloric stenosis and gastroesophageal reflux. As a general rule, gastroesophageal reflux can be managed medically. However, if medical management fails and the infant is failing to gain weight, bleeding, or aspirating, a surgical antireflux operation, such as a fundoplication, may be warranted. Other causes of vomiting in babies this age include Hirschsprung's disease, esophageal or intestinal webs, infection, increased intracranial pressure, and metabolic defects.

- **Beyond the neonatal period**, consider intussusception, appendicitis, and bowel obstruction caused by malrotation, incarcerated or strangulated hernia, duplication cysts, or Meckel's diverticulum.

  Moir CR: Abdominal pain in infants and children. Mayo Clin Proc 71:984–989, 1996

41. **What are the common causes of rectal bleeding in the pediatric age group? How do they present?**
    - **Fissures**. This is probably the most common cause. Often there is a history of constipation or passing a large, hard stool. The blood typically is bright red and found in streaks on the outside of the stool or on the toilet tissue. The diagnosis can be made by anal examination under a good light source. Treatment consists of sitz baths and lubrication of the rectal area with petroleum jelly. If the child suffers from constipation, address this as well.
    - **Juvenile polyps**. These occur in older infants and children in the lower part of the colon. They may be palpated on digital rectal examination and may bleed, especially if they break free. They are not premalignant, but they may serve as a lead point for intussusception.
    - **Meckel's diverticulum**. Remember the rule of 2s! Two percent of the population is born with a Meckel's diverticulum. It is usually located about 2 feet proximal to the terminal ileum. Also, only 2% of people with a Meckel's diverticulum have any clinical problems. Meckel's diverticuli usually contain ectopic gastric mucosa, and the acid secretion produces erosion at the junction of the normal ileal mucosa and the Meckel's mucosa. It may present with painless rectal bleeding, perforation with peritonitis, diverticulitis, or intussusception.
    - **Henoch-Schönlein purpura**. This type of vasculitis can cause symptoms ranging from painless rectal bleeding to abdominal pain and hematuria. The associated submucosal hemorrhage may also serve as a lead point for intussusception.
    - **Other causes**. Intestinal vascular malformations, intussusception, inflammatory bowel disease, duplications, swallowed blood, bleeding peptic ulcer disease, bleeding varices, and trauma.

42. **A 3-year-old child swallowed a safety pin that she found on the floor. You have located the object in her stomach on plain films, and the pin appears to be open. What do you do now?**
    Most foreign bodies that reach the stomach will pass completely through the gastrointestinal tract and be evacuated in the stool. Even an open safety pin may be allowed to pass. It is advisable to repeat an abdominal radiograph in about 5 days to be sure the pin has moved. Occasionally, a foreign body may get stuck at the junction of the duodenum and jejunum at the ligament of Treitz. These are usually long, thin objects such as bobby pins or long nails. Since perforation may occur, objects that "catch" beyond the pylorus should be removed surgically. Occasionally, objects get caught in the appendix, necessitating appendectomy. Obtain an x-ray in all children who have a history of swallowing a foreign body, both for the already mentioned reasons and to make sure that it is not lodged above the level of the thoracic inlet, where it could be aspirated if the child coughs.

43. **What is a vascular ring?**
    This is a congenital condition that causes airway or esophageal obstruction. The obstruction is usually at the level of the trachea, but a ductus arteriosus or a pulmonary artery sling can also compress the bronchi. Many of these rings are caused by failure of involution of various segments of the six embryologic aortic arches. Infants who present with stridor, recurrent pneumonia, or a history of noisy breathing since birth should prompt the consideration of this diagnosis.

44. **What is the difference between a pilonidal dimple and a pilonidal sinus?**
    Both are located in the midline in the sacrococcygeal area. Close inspection reveals that the dimple does not have a **central pore**, while the sinus does. The sinus is a tract lined by stratified

squamous epithelium that extends toward the spinal canal, but not into it. The sinus is asymptomatic until it becomes infected or obstructed, usually in adolescence. Predisposing factors are male sex, being overweight or hirsute, and a sedentary lifestyle. Once infection occurs, an abscess forms and expands deep to the skin surface. Patients usually report low back pain that is worse with sitting. They may also report localized tenderness. On examination, you will note a tender, indurated area in the sacrococcygeal region.

45. **How is a pilonidal abscess treated?**
Because these lesions typically expand inward, they must be incised and drained. Probe the abscess cavity to break up any loculations, and remove hair because it acts as a foreign body. Following incision and drainage, sitz baths and oral antimicrobial therapy (targeting staphylococcus, anaerobes, and fecal flora) are recommended. Once the inflammation has resolved, elective incision of the entire cyst and its sinus tracts is recommended.

46. **What is omphalitis?**
Omphalitis is an infection of a newborn's umbilical cord stump and the surrounding tissues, usually occurring in the first 2 weeks of life. Often, the infant initially presents with purulent, foul-smelling drainage from the umbilical stump and surrounding abdominal erythema, indicative of cellulitis. If the infection is not diagnosed and treated early, it can lead to more serious problems, such as peritonitis, liver abscess, or sepsis. The usual bacterial pathogens are *Streptococcus pyogenes*, *Staphylococcus aureus*, group B streptococcus, and gram-negative rods.

47. **How is omphalitis treated?**
If the findings are not clearly suggestive of omphalitis (i.e., there is minimal drainage or erythema), the infant can be treated at home with good skin and cord care (cleaning the cord with each diaper change and using topical antibiotics). Re-evaluation in 24 hours is recommended. Parents should be instructed to return for re-examination if the child has a change in feeding, activity, or disposition. If the infant appears toxic with obvious signs of omphalitis, he or she should be presumed to have a serious systemic infection. In this case, obtain appropriate laboratory evaluation for sepsis, admit, and treat with IV antibiotics.

48. **Why have physicians typically been taught not to use analgesics in patients being evaluated for abdominal pain?**
For almost a century, the teaching was to avoid pain relief for patients with abdominal pain to keep from masking the "true examination." When this idea was originally taught at the turn of the century (the 19th century, that is!), the clinician had only a physical examination and history upon which to base a diagnosis. To increase diagnostic accuracy, serial examinations were performed. In addition, few analgesics were available, and none of them were reversible. Given the limitations of the era, the rule of "no analgesics in abdominal pain" made sense. None of it, however, was evidence-based.

Fortunately, we now have many methods for evaluating abdominal pain, and the old teaching should be reassessed. Although history and physical examination remain foremost in the process of diagnosing the cause of abdominal pain, laboratory and radiologic evaluation allow physicians to assess the anatomy prior to surgery. And the analgesic options are better understood, often reversible, and more effective.

49. **Your 10-year-old patient with presumed appendicitis is in extreme pain. His tearful mother is asking if there is anything you can give him to make him feel better. The surgeons won't be available to examine him for another hour. What should you do?**
Providing pain relief for patients with abdominal pain is becoming more accepted because of increasing evidence. Studies in adults have shown that administration of opiates decreases

self-reported pain scores but does not hide evidence of peritoneal irritation. Studies in children are limited by small numbers of patients and serial observations by the same examiners, but suggest that opiate administration provides pain relief without adversely affecting the examination or the ability to diagnose children with surgical conditions.

Despite the growing evidence that opiate administration will not affect diagnostic accuracy, many experienced surgeons prefer to examine patients prior to administration of pain medication. It is important to respect the practice in your institution, while remaining aware of the current literature. Reassure your patient's mother that you will address the issue, and give your surgical colleagues a call to let them know your plan.

Kim MK, Galustyan S, Sato TT, Bergholte J, Hennes HH: Analgesia for children with abdominal pain: A survey of pediatric emergency physicians and pediatric surgeons. Pediatrics 111:1122–1126, 2003.

Kim MK, Strait RT, Sato TT, Hennes HM: A randomized clinical trial of analgesia in children with acute abdominal pain. Acad Emerg Med 9:281–287, 2002.

Kokki H, Lintula H, Vanamo K, Heiskanen M, Eskelinen M: Oxycodone vs placebo in children with undifferentiated abdominal pain. Arch Pediatr Adolesc Med 159:320–325, 2005.

CHAPTER 45

NEUROSURGICAL EMERGENCIES

Fred A. Fow, MD

1. **What is the basic pathophysiology of increased intracranial pressure?**
The theory is: The skull is a rigid compartment of fixed volume. Its three constituent parts are brain tissue, blood, and cerebrospinal fluid (CSF). Any increase in the volume of one of these constituents without a decrease in the volume of one or both of the other constituents must result in an increase in intracranial pressure (ICP) (modified Monro-Kelli hypothesis).

   Greenes DS: Neurotrauma. In Fleisher GR, Ludwig S, Henretig F (eds): Textbook of Pediatric Emergency Medicine, 5th ed. Philadelphia, Lippincott Williams & Wilkins, 2006, pp 1361–1388.

2. **How does increased ICP affect cellular survival?**
Cellular survival depends on cerebral blood flow delivering oxygen to meet cellular metabolic demand. Cerebral blood flow is related to cerebral perfusion pressure. Cerebral perfusion pressure (CPP) in turn is affected by changes in mean arterial pressure (MAP) or intracranial pressure ICP (CPP = MAP − ICP). Cerebrovascular autoregulation (reflex vasoconstriction/vasodilatation) allows cerebral blood flow to be maintained despite changes in cerebral perfusion pressure. Autoregulation prevents decreases in cerebral blood flow while MAP is greater than 60 mmHg and while ICP is < 40 mmHg. Outside these ranges, cerebral blood flow and oxygen delivery drop in a passively dependent fashion, resulting in cellular injury.

   Greenes DS: Neurotrauma. In Fleisher GR, Ludwig S, Henretig F (eds): Textbook of Pediatric Emergency Medicine, 5th ed. Philadelphia, Lippincott Williams & Wilkins, 2006, pp 1361–1388.

3. **What are the symptoms of increased ICP?**
   - Headache
   - Intellectual impairment
   - Stiff neck
   - Diplopia
   - Visual loss
   - Irritability
   - Vomiting

   Steele DW: Neurosurgical emergencies, nontraumatic. In Fleisher GR, Ludwig S, Henretig F (eds): Textbook of Pediatric Emergency Medicine, 5th ed. Philadelphia, Lippincott Williams & Wilkins, 2006, pp 1717–1725.

4. **What are the signs of increased ICP?**
   - Papilledema
   - Hyperresonance to percussion (cracked pot sound or MacEwen's sign)
   - Optic nerve atrophy
   - Cranial nerve palsies
   - Scalp vein enlargement, increased head size, suture separation, bulging fontanel
   - Cranial nerve IV: head tilt
   - Cranial nerve VI: sunset eyes
   - Decorticate or decerebrate posturing

- Altered mental status or level of consciousness
- Meningismus
- Hemiparesis
- Retinal hemorrhage
- Bradycardia, systemic hypertension, and irregular respirations (Cushing's triad)

Steele DW: Neurosurgical emergencies, nontraumatic. In Fleisher GR, Ludwig S, Henretig F (eds): Textbook of Pediatric Emergency Medicine, 5th ed. Philadelphia, Lippincott Williams & Wilkins, 2006, pp 1717–1725.

5. **What are the causes of increased ICP?**
   1. Increased CSF volume (hydrocephalus)
      Decreased absorption (communicating and noncommunicating hydrocephalus)
      - *Congenital*—Arnold-Chiari malformation, Dandy-Walker cyst, vein of Galen arteriovenous malformation
      - *Acquired*—Meningitis, tumor, leukemia, inflammatory response to intracranial hemorrhage
      Increased production
      - Choroid plexus papilloma—Rare
   2. Increased brain volume (cerebral edema)
      - Vasogenic—Tumor, abscess, hemorrhage
      - Cytotoxic—Hypoxia, ischemia, infection
      - Interstitial—Blockages in CSF absorption
   3. Mass lesions
      - Tumor
      - Abscess
      - Arteriovenous malformation
   4. Idiopathic (pseudotumor cerebri)

   Madikians A, Conway EE: Cerebrospinal fluid shunt problems in pediatric patients. Pediatr Neurosurg 26:613–620, 1997.

6. **Describe the initial management of increased ICP.**
   - Maintenance of airway, breathing, and circulation (**ABCs**) is paramount.
   - In the patient with suspected cervical spine trauma, **immobilization** is mandatory until cervical spine injury and spinal cord injury can be ruled out clinically and radiographically.

7. **What are the relevant features of airway management in patients with increased ICP?**
   - **Endotracheal intubation** allows for airway maintenance, protection from aspiration, maximal oxygenation, and control over ventilation. Rapid sequence induction (RSI) may help to prevent elevations in ICP and aspiration during intubation. The physician should be experienced in endotracheal intubation and have familiarity with RSI and with the specific indications and contraindications to the use of any of the agents used in RSI.
   - **Hyperventilation** causes cerebrovascular constriction, reducing cerebral blood volume and hence reducing ICP. Hyperventilation should be reserved for cases of impending herniation, as evidenced by severe alterations in mental status and vital signs changes or cases of increased ICP resistant to other modalities of treatment. Excessive or prolonged hyperventilation may result in cerebral ischemia and should be avoided.

8. **Which medications are recommended in the treatment of increased ICP?**
   - **Mannitol** may be used acutely to draw fluid from brain tissue in cases of impending herniation or cases of increased ICP resistant to other treatment modalities.
   - **Hypertonic saline** has been demonstrated to be an acceptable alternative to mannitol.

- **Dexamethasone** acts more slowly, but may be employed to reduce tissue edema, such as that accompanying tumor, brain abscess, and nontraumatic hemorrhage.
- **Acetazolamide** can be given to reduce CSF production but also has limited acute effect.

Adelson PD: Guidelines for the acute medical management of severe traumatic brain injury in infants, children and adolescents. Chapter 17. Critical pathway for the treatment of established intracranial hypertension in pediatric traumatic brain injury. Crit Care Med 4(3 Suppl):565–567, 2003.

Greenes DS: Neurotrauma. In Fleisher GR, Ludwig S, Henretig F (eds): Textbook of Pediatric Emergency Medicine, 5th ed. Philadelphia, Lippincott Williams & Wilkins, 2006, pp 1361–1388.

Steele DW: Neurosurgical emergencies, nontraumatic. In Fleisher GR, Ludwig S, Henretig F (eds): Textbook of Pediatric Emergency Medicine, 5th ed. Philadelphia, Lippincott Williams & Wilkins, 2006, pp 1717–1725.

9. **What steps can be taken to reduce metabolic demand?**
   - Adequate sedation helps to reduce oxygen demand and avoid any unwanted increases in ICP due to agitation.
   - Benzodiazepines, narcotics, and propofol should be used with caution because they may lower blood pressure and adversely affect cerebral perfusion pressure.
   - Barbiturate coma with pentobarbital reduces cerebral metabolic demand and ICP but requires aggressive pulmonary and hemodynamic management. As such, it is reserved for patients in whom other methods of ICP reduction have failed.
   - Paralysis may decrease oxygen consumption; however, this makes neurologic assessment, including recognition of seizures, problematic. Adequate sedation can obviate the need for paralysis. Avoidance of hyperthermia and of stimulation is also indicated.

Adelson PD: Guidelines for the acute medical management of severe traumatic brain injury in infants, children and adolescents. Chapter 17. Critical pathway for the treatment of established intracranial hypertension in pediatric traumatic brain injury. Crit Care Med 4(3 suppl):565–567, 2003.

Greenes DS: Neurotrauma. In Fleisher GR, Ludwig S, Henretig F (eds): Textbook of Pediatric Emergency Medicine, 5th ed. Philadelphia, Lippincott Williams & Wilkins, 2006, pp 1361–1388.

KEY POINTS: INCREASED INTRACRANIAL PRESSURE ✔

1. The first and most important step in the treatment of increased ICP, regardless of its cause, is maintenance of the ABCs.

2. Rapid sequence induction and endotracheal intubation allow for airway protection and help prevent elevation of ICP during intubation.

3. Hyperventilation should be reserved for cases of impending herniation.

4. Avoid excessive or prolonged hyperventilation.

5. Early recognition of signs and symptoms of increased ICP is very important if serious complications are to be avoided.

10. **What are the complications of CSF shunt placement in pediatric patients?**
    Shunt failure occurs in 30–40% of shunt placements within the first year of placement, 15% in the second year, and 1–7% per year thereafter.
    - **Shunt malfunction** is the most common complication of shunt placement. This is often a problem of underdrainage due to distal or proximal obstruction, but overdrainage can also occur. **Obstruction** can result from shunt infection, catheter blockage, valve problems, catheter disconnection, or catheter migration.

- **Shunt infection** occurs in 3–30% of shunt placements. Shunt failure as a result of malfunction or infection occurs in 30–40% of shunt placements within the first year of placement, 15% in the second year, and 1–7% per year thereafter.
- **Other complications** include scrotal or inguinal migration, small bowel obstruction, intussusception, omental cyst torsion, persistent hiccup, abdominal pseudocyst, volvulus, colon perforation, diaphragm perforation, intra-abdominal organ perforation, and subdural hemorrhage (from overdrainage and tearing of bridging veins or from surgery).

Garton HJ: Hydrocephalus. Pediatr Clin North Am 51:305–325, 2004.
Kestle JR: Pediatric hydrocephalus: Current management. Neurol Clin 21:883–895,vii, 2003.
Madikians A: Cerebrospinal fluid shunt problems in pediatric patients. Pediatr Neurosurg 26:613–620, 1997.

11. **What is the utility of "pumping a shunt" to test whether it is functioning properly?**
Evacuation and refill of the shunt reservoir by pumping the reservoir is one way of assessing the respective distal and proximal patency of the shunt. Unfortunately, by itself, this test has insufficient testing characteristics upon which to base the clinical decision to operate or not operate on a patient with a suspected shunt malfunction.

Garton HJ: Hydrocephalus. Pediatr Clin North Am 51:305–325, 2004.
Piatt JH: Physical examination of patients with cerebrospinal fluid shunts: Is there useful information in pumping the shunt? Pediatrics 89:470–473, 1992.
Piatt JH: Pumping the shunt revisited. A longitudinal study. Pediatr Neurosurg 25:73–76, 1996.

12. **Describe the approach to diagnosing CSF shunt malfunction.**
A patient with a CSF shunt with signs or symptoms of increased ICP, increasing or new seizures, or CSF swelling along the shunt path should be evaluated with a **shunt survey** (plain radiography of the shunt throughout its length) and **noncontrast head computed tomography (CT).**
Neck pain, syringomyelia, and lower cranial nerve palsy in myelodysplastic patients, and Parinaud syndrome (paralysis of conjugate upward eye movement without paralysis of convergence) in those with a history of neoplasm, may be other cues to shunt malfunction necessitating the same workup. The shunt survey helps to delineate the location and configuration of the shunt and to identify any disconnection.

13. **What is the value of head CT in evaluating for shunt malfunction?**
CT shows the size of the CSF ventricles, indicating how well CSF is being drained by the shunt, and provides a more detailed look at the brain anatomy and shunt placement. *Prior head CT is important for comparison of current ventricular size to baseline.* Although head CT is central to the evaluation of the patient with suspected shunt malfunction, it has its own limitations. In one report, 24% of patients with surgically proven shunt malfunction had CT readings that made no mention of shunt malfunction. In another study, 16% of such patients had studies that were interpreted as unchanged from baseline. In cases where shunt malfunction is suspected, CT is not a substitute for neurosurgical consultation.

Fein JA, Cronan KM, Posner JC: Approach to the care of the technology-assisted child. In Fleisher GR, Ludwig S, Henretig F (eds): Textbook of Pediatric Emergency Medicine, 5th ed. Philadelphia, Lippincott Williams & Wilkins, 2006, pp 1737–1758.
Garton HJ: Hydrocephalus. Pediatr Clin North Am 51:305–325, 2004.
Lee TL: Unique clinical presentation of shunt malfunction. Pediatr Neurosurg 30:122–126, 1999.
Srivastava R: Hospitalist care of the medically complex child. Pediatr Clin North Am 52:1165–1187, 2005.

14. **What is the treatment of CSF shunt malfunction?**
First, the ABCs. Then, measures to reduce ICP and metabolic demand (see questions 6 and 7). Specific pharmacologic interventions usually applicable here are acetazolamide and dexamethasone. More definitive therapy includes removal of CSF via shunt tap (effective with

distal obstruction only) or burr hole puncture (only in the case of proximal obstruction refractory to medical management and with life-threatening symptoms), and definitive shunt revision by a neurosurgeon.

Fein JA, Cronan KM, Posner JC: Approach to the care of the technology-assisted child. In Fleisher GR, Ludwig S, Henretig F (eds): Textbook of Pediatric Emergency Medicine, 5th ed. Philadelphia, Lippincott Williams & Wilkins, 2006, pp 1737–1758.

15. **What is the slit ventricle syndrome? How is it managed?**
This describes patients who have intermittent signs and symptoms of increased ICP despite small or unchanged ventricular size. Symptoms may arise from intermittent obstruction as the ventricular walls collapse around the catheter and obstruct drainage. As the ventricles fill with CSF, ICP rises. This opens the ventricles, allowing the shunt to function again. As might be expected, symptoms are worse when standing and are alleviated by lying down. Analgesia and a short course of steroids may be useful. Neurosurgical intervention is sometimes necessary.

Kestle JR: Pediatric hydrocephalus: Current management. Neurol Clinics 21:883–895, 2003.
Madikians A: Cerebrospinal fluid shunt problems in pediatric patients. Pediatr Neurosurg 26:613–620, 1997.

16. **When is shunt infection most likely to occur?**
Most shunt infections occur soon after shunt placement. Half occur within 2 weeks, 70–80% within 2 months, and 80–90% within 4 months.

Srivastava R: Hospitalist care of the medically complex child. Pediatr Clin North Am 52:1165–1187, 2005.

17. **List the symptoms and signs of shunt infection.**
Signs and symptoms of shunt infection include fever, cellulitis, headache, irritability, nausea, vomiting, lethargy, mental status change, feeding problems, bulging fontanel, seizure, diarrhea, ileus, abdominal tenderness (peritonitis), and shunt malfunction. Meningismus may be absent.
Sites of infection include the shunt lumen, the extraluminal ventricles, and the proximal and distal surgical sites. Abdominal pseudocysts can result from infection or become secondarily infected.

Srivastava R: Hospitalist care of the medically complex child. Pediatr Clin North Am 52:1165–1187, 2005.

18. **What are the typical CSF findings in shunt infection?**
CSF pleocytosis is often present in shunt infections, although it can be seen as a result of inflammation rather than infection in the early postoperative period, when many infections occur. In addition, the pleocytosis may be modest, as bacteria such as coagulase-negative staphylococcus, a common pathogen in shunt infections, may be protected from the body's immune response. Some evidence suggests that the combination of fever and CSF neutrophilia ($>$ 10% neutrophils) is highly specific (99%) and has high positive and negative predictive values (93% and 95%, respectively) for detecting or excluding shunt infection.

Lan CC: Early diagnosis of ventriculoperitoneal shunt infections and malfunctions in children with hydrocephalus. J Microbiology Immunol Infect 36:47–50, 2003.
McClinton D: Predictors of ventriculoperitoneal shunt pathology. Pediatr Infect Dis J 20:593–59, 2001.
Shah SS: Device related infections in children. Pediatr Clin North Am 52:1189–1208, 2005.

19. **Can a patient have a shunt infection with normal spinal fluid collected by lumbar puncture?**
Yes. If the ventricles are not communicating with the lumbar spinal fluid, ventriculitis may not be detectable by collection of lumbar spinal fluid.

Shah SS: Device related infections in children. Pediatr Clin North Am 52:1189–1208, 2005.

20. **Does bacteremia commonly accompany ventriculoperitoneal shunt infection?**
No. Bacteremia is unusual in cases of ventriculoperitoneal shunt infection. The shunt is not directly connected with the vascular system. Also, patients requiring shunt placement appear to have impaired CSF reabsorption into the venous system.

Shah SS: Device related infections in children. Pediatr Clin North Am 52:1189–1208, 2005.

21. **Which organisms cause shunt infections, and what is the treatment for shunt infection?**
Staphylococcus epidermidis and *S. aureus* (including methicillin-resistant strains) account for approximately 70% of infections and are the most likely pathogens in the early postoperative period, responsible for 85% of infections occurring in the first 15 days after shunt placement. Such infections are thought to result from intraoperative contamination.
   Gram-negative pathogens, including *Pseudomonas aeruginosa*, account for about 15% of infections. Infection with gram-negative organisms is more likely to occur outside the initial postoperative period. Such infections are thought to result from ascending infection from the distal portion of the shunt.
   Initial empiric treatment may include vancomycin to cover *S. epidermidis* and *S. aureus* (including methicillin-resistant strains) plus ceftazidime or a fluoroquinolone to cover gram-negative organisms, including *Pseudomonas aeruginosa*.

Shah SS: Device related infections in children. Pediatr Clin North Am 52:1189–1208, 2005.

22. **What are some historical clues to identifying a patient with a brain tumor?**
The diagnosis of brain tumor is often delayed because presenting symptoms are nonspecific and common to other childhood illnesses and conditions. Clues from the history that should prompt consideration of further evaluation, such as intracranial imaging, include vomiting (especially without fever, abdominal pain, or alteration in bowel pattern), headache, vision change (loss, diplopia, or blurriness), loss of milestones, seizures, neuroendocrine dysfunction, motor weakness, sensory change, speech problems, abnormal infantile hand preference, and neck pain or torticollis.
   Less specific clues include irritability, listlessness, failure to thrive, behavioral disturbances, and appetite disturbances.

23. **What clues from the physical examination may suggest a brain tumor?**
Focal neurologic deficits, including cranial neuropathy, visual abnormalities (loss of visual acuity, field loss, afferent papillary defect, or nystagmus), ataxia, loss of coordination or balance, upper motor neuron signs (hyperreflexia, clonus, and paraparesis), weakness, sensory change, funduscopic evidence of increased ICP, and macrocephaly, are important to recognize and warrant investigation. A few specific syndromes of note include Parinaud syndrome (paresis of upward gaze, pupillary dilatation reactive to accommodation but not to light, nystagmus to convergence or retraction and eyelid retraction) suggestive of pineal region tumor and diencephalic syndrome (infantile failure to thrive, emaciation, increased appetite, and euphoric affect).

Dobrovoljac M, Hengartner H, Boltshauser E, et al: Delay in the diagnosis of paediatric brain tumours. Eur J Paediatr 161:663–667, 2002.
Kottesch JF, Ater J: Brain tumors in childhood. In Kliegman RM, Behrman RE, Jenson HB (eds): Nelson Textbook of Pediatrics, 17th ed, 2004. Philadelphia, Saunders, pp 1702–1709.
Ullrich NJ: Pediatric brain tumors. Neurol Clin 21:897–913, 2003.

24. **Headache is a very common pediatric symptom. What are the historical features of headache that should prompt concern for brain tumor?**
Recurrent morning headaches; headaches awakening the child from sleep; intense, prolonged, incapacitating headaches; and changes in headache quality, frequency, and pattern are the

classic distinguishing features of "brain tumor headaches" described by Honig and Charney in 1982. Other features of headache that should raise concern are associated vomiting; exacerbation by bending, coughing, laughing, or the Valsalva maneuver; and posterior headache.

Honig P, Charney EB: Children with brain tumor headaches—distinguishing features. Am J Dis Child 136:122–124, 1982.

Piatt JH: Recognizing neurosurgical conditions in the pediatrician's office. Pediatr Clin North Am 51: 327–357, 2004.

KEY POINTS: CHARACTERISTICS OF BRAIN TUMOR HEADACHES ✔

1. Recurrent morning headaches

2. Prolonged incapacitating headaches

3. Changes in headache quality, frequency, and pattern

25. **What are the predisposing factors that may lead to brain abscess?**
Hematogenous spread is the most common source of brain abscess in children. Cyanotic congenital heart disease is an important risk factor in this regard. Endocarditis (especially left-sided and acute), deep neck vein phlebitis from parapharyngeal infection (Lemierre disease), and chronic pyogenic lung disease are also potential sources. Other sources of hematogenous spread include focal suppurative infections of bone, teeth, or the abdomen. Brain abscess can follow endoscopy as a result of spinal venous plexus contamination. Contiguous spread is the second most common source of brain abscess and can occur from infections of the middle ear, sinus, orbit, face, or scalp. Most patients with bacterial meningitis do not develop brain abscess. Penetrating skull injury, open skull fracture, recent neurosurgery, intracerebral hematoma, and neoplasm are other possible sources for brain abscess.

26. **What are the possible factors leading to subdural empyema and epidural abscesses?**
   - **Subdural empyema:** In young children, the usual source for subdural empyema is direct spread of infection from the meninges. In older children and adolescents, the usual source is contiguous spread through linking emissary veins from extracranial sites following otitis media, sinusitis, or osteomyelitis of the skull. Other causes cited include infection related to prior craniotomy, skull trauma, ventriculoperitoneal shunt, preexisting hematoma, halo-pin traction, hematogenous spread (such as from the lung), or endoscopic procedures.
   - **Epidural abscess:** Cranial epidural abscess is rare. Its usual source is contiguous spread of infection from sinusitis, otitis media, orbital cellulitis, or osteomyelitis of the skull, or following neurosurgical procedures or penetrating skull injuries. Epidural abscess has also been reported as a complication of fetal scalp monitoring.

   The source for spinal epidural abscess is usually hematogenous spread of infection from skin, soft tissue, bone, or the respiratory or urinary tract. Direct extension from local osteomyelitis, retropharyngeal, retroperitoneal, or abdominal abscess is another potential source. Penetrating injury and spinal surgery are also potential sources.

Yogev R: Focal suppurative infections of the central nervous system. In Long SS, Pickering LK, Prober CG (eds): Principles and Practice of Pediatric Infectious Diseases. New York, Churchill Livingstone, 2003, pp 302–312.

27. **What are some of the clues that can help identify brain abscesses?**
Unfortunately, the presentation of brain abscess in children is often nonspecific initially.
Common initial symptoms include headache, fever, and vomiting. Seizures, mental status
change, coma, focal neurologic deficits, papilledema, meningeal signs, and hemiparesis are
other clues. Unfortunately, most of these occur in less than half of patients with brain abscess
and may not manifest themselves initially. As unilateral headache is unusual in children, its
presence should also raise concern for the presence of brain abscess.

Yogev R: Focal suppurative infections of the central nervous system. In Long SS, Pickering LK, Prober CG
(eds): Principles and Practice of Pediatric Infectious Diseases. New York, Churchill Livingstone, 2003,
pp 302–312.

28. **Describe the laboratory findings in focal suppurative intracranial infections.**
Common blood test indicators of infection and inflammation, such as leukocytosis, left shift,
and elevated erythrocyte sedimentation rates (ESR) and CRP levels, are of limited usefulness in
diagnosing or excluding the presence of suppurative intracranial infections. An elevated CRP
level may be a better indicator of infection in this setting than leukocytosis or elevated ESR;
however, elevated CRP levels, like elevated WBC counts and ESR, are not specific to intracranial
infection, limiting its use. Although blood cultures are positive in only about 10% of cases,
they should be considered.

CSF can be normal or nonspecifically abnormal (mild to moderately elevated WBC count,
neutrophil predominance, low glucose and elevated protein levels). The rate of positive cultures in
brain abscess may be as low as 10%; the exceptions are concurrent meningitis or abscess rupture
into the subarachnoid space. Moreover, if focal intracranial infection is suspected, lumbar puncture
is contraindicated until CT or magnetic resonance imaging (MRI) has excluded increased ICP.

Yogev R: Focal suppurative infections of the central nervous system. In Long SS, Pickering LK, Prober CG
(eds): Principles and Practice of Pediatric Infectious Diseases. New York, Churchill Livingstone, 2003,
pp 302–312.

29. **What is the diagnostic modality of choice for focal suppurative central nervous
system (CNS) infections?**
CT (contrast-enhanced) or MRI is mandatory if the clinician is considering a focal
suppurative CNS infection. MRI is superior to CT for both intracranial and spinal
investigation. Consultation with a radiologist is helpful in choosing the correct study for
a specific patient.

Stevens JM, Hall-Craggs MA, "Kling" Chong WK, et al: Cranial and intracranial pathology (2): Infections;
AIDS; inflammatory, demyelinating and metabolic diseases. In Grainger & Allison's Diagnostic Radiology:
A Textbook of Medical Imaging, 4th ed. New York, Churchill Livingstone, 2001, pp 2377–2391.
Yogev R: Focal suppurative infections of the central nervous system. In Long SS, Pickering LK, Prober CG
(eds): Principles and Practice of Pediatric Infectious Diseases. New York, Churchill Livingstone, 2003,
pp 302–312.

30. **What is the treatment for focal suppurative CNS infections?**
The ABCs are the first priority, along with institution of measures to control increased ICP.
It is important to obtain the assistance of infectious disease and neurosurgical consultants.
Antibiotics are indicated in all cases. The initial choice of antibiotics may be driven by knowledge
of predisposing conditions and therefore likely pathogens. The extent of surgical treatment
will depend on the specific site of infection and other aspects of each individual case.
Corticosteroids may be indicated in limited instances for brain abscess, specifically in cases
where edema has resulted in increased ICP or neurologic deterioration.

Yogev R: Focal suppurative infections of the central nervous system. In Long SS, Pickering LK, Prober CG
(eds): Principles and Practice of Pediatric Infectious Diseases. New York, Churchill Livingstone, 2003,
pp 302–312.

31. **What are some causes of stroke in children?**

    General etiologic categories include cardiac abnormalities, hematologic abnormalities, coagulopathies, vascular anomalies, venous infarcts, metabolic disorders, vasculitides, vasospastic events, and trauma. Sickle cell disease and cardiovascular disease are the most common causes of childhood stroke. When considering hemorrhagic stroke alone, arteriovenous malformation is the most common cause.

    > Carlin TM, Chanmugam A: Stroke in children. Emerg Med Clin North Am 20:671–685, 2002.
    > Gorelick MH, Blackwell CD: Neurologic emergencies. In Fleisher GR, Ludwig S, Henretig F (eds): Textbook of Pediatric Emergency Medicine, 5th ed. Philadelphia, Lippincott Williams & Wilkins, 2006, pp 759–781.

32. **What is the initial evaluation for suspected stroke?**

    Noncontrast head CT is a reasonable first study in the emergency department (ED) because it will identify hemorrhage. Unfortunately, it may not detect an ischemic event in its early stages and provides limited evaluation of the posterior fossa. MRI is a better study in both regards and should be performed if the noncontrast CT is normal.

33. **What are the next steps in the diagnostic work-up for stroke?**

    The work-up that follows the initial evaluation above is directed at identifying the cause for the hemorrhage or ischemia. Such an evaluation may include additional brain imaging (magnetic resonance angiography/magnetic resonance venography/transfontanel Doppler), cardiovascular evaluation (electrocardiography, chest radiography, echocardiography, transesophageal echocardiography, bubble contrast echocardiography), and laboratory evaluation (complete blood count, electrolytes, drug screen, prothrombin time/partial thromboplastin time/international normalized ratio, anticardiolipin antibodies, lupus anticoagulants, ESR, antinuclear antibody, and screening for antithrombin III, protein C and protein S deficiencies, factor V Leiden mutation, and prothrombin 20210 polymorphism).

    > Carlin TM, Chanmugam A: Stroke in children. Emerg Med Clin North Am 20:671–685, 2002.
    > Gorelick MH, Blackwell CD: Neurologic emergencies. In Fleisher GR, Ludwig S, Henretig F (eds): Textbook of Pediatric Emergency Medicine, 5th ed. Philadelphia, Lippincott Williams & Wilkins, 2006, pp 759–781.

34. **What is the treatment for stroke?**

    The ABCs are the first priority. Control seizures and hyperthermia. Avoid free water overload if fluid resuscitation is required. Avoid hypoglycemia and hyperglycemia. Additional treatment depends on the type of stroke and specific etiology. Neurosurgical intervention may be necessary in cases of hemorrhagic stroke.

    > Carlin TM, Chanmugam A: Stroke in children. Emerg Med Clin North Am 20:671–685, 2002.
    > Gorelick MH, Blackwell CD: Neurologic emergencies. In Fleisher GR, Ludwig S (eds): Textbook of Pediatric Emergency Medicine, 5th ed. Philadelphia, Lippincott Williams & Wilkins, 2006, pp 759–781.

35. **What are the common signs and symptoms of nontraumatic spinal cord compression in the pediatric patient?**

    Back pain is an important clue. Weakness, increased or absent tendon reflexes, extensor Babinski reflex, symmetric loss of sensation with a sensory level, and sphincter abnormalities (late) are common signs of cord compression from a space-occupying lesion. Conus medullaris and cauda equina compression may also be associated with abnormalities in sensory-motor function, tendon reflexes, Babinski reflex, and sphincter function.

    > Rheingold SR, Lange, BJ: Oncologic emergencies. In Pizzo PA, Poplack DG (eds): Principles and Practice of Pediatric Oncology, 4th ed. Philadelphia, Lippincott Williams & Wilkins, 2002, pp 1177–1203.
    > Schiff D: Spinal cord compression. Neurol Clin 21:67–86, 2003.

36. **What is the ED approach to suspected nontraumatic spinal cord compression?**

A space-occupying lesion must be ruled out if spinal cord compression is suspected. As such, imaging is the cornerstone of the initial evaluation of such patients. Plain films are not sensitive enough in this setting. Emergent MRI is the preferred diagnostic tool. If a tumor is identified and there has been rapid progression of symptoms or there is a clear cord-level deficit, initiate high-dose corticosteroids without delay. Consultation with a neurosurgeon and an oncologist are crucial. Spinal epidural abscess and subdural abscess mandate the immediate involvement of a neurosurgeon as well.

Rheingold SR, Lange BJ: Oncologic emergencies. In Pizzo PA, Poplack DG (eds): Principles and Practice of Pediatric Oncology, 4th ed. Philadelphia, Lippincott Williams & Wilkins, 2002, pp 1177–1203.

Schiff D: Spinal cord compression. Neurol Clin 21:67–86, 2003.

CHAPTER 46

OPHTHALMOLOGIC EMERGENCIES

Kathy Palmer, MD

1. **What is an afferent pupillary defect?**
   The pupillary light reflex is a reflex arc through the midbrain involving crossover innervation. It is assessed with the swinging light test: Shining a light in one eye should result in constriction of both pupils. No change in pupillary size should be noted when the light swings toward the other pupil. If a patient has an afferent pupillary defect, both pupils dilate when the light swings to the affected eye. The abnormal pupil, called a Marcus Gunn pupil, can result from retinal artery or venous occlusions, retinal detachment, tumors, or ischemic optic neuropathy.

   Wright KW: Pupil and iris abnormalities. In Pediatric Ophthalmology for Pediatricians. Baltimore, Williams & Wilkins, 1999, pp 139–149.

2. **What is the Bruckner test? How is it performed?**
   The Bruckner test is a simultaneous bilateral red reflex test that elicits both a corneal light reflex and a red reflex. View the patient's eyes from about 2 feet away with a broad beam of light that encompasses both eyes. You should see both a red reflex and a small white light reflex in each eye. The key to a normal examination is symmetry. An absent or dull red reflex may indicate vitreous hemorrhage, cataract, hyphema, opacity of the cornea, enophthalmos (backward displacement of the globe in the orbit), or misalignment of the globe.

   Garcia SE, Hickey R, Santamaria JP: Pediatric ocular trauma. Pediatr Emerg Med Rep Oct:87–98, 1998.

3. **What is the differential diagnosis of papilledema?**
   Papilledema is caused by anything that increases intracranial pressure. It is usually bilateral.
   - Increased cerebrospinal fluid production
   - Decreased cerebrospinal fluid absorption
   - Intracranial mass
   - Obstruction of venous outflow
   - Obstructive hydrocephalus
   - Idiopathic intracranial hypertension (pseudotumor cerebri)

   Giovannini J: Papilledema: www.emedicine.com

4. **List and describe briefly the four types of orbital wall fractures.**
   - **Medial wall fractures** are caused by blows to the bridge of the nose. Physical findings include orbital emphysema, epistaxis, depressed nasal bridge, and enophthalmos (sunken eye). Excessive tearing may be seen if the lacrimal system is disrupted.
   - **Orbital floor ("blowout") fractures** result when an object larger than the orbital diameter, often in the inferior lateral orbital rim, impacts the bony orbit. The impact causes increased intraorbital pressure and rupture of the orbital floor, which often is associated with prolapse of orbital contents into the maxillary sinus. Entrapment of the inferior rectus muscle causes limitation of upward gaze. Infraorbital nerve injury causes hypesthesia of the ipsilateral cheek and upper lip. Traumatic optic neuropathy can complicate an orbital floor fracture with immediate loss of vision and afferent pupillary defect.
   - **Superior wall (orbital roof) fractures** are less common than medial or floor fractures but they are potentially life-threatening. They may be associated with central nervous system injury,

pneumocephalus, or intracranial foreign body. Potential complications include brain abscess and meningitis. Findings include rhinorrhea (cerebrospinal fluid leak) and superior and lateral subconjunctival hemorrhage.

- **Tripod fractures** involve the zygomatic arch and its lateral and inferior orbital rim articulations. Examination findings are similar to those of orbital floor fractures, along with limitation of mandibular movement and trismus.

  Garcia SE, Hickey R, Santamaria JP: Pediatric ocular trauma. Pediatr Emerg Med Rep Oct:87–98, 1998.
  Widell T: Fractures, orbital: www.emedicine.com

5. How are orbital fractures managed?

Therapeutic interventions for any orbital fracture include antibiotic prophylaxis, nasal decongestants, and ice packs; some fractures may require surgical intervention. Computed tomography of the orbit, including axial and coronal views, is useful in diagnosis and delineating the extent of injury. All patients should be cautioned to avoid blowing their nose. Consultation with an ophthalmologist is indicated.

  Levin AV: Eye trauma. In Fleisher GR, Ludwig S (eds): Textbook of Pediatric Emergency Medicine, 5th ed. Philadelphia, Lippincott Williams & Wilkins, 2000, pp 1485–1496.
  Widell T: Fractures, orbital: www.emedicine.com

6. What is the difference between monocular and binocular diplopia?

Binocular diplopia resolves when either eye is covered. With monocular diplopia, double vision is present even when one eye is covered.

7. What causes binocular and monocular diplopia?

The causes of binocular diplopia include blowout fracture, traumatic cranial nerve palsies, iris injuries, inflammation, neoplasm, and strabismus. The causes of monocular diplopia include uncorrected refractory error, cataract, displaced lens, and conversion disorder.

8. What are "raccoon eyes"? What causes them?

Raccoon eyes result from eyelid ecchymoses, which classically are associated with basilar skull fractures. Subcutaneous bleeding occurs in the area around the orbits.

9. List the eye emergencies that warrant ophthalmologic consultation.

- Ruptured globe
- Orbital hematoma
- Severe chemical burns
- Hyphema
- Retinal/vitreous detachment
- Intraocular foreign bodies
- Contact lens abrasions
- Complicated eyelid lacerations

10. What is the Seidel test? How is it performed?

A fluorescein strip touched to the lacerated area of the eye will show a stream of fluorescein, indicating an active leak of aqueous humor and full-thickness injury to the eye. A negative Seidel test does not exclude full-thickness injury because small injuries can self-seal. Full-thickness lacerations should be treated with a rigid eye shield and emergent ophthalmologic consultation.

11. While attempting to repair a superficial forehead laceration, some of the cyanoacrylate glue drips into the child's eye and his lashes are stuck together. How should this patient be managed?

Cyanoacrylate glue rarely causes a serious injury to the eye. Usually, the child manages to close the eye as the glue approaches and the lashes may be stuck together, but the eye is generally unharmed. The lashes can be separated by applying mineral oil or petroleum jelly to the glued area and allowing this to remain in place for 30–60 minutes. It is important to be patient and not to forcefully pull the lids apart. Use of gentle friction with a cotton swab may be helpful. Avoid the use of acetone to dissolve the glue as this could injure the eye. Ophthalmologic consultation is rarely needed.

12. **A teenager who was not wearing protective eyewear reports a "foreign body sensation" in his eye after hammering (metal on metal). How should this patient be managed?**

With this history, the emergency physician should be suspicious of an intraocular foreign body that penetrated the cornea or sclera. The physical examination of the eye can be deceiving because the globe heals quickly and a laceration may not be visualized. Subtle signs, such as red eye, pupil asymmetry, and decreased vision, may be noted. However, small particles that rapidly penetrate the eye may produce few or no signs, and a high index of suspicion is needed. Consult the ophthalmology service urgently. Consider computed tomography to look for a foreign body (not magnetic resonance imaging if the foreign body might be metallic).

Neylan V, Eilbert WP: Ocular emergencies. Foresight 43; 1998, pp 1–8.
Selbst SM: Pediatric emergency medicine legal briefs. Pediatr Emerg Care 18:133–136, 2002.

13. **How is a hyphema classified?**

A hyphema is a collection of blood in the anterior chamber of the eye caused by compression of the eyeball and tearing of the anterior ciliary body. Hyphemas are classified by estimating the volume of the anterior chamber of the eye that is occupied by blood:

Grade I: $< \frac{1}{3}$ Grade III: $> \frac{1}{2}$

Grade II: $\frac{1}{3} - \frac{1}{2}$ Grade IV: complete

The higher the grade of the hyphema, the greater the risk for rebleeding (15% in grade I, 60% in grades II and III).

Garcia SE, Hickey R, Santamaria JP: Pediatric ocular trauma. Pediatr Emerg Med Rep Oct:87–98, 1998.

14. **Who should you consider hospitalizing for treatment of a hyphema?**
   - Patients with hyphemas $> \frac{1}{3}$ of the anterior chamber
   - Patients with evidence of increased intraocular pressure
   - Patients with sickle cell disease
   - Patients in social situations that preclude close outpatient follow-up

Garcia SE, Hickey R, Santamaria JP: Pediatric ocular trauma. Pediatr Emerg Med Rep Oct:87–98, 1998.
Sheppard J: Hyphema: www.emedicine.com

15. **What is an "8-ball" hyphema?**

The entire anterior chamber of the eye is occupied by blood, resembling the 8-ball in pool.

16. **Why is a burn from an alkali more damaging to the eye than an acid burn?**

The pH of the chemical that splashes in the eye is related to severity of injury. Alkali solutions tend to be more damaging because they penetrate more deeply. Acidic solutions coagulate proteins in the superficial layers of the eye, forming a protective barrier against further penetration. The severity of the injury is also related to the volume and duration of exposure.

Garcia SE, Hickey R, Santamaria JP: Pediatric ocular trauma. Pediatr Emerg Med Rep Oct:87–98, 1998.
Chen A: Burns, ocular: www.emedicine.com

17. **Which corneal abrasions are most worrisome? Why?**

Corneal abrasions over the visual axis, abrasions in patients with a history of ocular herpes, and corneal abrasions in contact lens wearers. Abrasions caused by contact lens use predispose the patient to fungal and bacterial infections and corneal ulceration.

18. **Which of the following therapeutic interventions are indicated for the treatment of corneal abrasions?**

A. Eye patching
B. Topical mydriatics
C. Topical antibiotics
D. Topical nonsteroidal anti-inflammatory drugs
E. Topical anesthetics

Answer: C and D. Traditional therapies for corneal abrasions have included eye patching and topical mydriatics. Current recommendations are based upon the results of randomized controlled trials. These studies showed that:

1. Patching did not improve healing time or pain. Patching can also cause increased difficulty in walking in pediatric patients. It also decreases oxygen delivery, increases moisture, and thereby brings a risk of infection.
2. Topical mydriatics were used to treat pain from ciliary spasm. A randomized controlled trial showed that pain was similar with or without mydriatics.
3. Topical anesthetics have never been indicated after the initial eye examination.

Current treatment recommendations include the use of topical antibiotics and pain control with either topical or oral analgesics. Patients using topical nonsteroidal anti-inflammatory drugs (NSAIDs) reported greater relief from pain and other symptoms. Examples of topical NSAIDs include diclofenac (Voltaren) and ketorolac (Acular). Some clinicians use prophylactic topical antibiotics for treatment of corneal abrasions. Ointments are more lubricating than drops. Antipseudomonal coverage should be used in contact lens wearers, and lens use should be discontinued until the abrasion is healed and antibiotic therapy is complete.

Wilson SA: Management of corneal abrasions Am Family Physician 70:123–128, 2004.
Weaver CS, Terrell KM: Evidence based emergency medicine update. Do ophthalmic nonsteroidal anti-inflammatory drugs reduce the pain associated with simple corneal abrasions without delaying healing? Ann Emerg Med 41:134–140, 2003.

19. **What are the symptoms of retinal detachment?**

A retinal detachment is a separation between the sensory and pigment portions of the retina. Symptoms include "flashes," "floaters," and visual defects. Flashes of light are caused by traction at the peripheral retina. Floaters are caused by fibrous aggregates on the posterior portion of the vitreous that block light to the retina. Blurred vision and a dull red reflex are caused by vitreous hemorrhage. All patients who report flashes or floaters should be evaluated by an ophthalmologist to prevent progression of partial retinal tears to complete detachment. Traumatic damage to the retina often is located at the periphery of the retina, an area that is not easily examined with a direct ophthalmoscope. Any significant blunt eye trauma warrants evaluation by an ophthalmologist.

Garcia SE, Hickey R, Santamaria JP: Pediatric ocular trauma. Pediatr Emerg Med Rep Oct:87–98, 1998.
Larkin GL: Retinal detachment: www.emedicine.com

20. **What are the symptoms of lens dislocation?**

Symptoms of subluxation/dislocation of the lens include monocular diplopia, glare, and decreased visual acuity. A classic sign of lens dislocation is a tremulous iris. If the lens edge lies within the visual field, it may cause monocular diplopia or astigmatism. Lens subluxations may remain asymptomatic for weeks after the initial trauma, thereby making them difficult to diagnose. Rupture of the lens capsule rapidly results in cataract formation.

Eifrig C: Ectopia lentis: www.emedicine.com
Garcia SE, Hickey R, Santamaria JP: Pediatric ocular trauma. Pediatr Emerg Med Rep Oct:87–98, 1998.

21. **Which sports are associated with a high risk for eye injuries?**
    - Paintball and air rifle or BB gun
    - Basketball
    - Baseball/softball
    - Cricket
    - Lacrosse
    - Ice, field, and street hockey
    - Squash and racquetball
    - Fencing
    - Boxing, wrestling, and full-contact martial arts

    Committee on Sports Medicine and Fitness in Pediatrics: Protective eyewear for young athletes. Pediatrics 113:619–622, 2004.

22. **How are bungee cords related to eye emergencies?**
    Eye injuries resulting from bungee cords are becoming increasingly common. The bungee cords are elastic with metallic hooks at either end (sometimes padded). They are often used in occupational and recreational settings. They can snap back with tremendous force and cause blunt and penetrating trauma to the eye. In a study at Wills Eye Hospital in Philadelphia, the most common related injuries were hyphemas (63%), but 10% of patients had sustained open globe injuries and some required enucleation.

    Aldave AJ, Gertner GS, Davis GH, et al: Bungee cord associated ocular trauma. Ophthalmology 108:788–792, 2001.

23. **What are the current recommendations for use of protective eyewear in athletes?**
    Appropriately fitted protective eyewear has been shown to decrease the incidence of injury by 90%. The American Academy of Pediatrics and the American Academy of Ophthalmology recommend eye protection for all athletes and mandate it in functionally one-eyed patients and in patients whose ophthalmologist recommends eye protection after surgery or trauma. *Functionally one-eyed* is defined as best corrected visual acuity of less than 20/40 in the weaker eye.

    Recommendations for the appropriate protective eyewear for each sport can be found in the American Academy of Pediatrics policy referenced below and on the website for the Protective Eyewear Certification Council.

    Committee on Sports Medicine and Fitness in Pediatrics: Protective eyewear for young athletes. Pediatrics 113:619–622, 2004.
    Protective Eyewear Certification Council. Available at: www.protecteyes.org
    Prevent Blindness America. Available at: www.preventblindness.org

24. **What is the best solution to use for ocular decontamination after a chemical injury?**
    Traditional first aid teaches that tap water is an acceptable irrigant for immediate treatment of a foreign body or chemical in the eye. In the emergency department setting, the most common irrigant is normal saline solution (pH, 4.5–6.0). Other acceptable alternatives include lactated Ringers solution (pH, 6.2–7.5), buffered normal saline (pH, 7.4), and balanced salt solution plus (BSS Plus; pH, 7.4). Theoretically, irrigation solutions with a more neutral pH will provide less discomfort during prolonged irrigations.

    Saidinejad M: Ocular irrigant alternatives in pediatric emergency medicine. Pediatr Emerg Care 21:23–26, 2005.

KEY POINTS: EYE TRAUMA ✓

1. Always attempt to document the visual acuity in assessing a patient with a complaint related to the eye.

2. Emergent consultation with an ophthalmologist is indicated for any patient with a potentially ruptured globe. Place a rigid eye shield and keep the patient calm and receiving nothing by mouth.

3. Appropriately fitted protective eyewear can reduce the risk of ocular injury by 90%.

4. Patients with hyphemas should have the head of their bed elevated to facilitate settling of blood in the anterior chamber.

5. Patients with potential orbital fractures should be cautioned to refrain from blowing their nose.

CHAPTER 47

ORTHOPEDIC EMERGENCIES

Fred A. Fow, MD

1. **Describe the presentation of osteomyelitis.**

   Fever, pain, and decreased use of the involved extremity are common manifestations of osteomyelitis. There may be accompanying signs of systemic illness, such as anorexia, malaise, and vomiting. Infants may exhibit decreased feeding, irritability, or listlessness. Pain may be manifested in neonates as pseudoparalysis. Examination findings include focal swelling, warmth, tenderness, and erythema, often metaphyseal in location. Neonates and younger children are more prone than older patients to present with secondary joint involvement. Proximal humerus and proximal femur infections involve the joint as a result of their intracapsular location. When there is limited soft tissue involvement tenderness may be out of proportion to the soft tissue findings. A patient may present with symptoms of severe illness, including signs of generalized sepsis and shock.

   Other diagnoses to consider in the patient with suspected osteomyelitis include cellulitis, pyomyositis, necrotizing fasciitis, septic arthritis, toxic synovitis, thrombophlebitis, trauma, rheumatologic diseases, Ewing's sarcoma, osteosarcoma, and leukemia.

   Frank G, Mahoney HM, Eppes SC: Musculoskeletal infections in children. Pediatr Clin North Am 52:1083–1106, 2005.
   Gutierrez KM: Bone and joint infections. In Long SS, Pickering LK, Prober CG (eds): Principles and Practice of Pediatric Infectious Disease, 2nd ed. Philadelphia, Churchill Livingstone, 2003, pp 467–474.

2. **How are most cases of osteomyelitis acquired? Direct inoculation? Hematogenous spread? Contiguous spread?**

   The most common source for osteomyelitis is hematogenous spread. Direct inoculation into the bone is less common, as is local invasion from a contiguous infection.

   Gutierrez KM: Bone and joint infections. In Long SS, Pickering LK, Prober CG (eds): Principles and Practice of Pediatric Infectious Disease, 2nd ed. Philadelphia, Churchill Livingstone, 2003, pp 467–474.
   Kaplan SL: Osteomyelitis in children. Infect Dis Clin North Am 19:787–797, 2005.

3. **What laboratory tests are helpful in the diagnosis of osteomyelitis?**

   Reasonable screening laboratory tests to obtain in suspected cases of osteomyelitis include complete blood count (CBC), erythrocyte sedimentation rate (ESR), and C-reactive protein (CRP). ESR and CRP are more sensitive indicators than white blood cell (WBC) count. ESR is elevated in up to 90% of cases of hematogenously acquired osteomyelitis. CRP is elevated in up to 98% of cases. Blood cultures should be obtained and are positive in 50–80% of cases of hematogenously acquired osteomyelitis. The highest yield for isolating a causative organism is achieved when bone aspirate, joint aspirate, and blood are collected for culture. With the exception of patients who are clinically unstable, these cultures should be obtained before initiation of parenteral antibiotics.

   Look for emerging literature on the usefulness of polymerase chain reaction in identifying infections secondary to *Bartonella henselae* and *Kingella kingae*.

4. **What imaging studies are indicated when osteomyelitis is suspected?**

   - **Plain radiography** is a reasonable initial imaging choice in the emergency department (ED) evaluation of a patient with suspected osteomyelitis. This may rule out fracture, tumor, or other concerns. Its usefulness is limited, however, because bony changes (lytic lesions, periosteal elevation, and periosteal new bone formation) may not appear until 10–20 days after symptoms begin. Changes to adjacent soft tissues (deep soft tissue swelling and loss of normal tissue planes) may occur much earlier, as early as several days after symptoms begin.

- **Technetium 99 bone scanning** is more sensitive in the early diagnosis of osteomyelitis than plain radiography, with reported sensitivities of 80–100%. However, results of bone scanning can be normal in up to 20% of cases in the first few days of illness. Its specificity in differentiating osteomyelitis from other differential diagnostic considerations (malignancy, soft tissue cellulitis, septic arthritis, trauma, fracture, and infarction) is also limited.

- **Magnetic resonance imaging (MRI)** (Fig. 47-1) appears to be the imaging study of choice for evaluating the patient with suspected osteomyelitis. Sensitivity ranges from 92% to 100%.

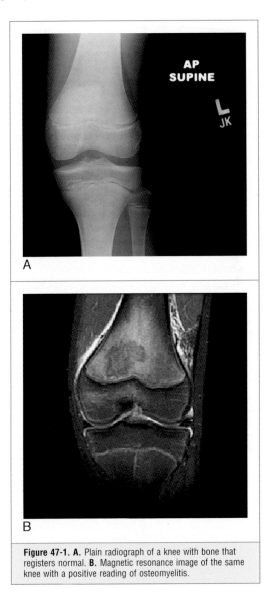

Figure 47-1. A. Plain radiograph of a knee with bone that registers normal. **B.** Magnetic resonance image of the same knee with a positive reading of osteomyelitis.

MRI helps differentiate osteomyelitis from cellulitis and demonstrate myositis or pyomyositis contiguous to the site of bone involvement. As with bone scanning, malignancy, fracture, and infarction can appear similar to osteomyelitis on MRI.

Special considerations apply for neonatal, pelvic, and vertebral osteomyelitis and osteomyelitis acquired in a nonhematogenous fashion.

Gutierrez KM: Bone and joint infections. In Long SS, Pickering LK, Prober CG (eds): Principles and Practice of Pediatric Infectious Disease, 2nd ed. Philadelphia, Churchill Livingstone, 2003, pp 467–474.

Kaplan SL: Osteomyelitis in children. Infect Dis Clin North Am 19:787–797, 2005.

5. **Which organisms are commonly seen in osteomyelitis?**
Staphylococcus aureus is the most common causative organism. Other common organisms include *Streptococcus pneumoniae, Streptococcus pyogenes*, and *Kingella kingae*. In addition to *Staphylococcus aureus*, group B streptococci and enteric gram-negative organisms are important organisms to consider in neonates with osteomyelitis. Other special considerations include *Neisseria gonorrhoeae* in sexually active adolescents; anaerobes in cases associated with sinusitis, mastoiditis, or dental abscess; *Serratia* spp. and *Aspergillus* spp. in patients with granulomatous disease; coagulase-negative staphylococci in patients who have undergone medical procedures; *Salmonella* spp. and gram-negative enteric organisms in patients with hemoglobinopathies; *Pseudomonas aeruginosa* in puncture wounds to the foot; *Bartonella henselae* in kitten exposures; and *Coxiella burnetii* in cases of exposure to farm animals. *Haemophilus influenzae* type B is only rarely seen since the advent of the *H. influenzae* type B vaccine but remains a consideration in an unimmunized child.

The increasing prevalence of methicillin-resistant *Staphylococcus aureus* (MRSA) is worthy of particular attention and concern. MRSA can be particularly virulent and is associated with multiple sites of bone involvement, myositis, pyomyositis, intraosseous, and subperiosteal abscess formation, pulmonary involvement, and vascular complications (such as deep vein thrombosis and septic pulmonary emboli). These patients may be quite ill and require admission to the intensive care unit.

Mycobacterial and fungal infections are rare causes of osteomyelitis.

Frank G, Mahoney HM, Eppes SC: Musculoskeletal infections in children. Pediatr Clin North Am 52:1083–1106, 2005.

Gutierrez KM: Bone and joint infections. In Long SS, Pickering LK, Prober CG (eds): Principles and Practice of Pediatric Infectious Disease, 2nd ed. Philadelphia, Churchill Livingstone, 2003, pp 467–474.

Kaplan SL: Osteomyelitis in children. Infect Dis Clin North Am 19:787–797, 2005.

6. **What historical features should raise suspicion for osteomyelitis (and/or septic arthritis) from *Kingella kingae*?**
Kingella kingae plays an important role in osteomyelitis and septic arthritis in children. Infection with this organism typically occurs in children younger than 2 years of age and often follows an upper respiratory tract infection, pharyngitis, or stomatitis. It may be seasonal in occurrence (late summer through winter). An outbreak of invasive infections from this organism has been reported in a daycare population.

Frank G, Mahoney HM, Eppes SC: Musculoskeletal infections in children. Pediatr Clin North Am 52:1083–1106, 2005.

Gutierrez KM: Bone and joint infections. In Long SS, Pickering LK, Prober CG (eds): Principles and Practice of Pediatric Infectious Disease, 2nd ed. Philadelphia, Churchill Livingstone, 2003, pp 467–474.

Kaplan SL: Osteomyelitis in children. Infect Dis Clin North Am 19:787–797, 2005.

Yagupsky P, Dagan R, Howard CB, et al: Clinical features and epidemiology of invasive *Kingella kingae* infections in southern Israel. Pediatrics 92:800–804, 1993.

7. **How should synovial fluid be handled to improve isolation of _Kingella kingae_?**

   Recovery of _K. kingae_ is improved when synovial fluid aspirate or bone aspirate is collected in aerobic blood culture medium.

   Kaplan SL: Osteomyelitis in children. Infect Dis Clin North Am 19:787–797, 2005.
   Ross JJ: Septic arthritis. Infect Dis Clin North Am 19:799–817, 2005.

8. **How is osteomyelitis treated?**

   Antibiotic treatment should be initiated as soon as appropriate cultures have been collected. Regardless of the patient's age, treatment should address the likelihood of infection with _Staphylococcus aureus_. Given the increasing prevalence of MRSA in many communities, coverage of MRSA in particular is very important. Many MRSA isolates are susceptible to clindamycin. In children, adolescents, and infants over 2 months of age, clindamycin is a good choice for initial antimicrobial coverage. Isolate testing for inducible resistance to clindamycin should be performed, since isolates demonstrating inducible resistance may not respond to treatment. Vancomycin provides excellent coverage for MRSA. However, because of concerns about widespread use of vancomycin resulting in increasing antimicrobial resistance, it should be reserved for patients who are moderately to severely ill or who live in communities where significant resistance to clindamycin has been demonstrated. In infants younger than 2 months of age, additional antimicrobial coverage for Group B Streptococcus and enteric gram-negative becteria is important. In this age group clindamycin or vancomycin plus cefotaxime or gentamycin would be appropriate initial antimicrobial choices.

   Special circumstances (noted in question 5) warrant consideration of antimicrobial coverage specific to the likely pathogens in such cases.

   An orthopedic surgeon should be involved in cases of suspected or confirmed osteomyelitis. Surgical treatment is indicated in a number of circumstances. Moreover, surgical tissue is often helpful in identifying a causative organism to guide antimicrobial treatment.

   Frank G, Mahoney HM, Eppes SC: Musculoskeletal infections in children. Pediatr Clin North Am 52:1083–1106, 2005.
   Gutierrez K: Bone and joint infections in children. Pediatr Clin North Am 52:779–794, 2005.
   Gutierrez KM: Bone and joint infections. In Long SS, Pickering LK, Prober CG (eds): Principles and Practice of Pediatric Infectious Disease, 2nd ed. Philadelphia, Churchill Livingstone, 2003, pp 467–474.
   Kaplan SL: Osteomyelitis in children. Infect Dis Clin North Am 19:787–797, 2005.

9. **Describe the signs and symptoms of septic arthritis.**

   Pain and decreased use of the involved limb are common symptoms of septic arthritis. Hip, knee, and ankle joints account for about 80% of cases of septic arthritis. Fever, malaise, and anorexia are seen in most patients. The involved joint is often held in a position of comfort. In the knee this is usually flexion. In the hip it is usually flexion, abduction, and external rotation. Passive range of motion away from the position of comfort is resisted and is painful. In joints other than the hip, tenderness, swelling, warmth, and erythema are usually seen and an effusion may be palpable. As in osteomyelitis, neonates may present with pseudoparalysis and tenderness of the affected limb.

   Other diagnoses to consider in the patient with suspected septic arthritis include traumatic joint pain, transient synovitis ("toxic synovitis"), reactive arthritis, Lyme arthritis, juvenile rheumatoid arthritis, acute rheumatic fever, osteomyelitis, pyomyositis, necrotizing fasciitis, tumor, slipped capital femoral epiphysis, and Legg-Calvé-Perthes disease.

   Frank G, Mahoney HM, Eppes SC: Musculoskeletal infections in children. Pediatr Clin North Am 52:1083–1106, 2005.
   Gutierrez KM: Infectious and inflammatory arthritis. In Long SS, Pickering LK, Prober CG (eds): Principles and Practice of Pediatric Infectious Disease, 2nd ed. Philadelphia, Churchill Livingstone, 2003, pp 475–481.
   Ross JJ: Septic arthritis. Infect Dis Clin North Am 19:799–817, 2005.

10. **What laboratory tests help diagnose septic arthritis?**

WBC counts, ESR, and CRP levels are usually elevated in cases of septic arthritis. The WBC count appears to be less useful than ESR in differentiating septic arthritis from transient synovitis. In cases of septic arthritis, the ESR is usually greater than 20 mm/hr. Mean ESR ranges from 44 to 65 mm/hr. The mean CRP level is 85 mg/L. Blood culture and synovial fluid analysis (cell count, Gram stain, and culture) are essential in the evaluation of children with suspected septic arthritis. Ideally, these tests should be performed before the administration of antibiotics. They yield an organism in up to 40% and up to 50–60% of cases, respectively, and when combined, they yield an organism in up to 60–70% of cases. The yield of synovial cultures may be improved by inoculation of the fluid into blood culture media. Typical synovial fluid WBC count is over 50,000 cells/mm^3, with a predominance of polymorphonuclear cells (> 75–90%). Unfortunately, cell counts less than 50,000 cells/mm^3 can be seen in cases of septic arthritis, and counts over 50,000 cells/mm^3 are seen in juvenile rheumatoid arthritis. Synovial fluid glucose and protein levels are not reliable enough to differentiate septic arthritis from other infectious or inflammatory processes.

11. **Which imaging studies can help make the diagnosis of septic arthritis?**

The initial imaging choice in the ED is plain radiography. Soft tissue swelling, joint space widening, and changes suggestive of osteomyelitis may be seen. In the hip, capsular swelling and loss of the gluteal fat planes may be seen as early evidence of infection in the joint. If hip infection is suspected, ultrasonography may be performed and ultrasonographically guided joint aspiration performed. Bone scanning and MRI are both sensitive modalities for detecting joint infection. MRI has the added advantage of delineating changes in the adjacent soft tissues and bone.

Frank G, Mahoney HM, Eppes SC: Musculoskeletal infections in children. Pediatr Clin North Am 52:1083–1106, 2005.

Greenspan A, Tehranzadeh J: Imaging of infectious arthritis. Radiol Clin North Am 39:267–276, 2001.

Gutierrez KM: Bone and joint infections. In Long SS, Pickering LK, Prober CG (eds): Principles and Practice of Pediatric Infectious Disease, 2nd ed. Philadelphia, Churchill Livingstone, 2003, pp 475–481.

Hughes JG, Vetter EA, Patel R, et al: Culture with BACTEC Peds Plus/F bottle compared with conventional methods for detection of bacteria in synovial fluid. J Clin Microbiol 39:4468–4471, 2001.

Ross JJ: Septic arthritis. Infect Dis Clin North Am 19:799–817, 2005.

Zawin JK: Joint effusion in children with an irritable hip: US diagnosis and aspiration. Radiology 187:459–463, 1993.

12. **Which organisms are commonly seen in septic arthritis?**

The organisms commonly responsible for septic arthritis are much the same as those commonly associated with osteomyelitis (see question 5). *Neisseria gonorrhoeae* should be considered in neonates and in sexually active patients, especially those with multifocal joint involvement. *Candida* spp. should be considered in neonates. Antibiotic considerations for initial empiric treatment of septic arthritis are similar to those in osteomyelitis (see question 8).

Frank G, Mahoney HM, Eppes SC: Musculoskeletal infections in children. Pediatr Clin North Am 52:1083–1106, 2005.

Gutierrez K: Bone and joint infections in children. Pediatr Clin North Am 52:779–794, 2005.

Gutierrez KM: Bone and joint infections. In Long SS, Pickering LK, Prober CG (eds): Principles and Practice of Pediatric Infectious Disease, 2nd ed. Philadelphia, Churchill Livingstone, 2003, pp 475–481.

Ross JJ: Septic arthritis. Infect Dis Clin North Am 19:799–817, 2005.

13. **What is the treatment for septic arthritis?**
Optimal treatment involves antibiotics and joint drainage. Early consultation with an orthopedic surgeon is mandatory. Emergent surgical drainage of infected hip and neonatal shoulder infections is appropriate, whereas repeated nonsurgical aspiration may be reasonable for other joints. There is recent evidence that a short course of steroids may improve residual function and shorten the duration of acute symptoms.

Frank G, Mahoney HM, Eppes SC: Musculoskeletal infections in children. Pediatr Clin North Am 52:1083–1106, 2005.

Odio CM, Ramirez T, Arias G, et al: Double blind, randomized, placebo-controlled study of dexamethasone therapy for hematogenous septic arthritis in children. Pediatr Infect Dis J 22:883–888, 2003.

Ross JJ: Septic arthritis. Infect Dis Clin North Am 19:799–817, 2005.

14. **Reactive arthritis is in the differential diagnosis for the patients described above. What are the common organisms responsible for reactive arthritis?**
Salmonella, Shigella, and *Campylobacter* spp. and *Yersinia enterocolitica* from the gastrointestinal tract; *N. gonorrhoeae* and *Chlamydia trachomatis* from the genitourinary tract; and *Streptococcus pyogenes, Mycoplasma pneumoniae,* and *N. meningitidis.* Both *Neisseria* spp. and *Streptococcus pyogenes* can also cause septic arthritis.

Frank G, Mahoney HM, Eppes SC: Musculoskeletal infections in children. Pediatr Clin North Am 52:1083–1106, 2005.

Gutierrez K: Bone and joint infections in children. Pediatr Clin North Am 52:779–794, 2005.

15. **Describe the typical presentation and evaluation of suspected pyomyositis.**
Unfortunately, the diagnosis of pyomyositis is often not made until symptoms have been present for several weeks. Initial symptoms include crampy local muscle pain, most commonly involving the thigh, calf, buttock, upper extremity, and iliopsoas muscles. Early in the course of the infection local edema is present, although the overlying skin is often normal. The edema has been described as having a woody or rubbery feel. Over time, induration, edema, erythema, and tenderness increase. Fever, increasing constitutional symptoms, toxicity, and signs of sepsis may develop if the infection progresses and is untreated.

Leukocytosis and elevated CRP levels and ESR may develop as the infection progresses. Blood cultures should be collected. Creatine kinase level is often normal, however. Ultrasonography, computed tomography (CT), and MRI may demonstrate the presence of pyomyositis. MRI is more sensitive than CT.

Frank G, Mahoney HM, Eppes SC: Musculoskeletal infections in children. Pediatr Clin North Am 52:1083–1106, 2005.

Small LN, Ross JJ: Tropical and temperate pyomyositis. Infect Dis Clin North Am 19:981–989, 2005.

16. **How is pyomyositis treated?**
The organisms most commonly responsible for pyomyositis are *Staphylococcus aureus* and *Streptococcus pyogenes* (often associated with varicella infection). As is the case in osteomyelitis and septic arthritis, MRSA must be considered in these patients and antimicrobial treatment directed appropriately. When an identifiable abscess is present, drainage is indicated. In the interest of isolating an organism, consider delaying the initiation of antibiotics until drained fluid can be collected for culture, in stable patients. More extensive surgical intervention may be necessary if there is muscle necrosis.

Frank G, Mahoney HM, Eppes SC: Musculoskeletal infections in children. Pediatr Clin North Am 52:1083–1106, 2005.

Small LN, Ross JJ: Tropical and temperate pyomyositis. Infect Dis Clin North Am 19:981–989, 2005.

17. **Describe the typical presentation and evaluation of suspected necrotizing fasciitis.**

Patients with necrotizing fasciitis often have soft tissue swelling and pain near a site of trauma. Initially, pain with manipulation may be out of proportion to the skin findings seen. Induration and edema follow, then blistering and bleb formation. The skin becomes dusky and drains fluid. Subcutaneous pain and tenderness become severe, again often out of proportion to the appearance of the overlying skin. There is often high fever and signs of systemic illness. The process may be quite fulminant, accompanied by toxic shock syndrome and multiorgan failure.

Laboratory evaluation and imaging, particularly MRI, may be helpful in establishing the diagnosis. However, because of the rapidly progressive nature of necrotizing fasciitis, laboratory evaluation and imaging should not delay initiation of treatment. Collect wound, tissue, and blood cultures (aerobic and anaerobic).

Frank G, Mahoney HM, Eppes SC: Musculoskeletal infections in children. Pediatr Clin North Am 52:1083–1106, 2005.

18. **What is the treatment for necrotizing fasciitis?**

The most important aspect of treatment for necrotizing fasciitis is immediate surgical debridement. Seek surgical consultation as soon as possible. Antibiotic treatment should be directed at the likely causative organisms, including *Streptococcus pyogenes* and *Staphylococcus aureus* (including MRSA). A reasonable antibiotic choice would be clindamycin plus oxacillin. Add vancomycin in patients who are very ill. Ampicillin-sulbactam and piperacillin-tazobactam are other possible antimicrobial choices. In areas where MRSA is prevalent, treatment should also include vancomycin. It cannot be overemphasized, however, that antibiotic treatment alone is insufficient treatment for this severe, rapidly progressive, and often life-threatening infection.

Darmstadt GL: Subcutaneous tissue infections and abscesses. In Long SS, Pickering LK, Prober CG (eds): Principles and Practice of Pediatric Infectious Disease, 2nd ed. Philadelphia, Churchill Livingstone, 2003, pp 449–457.

Frank G, Mahoney HM, Eppes SC: Musculoskeletal infections in children. Pediatr Clin North Am 52:1083–1106, 2005.

Miller LG: Necrotizing fasciitis caused by community-associated methicillin-resistant *Staphylococcus aureus* in Los Angeles. N Engl J Med 352:1445–1453, 2005.

19. **What concerns should the ED physician have when a child younger than 4 years presents with back pain?**

Back pain is not a common symptom in young children, nor is it a particularly common expression of functional pain in young children. Concerning signs and symptoms in a young child with back pain include refusal to walk, limited range of motion in the back, persistent or increasing pain despite analgesics, anti-inflammatory agents and rest, fever, weight loss, signs of systemic illness, and abnormal neurologic signs. Serious causes to be considered in the young child include discitis, vertebral osteomyelitis, and tumors.

American Academy of Orthopaedic Surgeons: Slipped capital femoral epiphysis. In American Academy of Orthopaedic Surgeons: Orthopaedic Knowledge Update: Pediatrics. Rosemont, Illinois, American Academy of Orthopaedic Surgeons, 1996, pp 151–159.

Payne WK, Ogilvie JW: Back pain in children and adolescents. Pediatr Clin North Am 43:899–918, 1996.

KEY POINTS: ORTHOPEDIC EMERGENCIES ✓

1. MRSA is an important organism to consider in bone, joint, and soft tissue infections. Provide adequate antimicrobial coverage if it is prevalent in your area.

2. Overlying skin findings may not be very remarkable early in the course of pyomyositis and necrotizing fasciitis.

3. Surgical debridement without delay is the most important aspect of the treatment of necrotizing fasciitis.

4. Back pain in a young child warrants serious consideration.

---

20. How do children with slipped capital femoral epiphysis present?

Slipped capital femoral epiphysis (SCFE) usually occurs during the rapid growth phase of adolescence and tends to occur more often in obese children. Males are affected almost twice as often as females. Black adolescents are affected about twice as often as white adolescents. SCFE may be chronic, acute, or acute superimposed on chronic in its presentation. Obesity is a risk factor in the development of SCFE. The presentation of SCFE is bilateral in approximately 20% of cases. Patients with SCFE will often have pain in the anterior hip, groin, medial thigh, or knee and will also demonstrate limitation of hip motion. Because SCFE can present with knee pain, the presence of knee pain in a child or adolescent mandates a thorough examination of the hip. Patients who are ambulatory have an antalgic gait with external rotation of the affected leg. Passive internal rotation of the hip is painful, and passive hip flexion is associated with compensatory external rotation.

American Academy of Orthopaedic Surgeons: Slipped capital femoral epiphysis. In American Academy of Orthopaedic Surgeons: Orthopaedic Knowledge Update: Pediatrics. Rosemont, Illinois, American Academy of Orthopaedic Surgeons, 1996, pp 151–159.

Canale ST: Fractures and dislocations in children. In Canale ST (ed): Campbell's Operative Orthopaedics, 10th ed. Philadelphia, Mosby, 2003, pp 1481–1503.

Kienstra A; Macias C: Slipped capital femoral epiphysis: www.uptodate.com

21. What is the approach to the patient with suspected SCFE in the ED?

Plain radiography is the first step in the evaluation of patients with suspected SCFE. Films show displacement of the femoral capital epiphysis from the metaphysis through the growth plate. If the slip is chronic, metaphyseal remodeling may be seen. The anteroposterior view often demonstrates the presence of the slip. A line drawn tangent to the superior femoral neck should intersect the lateral aspect of the femoral head (Klein's line). In SCFE this line passes more lateral on the capital epiphysis. Cross-table lateral radiography of the hip can help define the extent of posterior epiphyseal displacement. A frog-leg view of the pelvis may reveal a subtle slip, however, movement of the hip for radiography should be avoided as it may cause further slippage. Although a slip may be symptomatic on one side only, it is often present bilaterally on plain radiography. Because as many as 40% of patients have slips bilaterally, comparing sides on plain films may give false reassurance and result in failure to diagnose both slips.

Once the diagnosis is strongly suspected, the patient should avoid weight-bearing and an urgent orthopedic consultation should be obtained.

American Academy of Orthopaedic Surgeons: Slipped capital femoral epiphysis. In American Academy of Orthopaedic Surgeons: Orthopaedic Knowledge Update: Pediatrics. Rosemont, Illinois, American Academy of Orthopaedic Surgeons, 1996, pp 151–159.

Canale ST: Fractures and dislocations in children. In Canale ST (ed): Campbell's Operative Orthopaedics, 10th ed. Philadelphia, Mosby, 2003, pp 1481–1503.

22. **What is the etiology of "growing pains"?**

Growing pains do not correlate with growth spurts and do not affect growth. They do not occur at the growth plate regions. Possible causes include fatigue, abnormal posture, restless legs syndrome, and overuse. Growing pains are often seen in children with other types of recurrent pain, such as headaches and abdominal pain. They are slightly more common in girls.

Wilking A: Growing pains. Available at: www.uptodate.com

23. **What are some of the features of growing pains?**

- Pain occurs most commonly in the lower extremities and is bilateral.
- Pain occurs in the evening hours and is often better by morning.
- Pain can become severe and is relieved by acetaminophen or ibuprofen.
- The physical examination is normal.
- There is often a family history of growing pains.
- Pain is chronic and may last for years.

Wilking A: Growing pains. Available at: www.uptodate.com

CHAPTER 48

OTORHINOLARYNGOLOGY EMERGENCIES

Frances M. Nadel, MD, MSCE, and Douglas M. Nadel, MD

EPISTAXIS

1. **From what part of the nose do most nosebleeds originate?**
   The vast majority of nosebleeds in children arise anteriorly (90%). On the anterior part of the septum, many capillaries converge, giving rise to Kiesselbach's plexus. Anterior nosebleeds tend to be slow and persistent. Posterior nosebleeds usually originate from branches of the sphenopalatine artery and ethmoidal arteries. As a result, the bleeding is more profuse.

   McGarry G: Nosebleeds in children. Clin Evid 10:437–440, 2003.

2. **What factors often contribute to nosebleeds in otherwise normal children?**
   Desiccation of the fragile nasal mucosa makes the tissue more friable. Inflammation from a viral upper respiratory tract infection or allergies can also make the mucosa more likely to bleed. Finally, local trauma from nose picking is usually a major contributor.

   McGarry G: Nosebleeds in children. Clin Evid 10:437–440, 2003.

3. **How can one elicit a truthful answer about nose picking?**
   Ask the child which finger she uses to pick her nose.

4. **What is "rhinitis sicca"?**
   This refers to the drying of the nasal mucosa, which may make it more susceptible to bleeding. This often occurs during winter months, when dry hot air systems are being used to heat one's house.

5. **Though most nosebleeds occur from the benign local conditions listed above, what else should be considered in the differential diagnosis of nosebleeds?**
   See Table 48-1.

6. **What historical factors make one suspicious for a systemic cause of a nosebleed?**
   Children with a history of bleeding from other sources, easy bruising, weight loss, or other constitutional symptoms, a family history of a bleeding disorder, and severe or recurrent nosebleeds may need more extensive workup or subsequent follow-up.

   Sandoval C, Dong S, Visintainer P, et al: Clinical and laboratory features of 178 children with recurrent epistaxis. J Pediatr Hematol Oncol 24:47–49, 2002.

7. **What steps should be taken for a patient who has a nosebleed in the emergency department (ED)?**
   Calming the patient and family is often the most important step. For an anterior bleed, insert a roll of cotton saturated with a topical decongestant (oxymetazoline or adrenaline) in the affected side and squeeze the nose gently for 5 minutes to compress the cotton against the septum. If the bleeding site is visible, it can then be cauterized with silver nitrate. Adding a

TABLE 48-1. DIFFERENTIAL DIAGNOSIS OF EPISTAXIS

Local predisposing factors

Trauma

    Facial trauma

    Direct nasal trauma

    Nose picking

Local inflammation

    Acute viral upper respiratory tract infection (common cold)

    Bacterial rhinitis

    Nasal diphtheria (rare)* }   Usually a blood-tinged discharge

    Congenital syphilis

    Hemolytic streptococci

    Foreign body

    Acute systemic illnesses accompanied by nasal congestion:

        measles, infectious mononucleosis, acute rheumatic fever

    Allergic rhinitis

    Nasal polyps (cystic fibrosis, allergic, generalized)

    Staphylococcal furuncle

    Sinusitis

Cocaine or heroin sniffing

Telangiectasias (Osler-Weber-Rendu disease)

Juvenile angiofibroma*

Other tumors, granulomatosis (rare)*

Rhinitis sicca

Systemic predisposing factors

Hematologic diseases*

    Platelet disorders

        Quantitative: idiopathic thrombocytopenic purpura, leukemia, aplastic anemia

        Qualitative: von Willebrand's disease, Glanzmann's disease, uremia

    Other primary hemorrhagic diatheses: hemophilias, sickle cell anemia

    Clotting disorders associated with severe hepatic disease, disseminated intravascular coagulopathy, vitamin K deficiency

Drugs: aspirin, nonsteroidal anti-inflammatory drugs, warfarin, rodenticide, valproate

Vicarious menstruation

Hypertension*

    Arterial (unusual cause of epistaxis in children)

    Venous: superior vena cava syndrome or with paroxysmal coughing seen in pertussis and cystic fibrosis

*Life-threatening condition.
Adapted from Nadel FN, Henretig FM Epistaxis. In: Textbook of Pediatric Emergency Medicine, 5th ed. Fleisher GR, Ludwig S, Henretig, FM (eds). Philadelphia, Lippincott Williams & Wilkins, 2006, pp 417–425.

topical anesthetic to the cotton ball greatly decreases the amount of discomfort of cautery. If the bleeding cannot be stopped with cautery, the nose should then be packed. Bleeding that cannot be stopped with these measures should be evaluated by an otolaryngologist without delay.

8. **What findings would make you more suspicious for a posterior nosebleed?**
Suspect a posterior nosebleed when no obvious site is visible anteriorly. Bleeding from both nostrils and blood in the posterior pharynx suggest a posterior nosebleed, but can occur from brisk anterior epistaxis. Continued bleeding despite adequate anterior pressure is also concerning. Posterior nasal bleeding is rare in children.

Alvi A, Joyner-Triplett N: Acute epistaxis. How to spot the source and stop the flow. Postgrad Med 99:83–90, 94–96, 1996.

9. **A teenage male presents with recurrent, profuse unilateral epistaxis. He reports that this same side of his nose has been progressively obstructed for 2 months. What other diagnosis should you consider?**
Teenage males may develop **juvenile nasopharyngeal angiofibroma**. These uncommon tumors arise from the sphenopalatine region and can present with severe epistaxis. The diagnosis is made with nasal endoscopy or computed tomography (CT). These patients need a referral to an otolaryngology specialist for further surgical management.

10. **A teenager presents with her fifth nosebleed in as many months. Her history and physical examination are otherwise unremarkable. What additional information regarding her nosebleeds may be helpful?**
One should ask her the timing of nosebleeds in relation to her menstrual cycle. Some girls may experience "vicarious menstruation" in which they have a nosebleed at the same time as their menses.

RETROPHARYNGEAL ABSCESS

11. **What are the common signs and symptoms of a retropharyngeal abscess?**
Commonly, there is a recent history of an upper respiratory tract infection, fever, and poor oral intake. Patients may be drooling, have a stiff neck, and have tender cervical adenopathy. Respiratory symptoms of stridor, stertor, or dyspnea are usually late findings and are rarely described in the most current series of patients. A midline mass can sometimes be seen in the posterior pharynx.

Craig FW, Schunk JE: Retropharyngeal abscess in children: Clinical presentation, utility of imaging, and current management. Pediatrics 111:1394–1398, 2003.

12. **Why is it unusual to see retropharyngeal abscess in children > 4 years old?**
The retropharyngeal nodes of Rouvier usually involute around 5 years of age, making retropharyngeal abscess (RPA) a rare disease in older children.

13. **What is a parapharyngeal abscess?**
A parapharyngeal or lateral space infection develops in the lateral aspect of the neck. This space is shaped like an inverted cone. It is divided into an anterior compartment, which contains no vital structures and is closely related to the tonsillar fossa. The posterior compartment contains some of the cranial nerves and the carotid sheath. Infection in the lateral space results from dental infection, pharyngitis, tonsillitis, parotitis, and mastoiditis.

Parapharyngeal abscesses are less common than RPA. Symptoms are very similar to those seen in RPA.

14. **List the mechanisms of infection of the retropharyngeal space.**
    Usually, bacteria in the pharynx spread via lymphatic channels to the nodes of Rouvier, where they multiply and suppurate. Other possible mechanisms include oral trauma (causing a mucosal tear), hematogenous spread during bacteremia, or, rarely, extension from vertebral osteomyelitis.

15. **Which pathogens are common in RPA?**
    RPA is usually a polymicrobial infection and may include *Streptococcus* spp., *Staphylococcus aureus,* and anaerobes. *Haemophilus influenzae* type B has become a less common pathogen since the introduction of the *Hib* vaccine. Less commonly, gram-negative organisms such as *Klebsiella* and *Salmonella* spp. have been cultured.

    Brook I: Microbiology and management of peritonsillar, retropharyngeal, and parapharyngeal abscesses. J Oral Maxillofac Surg 62:1545–15650, 2004.

16. **How wide is the normal retropharyngeal space on a lateral neck radiograph in children?**
    Prevertebral soft tissues at the level of C3 should measure less than two thirds of the anterior-posterior width of the body of the third cervical vertebrae. This space is markedly widened in a child with retropharyngeal abscess (Fig. 48-1).

    Jasin ME, Osguthorpe JD: The radiographic evaluation of infants with stridor. Otolaryngol Head Neck Surg 90:736–739, 1982.

17. **List the causes of a false-positive lateral neck radiograph.**
    - Neck not in full extension
    - Radiography done during expiration
    - Not a true lateral position
    - Crying child

    Jasin ME, Osguthorpe JD: The radiographic evaluation of infants with stridor. Otolaryngol Head Neck Surg 90:736–739, 1982.

18. **How does CT assist in RPA management?**
    CT with contrast is the most reliable test in the initial evaluation. A hypodense region with rim enhancement is virtually diagnostic for an abscess, while a more heterogeneous mass without rim enhancement suggests retropharyngeal cellulitis only. However, the CT results should be clinically correlated because the false-positive and false-negative rates may be as high as 15%. CT can help demonstrate the extent of infection and the potential of airway compromise. The scan also helps the otolaryngologist decide whether intraoral drainage is feasible or whether an external approach is necessary.

    Craig FW, Schunk JE: Retropharyngeal abscess in children: Clinical presentation, utility of imaging, and current management. Pediatrics 111:1394–1398, 2003.

    Wetmore RF, Mahboubi, Soyupak SK. Computed tomography in the evaluation of pediatric neck infections. Otolaryngol Head Neck Surg 119:624–627, 1998.

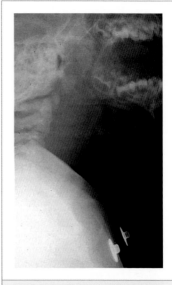

Figure 48-1. Widened retropharyngeal space on a lateral neck radiograph of a child with retropharyngeal abscess.

19. **Do most patients with RPA require surgery?**
The management of RPA varies greatly in the literature and by surgeon. Though it was previously the standard to drain all abscesses, more clinicians are willing to attempt a trial of IV antibiotics alone on patients with retropharyngeal cellulitis or small RPA without airway compromise.

   Lalakea M, Messner AH: Retropharyngeal abscess management in children: Current practices. Otolaryngol Head Neck Surg 121:398–405, 1999.

20. **How far inferiorly does the retropharyngeal space extend in the neck?**
The retropharyngeal space extends from the base of the skull to the level of the second thoracic vertebrae. The abscess can rupture into the prevertebral space, which communicates with the mediastinum and descends as far as the psoas muscles.

21. **List some of the complications of an RPA.**
Earlier recognition and treatment and improved diagnostic strategies have greatly reduced the morbidity and mortality of RPAs. However, a large RPA may obstruct the airway at the pharyngeal, laryngeal, or tracheal level, and a tracheostomy may be necessary. Aspiration of purulent fluid may occur from rupture of the abscess. Sepsis, mediastinitis, jugular vein thrombosis, Lemierre's syndrome, carotid arteritis with subsequent rupture are rare complications.

22. **What findings may herald a carotid artery rupture?**
A pulsatile ecchymotic mass may be found anterior to the sternocleidomastoid muscle. Bleeding from the ear, nose, or mouth may occur.

KEY POINTS: DANGERS OF DEEP NECK INFECTIONS ✓

1. Localized infections in the head and neck can spread regionally.
2. Intracranial extension may present with prolonged symptoms, change in mental status, or focal neurologic deficit.
3. Mediastinal extension can also be associated with prolonged symptoms, poor response to therapy, respiratory symptoms, and sepsis syndrome.

MASTOIDITIS

23. **Define mastoiditis.**
Mastoiditis is an infection of the mastoid air cells. Technically, a simple case of acute otitis media leads to some inflammation of the air cells, but true coalescent mastoiditis implies bony destruction.

24. **Why is it unusual to see mastoiditis in children less than 1 year old?**
The mastoid air cells are not yet pneumatized.

25. **How does a patient who has acute mastoiditis present?**
Patients commonly present with persistent symptoms of acute otitis media, such as ear pain or drainage. Fever is common. On physical examination, the ear may protrude away from the head, and in younger children the ear is pushed down and out (Fig. 48-2). The postauricular skin is often tender, erythematous, fluctuant, or edematous. Otoscopy shows findings

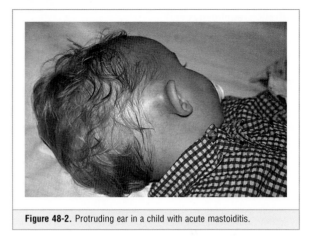

Figure 48-2. Protruding ear in a child with acute mastoiditis.

consistent with acute otitis media. One may see sagging of the posterosuperior external ear canal due to periosteal thickening.

Nussinovitch M, Yoeli R, Elishkevitz K, Varsano I: Acute mastoiditis in children: Epidemiologic, clinical, microbiologic, and therapeutic aspects over past years. Clin Pediatr 43:261–267, 2004.

26. **What are the common pathogens seen in acute mastoiditis?**
Streptococcus pneumoniae, Streptococcus pyogenes, and S*taphylococcus aureus* are common pathogens. Anaerobic enteric bacteria and *Pseudomonas* spp. are more often seen in subacute or chronic disease. *H. influenza* is a rare pathogen.

Nussinovitch M, Yoeli R, Elishkevitz K, Varsano I: Acute mastoiditis in children: Epidemiologic, clinical, microbiologic, and therapeutic aspects over past years. Clin Pediatr 43:261–267, 2004.

27. **What study would assist in the diagnosis and management of coalescent mastoiditis?**
CT with contrast can confirm your clinical diagnosis as well as show whether there is a subperiosteal abscess, intracranial extension, or sigmoid sinus thrombosis.

Antonelli PJ, Garside JA, Mancuso AA, et al: Computed tomography and the diagnosis of coalescent mastoiditis. Otolaryngol Head Neck Surg 120:350–354, 1999.

28. **List some of the central nervous system complications of mastoiditis.**
The temporal bone's proximity to many important intracranial structures can lead to serious complications. Intracranial extension can include meningoencephalitis and intracerebral, epidural, or subdural abscesses. Progressive thrombophlebitis may lead to sigmoid or lateral sinus thrombosis. Any child with mastoiditis with focal neurologic symptoms should receive an immediate evaluation for intracranial spread. Other concerning findings include toxic appearance, stiff neck, persistent fever despite adequate antibiotic treatment, headache, vomiting, or unusual behavior.

Go C, Bernstein JM, de Jong AL, et al: Intracranial complications of acute mastoiditis. Int J Pediatr Otorhinolaryngol 52:143–148, 2000.

29. **What is a Bezold's abscess?**
This is a type of mastoiditis that has ruptured through the mastoid tip and formed an abscess within the sternocleidomastoid muscle.

30. **What is Gradenigo's syndrome?**
Gradenigo's syndrome occurs from inflammation of the petrous apex of the temporal bone (petrositis), affecting cranial nerves V and VI. It presents as a suppurative otitis, pain around the eye and ear, abducens nerve paralysis (inability to move the eye laterally), and diplopia. Additional symptoms are facial paresis, vertigo, and fever.

POSTOPERATIVE TONSILLECTOMY BLEEDING

31. **What are the two types of postoperative tonsillectomy bleeding?**
A common dictum states that bleeding occurs "in 7 minutes or 7 days":
- **Primary hemorrhage** occurs within 24 hours of surgery. This type of bleed is usually detected in the postoperative care unit and rarely will present to the ED.
- **Secondary or delayed hemorrhage** occurs anytime thereafter. It most commonly occurs 7–10 days after surgery but can occur as early as 3 days and as late as 21 days.

    Liu JH, Anderson KE, Willging JP, et al: Posttonsillectomy hemorrhage: What is it and what should be recorded? Arch Otolaryngol Head Neck Surg 127:1271–1275, 2001.

32. **What percentage of children has delayed hemorrhage?**
About 3% of children have delayed posttonsillectomy hemorrhage. Active bleeding or the presence of a clot in the tonsillar fossa requires a return to the operating room for hemostasis.

    Liu JH, Anderson KE, Willging JP, et al: Posttonsillectomy hemorrhage: What is it and what should be recorded? Arch Otolaryngol Head Neck Surg 127:1271–1275, 2001.

33. **Does posttonsillectomy bleeding occur more often in redheads, during a full moon, on Friday the 13th, or in patterns of three?**
No—at least not in Philadelphia.

    Kumar VV, Kumar NV, Isaacson G: Superstition and post-tonsillectomy hemorrhage. Laryngoscope. 114:2031–2033, 2004.

34. **How does the normal healing eschar of oropharyngeal tissue look?**
The healing operative site will be covered with a grayish-white exudate. Beneath the exudate there is usually beefy-red granulation tissue. A blood clot will appear dark red, purple, or black and may be located inferiorly near the tongue.

35. **What is the significance of seeing a clot on inspection of the oropharynx?**
A blood clot not only shows you where the offending vessel is located, it also indicates that the vessel is in the earliest stages of hemostasis and can continue to bleed if provoked. *This blood clot should never be removed in the ED as brisk bleeding and loss of the airway can ensue!*

36. **Why do children die from postoperative bleeding?**
The usual mechanism of death is aspiration of blood, though some may die from hemorrhagic shock.

37. **How should you manage a patient who is actively bleeding after tonsillectomy in the ED?**
Assess the ABCs, with particular attention to obstruction of airway due to blood, as well as circulatory compromise due to blood loss. It is important to calm the patient and the family. Examination will show if any active bleeding is present. Any clot in the tonsillar fossa should be left undisturbed! For severe, active bleeding, the site should be tamponaded with gauze and digital pressure until the otolaryngologist arrives.

38. **Is postadenoidectomy bleeding treated differently?**
Bleeding from the adenoid bed poses less of a threat because the nasopharynx is supplied with fewer blood vessels than the tonsillar bed. Nonetheless, persistent nasopharyngeal hemorrhage still requires surgical intervention.

KEY POINTS: MANAGEMENT OF BLEEDING AFTER TONSILLECTOMY AND ADENOIDECTOMY ✓

1. Attend to the ABCs.

2. Restore intravascular volume.

3. If there is a clot, leave it alone.

4. For severe active bleeding, tamponade the site with digital pressure.

PERITONSILLAR ABSCESS

39. **What is quinsy?**
Quinsy is derived from the Latin word for "sore throat" (*cynanche)* and refers to a peritonsillar abscess (PTA).

40. **Define the classic presentation of PTA.**
PTAs are most commonly seen in late adolescence, but have been rarely reported in young infants. Patients often present with a muffled voice, trismus, and odynophagia. Other symptoms may include fever, worsening sore throat, ear pain, and neck pain.

41. **Which way does the uvula point when there is a PTA?**
The abscess pushes the uvula away to the contralateral side of the oropharynx.

42. **What other physical examination findings may you find?**
The tonsils and pharynx will be erythematous and there may be an exudate on the tonsils, as in straightforward tonsillitis. One tonsil may be larger than the other, but by itself this asymmetry does not suggest PTA. A PTA should be suspected when the soft palate is red and bulging on one side while the uvula is deviated to the contralateral side. Often there is ipsilateral cervical adenopathy and trismus.

43. **What should be considered in your differential diagnosis of a PTA?**
It is often difficult to differentiate a peritonsillar cellulitis from an abscess. The significant asymmetry of tonsil size, the presence of uvular deviation, and palatine fullness are more consistent with a PTA. Children with mononucleosis also have very enlarged tonsils with exudate, though they are usually symmetrically enlarged. It is unusual for tonsillitis from other viruses to be confused with a PTA. If the patient has significant respiratory symptoms, one may be concerned about epiglottitis or RPA. Since the introduction of the Hib vaccine, epiglottitis is extremely rare. Though not always true, children with RPAs or epiglottitis are usually younger than 4 years of age, whereas PTAs are usually seen in teenagers.

44. **What are the common pathogens in PTA?**

As one would imagine, *Streptococcus pyogenes* is the most common pathogen. *Staphylococcus aureus* and oral anaerobes are common pathogens as well.

Brook I: Microbiology and management of peritonsillar, retropharyngeal, and parapharyngeal abscesses. J Oral Maxillofac Surg 62:1545–1550, 2004.

45. **How is a PTA treated?**

When physical examination suggests a PTA, the peritonsillar space should be aspirated by an otolaryngologist. Aspiration of pus confirms the diagnosis and often gives the patient immediate symptomatic relief. Some practitioners prefer a course of IV antibiotics, with aspiration reserved for treatment failures. Once drained, PTA is treated just like acute tonsillitis: with antibiotics, hydration, and analgesics. Repeated aspirations are occasionally necessary. Penicillin usually provides adequate coverage. For patients who are allergic or have not responded to penicillin, clindamycin provides excellent coverage. Route of administration will depend on the patient's general appearance and ability to swallow.

Johnson RF, Stewart MG, Wright CC: An evidence-based review of the treatment of peritonsillar abscess. Otolaryngol Head Neck Surg 128:332–343, 2003.

46. **List the four findings of Lemierre's syndrome.**
   - Pharyngitis/tonsillitis
   - Septicemia with at least one positive blood culture, usually of *Fusobacterium necrophorum*
   - Evidence of internal jugular thrombosis
   - Metastatic focus of infection, often pulmonary

47. **What findings would make you suspect Lemierre's syndrome?**

Patients with recent or prolonged pharyngitis who have persistent fever, lateral neck pain/swelling, myalgias/arthralgias, and pulmonary decompensation should arouse suspicion.

Venglarcik J: Lemierre's syndrome. Pediatr Infect Dis J 22:921–923, 2003.

CHAPTER 49

UROLOGIC EMERGENCIES

Kate M. Cronan, MD, FAAP

1. **How is the diagnosis of testicular torsion made?**
   A torsed testis is typically swollen and tender and lies higher in the scrotum than that on the contralateral side. Erythema of the scrotal skin may or may not be present. Edema increases with time. In the case of complete torsion, the cremasteric reflex is absent. The presence of a brisk cremasteric reflex with a 2- to 3-cm testicular shift makes the diagnosis of testicular torsion very unlikely. Pain may be referred to the abdomen. Systemic symptoms (nausea, vomiting, diaphoresis) may also occur. Color Doppler ultrasonography has become the imaging study of choice. Its availability increases its value as compared with scintigraphy. No clinical findings, laboratory tests, or radiographic studies can approach the sensitivity of surgical exploration.

2. **How is testicular torsion differentiated from torsion of the appendix testis?**
   Although it can happen at any age, torsion of the appendix testis is most common from ages 7 through 12 years. Pain in torsion of the appendix testis is reportedly not as severe as that seen in testicular torsion. Classically, the **blue dot sign** on the scrotum indicates the site of the infarcted appendage, although as edema increases this may become obscured. In the early stages, pain may be localized initially to the upper pole of the testis, with the remainder of the testis nontender. Doppler ultrasonography reveals normal or increased blood flow to the affected testis in the case of torsion of the appendix testis, whereas arterial blood flow is absent or diminished in the case of testicular torsion. None of these studies is perfect, and changes in blood flow may be missed, especially in the case of intermittent torsion. Treatment for torsion of the torsed appendix includes analgesics or anti-inflammatory medications and rest. Pain should resolve in 2–5 days.

3. **Why does epididymitis occur more frequently in adolescent males?**
   Epididymitis indicates the presence of inflammation of the epididymis. It generally results from infection, which may lead to an enlarged and tender epididymis on palpation. Patients may also have evidence of urinary tract infection (UTI), including dysuria and frequency. Most cases in young men are caused by sexually transmitted organisms, predominantly *Chlamydia trachomatis*, followed by *Neisseria gonorrhoeae* and *Ureaplasma urealyticum*. These organisms are common among adolescent boys. Patients should be treated for both chlamydia and gonorrhea. Epididymitis is extremely rare among prepubertal boys; if it is diagnosed, further investigation is warranted to rule out structural abnormalities of the urinary tract.

4. **Can epididymitis be treated on an outpatient basis?**
   Patients who are febrile and toxic-appearing should be admitted to the hospital for treatment with IV antibiotics, and possibly for further diagnostic tests to exclude a scrotal or testicular abscess (e.g., testicular ultrasonography). Otherwise, outpatient therapy is appropriate. Treatment for sexually transmitted disease–related epididymitis includes a single dose of ceftriaxone, 250 mg intramuscularly, and doxycycline, 100 mg orally twice daily for 7–10 days. Also evaluate and treat the patient's sexual partner(s).

5. **Describe the difference between phimosis and paraphimosis.**
Both of these conditions are seen in the uncircumcised male. *Phimosis* occurs when the distal foreskin is too tight to retract over the glans penis. *Paraphimosis* occurs when the foreskin is left in the retracted position, becomes swollen and edematous, and is then unable to be reduced (Fig. 49-1). Phimosis is not generally a problem in children, and is normal in boys younger than 6 months. Frequent retraction of the foreskin should not routinely be attempted in infants. In contrast, paraphimosis should be reduced. This is generally accomplished by application of lidocaine gel to the swollen foreskin, followed by steady pressure on the glans. Then pull the foreskin forward while pushing the glans backward with the thumb, as you would to turn a sock inside out. A dorsal penile block with local anesthetic may make the patient more comfortable, but it is generally not needed.

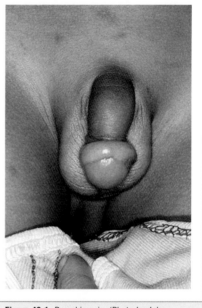

Figure 49-1. Paraphimosis. (Photo by John Lorselle, MD, with permission.)

6. **What is balanoposthitis?**
Balanoposthitis occurs in uncircumcised boys. It is an infection of the foreskin that may also affect the glans. If the foreskin is irritated as the result of poor hygiene, a break in the skin may occur, allowing bacteria to establish cellulitis. Treatment includes warm soaks and oral antibiotics (amoxicillin). Voiding may be more comfortable while the patient is sitting in a tub of warm water. True phimosis may occur as a complication, resulting from scarring after the inflammatory reaction. Circumcision may be necessary to avoid recurrent infections. The term *balanitis* is used to describe an infection involving only the glans penis.

7. **What are other causes of penile swelling in children?**
Penile swelling is usually painful and results from infection, sickling of red blood cells, or trauma. Other considerations in the presence of isolated, nontender penile swelling include insect bite (look for the lesion), allergic reaction, or more generalized edematous states, including renal, cardiac, or hepatic problems.

8. **How do a "communicating" and a "noncommunicating" hydrocele differ?**
A hydrocele is an accumulation of fluid within the tunica vaginalis surrounding the testis. Although it may arise in the case of torsion, trauma, tumor, or epididymitis, a simple hydrocele may be present in the absence of any underlying testicular abnormality. Infants may be left with a simple noncommunicating hydrocele when fluid is trapped around the testis after the *processus vaginalis has closed* during development. The baby presents with painless scrotal swelling of constant size. Management consists of observation only, as most are resorbed by the age of 12–18 months.
If the history is of scrotal swelling that "comes and goes," especially with crying or exertion, the same fluid may be present, but *the processus vaginalis has not closed*. This allows

"communication" between the scrotum and the abdominal cavity. Treatment in this case is surgical exploration with ligation of the processus vaginalis and drainage of the hydrocele.

Brenner J, Ojo A: Causes of painless scrotal swelling in children and adolescents: www.uptodate.com

9. **In an infant, how can a hydrocele be differentiated from an inguinal hernia?**
   The history given with an *inguinal hernia* is generally that the parents have observed a nonpainful, nonerythematous scrotal and inguinal swelling in males, or inguinal swelling in females. The swelling typically occurs when the baby is crying or straining. Sometimes bowel sounds can be heard over the mass. In contrast, the swelling of a *hydrocele*, though it may extend toward the inguinal canal, should not be felt as a mass at the internal inguinal ring.
   Transillumination with a high-intensity light does *not* definitively make the distinction. Although the mass of a hydrocele generally does transilluminate, transillumination of a hernia can be variable.

10. **What should be done to reduce an inguinal hernia?**
    First determine that the testes are bilaterally descended. Apply steady, gentle pressure to the mass in the direction of the inguinal ring. Often the mass will slip easily back into the abdominal cavity. It may take several minutes of steady pressure to accomplish this goal. If the hernia remains difficult to reduce, it may be necessary to sedate the child (e.g., with midazolam), and place him or her in the Trendelenburg position. This may be enough to allow the child to relax and the hernia to reduce.

11. **What is a ureterocoele?**
    A ureterocele is a dilation of the distal ureter that produces a cystic structure within the bladder. Ureteroceles can prolapse out of the bladder neck, and in doing so may cause bladder outlet obstruction. In a female, a ball valving ureterocele is the most common cause of bladder outlet obstruction. These patients will present with a painless pink cystic structure that is bulging out between the labia. This may be reduced by placing a feeding tube within the bladder. Ureteroceles should be managed by urologists, who will usually opt to carry out an endoscopic puncture and decompression of the obstructed system.

12. **How can one distinguish between a prolapsed ureterocoele and a prolapsed urethra?**
    The differentiation of a prolapsed ureterocele and urethral prolapse can usually be made by physical examination. A urethral prolapse appears as a red or purplish doughnut-shaped mass. It is usually not tender and is 1–2 cm in diameter. A small central dimple indicates the lumen of the urethra. Rarely, there may be a dark ring of necrotic tissue around the edge of the prolapse. In contrast, the prolapsed ureterocele is a cystic swelling of the terminal ureter and appears as a cystic mass protruding from the urethra. They are frequently associated with ureteral duplication.

13. **What is the most common cause of severe obstructive uropathy in children?**
    Posterior urethral valves is most common and occurs only in boys. If the condition is not diagnosed in utero, the infant presents with a palpably distended bladder and a weak urinary stream. Urgent urologic consultation is indicated.

14. **What is the first evaluation to do for a patient with "blood in the urine"?**
    Confirm that the red urine actually contains blood. Urine can appear red as the result of ingestion of a number of foods (blackberries, beets, red Kool-Aid drink, Fruit Loops cereal), substances (aniline dyes, urates), or drugs (phenazopyridine, phenolphthalein). A urine dipstick test can quickly and easily determine whether blood is present. If the result is positive, send the urine for microscopic analysis to determine the presence or absence of red blood cells. Myoglobin

will also give a positive result for blood on the dipstick. The presence of > 5–10 red blood cells/high-powered field should be considered hematuria, often warranting further work-up.

15. **Describe the differences among bacteriuria, cystitis, pyelonephritis, and urethritis.**
Bacteriuria refers to the presence of bacteria anywhere in the urinary tract. It may or may not cause symptoms.

Cystitis and pyelonephritis are part of the continuum of UTIs. **Cystitis** is bacteriuria with invasion of the bladder mucosa. Patients with cystitis present with urgency, frequency, and dysuria, and may on occasion develop a low-grade fever.

Pyelonephritis occurs when the UTI has localized within the renal parenchyma and causes systemic symptoms; thus, it is the most serious of UTIs. Children present with fever (temperature often > 39° C) pyuria, and bacteruria, often accompanied by nausea, vomiting, leukocytosis, flank pain, and tenderness.

Urethritis indicates inflammation or an infection localized to the urethra. There is usually a discharge, and in adolescents, urethritis generally is a manifestation of a sexually transmitted disease (*C. trachomatis* or *N. gonorrhoeae* infection). Urethritis can also result from noninfectious causes, including local irritation from detergents, fabric softeners, soaps, or bubble baths, as well as minor injury.

16. **What are the most common organisms in UTI?**
Most common are the enteric organisms, with *Escherichia coli* isolated in about 90% of cases. Other less common organisms include *Enterobacter*, *Klebsiella*, and *Proteus* spp. *Enterococcus* sp. occasionally is isolated in patients of any age. *Staphylococcus saprophyticus* and *Staphylococcus epidermidis* are seen in adolescents, while group B streptococci are found in infants and during pregnancy. In immunocompromised and chronically ill patients, as well as patients with anatomic abnormalities or indwelling catheters, *Pseudomonas aeruginosa*, *C. albicans*, and *Staphylococcus aureus* account for a small percentage of UTIs.

17. **Which age groups most commonly get UTIs?**
Overall, UTIs are more common in neonates and infants and in sexually active adolescent females. As many as 3–5% of febrile young infants presenting to the emergency department (ED) have a UTI. In neonates and infants under the age of 6 months, males have a higher incidence, perhaps because of a higher incidence of anomalies of the urinary tract. After this age, UTI becomes less common in males and is rare beyond the age of 1 year. In contrast, girls have a rate of UTI as much as tenfold higher than that of boys between the ages of 6 months and 2 years, with the risk being greater in the first year than in the second.

18. **List the variables that have optimal diagnostic accuracy in diagnosing UTI in young females.**
   - Age < 1 year
   - Temperature > 39° C
   - White race
   - Fever for > 2 days
   - Absence of another source of fever on history or examination
   Note: Three or more of the above have the best accuracy in making the diagnosis.

   Gorelick MH, Hoberman A, Kearney D, et al: Validation of a decision rule identifying febrile young girls at high risk for urinary tract infection. Pediatr Emerg Care 19:162, 2003.

19. **How does the clinical presentation of UTI vary with the age of the patient?**
Neonates and very young infants with UTI may present with fever or with nonspecific symptoms, including poor feeding, vomiting, diarrhea, irritability, jaundice, and even seizures. This is clearly why assessment of the urine is an integral part of the "full sepsis work up" performed on infants with any of these presenting symptoms.

Older infants and children up to the age of 2 years often have fever, and parents may notice such urinary symptoms as change in voiding pattern or foul-smelling urine. *Preschool and school-age children* describe specific urologic symptoms, such as frequency, urgency, dysuria, and enuresis. They may also report less specific symptoms, including abdominal pain and vomiting.

KEY POINTS: CLINICAL PRESENTATION OF UTI BY AGE ✓

1. **Neonates:** Nonspecific symptoms, fever

2. **Infants up to age 2 years:** Fever, voiding issues, foul-smelling urine

3. **Preschool and school-age children:** Dysuria, frequency, urgency, abdominal pain

20. **When should I get a catheterized specimen as opposed to a "clean-catch" specimen?**
    The external genitalia should be examined for signs of inflammation or infection. Obtain a catheterized specimen (or in some instances a specimen by suprapubic tap) in any patient who lacks bladder control (e.g., infants and toddlers), has evidence of vaginitis, or is unable to provide an adequate midstream specimen. Putting a urine "bag" on any infant or toddler is not helpful if the specimen is being collected for culture because the urine will probably be contaminated with perineal flora, no matter how much preparation is done. This type of collection is reliable only if the culture has no growth. If you suspect that a child has a UTI, it is worth getting the most accurate specimen possible.

21. **What is the significance of a positive test result for nitrites on the urine dipstick?**
    Most urinary pathogens (with the exception of enterococcus) are able to reduce urine nitrates to nitrite. Hence, a positive test result indicates the presence of pathogenic bacteria.

22. **What is the significiance of a positive leukocyte esterase test result?**
    Leukocytes are able to convert indoxyl carboxylic acid to an indoxyl moiety. This test is highly specific for pyuria.

23. **How should dipstick indicators be used to screen for UTI?**
    Many studies have been published regarding the usefulness of these tests in diagnosing UTI. Most of the studies have been performed in adult patients, and results of studies in children frequently differ. A meta-analysis by Gorelick and Shaw concludes that the presence of nitrites or leukocyte esterase or both on a dipstick test is almost as sensitive as a Gram stain in detecting UTI in children.

    Gorelick MH, Shaw KN: Screening tests for urinary tract infection in children: A meta-analysis. Pediatrics 104:e54, 1999.

KEY POINTS: SCREENING FOR INFECTION VIA URINE DIPSTICK ✓

1. **Nitrite positive:** Indicates pathogenic bacteria (does not screen for enterococcus)

2. **Leukocyte esterase positive:** Specific for pyuria

24. **Do white blood cells in the urine always signify a UTI?**

No, not always. Pyuria can be found in the absence of bacteriuria (i.e., "sterile pyuria"). Vaginitis can cause the leukocyte esterase test result to be positive, but does not necessarily mean the patient has a UTI. Moreover, an inflammatory process in the abdomen (e.g., appendicitis, inflammatory bowel disease, pelvic inflammatory disease) can cause white blood cells to appear in the urine. A recent meta-analysis shows that the presence of white blood cells in the urine (either spun or unspun) is only about 75% sensitive for UTI.

25. **Is a gram stain of the urine helpful?**

The presence of any bacteria on Gram stain of an uncentrifuged urine specimen is about 93% sensitive for detection of UTI, compared with culture as the reference standard. It does, however, require trained personnel to prepare the sample and read the results, and may not be available to the emergency physician at all times. Fortunately, dipstick analysis has been shown to be almost as sensitive in detecting UTI and is a readily available, quick, easy, and inexpensive alternative.

Gorelick MH, Shaw KN: Screening tests for urinary tract infection in children: A meta-analysis. Pediatrics 104:e54, 1999.

26. **When should you order a urine culture?**

Opinions differ, and there are no clear-cut answers to this question. Practice parameters developed by the American Academy of Pediatrics (AAP) in 1999 recommend culture for infants and young children 2 months to 2 years of age with unexplained fever. An evidence-based review of the recent literature suggests that for children younger than 36 months of age who present with fever without source or UTI symptoms (e.g., dysuria, vomiting, abdominal pain), a urine culture should be obtained by using an age-appropriate method. If the child is 3 years of age or older, a culture should be sent if the urine dipstick result is positive for nitrite or leukocyte esterase, or if the patient is symptomatic (even with a negative dipstick result).

27. **Which patients should be treated with antibiotics?**

Patients of any age should be treated presumptively if the dipstick result is positive for moderate leukocyte esterase or nitrite, if they have symptoms of UTI, or if follow-up is in question. For patients with a negative dipstick result (or trace leukocyte esterase but otherwise negative results), no symptoms other than fever, and good follow-up, it is prudent to defer treatment while awaiting results of culture. Febrile infants younger than 1 month of age should be treated empirically with antibiotics because of the risk of serious bacterial illness. Infants 1–2 months of age should undergo thorough evaluation and be treated if there is evidence of UTI.

28. **What should be the duration of treatment for UTI?**

A 10-day course is recommended for antibiotic therapy in children. High failure rates have been documented for shorter courses of treatment.

29. **Which patients with UTI should be admitted for parenteral antibiotics?**

AAP Practice Parameters recommend parenteral therapy for infants and young children with suspected UTI who are "toxic, dehydrated, or unable to retain oral intake." Those who "may not appear ill but who have a culture confirming the presence of UTI" should have antimicrobial therapy initiated either parenterally or orally. Additional considerations in the decision to admit a patient include the presence of underlying urologic abnormalities, identification of a urinary pathogen resistant to oral antibiotics, and issues regarding adherence with outpatient therapy. Indication for parenteral therapy based on patient age varies in the literature, with some authors recommending IV antibiotics for patients younger than 3 to 6 months of age, and some extending the recommendation to 1 year of age.

Hoberman A, Wald ER: Treatment of urinary tract infections. Pediatr Infect Dis J 18:1020–1021, 1999.
American Academy of Pediatrics: www.aap.org

30. **Define urinary retention.**
    Urinary retention is the inability to pass urine from the bladder through the urethra. Since urine is being produced normally, the bladder may become largely distended, causing substantial discomfort to the patient.

31. **What causes urinary retention in infants?**
    In the infant, most urinary retention is the result of obstruction. In males, the most common cause is posterior urethral valves; other causes include urethral polyps, strictures, diverticula, and, rarely, meatal stenosis. Urinary retention has been noted as a complication of the Plastibell device used for circumcision. Female infants may experience a prolapsing ureterocele, urethral prolapse, or a foreign body. Neurologic urinary retention may result from a spinal cord lesion.

32. **How can sexual abuse contribute to urinary retention?**
    The emergency physician should always be aware that urinary retention or dysfunctional voiding may on rare occasions be the presenting symptom of sexual abuse. Children who have been sexually abused are often very fearful of any processes involving the genitalia, and seek to avoid that portion of their anatomy. Furthermore, abusive acts may result in genital or urethral trauma or infection. Ask appropriate questions if no other cause for urinary retention can be found.

33. **What should be done in the ED about urinary retention?**
    The approach depends on the cause. Refer newborn infants with ineffective voiding to a urologist for further evaluation. While waiting for the consultant, obtain a basic metabolic panel to check electrolytes, blood urea nitrogen (BUN), and creatinine. A suprapubic tap may be necessary to obtain a specimen for urinalysis. Consult a neurologist if a spinal cord lesion is suspected on the basis of physical examination. Older children who have previously voided normally may be catheterized for urinalysis if they are unable to void. Treat infections with appropriate antibiotics. Retention from trauma to the urethra should be treated with frequent sitz baths (at least three times per day). Medications causing retention should be discontinued if possible. Urinary retention suspected to be of psychosomatic origin or as the result of sexual abuse should be referred to psychiatric and sexual abuse management specialists as appropriate. If the patient is unable to void, catheterization may be necessary.

34. **What causes renal stones in children?**
    Renal stones (calculi) are uncommon in children and adolescents. Seven percent of urinary calculi occur in children younger than 16 years of age. The cause of calculi depends on geography. In the United States, most stones are attributed to metabolic causes, and most contain calcium. Infectious stones are more common in European children, and uric acid stones occur in southeast Asian children. Boys and girls are equally likely to be affected, and 94% of stones occur in white persons.

    Cronan K, Kost S: Renal emergencies. In Fleisher G, Ludwig S, Henretig F (eds). Textbook of Pediatric Emergency Medicine, 5th ed. Philadelphia, Lippincott Williams & Wilkins, 2006, pp 913–914.

35. **What are the symptoms of urolithiasis in children?**
    Unlike the classic presentation of excruciating abdominal pain seen in adults, symptoms in children can be far less specific. The patient may appear uncomfortable and may report flank pain, abdominal pain, or costovertebral angle tenderness. Intense pain may cause an elevation in heart rate and blood pressure. Almost all children have some degree of hematuria, which may be microscopic or macroscopic. They may also have symptoms of dysuria, urinary frequency, or urinary retention. The etiology of these symptoms needs to be distinguished from UTI.

36. **How is the diagnosis of urolithiasis confirmed?**
The first test to obtain is a urinalysis, to look for hematuria and for crystals in the urinary sediment. In recent years, spiral computed tomography has become the accepted gold standard study for the detection of urolithiasis, albeit at the expense of a higher dose of radiation exposure.

37. **What treatment for urolithiasis should be initiated in the ED?**
The foremost issue that must be addressed in the ED is pain management. Nonsteroidal anti-inflammatory drugs may be adequate if the patient is able to tolerate oral intake, but IV ketorolac offers excellent pain relief and may reduce the need for narcotics. Obtain urologic consultation in any patient with evidence of obstruction since endoscopic stenting may be indicated. Initiate IV hydration and strain the urine to collect any particles for laboratory analysis. Prescribe antibiotics if there is an associated UTI.

38. **Which patients with urolithiasis need to be admitted?**
Any patient with evidence of obstruction should be admitted with urologic consultation, since immediate intervention (e.g., endoscopic stenting or ureteroscopy with stone extraction) is necessary to relieve the obstructing stone. Also consider admission for patients with severe pain requiring parenteral analgesia, vomiting or dehydration, and inability to tolerate oral hydration. Patients with renal insufficiency, structural abnormalities of the genitourinary tract, or a solitary kidney should also be admitted.

Bartosh S: Medical management of pediatric stone disease. Urol Clin North Am 31: 575–588, 2004.

39. **What are the presenting symptoms of uretero pelvic junction obstruction in older children?**
Uretero pelvic junction obstruction presents more commonly on the left side and is bilateral in 10% of cases. The male-to-female ratio is 2:1. There is a history of episodic pain that can occur in the abdomen, flank, or back. Nausea and vomiting may occur. The episodes of pain last from 30 minutes to several hours. Examination may reveal an enlarged kidney and tenderness.

40. **What is the most common cause of acute glomerulonephritis?**
There are numerous causes of acute glomerulonephritis, but in children the most common is **postinfectious** or **poststreptococcal nephritis**. It is a syndrome that occurs predominantly in school-aged children, and is characterized by the sudden appearance of either grossly bloody or tea-colored urine, peripheral edema, and decreased urine output. Patients generally present 1–2 weeks after having had a sore throat, sometimes 2–3 weeks after a case of impetigo. Other infectious causes include viral upper respiratory tract infections or mononucleosis syndromes.

41. **What are the physical findings in acute glomerulonephritis?**
In addition to dark or bloody urine, peripheral edema develops. The edema is firm, and initially appears around the eyes. Weight gain is frequently noted. Patients may have mildly elevated blood pressure. Some children have no symptoms other than abnormally colored urine. In others, hypertension can be significant and lead to complications requiring emergency intervention.

42. **What laboratory tests should I order for suspected acute glomerulonephritis?**
The most important test is the urinalysis, with a microscopic examination of the urine. Dysmorphic red blood cells and red blood cell casts are diagnostic of this condition. Significant proteinuria is also characteristic. White blood cells may be present, and since hematuria and proteinuria may be presenting signs of a UTI, a urine culture should be included in the initial evaluation. Other studies include complete blood count with differential, platelet count,

erythrocyte sedimentation rate, serum electrolytes, calcium, BUN, creatinine, total protein, albumin, and complement (C3 and C4). Antistreptolysin O titer should be tested if poststreptococcal acute glomerulonephritis is considered; antinuclear antibody and anti–double-stranded DNA should be done in the case of systemic lupus erythematosus. Order prothrombin time and partial thromboplastin time if there is concern about a bleeding diathesis. A throat culture may reveal group A streptococcal infection, and chest radiography may be important to evaluate heart size in a hypertensive patient.

43. **What are the goals of ED management of acute glomerulonephritis?**
The goal is aggressive treatment of life-threatening complications, particularly hypertension, congestive heart failure (CHF), and hyperkalemia. If the blood pressure is elevated but the patient is asymptomatic, oral antihypertensives (sublingual nifedipine or captopril) may be adequate. In the patient with acute neurologic changes, antihypertensives (diazoxide or hydralazine) should be given intravenously. Treat CHF by keeping the head of the bed elevated, providing supplemental oxygen, and promoting diuresis with furosemide (0.5–1.0 mg/kg via IV route). Tailor fluid management to restrict volume and sodium, to replace only insensible losses plus urine output. Do not give potassium until the patient's urine output is established and hyperkalemia is resolved.

44. **What is the most common cause of nephrotic syndrome in children?**
Nephrotic syndrome is a constellation of findings, including edema, proteinuria, hypoalbuminemia, and hyperlipidemia. It can occur in children as a primary renal disorder, or secondary to systemic disease, environmental toxins (heavy metals, bee venom), or medications. About 80% of pediatric cases occur between the ages of 2 and 5 years and are associated with "minimal change" or "nil disease" when renal biopsy specimens are examined.

45. **How is the diagnosis of nephrotic syndrome made?**
After physical examination, evaluate urine for the presence of protein. Measure total serum protein, albumin, and cholesterol levels. Typical values in nephrotic syndrome are a urinary protein of 3–4+ on dipstick, serum albumin level < 3 g/dL, and elevated cholesterol level. Other laboratory values that may be important for management include the hematocrit (which may be elevated secondary to intravascular volume depletion), electrolytes (sodium is often low); and BUN/creatinine (BUN level may initially be elevated, reflecting the lowered intravascular volume; creatinine level may be normal or elevated depending on whether there is primary renal damage).

46. **What management decisions need to be made in the ED for a child with nephrotic syndrome?**
Complications requiring emergency management include the progression from hypovolemia to shock, hypercoagulability, and pleural effusions and ascites leading to difficulty walking, abdominal pain, or respiratory distress. The child must be evaluated for peritonitis, usually due to *Streptococcus pneumoniae*. Give normal saline boluses (20 mL/kg) to restore circulation, if needed. For symptomatic massive edema, furosemide can be given orally, or in extreme cases, albumin followed by IV furosemide. Rarely is paracentesis necessary. Deep venipunctures should be avoided because of the increased risk of thromboembolic events.

47. **What is the treatment for nephrotic syndrome?**
Steroids (prednisone) at 2 mg/kg/d. Start antibiotics (after blood culture is obtained) if the child is febrile or there is another reason to suspect bacterial infection.

48. **Should all patients with nephrotic syndrome be admitted?**
Most should be, including those newly diagnosed, those in whom there is a possibility of infection, and any who are symptomatic from dehydration or edema. Consult a pediatric nephrologist regarding steroid therapy and indications for renal biopsy.

49. **What is the treatment for priapism?**

Priapism (prolonged painful penile erection without sexual stimulation) may be caused by trauma or leukemic infiltration. However, most commonly it is seen in males with sickle cell disease. Erythrocyte sickling leads to sludging in the erectile portion of the corporal bodies. Stasis yields hypoxia and more sickling occurs. The most effective treatment consists of hydration and irrigation of the corporal bodies using saline with vasoactive substances. Transfusion of packed red blood cells is reserved for refractory cases. Urologic consultation should be obtained.

ABDOMINAL TRAUMA

Ronald A. Furnival, MD

1. **What are the most common mechanisms of injury for pediatric patients with abdominal trauma?**
    Across the United States, more than 85% of pediatric patients with abdominal trauma are injured from blunt mechanisms, most commonly motor vehicle collisions (as passengers or pedestrians), and from falls. In some urban emergency departments (EDs), penetrating injuries from gunshots or stab wounds in adolescents account for up to 40% of pediatric abdominal injuries.

2. **Is the age of a patient a factor for some abdominal injuries?**
    Yes. Young infants have a larger portion of the liver and spleen exposed below a more flexible rib cage, placing those organs at greater risk for injury with upper abdominal and lower thoracic trauma. Infants and preschool children may be victims of child abuse, with liver, pancreatic, and duodenal injuries resulting from a direct blow to the abdomen. In addition, young preschool children involved in auto crashes may have injuries related to lap belts.

3. **What is the "lap-belt complex" seen with motor vehicle crash victims?**
    This complex of injuries results during an automobile crash when the seat belt rides up from the pelvic bones and over the softer abdominal viscera in an improperly restrained child not sitting in a car seat or booster seat. Young children may have some or all of the lap-belt complex. A visible abdominal wall bruise or mark from the lap belt may be present. A perforated or ischemic colon is a unique injury associated with lap belts, and splenic injury as well as associated spinal injury or vertebral fracture (lumbar fracture) also are possible. The lap-belt complex is the most common cause of blunt pediatric bowel injury.

    Lutz N, Nance ML, Kallan MJ, et al: Incidence and clinical significance of abdominal wall bruising in restrained children involved in motor vehicle crashes. J Pediatr Surg 39:972–975, 2004.
    Sokolove PE, Kupperman N, Holmes JF. Association between the "seat belt sign" in intra-abdominal injury in children with blunt torso trauma. Acad Emerg Med 2005; 12:808–813.

4. **Which injuries may result from a direct blow to the midabdomen, such as from a bicycle handle bar or abuse?**
    Duodenal hematoma, pancreatic trauma, and injury to the left lobe of the liver have been associated with handle bar injury. Infants and preschool children may also be victims of child abuse, with a potentially delayed presentation of the above injuries from a fist to the upper abdomen.

    Gaines BA, Shultz BS, Morrison K, Ford HR: Duodenal injuries in children: Beware of child abuse. J Pediatr Surg 39:600–602, 2004.
    Nadler EP, Potoka DA, Shultz BL, et al: The high morbidity associated with handlebar injuries in children. J Trauma 58:1171–1174, 2005.

5. **When is it appropriate to assess for abdominal injury in the pediatric patient with multiple trauma?**
    As outlined by the Advanced Trauma Life Support program, the pediatric patient with multiple injuries must initially have a **primary survey** of the ABCs to identify and begin therapy for immediately life-threatening injuries. Once the primary survey is completed, the **secondary survey** to identify any additional injuries, including the abdominal evaluation, should begin. The secondary survey may include laboratory testing and imaging studies for the diagnosis of all injuries.

American College of Surgeons' Advanced Trauma Life Support program. Available at: www.facs.org/trauma/atls/index.html

6. **What physical examination findings are useful for identifying abdominal injuries?**
The physical examination during the secondary survey is intended to recognize that an intra-abdominal injury exists, rather than to identify a specific diagnosis. Physical findings, including absent or diminished bowel sounds, evidence of peritoneal irritation with involuntary guarding or rebound, abdominal distention, abdominal wall abrasions or bruising, abdominal or flank tenderness, lower chest wall injury, or unexplained hypotension, may indicate the presence of an intra-abdominal injury. Gently palpate the pelvic bones for tenderness or instability since pelvic fractures have been associated with an increased risk of intra-abdominal injury. Inspect the perineum for injury, including extravasation of blood or urine. Finally, perform a rectal examination for palpable mass, lacerations, pelvic brim fracture, or blood.

Perform **serial** abdominal examinations to look for evidence of delayed clinical deterioration. (The pediatric patient with a small bowel perforation may develop physical findings 6–24 hours after injury.) Look for increasing abdominal girth and tenderness. Serious abdominal injury is possible even without bruises on the abdomen.

7. **What is the appropriate management of a child with a normal abdominal examination who appears to be at low risk for injury?**
The patient with stable vital signs, normal mental status, normal results on screening laboratory tests, and a normal abdominal examination on serial evaluations may be discharged from the ED after a period of observation.

Cotton BA, Beckert BW, Smith MK, et al: The utility of clinical and laboratory data for predicting intra-abdominal injury among children. J Trauma 56:1068–1075, 2004.

Holmes JF, Sokolove PE, Brant WE, et al: Identification of children with intra-abdominal injuries after blunt trauma. Ann Emerg Med 39:500–509, 2002.

8. **Why is gastric distention following abdominal trauma concerning?**
Children often develop gastric distention after abdominal trauma from crying and swallowing air. This can interfere with respiration by altering motion of the hemidiaphragm. Young children are primarily diaphragmatic breathers, so this can be serious. Also, gastric dilatation increases the risk of vomiting. Children often have a full stomach when injured, and vomiting could lead to aspiration of stomach contents. Gastric distention also makes abdominal examination difficult. Place a nasogastric tube to decompress the stomach.

9. **What is the treatment for the child with an apparent abdominal injury and clinical instability?**
The initial care for the unstable pediatric patient with abdominal trauma must begin with the ABCs. Once airway and breathing are secure, circulation is addressed with an initial infusion of an isotonic crystalloid solution (normal saline or lactated Ringer's solution) of up to 40–60 mL/kg via the IV route. For the patient who continues to be unstable, a transfusion with packed red blood cells is indicated. If the transfusion requirement exceeds 40 mL/kg during the initial resuscitation, or with separate transfusions during the hospital course, surgical exploration must be considered for ongoing bleeding. Intra-abdominal hemorrhage is the primary cause of early death in pediatric abdominal trauma.

10. **Which laboratory studies are useful for evaluating patients with abdominal trauma?**
An initial hemoglobin/hematocrit (or as part of a complete blood count) can serve as a baseline; subsequent decreases may be evidence of internal bleeding. Hematuria, either gross or microscopic (> 5 red blood cells/high-powered field) on urinalysis, may indicate the presence of genitourinary or other internal organ injury. About 30% of pediatric trauma patients with hematuria have liver or

splenic injury, demonstrating the utility of hematuria as a nonspecific marker for intra-abdominal injury. The liver function tests aspartate aminotransferase (AST) and alanine aminotransferase (ALT) have been valuable markers of injury in several studies, with levels exceeding 200 and 100 IU/L, respectively, an indicator of possible liver injury. A serum amylase level may also serve as a marker for pancreatic or bowel injury, but given the low sensitivity and specificity of the initial value, serial levels are more useful as evidence of evolving pancreatic injury.

Additional laboratory studies should include a type and crossmatch for the patient requiring (or who may require) blood transfusion for hemodynamic instability, a serum pregnancy test for the adolescent female trauma patient, blood gases for the patient requiring respiratory support, and coagulation studies for the multiply injured patient with concomitant head injury. Some recommend an alcohol and drug screen for adolescent trauma victims.

Cotton BA, Beckert BW, Smith MK, et al. The utility of clinical laboratory data for predicting intrabdominal injury among children. J Trauma 56:1068–1074, 2004.

11. **What is the role of computed tomography (CT) for pediatric abdominal trauma?**
For the clinically stable pediatric patient with blunt trauma (those without any of the clinical indications for laparotomy), CT continues to be the **gold standard** for abdominal injury diagnosis, with sensitivity, specificity, and accuracy all exceeding 95%. Advantages of CT over other imaging modalities include the ability to noninvasively assess anatomic organ injury, perfusion, renal function, and the retroperitoneal space and lower chest. CT seldom affects the decision for laparotomy for solid organ injury, which is usually based upon the patient's clinical condition, but CT does have a greater role in decision making for hollow viscous injuries, which are often clinically subtle.

Disadvantages of CT include a limited utility for the unstable patient (it is difficult to resuscitate an unstable patient in a CT suite), radiation exposure for the patient (and caregivers), and limited (60–80%) sensitivity for the diagnosis of pancreatic or bowel injury. Some believe CT scans are overused and that better decision rules are needed to limit these studies in children.

Fenton SJ, Hansen KW, Meyers RL, et al. CT scan and the pediatric trauma patient—are we overdoing it. J Pediatr Surg 398:1877–1881, 2004.
Peters E, LoSasso B, Foley J, et al. Blunt bowel and mesenteric injuries in children: Do nonspecific computed tomography findings reliably identify these injuries. Pediar Crit Care Med 7:551–556, 2006.

12. **What is the role of ultrasonography (US) for pediatric abdominal trauma?**
A number of studies of adults, and a few involving pediatric patients, advocate US over CT for the initial evaluation of blunt abdominal trauma. US is primarily used to identify the presence of intra-abdominal fluid, usually a hemoperitoneum in the patient with blunt trauma, with sensitivity and specificity approaching 90%. The chief advantage of US over CT is the ability to perform an **evaluation in the trauma suite** during the initial resuscitation, even for the unstable patient, in a rapid (generally < 5 minutes) and noninvasive manner.

Since the presence of hemoperitoneum is an indirect marker of organ injury, and is not an indication for laparotomy in pediatric trauma, most authors recommend follow-up with CT or other imaging for the patient at risk for an intra-abdominal injury. Other disadvantages of US include the need for additional imaging for the patient with multiple injuries (i.e., head or thoracic CT) and a limited ability to diagnose solid organ, hollow viscous, or bony injuries.

Holmes JF, Gladman A, Chang CH. Performance of abdominal ultrasonography in pediatric blunt trauma patients: a meta-analysis. J Pediatr Surg 42:1588–1594, 2007.
Mutabagani KH, Coley BD, Zumberge N, et al: Preliminary experience with focused abdominal sonography for trauma (FAST) in children: Is it useful? J Pediatr Surg 34:48–54, 1999.
Patel JC, Tepas JJ: The efficacy of focused abdominal sonography for trauma (FAST) as a screening tool in the assessment of injured children. J Pediatr Surg 34:44–47, 1999.

13. **So which is better, CT or US?**
Good question. If the accurate diagnosis of all intra-abdominal injuries is necessary for nonoperative management of the patient with blunt trauma, as some authors contend, then

CT has the clear advantage. However, if the patient is clinically unstable and cannot leave the resuscitation suite, US has the advantage. For the stable patient with a possible intra-abdominal injury, the benefit of US versus CT on clinical decision making, management outcome, and medical cost has yet to be fully defined.

14. **What is FAST? Is it useful in children?**
FAST is focused abdominal sonography for trauma. The FAST exam is helpful to identify intrabdominal free fluid and parenchymal injury. It is advantageous because it is a rapid, convenient, inexpensive tool that does not expose a child to radiation. It is done at the bedside in some emergency departments, so the patient does not need to be transported. There are few studies to evaluate its utility in children. One study found FAST to be inadequate to independently identify intraabdominal trauma, since free fluid may not be seen in many cases of blunt abdominal trauma. Other studies imply the FAST exam should be used as a screening tool and, if positive, a CT scan is needed to better identify in a hemodynamically stable patient.

Coley BD, Mutabagani KH, Martin LC, et al. Focused abdominal sonography for trauma (FAST) in children with blunt abdominal trauma. J Trauma 48: 902–906, 2000.

Eppich WJ, Zonfrillo MR. Emergency department evaluation and management of blunt abdominal trauma in children. Curr Opin Pediatr 19: 265–269, 2007.

15. **What are the indications for laparotomy for pediatric abdominal trauma?**
See Table 50-1.

TABLE 50-1. INDICATIONS FOR AN EMERGENT LAPAROTOMY FOR THE PEDIATRIC TRAUMA PATIENT

- Vital sign instability, despite fluid resuscitation, or blood transfusion requirement totaling > 40 mL/kg *during the hospital course*
- Peritoneal irritation on physical examination
- Gunshot wound to the lower chest or abdomen
- Stab wound of the abdomen, with vital sign instability, peritoneal irritation, or clinical evidence of organ injury
- Rectal or vaginal laceration
- Evisceration of abdominal contents
- Evidence of intestinal perforation (e.g., pneumoperitoneum on imaging studies, fecal content on diagnostic peritoneal lavage
- Evidence of renal vascular injury on imaging studies (controversial)

---

16. **What is meant by the nonoperative management of blunt abdominal trauma in children?**
Despite the long list of indications for laparotomy mentioned above, operative intervention is infrequently required for pediatric blunt abdominal trauma, and nonoperative management is the current standard of care for the majority of patients. With few exceptions, the need for an operation rests entirely with the **patient's clinical condition**, rather than with specifics of the intra-abdominal organ injuries or the grade or severity of organ injury. Studies indicate that appropriately selected patients (i.e., those without surgical indications) have excellent overall outcomes, low transfusion rates, and few complications.

However, nonoperative does not mean nonaggressive or nonsurgical management. These patients must be closely monitored, often in the intensive care unit, with surgical supervision and adequate laboratory, blood bank, radiologic, nursing, and medical support. An aggressive and continuing reevaluation of the patient's clinical condition is mandatory, with surgical exploration for any evidence of deterioration.

Stylianos S. Outcomes from pediatric solid organ injury; role of standardized care guidelines. Curr Opin Pediatr 17:402–406, 2005.

Venkatsh KR, McQuay N Jr. Outcome of management in stable children with intra-abdominal free fluid without solid organ injury after blunt abdominal injury. J Trauma 62:216–220, 2007.

17. **How often do pediatric patients require operative versus nonoperative management of blunt abdominal injuries?**
A number of studies dating back to the 1980s note that over 90% of pediatric patients with abdominal trauma may be successfully managed with nonoperative care. Delayed laparotomy rates at most centers have been $< 1\%$, usually for recognition of an initially occult bowel injury, or for late intra-abdominal bleeding. Laparoscopic repair of bowel injuries in hemodynamically stable children seems to be less invasive and decreases hospital stay.

Studies show that splenectomy after injury is more likely at general hospitals than children's hospitals, and more likely in non-trauma centers.

Bowman SM, Zimmerman FJ, Christakis DA, et al. Hospital characteristics associated with the management of pediatric splenic injuries. JAMA 294:2611–2617, 2005.

Davis DH, Localio AR, Stafford PW, et al. Trends in operative management of pediatric splenic injury in a regional trauma system. Pediatrics 115:89–94, 2005.

Holmes JH, Wiebe DJ, Tataria M, et al. The failure of non-operative management in pediatric solid organ injury; a multi-institutional experience. J Trauma 59:1309–1313, 2005.

Streck CJ, Lobe TE, Pietsch JB, et al. Laproscopic repair of traumatic bowel injury in children. J Pediatric Surg 41:1864–1869, 2006.

KEY POINTS: ABDOMINAL TRAUMA ✓

1. Nonoperative management is appropriate for $> 90\%$ of pediatric patients with an abdominal injury.

2. Clinical instability is the most important indication for an emergent laparotomy in the child with an abdominal injury.

3. Hemoperitoneum in the stable pediatric trauma patient is not an indication for laparotomy.

4. Physical examination findings in the child with a bowel perforation may be clinically silent for 6–24 hours.

5. Laboratory tests (hematocrit, urinalysis, aspartate aminotransferase, alanine aminotransferase) are excellent adjuncts to the physical examination to screen for an abdominal injury in the stable pediatric patient.

18. **What is the clinical approach to penetrating abdominal trauma?**
Because of their high velocity and penetrating ability, $> 90\%$ of gunshot wounds to the abdomen will result in organ injury requiring laparotomy. Stab wounds are typically of lower velocity, with less penetrating ability, and can be managed more selectively. Triple-contrast CT, laparoscopy, clinical observation, or local wound exploration have all been advocated to identify peritoneal penetration or intra-abdominal organ injury in the stable stab wound victim. Evidence of clinical instability, peritoneal irritation, pneumoperitoneum, hematuria, or rectal blood are all absolute indications for laparotomy for either the gunshot or stab wound patient.

CHAPTER 51

BURNS AND SMOKE INHALATION

John M. Loiselle, MD

BURNS

1. **How common are burns and fire-related deaths among children?**
   Injury-related deaths are the leading cause of death in children ages 1–14 years. Centers for Disease Control and Prevention statistics from 2002 rate fire- or burn-related injuries as the third leading cause of injury-related deaths in this age group, behind motor vehicle–related deaths and drowning. Burns and fire-related injuries were responsible for 480 childhood deaths in the United States in 2002 and more than 1600 hospitalizations.

   National Center for Injury Prevention and Control: www.cdc.gov/ncipc

2. **What functions of the skin do burns affect?**
   - Temperature control
   - Protection from infection
   - Pain and sensation
   - Fluid homeostasis

3. **How are different depths of burns classified?**
   See Table 51-1.

TABLE 51-1. CLASSIFICATION OF BURN DEPTH			
Wound Depth	**Layer Involved**	**Clinical Findings**	**Common Causes**
First-degree (superficial)	Epidermis	Erythema	Sun exposure
Second-degree (partial-thickness)	Dermis	Erythema, blistering	Hot liquids
Third-degree (full-thickness)	Subcutaneous tissue	Pale or charred, waxy or leathery, does not bleed, insensate	Flame
Fourth-degree	Fascia, muscle, or bone	Tissue loss	Flame or high-voltage electricity

Data from Sheridan R: Outpatient burn care in the emergency department. Pediatr Emerg Care 21:449–456, 2005.

4. **What are the common sources of burns in children?**
   The cause of burns in children varies with the setting in which they are evaluated and the age of the child (Table 51-2). Common burns treated in an emergency department (ED) differ from those requiring hospitalization. Contact and scald burns make up a higher proportion of burns treated on an outpatient basis. The true pattern of burn injuries in children, including those not seeking medical care, may be substantially different. Scald burns predominate in the younger age group. Most of these occur when the child pulls over a hot liquid from the surface of a table or stove. Burns due to flames account for most hospital admissions in older children.

   Banco L, Lapidus G, Zavoski, et al: Burn injuries among children in an urban emergency department. Pediatr Emerg Care 10:98–101, 1994.
   Morrow SE, Smith DL, Cairns BA: Etiology and outcome of pediatric burns. J Pediatr Surg 31:329–333, 1996.

TABLE 51-2. COMMON SOURCES OF BURNS IN CHILDREN			
Hospitalized Patients (%)		Emergency Department Patients (%)	
Flames	36	Contact	43.1
Scald	35	Scald	33.9
Immersion	14	Flame	11.0
Contact	9	Cigarette	5.5
Chemical	3.5	Electrical	2.8
Electrical	1.5	House fire	0.9
Other	2.7		

5. **How long must the skin be in contact with hot water to cause a burn?**
   The actual duration of contact and water temperature required to cause a partial-thickness burn depend on the location and thickness of the skin. Partial-thickness burns on the soles of the feet require a longer period of contact with the water because of the thick layer of skin. Scald burns occur more rapidly in the skin of young children than in adults, and partial- or full-thickness burns can occur in less time than listed below:

Temperature	Time
160°F	1 seconds
150°F	2 seconds
140°F	5 seconds
130°F	30 seconds
120°F	300 seconds

   Tepas JJ III, Fallat ME, Moriarty TM: Trauma. In Gausche-Hill M, Fuchs S, Yamamoto L (eds): The Pediatric Emergency Medicine Resource, 4th ed. Boston, Jones and Bartlett, 2004, pp 268–323.

6. **Why is it important to interview the paramedics who arrive with fire victims?**
   Paramedics can provide the answers to questions that influence therapy as well as prognosis. Important questions include the following:

- Did the fire occur in an open or enclosed area?
- Where was the child found?
- What was the duration of exposure to smoke?
- Did the child lose consciousness?
- How long was the transport?
- What therapy was instituted?
- Are trauma or associated injuries suspected?
- What materials were at the fire scene?
- Is additional toxic fume exposure a concern?

7. **Name the methods commonly used to estimate the percentage of body surface area (BSA) damaged by burns in a child.**
   The distribution of BSA is different in children and adults. The standard "rule of nines" used in adults is not as accurate in children. The young child has a greater proportion of the BSA in the head and less in the lower extremities. Nagel and Schunk demonstrated that the entire palmar surface of a child's hand (including the fingers) is approximately 1% of BSA. The Lund and Browder chart (Fig. 51-1) provides useful estimates of larger contiguous burn areas in children younger than 10 years of age. First-degree burns are not generally included in the calculation of total BSA burned.

   Lund C, Browder N: The estimation of areas of burns. Surg Gynecol Obstet 79:352–358, 1944.
   Nagel TR, Schunk JE: Using the hand to estimate the surface area of a burn in children. Pediatr Emerg Care 13:254–255, 1997.

8. **What is the initial treatment of major burns in a child?**
   1. Address and stabilize the airway, breathing, and circulation.
   2. Remove clothing and any remaining hot or burning material.
   3. Obtain IV access and begin fluid resuscitation, as needed, for severe burns.
   4. Administer pain medication.
   5. Monitor and maintain core temperature.
   6. Assess the extent and depth of burns.
   7. Irrigate with lukewarm sterile saline.
   8. Gently remove devitalized tissue with sterile gauze.
   9. Perform escharotomies, as needed, for full-thickness circumferential burns.
   10. Apply topical antibiotics to partial-thickness burns.
   11. Cover large burn areas with sterile sheets.
   12. Administer tetanus prophylaxis as indicated.
   13. Consider transfer to a burn center

   Tepas JJ III, Fallat ME, Moriarty TM: Trauma. In Gausche-Hill M, Fuchs S, Yamamoto L (eds): The Pediatric Emergency Medicine Resource, 4th ed. Boston, Jones and Bartlett Publishers, 2004, pp 268–323.

KEY POINTS: MAJOR THREATS TO CHILDREN WITH EXTENSIVE BURN INJURIES ✔

1. Hypothermia

2. Hypovolemia

3. Infection

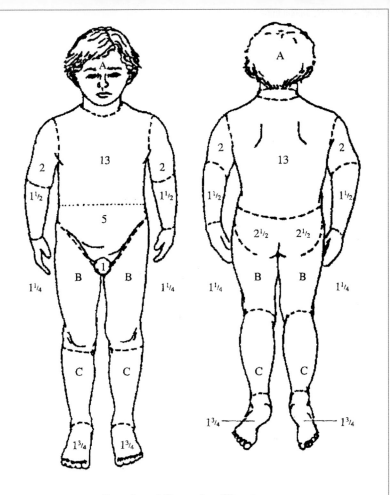

Lund and Browder Chart

Age (years)	0	1	5	10	15	Adult
A: Half of head	9 ½	8 ½	6 ½	5 ½	4 ½	3 ½
B: Half of thigh	2 ¾	3 ¼	4	4 ¼	4 ½	4 ¾
C: Half of leg	2 ½	2 ½	2 ¾	3	3 ¼	3 ½

Total area burned = second-degree surface area and third-degree surface area

Initial fluid maintenance: Ringer's lactate solution* given at:

$$\frac{\text{Surface area burned (kg)} \times \text{weight (kg)}}{4} = \text{mL/hr}$$

*Some authors recommend adding sodium bicarbonate or 5% albumin to the solution.

Figure 51-1. Lund and Bowder charts are somewhat more accurate to estimate the percentage of body surface than the rule of nines. Compared with adults, children have larger heads and smaller legs. Other areas are relatively stable through life. (From Roberts JR, Hedges JR: Clinical Procedures in Emergency Medicine, 2nd ed. Philadelphia, W.B. Saunders, 1991, pp 614–615.)

9. **Name some recommended topical therapies for burns.**
   Multiple creams and ointments are appropriate for the treatment of burns. They should
   perform several functions, including minimizing bacterial colonization, preventing desiccation,
   and reducing pain. Superficial burns require only a moisturizer. Commonly used topical
   therapies include:
   - Bacitracin ointment—burns on the face
   - Erythromycin ophthalmic ointment—burns around the eye
   - 1% silver sulfadiazine cream—burns on the body
   - 11.1% mafenide acetate (Sulfamylon)—burns on the external ear. Mafenide acetate
     penetrates the burn eschar to reach and protect the cartilage of the ear.
   - Synthetic membranes are also available to cover burn wounds. These dressings do not
     require daily changes but are much more expensive.

   Monafo WW: Current concepts: Initial management of burns. N Engl J Med 335:1581–1586, 1996.

10. **How should blisters be treated?**
    Intact blisters maintain a sterile environment below the surface, while unroofing the blisters
    allows for easier cleaning. Nonviable skin from a ruptured blister that is allowed to remain in
    the burn provides a medium for bacterial growth. Blisters should never be aspirated as this
    predisposes to infection by disrupting the sterile environment and can introduce bacteria into
    the wound. The treatment is controversial, but in general, small blisters should be allowed
    to remain intact. Open blisters, large blisters likely to rupture, and those crossing joints should
    be unroofed and debrided. The burn is then cleaned with mild soap and water.

    Reed JL, Pomerantz WJ: Emergency management of pediatric burns. Pediatr Emerg Care 21:118–129,
    2005.

11. **What is the approach to fluid management of a child with severe burn
    injuries?**
    Fluid resuscitation is typically required in children with partial- or full-thickness burns
    covering 15% or more of the total BSA. Fluid administration initially consists of lactated Ringer's
    solution or normal saline as needed for shock. Early fluid replacement can be estimated by
    following one of two formulas. The Parkland formula dictates that 4 mL/kg/% BSA burned
    should be administered over the first 24 hours. Half of the total volume is infused over the
    first 8 hours and half over the next 16 hours. Maintenance requirements should be added for
    children younger than 5 years of age. The Carvajal formula recommends 5000 mL/m^2/% BSA
    burned. Half is given in the first 8 hours and the other half in the next 16 hours. Maintenance
    fluids of 2000 mL/m^2/d are added to the total. Initial resuscitation is followed by an infusion
    of 5% dextrose in one-fourth normal saline solution titrated to maintain urine output at
    0.5–1 mL/kg/hr. Overhydration is poorly tolerated and may contribute to development of
    acute pulmonary edema. Placement of a central venous pressure monitor or Swan-Ganz
    catheter should be considered in severe cases.

    Joffe MD: Burns. In Fleisher GR, Ludwig S, Henretig FM (eds): Pediatric Emergency Medicine, 5th ed.
    Philadelphia, Lippincott Williams & Wilkins, 2006, pp 1521–1522.

12. **What are the indications for referral to a regional burn center?**
    - Burns accompanied by respiratory injuries or major trauma
    - Major chemical or electrical burns
    - Partial-thickness and full-thickness burns covering over 10% BSA in children under 10 years
      of age, or over 20% in children older than 10 years
    - Full-thickness burns over 2% BSA
    - Burns that involve the face, hands, feet, genitalia, perineum, or major joints
    - Burn injury in patients with preexisting medical conditions affecting management or
      prognosis

■ Burn injury in patients requiring special social, emotional, or long-term rehabilitative intervention

Committee on Trauma, American College of Surgeons: Resources for optimal care of the injured patient: 1999. Chicago, American College of Surgeons, 1999, p 55.

13. **A 15-year-old male presents with circumoral burns consistent with frostbite injury. What should you suspect?**
This boy has burns that are suspicious for inhalant abuse. Other cutaneous findings may include a rash or paint stains around the mouth and nose. Inhalation of fluorinated hydrocarbons can cause local burns to the face and upper airways. General toxicity of inhalants involves the pulmonary, central nervous, cardiac, and renal systems. Abusers are at risk for dysrhythmias and seizures. Inhalant abuse is often associated with alcohol and other drugs of abuse. Standard urine toxicology screens do not detect inhalants. Gas chromatography can occasionally be useful, but is not routinely available.

Lorenc JD: Inhalant abuse in the pediatric population: A persistent challenge. Curr Opin Pediatr 15:204–209, 2003.

14. **Describe the patterns of burns commonly associated with child abuse.**
   ■ **Immersion burns**. This pattern of injury occurs as the result of a body part being dipped in a hot liquid. These burns are often circumferential with a sharply demarcated border. Burns in a glove-and-stocking distribution are a classic example.
   ■ **Doughnut burn**. This term describes the sparing of the central area of the buttocks when it is held in contact with the cooler ceramic of the bathtub floor. The surrounding areas of skin remain in contact with the water and sustain more severe burns. Burns involving the genitals, the buttocks, or perineum are unlikely to be accidental.
   ■ **Contact burns on the dorsum of the hands**. Children are more likely to sustain accidental burns by reaching for hot objects and grasping them with the palmar surface.
   ■ **Markings consistent with an object**, such as a cigarette or iron, held to the skin.
   In addition, burns that are inconsistent with the history or are attained in a manner beyond the developmental capacities of the child deserve further investigation.

SMOKE INHALATION

15. **Name three potential causes of loss of consciousness in a fire victim.**
   ■ Carbon monoxide poisoning
   ■ Head trauma
   ■ Severe hypovolemia

16. **What are the indications for intubation of the trachea of a fire victim?**
   ■ **Early-onset stridor.** The presence of stridor or hoarseness suggests upper airway injury that can be expected to progress. Laryngeal edema does not peak until 2–8 hours after exposure. Intubation for this cause frequently requires an endotracheal tube with a smaller internal diameter than standard calculations suggest because of airway swelling.
   ■ **Severe burns of the face or mouth.** Patients are at significant risk for upper and lower airway injury.
   ■ **Progressive respiratory insufficiency.** Respiratory insufficiency may be diagnosed clinically or by the finding of a widening arterial-alveolar gradient or rising levels of partial pressure of carbon dioxide. Hypercarbia may result from depressed mental status, pain associated with chest wall movement, restriction of chest wall movement secondary to burns, pulmonary restrictive or obstructive injury, or upper airway swelling and obstruction.
   ■ **Inability to protect the airway due to coma or profuse tracheobronchial secretions.**

- **Carboxyhemoglobin levels > 50.** Intubation and active ventilation provide increased oxygen concentrations and help to decrease levels more rapidly.

The presence of soot in the nares or carbonaceous sputum in isolation is not an indication for intubation.

17. **What acute findings are common on the chest radiograph of a child with smoke inhalation?**
Initial chest radiographs are usually normal. Radiographic findings lag behind physical symptoms. Chest radiographs are thus an insensitive means of determining lung injury and rarely dictate ED management. A normal chest radiograph does not exclude the presence of significant pulmonary injuries. Early findings are suggestive of severe injury. Diffuse interstitial infiltrates are consistent with significant smoke inhalation. Focal infiltrates in the first 24 hours indicate atelectasis. Bronchopneumonia as the result of smoke inhalation does not typically occur until 3–5 days after injury. Pulmonary edema typically follows aggressive fluid resuscitation and does not appear until 6–72 hours after exposure. Pneumothorax is often the result of barotrauma after intubation and positive-pressure ventilation.

Clark WR, Bonaventura M, Myers W: Smoke inhalation and airway management at a regional burn unit: 1974 to 1983. Part I. Diagnosis and consequences of smoke inhalation. J Burn Care Rehabil 10:52–62, 1989.

18. **What precautions must be taken when interpreting an arterial blood gas sample from a victim of smoke inhalation?**
Partial pressure of oxygen in arterial blood (PaO_2) measures only dissolved oxygen in the blood. It is unaffected by the presence of carbon monoxide. PaO_2, therefore, provides a falsely reassuring measure of oxygenation. In addition, it is important to know whether the blood gas report includes a measured or calculated oxygen saturation. A calculated oxygen saturation does not take into account the presence of carboxyhemoglobin, whereas a measured oxygen saturation does. A calculated oxygen saturation registers falsely elevated readings in the setting of carbon monoxide poisoning.

19. **Describe the pathophysiologic effects of carbon monoxide toxicity.**
Carbon monoxide binds hemoglobin with 230 times the affinity of oxygen. The production of carboxyhemoglobin significantly reduces the oxygen-carrying capacity of blood. The binding of carbon monoxide to the hemoglobin molecule shifts the oxygen dissociation curve to the left. This shift inhibits the release of oxygen at the tissue level. Carbon monoxide also has toxic effects on the cellular level. Carbon monoxide binds cytochrome oxidase and effectively blocks cellular respiration. This blockade facilitates free radical production and disrupts mitochondrial function. The results are tissue hypoxia and metabolic acidosis.

20. **How is the half-life of carboxyhemoglobin affected at different oxygen concentrations?**
- **Room air (21%, 1 atmosphere [1 atm]):** Half-life of 4 hours
- **100% O_2 1 atm:** Half-life of 60–90 minutes
- **Hyperbaric oxygen (100% oxygen, 2.5 atm):** Half-life of 15–30 minutes

KEY POINTS: PATHOPHYSIOLOGIC EFFECTS OF SMOKE ✔ INHALATION

1. Airway burns and edema from superheated gases and particles

2. Hypoxia due to carbon monoxide

3. Disruption of cellular respiration by carbon monoxide and cyanide

4. Bronchospasm from gases and particulate matter

21. **How is a pulse oximeter reading affected by the presence of carboxyhemoglobin?**

    The pulse oximeter essentially measures the absorption of two separate wavelengths of light. These wavelengths correspond to the peak absorption spectra of oxygenated and deoxygenated hemoglobin. Carboxyhemoglobin absorbs light at a wavelength similar to oxygenated hemoglobin and therefore does not affect the overall reading. The result is a falsely high oxygen saturation reading. Pulse oximeter readings are unreliable measures of true oxygen saturation in patients with smoke inhalation.

    Bozeman WP, Myers RM, Barish RA: Confirmation of the pulse oximetry gap in carbon monoxide poisoning. Ann Emerg Med 30:608–611, 1997.

22. **What are the indications for hyperbaric oxygen therapy?**

    The use of hyperbaric oxygen in the setting of smoke inhalation is highly controversial. Although no randomized, controlled, prospective trials in humans demonstrate reduced mortality with hyperbaric oxygen therapy, animal studies have shown improved survival with treatment after smoke inhalation. When indications for a particular patient remain unclear, further consultation should be sought from hyperbaric experts. To be considered a candidate for hyperbaric oxygen therapy, the patient must be deemed stable enough for transport. The potential benefits should outweigh the risks of transferring the patient to the chamber, especially when long distances are involved.

    Juurlink DN, Buckley NA, Stanbrook MB, et al: Hyperbaric oxygen for carbon monoxide poisoning. The Cochrane Database of Systematic Reviews. CD002041, 2005.

23. **What are the criteria for hyperbaric oxygen therapy?**

    Generally Accepted Criteria
    - Syncope
    - Severe neurologic symptoms on presentation (seizures, focal neurologic findings, coma)
    - Myocardial ischemia diagnosed by history or electrocardiography
    - Cardiac dysrhythmias (ventricular, life-threatening)
    - Persistent neurologic symptoms and signs after several hours of 100% oxygen therapy at ambient pressure (mental confusion, visual disturbance, ataxia)
    - Pregnancy (symptomatic, carboxyhemoglobin level > 15%, evidence of fetal distress)

    Criteria for Consideration
    - Carboxyhemoglobin level > 20–25%
    - Abnormal results on neuropsychological examination
    - Age < 6 months with symptoms (lethargy, irritability, poor feeding) or involved in same exposure as adults with any of the above criteria
    - Children who have underlying diseases (i.e., sickle cell anemia) for whom hypoxia may have deleterious effects

    Liebelt EL: Hyperbaric oxygen therapy in childhood carbon monoxide poisoning. Curr Opin Pediatr 11:259–264, 1999.

24. **List the major therapeutic actions of hyperbaric oxygen.**
    - Rapidly reduces levels of carboxyhemoglobin through mass action
    - Inhibits lipid peroxidation, a process mediated by carbon monoxide that produces metabolites toxic to the brain
    - Directly oxygenates tissues by raising the partial pressure of oxygen to extremely high levels
    - Reduces cerebral edema
    - May be effective in reversing cyanide poisoning

25. **What is the evidence for cyanide toxicity in relation to house fires?**

A study performed in France measured cyanide concentrations in blood samples obtained from fire victims by ambulance physicians at the scene. Cyanide levels were found to be significantly higher than those in one control group of patients with no fire exposure and a second control group with isolated carbon monoxide poisoning. Mean cyanide levels in fire victims declared dead at the scene were over 110 μmol/L. Mean cyanide levels in survivors were 21.6 μmol/L. Lethal cyanide levels are generally considered those exceeding 40 μmol/L.

Baud FJ, Barriot P, Toffis V, et al: Elevated blood cyanide concentrations in victims of smoke inhalation. N Engl J Med 325:1761–1766, 1991.

26. **How are cyanide levels assessed for treatment?**

Treatment for cyanide poisoning is indicated in fire victims with evidence of significant smoke inhalation. Elevated lactate levels correlate with the presence of cyanide and are typically available sooner than a cyanide level.

27. **What treatments are available for cyanide poisoning?**

- **Sodium thiosulfate** can be administered intravenously as an infusion of a 25% solution of sodium thiosulfate at a dose of 1.65 mL/kg. It is the rate-limiting compound in the conversion of cyanide to thiocyanate, which is excreted harmlessly in the urine.
- **Amyl nitrate** and **sodium nitrate** convert hemoglobin to methemoglobin, which preferentially binds cyanide in the form of cyanmethemoglobin. This therapy is generally not recommended for smoke inhalation because it further reduces the level of normal hemoglobin in fire victims who already have a significant amount of dysfunctional hemoglobin.
- **Hydroxocobalamin** is used to treat cyanide poisoning in Europe but is not available for this use in the United States.

Kulig K: Cyanide antidotes and fire toxicology. N Engl J Med 325:1801–1802, 1991.

28. **What is the role of steroids in the setting of smoke inhalation?**

Steroids may benefit patients with acute bronchospasm due to smoke inhalation. No evidence indicates that steroids are beneficial in the acute treatment of airway edema or inflammatory processes due to smoke inhalation. Randomized trials have demonstrated an association of steroid use with worse outcomes in terms of infection and mortality.

Ruddy RM: Smoke inhalation injury. Pediatr Clin North Am 41:317–336, 1994.

29. **Where do most pediatric deaths from house fires occur?**

Most children (82%) die at the scene of the fire. About 7% die at a local hospital, and 11% die at a burn center.

Parker DJ, Sklar DP, Tandber D, et al: Fire fatalities among New Mexico children. Ann Emerg Med 22:517–522, 1993.

30. **What is the most effective measure in reducing mortality from burns and smoke inhalation?**

Anticipatory guidance and preventive care have the greatest potential to reduce deaths from burns and house fires. It is estimated that over 50% of fire-related deaths could be avoided with the proper use of smoke detectors. Over 90% of childhood deaths from fires occur in homes without properly functioning smoke detectors, and most children in house fires die from smoke inhalation rather than burns. Smoke detectors should be installed on every level of the house and tested regularly. Batteries should be replaced twice a year. Families should be educated about the planning of escape routes, evaluating fire risks in the house and in the use and storage of fire extinguishers. Careless (or any) cigarette use should be avoided. Lowering the setting on the water heater to deliver water at a maximum temperature of 120°F (48.8°C) substantially increases the time it takes for direct exposure to induce a full-thickness burn (see question 5). Boiling liquids should be placed on the back burners of the stove where they are out of the reach of young children. Children should be dressed in flame-retardant sleepwear.

WEBSITES

1. National Center for Injury Prevention and Control
www.cdc.gov/ncipc

2. Emergency Medical Services for Children
www.ems-c.org

CHAPTER 52

CHILD ABUSE

Stephen Ludwig, MD

1. **What four elements should you consider in making a diagnosis of suspected child abuse?**
   1. Detailed history of injury
   2. Physical findings and their correspondence with the history
   3. Laboratory and radiographic information
   4. Observed interaction between parent–child and health care team members
   Combining these four elements should help to determine whether you have sufficient grounds to institute a report of suspected abuse.

2. **What forms of abuse are defined by most state child abuse laws?**
   - Physical abuse
   - Physical neglect
   - Sexual abuse
   - Psychological/emotional abuse

3. **Which form of abuse is reported most often? What form occurs most often?**
   Although physical abuse is most often reported, with sexual abuse a close second, psychological abuse occurs most often and has the most disabling long-term consequences.

   Tenney-Soeiro R, Wilson C: An update on child abuse and neglect. Curr Opin Pediatr 16:233–237, 2004.

4. **What injury accounts for most deaths due to child abuse?**
   Head injury accounts for most child abuse–related deaths, including children who suffer direct trauma and shaking-impact injuries. Abdominal trauma causes most other child abuse–related deaths.

5. **Abuse occurs most often in which ethnic group?**
   The rate of abuse by ethnic groups roughly matches the ethnic distribution in the general population. Thus, white children are abused most often.

6. **True or false: Most cases of abuse are reported by medical professionals.**
   False. Most cases are reported by nonphysicians and non–health care institutions. Abuse is rarely reported by primary care physicians (probably less than 2% of reported cases nationwide).

7. **When did children first gain legal protection against abuse?**
   In the mid-to-late 1960s and early 1970s. Before passage of the first set of state child abuse laws, children had no legal protection from injury inflicted by parents.

8. **What has happened to the incidence of abuse over the past 20 years?**
   Three national incidence studies have been conducted in the United States during the past 20 years. They show a stepwise increase in the rates of abuse. From the mid-1980s to the present, physical abuse has doubled and sexual abuse has increased threefold.

9. **How many abuse victims are killed each year in the United States?**
   Approximately 1400 children annually. This rate has been fairly constant.

   Sirotnak AP, Grigsby T, Krugman RD: Physical abuse of children. Pediatr Rev 25:264–277, 2004.

10. **Can the color of bruises on a child's body be used to date the injury definitively?**
    Despite findings noted in most standard textbooks, the color of the bruise does not indicate
    the age. The color of a bruise is determined by location, nature of the traumatic force, amount
    of subcutaneous tissue, and other factors. Aging of bruises based on color is highly unreliable.

    Bariciak ED, Plint AC, Gaboury I, et al: Dating of bruises in children: An assessment of physician accuracy.
    Pediatrics 112:804–807, 2003.

11. **In a child with multiple bruises and normal neurologic examination, is computed tomography (CT) of the head indicated?**
    At least one study indicated a high yield of positive CT findings, even in children with normal
    neurologic examinations. CT screening appears to be more helpful than routine ophthalmologic
    examinations.

    Rubin DM, Christian CW, Bilaniuk LT, et al: Occult head injury in high-risk abused children. Pediatrics
    111:1382–1386, 2003.

12. **What is the most common skin lesion mistaken for abuse?**
    Mongolian spots, which most commonly occur on the back, at the base of the spine, and on the
    buttocks. However, they also may occur on other skin surfaces.

13. **What conditions may lead to easy bruisability?**
    Ehlers-Danlos syndrome and other connective tissue disorders may lead to easy bruisability.
    Hemophilia usually results in deep soft tissue and joint bleeding rather than superficial skin
    bruises. Idiopathic thrombocytopenia purpura and other platelet abnormalities lead to petechiae
    and mucous membrane bleeding rather than bruises. Henoch-Schönlein purpura also may be
    initially confused with bruising.

    Bechtel K: Identifying the subtle signs of pediatric physical abuse. Pediatr Emerg Med Rep 6:57–67, 2001.

14. **What developmental skill is associated with bruising?**
    Walking or learning to walk may be associated with bruises. However, bruises found on
    children who have not yet learned to walk should be considered a sign of possible abuse.
    Children who do not cruise or walk generally do not bruise.

    Sugar NF, Taylor JA, Feldman KW, et al: Bruises in infants and toddlers: Those who don't cruise rarely
    bruise. Arch Pediatr Adolesc Med 153:399–403, 1999.

15. **A 2-week-old infant, seen in the emergency department (ED) for crying, has several fractures at varying stages of healing. What may you conclude from these findings?**
    Although this scenario may indicate abuse, the young age of the infant and the possibility
    that fractures may have occurred in utero make a metabolic bone disease more likely.

16. **What findings make osteogenous imperfecta more likely than child abuse?**
    Blue sclera, dental abnormalities, hearing loss, wormian bones, and radiographs showing
    osteopenia and healing with abundant callus formation.

17. **Which specific fractures have a high probability of being caused by child abuse?**
    Rib fractures, metaphyseal chip fractures (Fig. 52-1), spine and scapula fractures, and complex
    skull fractures.

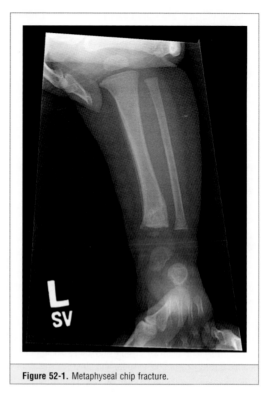

Figure 52-1. Metaphyseal chip fracture.

18. **Which specific fractures have a low specificity for abuse?**
Linear skull fractures, clavicle fractures, single-bone transverse fractures, and spiral fractures of the tibia (toddler's fracture).

19. **What type of force is consistent with the finding of a metaphyseal fracture?**
Metaphyseal fractures occur when an extremity is pulled in the direction of its long axis. Stress on the tight periosteal attachments along the metaphysis results in a chip or corner fracture.

20. **A child appears to be tender when his upper humerus is palpated. Plain radiographs fail to show any injury. What other studies may be helpful?**
Bone scanning or skeletal magnetic resonance imaging (MRI) scan may be more sensitive at demonstrating bony injury.

   Mandelstam SA, Cook D, Fitzgerald M, et al: Complementary use of radiologic skeletal survey and bone scintigraphy in detection of bony injuries in suspected child abuse. Arch Dis Child 88:387–390, 2003.

21. **What criteria should be used to order a skeletal survey for trauma?**
   - Young child (< 2 years) with multiple bruises
   - One fracture suspicious for abuse
   - Failure to thrive
   - Head injury

22. **What tests should be used to differentiate rickets from child abuse as the cause of skeletal abnormality?**
    - Bone density (appearance of bones)
    - Serum calcium and phosphorous
    - Serum alkaline phosphatase
    The best radiograph to demonstrate rickets is that of the distal radius and ulna (wrist).

23. **What history of injury matches a spiral fracture?**
    A spiral injury is caused by torque or twisting (Fig. 52-2). The extremity is twisted, or the child's body is twisted while the extremity is held in a fixed position. If the mechanism of injury does not match the nature of the injury, suspect abuse.

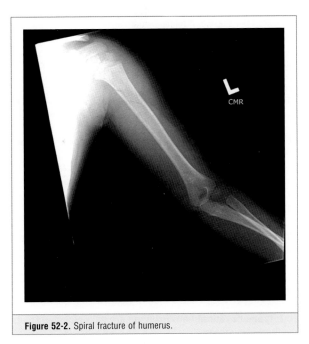

Figure 52-2. Spiral fracture of humerus.

24. **What study has the highest sensitivity and specificity for diagnosing a suspected skull fracture?**
    A skull radiograph best shows a skull fracture, although a CT scan of the head often reveals a fracture. If the fracture line is horizontal, it may be missed by the horizontal cuts of the CT scan. Documentation of skull fracture associated with abuse is one of the few indications for ordering skull radiography.

25. **A 6-month-old boy is brought to the ED for new onset of seizures. You note retinal hemorrhages. A CT scan of the brain is read as normal. What is your conclusion?**
    CT may not pick up all central nervous system (CNS) injuries. Your next step is to order an MRI. MRI may detect small punctate hemorrhages or subdural collections that are isodense on CT.

A new onset of seizures and retinal hemorrhages has a high probability of being caused by child abuse.

Care M: Imaging in suspected child abuse: What to expect and what to order. Pediatr Ann 31:651–659, 2002.

26. **What preimagery signs may be clues to shaken baby syndrome?**
Retinal hemorrhages are present in 75–80% of cases. Signs of external trauma are minimal or absent. The child may present with hypothermia or respiratory difficulties. Xanthochromic fluid may be present in the cerebral spinal fluid obtained to rule out sepsis. Bruising may be seen on the upper extremities or chest wall in the place where the child was grasped.

27. **True or false: Nonabusive head trauma may result in retinal hemorrhage.**
True. Other causes of trauma may be associated with retinal hemorrhage, but with much lower frequency than shaking. If retinal hemorrhages are present with no history of trauma, suspect an incorrect or hidden history.

Bechtel K, Stoessel K, Leventhal JM, et al: Characteristics that distinguish accidental from abusive injury in hospitalized young children with head trauma. Pediatrics 114:165–168, 2004.
Feldman K, Bethel R, Shugerman R, et al: The cause of infant and toddler subdural hemorrhage: A prospective study. Pediatrics 108:636–646, 2001.
Reese RM, Sege R: Childhood head injuries: Accidental or inflicted? Arch Pediatr Adolesc Med 154:11–15, 2000.

28. **True or false: In comparison between inflicted head trauma and noninflicted head trauma, the neurologic findings are similar.**
False. Children with inflicted head trauma have more severe head injury, which requires more ED management and longer hospital stays and is associated with poorer outcomes.

Bechtel K, Stoessel K, Leventhal JM, et al: Characteristics that distinguish accidental from abusive injury in hospitalized young children with head trauma. Pediatrics 114:165–168, 2004.

29. **How often have children with head trauma due to child abuse been injured only once?**
Rarely. Studies demonstrate that by the time head trauma due to child abuse is diagnosed, many earlier episodes probably have gone undiagnosed and unreported. Chronic effusions from old blood or cerebral atrophy may be present.

30. **What four types of retinal hemorrhages are associated with abuse?**
1. Simple flame hemorrhage
2. Dot-and-blot hemorrhage
3. Surface hemorrhage, obscuring vessels
4. Retinoschisis

31. **Which metabolic disease is associated with CNS hemorrhage?**
Glutaric acidemia has the features of CNS hemorrhage and retinal hemorrhage. Usually, other signs of metabolic derangement and mental retardation are present. Glutaric acidemia is extremely rare, unlike abuse.

32. **How can you tell a "bloody tap" from a CNS hemorrhage?**
The differentiation can be difficult. With a bloody lumbar puncture, the blood usually clears as you collect more fluid. When the collection tube is spun, the cerebrospinal fluid of the CNS hemorrhage is xanthochromic; the bloody tap is clear.

33. **What are the classic CT findings in shaken baby syndrome?**
The classic findings are subdural hemorrhage, particularly in the intrahemispheric fissure; injury to frontal or occipital lobe; loss of gray-white matter differentiation; and basal ganglia injury. Evidence of old CNS injury is another alerting sign.

34. **A child is taken to a babysitter. Six hours later the child collapses, has seizures, and is brought to the ED, where a serious head injury is found. The babysitter claims that the injury occurred at home before the parent dropped off the child. What is the likely determination?**
With the exception of an epidural hematoma, symptoms develop just after the trauma is inflicted. There is no lucid or normal interval. The findings suggest that the babysitter or someone in the babysitter's house inflicted the trauma.

35. **Do children with preexisting causes of hydrocephalus or abnormal brain anatomy have an increased risk for CNS bleeding?**
This area remains controversial. No data confirm or refute. However, some physicians believe that once the normal anatomic protective structures around the brain have been altered, the risk for bleeding is increased.

36. **Raccoon eyes are a sign of what kind of injury?**
Raccoon eyes are consistent with basilar skull fracture. More common than true raccoon eyes is bilateral infraorbital ecchymosis due to a midline forehead hematoma and tracking of blood into the infraorbital position.

37. **If a child is slapped forcefully, what skin finding is typical?**
A slap mark shows the outline of the shape of the fingers in petechiae or bruise lesions—not the imprint of the fingers themselves.

38. **What does a cigarette burn look like?**
Cigarette burns are often talked about but rarely seen. When a cigarette is extinguished on a child's skin, the mark should be circular and the width slightly larger than the cigarette (roughly 0.8–1 cm). The second-degree burn should be uniform throughout the circular lesion, and the edges of the circle are raised by 1–2 mm. Inadvertent contact between a child and a cigarette (nonintentional) produces a simple partial-thickness bullous lesion.

39. **At what temperature does water produce a burn in a child?**
There is a relationship between water temperature and time of exposure. Exposure for 20 seconds to 125°F water is sufficient to cause a second-degree or partial-thickness burn.

40. **What factors help to differentiate an inflicted bathtub scald burn from an accidental burn?**
If the child is of toilet-training age, if there was a delay ($>$ 1–2 hours) in seeking care, and if the person who brings the child to the ED is not the person who was supervising the child when the burn occurred, the likelihood of abuse increases.

Andronicus M, Oates RK, Peat J, et al: Non-accidental burns in children. Burns 24:552–558, 1998.

41. **If a child is immersed in hot water while wearing some articles of clothing, what should physical examination of the burn reveal?**
The clothed areas have increased burn severity because clothes hold the hot water closer to the skin. On the other hand, areas of thicker skin (e.g., palms and soles) may be relatively spared.

42. **What is a "boxed ear"? How do you recognize it?**
   A boxed ear is a common injury caused by abuse. It results when the child receives a blow to the side of the head, including the ear. The finding to look for is ecchymosis on the inside surface of the pinna. This area is not exposed to other forms of injury.

43. **What is "bottle-jamming"?**
   Trauma to the upper gum line and frenulum, which results when a frustrated parent forcefully jams a bottle into the child's mouth.

44. **A child with multiple bruises is brought to the ED. Other than documentation of normal coagulation, what laboratory studies should be obtained?**
   Assess amylase, lipase, and liver enzymes. Studies have shown that the rate of intra-abdominal injury is higher than what may be apparent. Also order a urinalysis to look for signs of renal bleeding.

45. **In checking a urinalysis, how many red blood cells should prompt the ordering of radiologic studies?**
   If there are more than 25–30 red blood cells per high-powered field, the rate of documentable renal pathology increases, and it is worth performing renal ultrasonography or CT of the abdomen.

46. **A 10-month-old baby is brought to the ED, essentially dead on arrival. No marks, bruises, or ecchymoses are found on the child's body, and there is no history of illness. Is sudden infant death syndrome the most likely diagnosis?**
   Most cases of sudden infant death syndrome (SIDS) occur at ages 2–5 months. Once a child is older than 6 months, you should be highly skeptical. Accurate diagnosis of SIDS requires a complete autopsy and death-scene investigation.

KEY POINTS: SUSPECTED CHILD ABUSE ✔

1. Child abuse occurs frequently and should be considered a possible mechanism in every traumatic injury.

2. Physicians and nurses are mandated to report the suspicion of abuse.

3. A level of suspicion is built by compiling elements of history, physical examination, laboratory, radiographic data, and observed interactions of the family.

4. Injuries that kill children are head injuries from both direct trauma and shaking, and abdominal injuries.

5. The more similar the family is to you in such characteristics as age, race, socioeconomic status, and education level, the more difficult it will be to suspect abuse.

47. **What metabolic disease may present to the ED as an apparent case of SIDS?**
   Deficiency of medium-chain acyl-CoA dehydrogenase, a defect in fatty acid metabolism.

48. **What are the characteristics of a parent who may be involved in Münchhausen syndrome by proxy?**
   - Mother
   - Medical background or experience as a patient

- Articulate and cooperative
- Unusual or unexplainable disorder that you are asked to diagnose
- Always present when episode, event, or finding is discovered
- Distant relationship with the child's father

49. **A child is brought to the ED for spitting up blood. The mother brings in a bib with a large blood spot. She reports that it has happened before and the child underwent an extensive workup at a nearby medical center. What should you do?**
Check the type of the blood on the bib to confirm that it is the same as the baby's. Get the records from the other hospital to see what the physician's impressions were. Check with the child's primary care physician. Collect as much background data as possible.

50. **What chief complaint is associated most often with Münchhausen syndrome by proxy?**
Complaints of apnea and near-SIDS have been documented as Münchhausen syndrome by proxy in many case series. It is an important element in the differential diagnosis of apnea or acute life-threatening events.

51. **A child comes alone to the ED with abdominal pain. She does not want her mother called for permission and states that she is afraid of her mother. Is this a case of child abuse?**
This is a difficult case. It may meet the criteria for emotional abuse, and you should attempt to report it. The diagnosis of abuse usually rests on documentation of an injury. You may need a mental health consultation to document the nature and extent of the fear.

52. **Does failure to thrive always indicate abuse or neglect?**
No. Some cases of failure to thrive are based on lack of proper child-rearing practices, others are due to an organic condition, and still others result from the combination of a child who is difficult to feed and a family without proper skills and resources. Cases that result from abuse, of course, must be reported.

53. **What forms of neglect are included in the definition of most state laws?**
- Physical neglect
- Educational neglect
- Medical neglect
- Emotional neglect
- Abandonment

54. **What are the indications for the immediate ED evaluation of a sexually abused child?**
If bleeding or other specific symptoms are present or if the suspected abuse has occurred in the past 72 hours, most specialists suggest that the child should be seen immediately. Otherwise, the patient and family may be referred to a special center for child sexual abuse.

55. **Should vaginal, pharyngeal, and rectal cultures be performed on every child undergoing a sexual abuse evaluation?**
Studies clearly show that cultures should be performed only if the child has symptoms (e.g., vaginal discharge, genital injury) and if the perpetrator or sibling of the patient has a sexually transmitted disease.

Atabaki S, Paradise JE: The medical evaluation of the sexually abused child: Lessons from a decade of research. Pediatrics 104:178–186, 1999.

56. **Does a Gram stain showing gram-negative intracellular diplococci indicate gonorrheal infection and possible sexual abuse?**
Although *Neisseria gonorrhoeae* has these characteristics, other normal flora may be visualized in the same way. A diagnosis of suspected sexual abuse should not be based on smear findings. Cultures are essential, and results must be confirmed by at least two different laboratory methods.

57. **Which sexually transmitted diseases are highly specific for sexual abuse?**
Gonorrhea and syphilis are transmitted sexually. If they are found in a prepubertal child beyond infancy, you can be almost certain that sexual abuse has occurred.

58. **Which sexually transmitted diseases are less specific because they have other modes of transmission?**
Herpes simplex virus, *Trichomonas* spp., condylomata, *Gardnerella* spp., and *Chlamydia* spp. may indicate sexual abuse, but all may be transmitted nonsexually and thus have lower specificity.

Centers for Disease Control and Prevention: Sexually transmitted diseases treatment guidelines. MMWR Morb Mortal Wkly Rep 55(No. RR-11):1–94, 2006.

59. **In examining a child for possible sexual abuse, how helpful is the width of the intralabial distance?**
Although at one time this finding was thought to be important, subsequent research has negated its diagnostic usefulness.

60. **A child comes to the ED for bloodstains in her underpants. Physical examination reveals a red doughnut-shaped mass just inferior to the clitoris. What is the likely diagnosis?**
Urethral prolapse, a finding often misidentified as child abuse. The mucosa of the urethra is friable and bleeds. It is treated with sitz baths and time. It has no association with sexual abuse.

61. **True or false: The physical examination of a recently sexually abused child will be abnormal.**
False. The physical examination of most sexually abused children is expected to be normal.

62. **Should the examination for child sexual abuse be performed under conscious sedation?**
It is important to gain the confidence of the child in order to perform the examination, whenever possible. Use of dissociative medication is to be avoided. When acute severe trauma must be ruled out, for example in the situation of ongoing vaginal bleeding, there is some justification for the examination under sedation or anesthesia.

63. **Should most child sexual abuse cases be initially evaluated in the ED?**
No. If abuse has occurred more than 72 hours prior to presentation of the child, then it is best to refer the child to a child sexual abuse center.

64. **What are the two types of child abuse cases in the court system? What are the differences?**
The two types are criminal and civil. Civil cases are brought in violation of specific child abuse laws. They require only proof that injury occurred through nonaccidental means. The ultimate penalty is removal of the child from the family. The rules of evidence tend to be more lenient. In criminal cases one must prove that a specific perpetrator committed a specific crime—a

violation of the crime code. The penalty is incarceration, and the rules of the courtroom are strictly enforced.

65. **What is a waiver trial?**
A trial in criminal or civil court in which the defendant or the party named in the civil case waives the right to trial by a jury. In such cases, decision making lies in the hands of the judge. Defendants who know the particular leanings of a judge or the projected reaction of the jury may find this choice to their advantage.

66. **What are the differences between a fact witness and an expert witness?**
A fact witness may testify to what he or she saw, heard, and did in a given case. An expert witness can interpret the facts of the case into an expert opinion. The expert may not have had first-hand contact with the child but bases opinions on record review.

67. **In testifying in a child abuse case, what is the role of the ED physician?**
The physician must be fair, objective, and reasonable in the presentation of facts and medical data. There is no room for testimony that presents feelings, sentiment, or emotion. The role of the emergency physician is to offer and explain medical information.

68. **What is the most important step in managing a child abuse case?**
The most important step is to have a high degree of suspicion for every traumatic injury; to build a level of suspicion with objective findings and observations; and, when the level of suspicion is high, to report all cases of suspected abuse.

CHAPTER 53

DENTAL INJURIES

Evaline A. Alessandrini, MD, MSCE, and Linda L. Brown, MD

1. **How frequently do health care practitioners encounter pediatric dental injuries?**
   Pediatric dental injuries occur in approximately 50% of all children at some time during
   childhood with either primary or secondary teeth. Most injuries occur during the summer
   months. Injuries to the primary teeth typically involve displacement in the alveolar bone.
   The incidence is equal in males and females, and most injuries are caused by falls, usually in
   the home. Injuries to the permanent dentition most often involve trauma to the hard dental
   structures. In this age group, males incur injuries more commonly than females. Trauma to
   the permanent dentition typically occurs on playgrounds, during sports events, or as a result
   of motor vehicle and pedestrian injuries.

   Dale RA: Dentoalveolar trauma. Emerg Med Clin North Am 18:521–538, 2000.
   Wilson S, Smith GA, Preisch J, Casamassimo PS: Epidemiology of dental trauma treated in an urban
   pediatric emergency department. Pediatr Emerg Care 13:12–15, 1997.

2. **What is the hardest substance in the human body?**
   Enamel, which covers the entire crown of the tooth.

3. **What are the other components of the tooth?**
   Other components of the crown of the tooth include dentin, a softer, microtubular structure,
   and pulp, which provides the tooth's neurovascular supply (Fig. 53-1). The root of the tooth,
   which anchors it to the alveolar bone, consists of cementum, the periodontal ligament, and
   the alveolar bone.

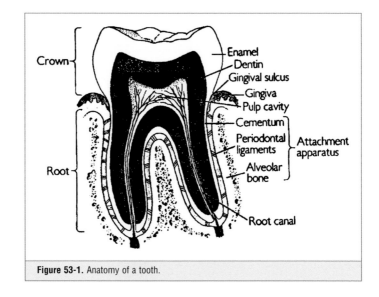

Figure 53-1. Anatomy of a tooth.

4. **Why is it important to distinguish primary from permanent teeth?**
   Management strategies for most dental injuries differ according to the type of tooth.

5. **How do I make the distinction?**
   - **Primary (deciduous) teeth** begin to erupt at about 6 months of age and are complete by 3 years. A full complement of primary teeth consists of 10 mandibular and 10 maxillary teeth, including four central incisors, four lateral incisors, four canines, and eight molars. Usually, mandibular teeth erupt before their maxillary counterparts (Fig. 53-2).
   - **Permanent teeth** typically begin to erupt at 5 years of age and are complete by 16 years of age. A full complement of permanent teeth consists of 16 mandibular teeth and 16 maxillary teeth, including four central incisors, four lateral incisors, four canines, eight bicuspids (premolars), and 12 molars (*see* Fig. 53-2).

   If in doubt, parents usually can distinguish the child's primary from permanent teeth. If a parent is unavailable, two other hints are helpful:
   - Primary teeth are often much smaller than permanent teeth.
   - The occlusive or chewing surface of the permanent tooth is ridged, whereas the occlusive surface of the primary teeth is smooth.

   Helpin ML, Alessandrini EA. Dental trauma. In Schwartz MW, Curry TA, Sargent AJ, et al (eds): Pediatric Primary Care: A Problem-oriented Approach, 3rd ed. St. Louis, Mosby Yearbook, 1997, pp 777–782.

   Nelson LP, Needleman HL, Padwa BL: Dental trauma. In Fleisher GR, Ludwig S, Henretig FM (eds): Textbook of Pediatric Emergency Medicine, 5th ed. Philadelphia, Lippincott Williams & Wilkins, 2006, pp 1507–1515.

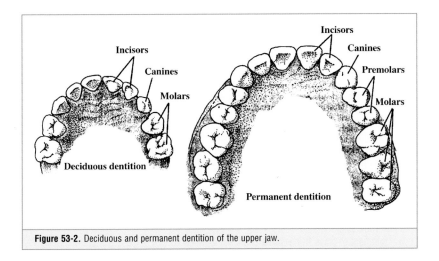

Figure 53-2. Deciduous and permanent dentition of the upper jaw.

6. **How do I accurately describe which tooth is injured?**
   The best and easiest way to describe an injured tooth is to divide the mouth into quadrants: right maxillary, right mandibular, left maxillary, and left mandibular. Then describe the type of tooth and the quadrant in which it is located. For example, the terms *right maxillary central incisor* and *left mandibular canine* denote both the type of tooth and the quadrant of the mouth in which it is found (*see* Fig. 53–2). Thus, you need not memorize the complex numbering or lettering systems.

7. **How are broken or fractured anterior teeth classified?**
   In the Ellis classification system, **class I fractures** involve only the enamel and result in jagged tooth edges but no other sequelae. **Class II fractures** break through both the enamel and dentin of the crown. The yellowish dentin is visible within the pearly white enamel. Class II fractures are often sensitive to heat, cold, and air. **Class III fractures** involve the pulp of the tooth. The pink and bleeding neurovascular bundle of the tooth is exposed, along with the dentin. Pain is often severe. **Class IV fractures** involve the root. The diagnosis must be confirmed by a dental radiograph or panoramic radiograph (Fig. 53-3).

   American Academy of Pediatric Dentistry. Clinical guideline on management of acute dental trauma. Chicago, American Academy of Pediatric Dentistry, 2004, p 8. Available at www.guideline.gov/summary/summary.aspx?view_id=1&doc_id=6278

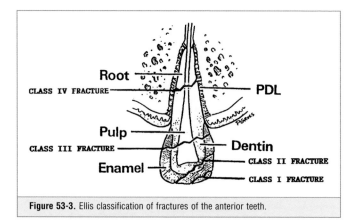

Figure 53-3. Ellis classification of fractures of the anterior teeth.

8. **How are fractured teeth treated? How soon does a dentist need to be consulted?**
   Treatment depends on the classification of the tooth fracture:
   - **Class I fractures** require filing of sharp tooth edges to prevent oral soft tissue injury. Patients can see a dentist for tooth bonding if cosmetic issues arise.
   - **Class II fractures** require prompt treatment. The fractured tooth should be covered with dental foil (aluminum foil with an adhesive coating) or a calcium hydroxide coating made with commercially available products, such as Dycal. A base and accelerator are mixed and applied to the dry tooth. The patient is instructed to eat a soft diet, take analgesics for pain, and see a dentist within 48 hours. Correct treatment of class II fractures decreases the need for root canal therapy.
   - Treatment of **class III fractures** is almost identical to that of class II fractures. Delay in dental treatment may result in severe pain and tooth abscess. Ultimately, the tooth requires total removal of pulpal tissue (root canal) with subsequent cosmetic tooth restoration.

   Flores MT: Traumatic injuries in the primary dentition. Dent Traumatol 18:287–298, 2002.
   Flores MT, Andreasen JO, Bakland LK, et al: Guidelines for the management of traumatic dental injuries. Dent Traumatol 17:145–148, 2001.

9. **How are root fractures diagnosed?**
   Classified by their location along the root, these fractures are identified as coronal, midroot, or apical, and are seen most commonly in teeth with complete root formation, approximately 2–3

years after eruption. The coronal fractures may be associated with crown displacement and, therefore, are usually the easiest to diagnose clinically. Such fractures with displacement often require immediate dental consultation for splinting. The midroot and apical fractures, however, may only be suspected by the presence of bleeding from the gingival sulcus after a traumatic event, and require follow-up intraoral dental radiographs for confirmation.

Nelson LP, Needleman HL, Padwa BL: Dental trauma. In Fleisher GR, Ludwig S, Henretig, FM (eds): Textbook of Pediatric Emergency Medicine, 5th ed. Philadelphia, Lippincott Williams & Wilkins, 2006, pp 1507–1515.

10. **When should I suspect an alveolar ridge fracture?**
Alveolar ridge fractures occur in less than 10% of all dentoalveolar injuries. They are most commonly associated with anterior teeth and may be either single or segmental. Identification of subtle fractures may be possible by palpating the gingiva and looking for any evidence of crepitus or step-offs. The most important management strategy involves the repositioning and splinting of the affected area; therefore, immediate dental consultation is often necessary. Oral antibiotics may also be utilized, although little evidence is available regarding the effectiveness of this strategy.

McTigue DJ: Diagnosis and management of dental injuries in children. Pediatr Clin North Am 47:1067–1084, 2000.

KEY POINTS: TOOTH FRACTURES ✓

1. Tooth fractures most commonly occur in the anterior dentition and have 3 classes: Class I involves enamel only; class II involves enamel and dentin; and class III involves enamel, dentin, and pulp.

2. Class II and III fractures receiving proper treatment within 48 hours will have excellent outcomes.

3. Alveolar ridge fractures should be suspected when palpation of the gingiva reveals crepitus or step-offs, there are large gingival lacerations, or several teeth are luxated en bloc.

11. **A 2-year-old patient struck his mouth on a coffee table. He reports pain with occlusion and chewing. Both maxillary central incisors are painful when percussed with a tongue blade, and the right one is slightly loose. What are the diagnosis and treatment?**
Children may sustain a tooth concussion after dental trauma. Tooth concussion is defined as a traumatic injury to the tooth and supporting structures without displacement or mobility. Signs and symptoms include exaggerated tooth sensitivity during percussion, chewing, occlusion, or mobility testing. Treatment includes a soft diet and analgesics for 7–10 days with dental follow-up to monitor tooth viability.

The loose right central incisor is called a tooth subluxation. *Subluxation* is defined as trauma to the tooth with minor mobility but no displacement. Signs and symptoms include tooth sensitivity to percussion, minor mobility on tooth examination, and blood in the gingival sulcus. Treatment is the same as for tooth concussion, but dental follow-up is more important—not only to monitor tooth viability but also to rule out a root fracture.

Flores MT: Traumatic injuries in the primary dentition. Dental Traumatol 18:287–298, 2002.

12. **What is a luxation injury? Define the five types.**

Luxation injuries result in physical displacement of the tooth within the alveolar socket, tearing of the periodontal ligament, and possible injury to the alveolar bone. Luxation injuries occur in any of five directions:

1. **Intrusion** describes a tooth impacted into the alveolar socket.
2. **Extrusion** describes a tooth that is vertically dislodged from the socket.
3. **Lingual luxation** is displacement of the tooth toward the tongue. It is common because of the frequency of injuries from an anterior force on the anterior teeth.
4. **Labial luxation** is tooth displacement toward the lips.
5. **Lateral luxations** occur within the plane of the tooth.

    www.iadt-dentaltrauma.org/Trauma/web

13. **How are luxation injuries of primary teeth treated?**

Although treatment of intrusions differ, treatment of the other four types of luxation injuries is the same. Most luxation injuries of **primary teeth** are treated with tooth extraction, particularly if the tooth is loose enough to become avulsed and possibly aspirated. In most circumstances, emergency physicians can extract primary teeth with firm pressure applied manually with the aid of gauze. If the tooth is not too loose, it may be repositioned within the alveolar socket and splinted. A dentist generally does this procedure within 48 hours.

Flores MT, Andreasen JO, Bakland LK, et al: Guidelines for the management of traumatic dental injuries. Dent Traumatol 17:145–148, 2001.

14. **How are luxation injuries of permanent teeth treated?**

Luxation injuries of the **permanent dentition** require immediate treatment, usually by a dentist, if malocclusion or significant tooth mobility is present. Otherwise, patients should seek dental care within 48 hours. Therapy for a luxated permanent tooth usually necessitates a local nerve block, followed by repositioning in the alveolar socket and splinting for 10–14 days or, if an alveolar fracture is present, 6 weeks. Temporary splinting may be done in the emergency department (ED) with a Coe pack. Zinc oxide and a catalyst are mixed, then applied to the dry injured tooth and one or two teeth on either side for stabilization. The mixture is carefully placed to the gingival line and between the teeth for best results and allowed to dry. The patient must see a dentist within 24 hours for more permanent splinting. In the meantime, the patient may take analgesics and is restricted to a soft diet.

Flores MT, Andreasen JO, Bakland LK, et al: Guidelines for the management of traumatic dental injuries. Dent Traumatol 17:145–148, 2001.

15. **How is an intrusion injury to a primary tooth treated?**

Patients who sustain an intrusion injury to a primary tooth can be treated in the ED with analgesics and a soft diet and instructed to see their dentist within the next 48 hours. Management of an intruded primary tooth varies. Some dentists obtain a dental radiograph. If the underlying tooth bud is uninjured, they allow the primary tooth to re-erupt. If the permanent tooth bud is injured, the intruded primary tooth is extracted. Others allow the tooth to re-erupt spontaneously. Ninety percent of all intruded primary teeth re-erupt after 6 months.

Kenny DJ, Barrett EJ, Casas MJ: Avulsions and intrusions: The controversial displacement injuries. J Can Dent Assoc 69:308–313, 2003.

16. **How is an intrusion injury to a permanent tooth treated?**

Patients with intruded permanent teeth can be managed conservatively in the ED and instructed to see their dentist within the next 48 hours. In adolescents and patients with more thorough development of the root, the injured tooth is submerged, realigned, and splinted, as described above. In younger patients with an immature root, the tooth usually is allowed to re-erupt spontaneously. If re-eruption has not occurred within 6 weeks, the intruded tooth is submerged, realigned, and splinted.

Kenny DJ, Barrett EJ, Casas MJ: Avulsions and intrusions: The controversial displacement injuries. J Can Dent Assoc 69:308–313, 2003.

17. **What affects the outcome for intruded permanent teeth?**
Intrusion injuries, with displacement of the tooth into the alveolar bone and crushing of the periodontal ligament, can result in significant long-term damage to the dentition. Intrusion injuries to permanent teeth can be especially difficult to manage. The most important factor in outcome has recently been reported to be the amount of intrusion present. Several studies have reported that intrusions < 3 mm have an excellent prognosis, while those > 6 mm have a universally poor outcome secondary to inflammatory root resorption and pulp necrosis.

Al-Badri S, Kinirons M, Cole B, Welbury R: Factors affecting resorption in traumatically intruded permanent incisors in children. Dent Traumatol 18:73–76, 2002.

Kinirons MJ, Sutcliffe J: Traumatically intruded permanent incisors: A study of treatment and outcome. Br Dent J 170:144–146, 1991.

18. **What is an avulsion injury?**
An avulsion injury is complete displacement of the tooth (crown and root) from the alveolar socket.

19. **What storage medium is best for an avulsed tooth?**
It is imperative to store the tooth in an appropriate solution to keep the periodontal ligament alive and to ensure successful reimplantation. Appropriate fluids, in descending order of preference, are milk, saliva, and saline. Adolescents may place the avulsed tooth under their tongue until they are seen by an emergency physician or dentist. This option is risky with younger children, who may swallow or aspirate the tooth. Hank's solution, a pH-balanced cell-culture fluid commercially marketed by 3M as Save-a-Tooth, can store an avulsed tooth and preserve the periodontal ligament for nearly 24 hours. It is useful for patients with multiple traumas who have more life-threatening injuries that must be addressed first.

Sigalas E, Regan JD, Kramer PR, et al: Survival of human periodontal ligament cells in media proposed for transport of avulsed teeth. Dent Traumatol 20:21–28, 2004.

20. **What is the procedure for reimplanting an avulsed permanent tooth?**
1. Hold the crown of the tooth, and rinse the root with Hank's solution or saline. To avoid injury to the periodontal ligament, do not handle or scrub the root of the tooth.
2. Insert the root of the tooth into the alveolar socket. The concave part of the tooth should face the tongue.
3. The tooth should be splinted for 10–14 days.
4. If the tooth has been avulsed for a while and the alveolar socket is filled with blood, it may be necessary to perform a local nerve block and irrigate the socket with saline prior to successful tooth reimplantation.
5. Soft diet, analgesics, and antibiotics (penicillin or amoxicillin) are then prescribed.

Helpin ML, Alessandrini EA: Dental trauma. In Schwartz MW, Curry TA, Sargent AJ, et al (eds): Pediatric Primary Care: A Problem-oriented Approach, 3rd ed. St. Louis, Mosby Yearbook, 1997, pp 777–782.

21. **Why is it so important to reimplant a permanent tooth within 30 minutes?**
There is a 90% likelihood of tooth survival if a permanent tooth is reimplanted within 30 minutes. Survival declines rapidly with time, by approximately 1% for each minute beyond 30 minutes. A tooth reimplanted after 2 hours is almost never viable.

Finucane D, Kinirons MJ: External inflammatory and replacement resorption of luxated, and avulsed replanted permanent incisors: A review and case presentation. Dent Traumatol 19:170–174, 2003.

Trope M: Clinical management of the avulsed tooth: Present strategies and future directions. Dent Traumatol 18:1–11, 2002.

22. **Why should an avulsed primary tooth never be reimplanted?**
An avulsed primary tooth should never be reimplanted because of a risk of ankylosis—a bony fusion of the tooth with the alveolar bone that may result in facial deformities. In addition, reimplantation of a primary tooth may interfere with eruption of the underlying permanent tooth. Temporary prosthetic devices can be made if a cosmetic effect is desired.

www.iadt-dentaltrauma.org/Trauma/web

KEY POINTS: TOOTH AVULSIONS ✔

1. Avulsed primary teeth should never be reimplanted because of the risk of ankylosis and resultant facial deformities.

2. Fluids suitable to store avulsed permanent teeth in descending order are milk, saliva, and saline.

3. An avulsed permanent tooth that is reimplanted within 30 minutes has a 90% survival rate.

4. The prognosis for avulsed permanent teeth is highly time-dependent, and reimplantation should be completed as soon as possible.

23. **When should a chest radiograph be obtained in patients with dental injury?**
If the patient has a fractured or avulsed tooth and the entire missing segment has not been found by the medical team, a chest radiograph should be obtained. Patients requiring lobectomies from aspirated teeth have been reported.

24. **When should prophylactic antibiotic therapy be prescribed for patients with dental injuries?**
Although this topic is controversial, most authorities agree that prophylactic penicillin, amoxicillin, or erythromycin (for penicillin-allergic patients) should be prescribed for 3–5 days in patients who have sustained an injury to the periodontal ligament. Examples include avulsed permanent teeth, significant luxation injuries, and alveolar ridge fractures. Several studies have suggested that this may decrease the risk of inflammatory root resorption and may, therefore, improve outcome.

Andreasen JO, Andreasen FM, Skeie A, et al: Effect of treatment delay upon pulp and periodontal healing of traumatic dental injuries—a review article. Dent Traumatol 18:116–128, 2002.
Finucane D, Kinirons MJ: External inflammatory and replacement resorption of luxated and avulsed replanted permanent incisors: A review and case presentation. Dent Traumatol 19:170–174, 2003.

25. **Summarize the appropriate timing of dental consultation for patients with dental trauma.**

Immediate Dental Consultation
- Avulsed permanent teeth
- Luxation injuries with malocclusion or significant tooth mobility

- Root fractures with crown displacement
- Alveolar ridge fractures

Urgent Dental Consultation (within 48 hours)
- Class II and III tooth fractures
- Tooth subluxation
- Tooth intrusion
- Luxation injuries not included above

Nonurgent Dental Consultation (within 1 week)
- Class I tooth fractures
- Tooth concussion

Andreasen JO, Andreasen FM, Skeie A, et al: Effect of treatment delay upon pulp and periodontal healing of traumatic dental injuries—a review article. Dent Traumatol 18:116–128, 2002.

KEY POINTS: PEDIATRIC DENTAL TRAUMA ✓

1. Each patient with dental trauma should foremost be considered a trauma patient like any other.

2. A unique consideration in the evaluation of children with dental injuries is the need to understand normal dental development as proper identification of primary versus permanent dentition may affect diagnosis and treatment.

3. Primary teeth may be distinguished from permanent teeth because they are usually found in children younger than 6 years of age, are smaller in size, and have a smooth, not ridged, occlusive surface.

4. It is possible to prevent many sports-related dental injuries with the use of properly fitted mouthguards.

26. **A mother brings her adolescent son for his yearly physical, and you learn he is very active in sports. What information should you give him regarding the prevention of sports-related dental injuries?**
Sports-related dental injuries occur frequently during adolescence. A 1995 study by Flanders showed that dental injuries were increased sixfold to eightfold in high school basketball players who did not wear mouthguards. To support this finding, it was noted that in football, where mouthguards are always worn, 0.07% of the injuries were orofacial, while in basketball, where mouthguards are not routinely worn, 34% of the injuries were orofacial.

Multiple types of these guards are available on the market, including stock, boil and bite, and custom-fitted. It is generally felt that the better-fitted mouthguards, primarily those that are custom-fitted, will be more comfortable and provide better protection against dental injuries.

Andreasen JO, Andreasen FM, Skeie A, et al: Effect of treatment delay upon pulp and periodontal healing of traumatic dental injuries—a review article. Dent Traumatol 18:116–128, 2002.

WEBSITES

1. www.iadt-dentaltrauma.org/Trauma/web

2. National Guideline Clearinghouse: American Academy of Pediatric Dentistry
   www.guideline.gov/summary/summary.aspx?view_id=1&doc_id=6278

3. American Dental Association: Mouthguards
   www.ada.org/public/topics/mouthguards_faq.asp

CHAPTER 54

EXTREMITY INJURIES

John M. Loiselle, MD

DEVELOPMENT

1. **How do the pediatric musculoskeletal system and its response to stress differ from those in the adult?**
   - The pediatric skeleton is less densely calcified than the adult version. It is composed of a higher percentage of cartilage. Pediatric bones are lighter and more porous than adult bones, with haversian canals making up a greater percentage.
   - The pediatric musculoskeletal system is an actively growing structure. Long bones contain growth plates or physes that are the primary site of this growth. The ends of the bone contain a chondro-osseous segment termed the *epiphysis* or secondary site of ossification.
   - The bones in a child are surrounded by a thick and very active periosteum. This structure provides additional support as well as a high capacity for remodeling injured bone.
   - The relative strengths of the different musculoskeletal components differ from child to adult. In the child, the ligaments and periosteum are stronger than the bone itself and less likely to give way under stress. The physis is the weak link. As a result, fractures tend to be relatively more common than sprains or ligamentous injuries in children than in adults.
   - The degree of ossification, the thickness of the periosteum, and the width of the growth plate vary with age. Therefore, the age of the child and the corresponding anatomy dictate the response of the musculoskeletal system to trauma.

KEY POINTS: UNIQUE CHARACTERISTICS OF THE PEDIATRIC MUSCULOSKELETAL SYSTEM ✔

1. Less densely calcified

2. Thick periosteum

3. Presence of the growth plate

4. Relatively strong ligaments

2. **What unique categories of fractures are commonly seen in pediatrics as a result of these differences?**
   - Physeal or Salter-Harris fractures
   - Plastic deformation fractures
   - Avulsion fractures

   Bachman D, Santora S: Orthopedic trauma. In Fleisher G, Ludwig S, Henretig FM (eds): Textbook of Pediatric Emergency Medicine, 5th ed. Philadelphia, Lippincott Williams & Wilkins 2006, pp 1525–1569.

3. **Describe the Salter-Harris classification of fractures.**
   - **Salter I:** A fracture within the growth plate. The fracture line itself is not visible on radiographs, but a widening of the physis or displacement of the epiphysis may be suggestive of such a fracture.
   - **Salter II:** A fracture that extends through the growth plate and metaphysis
   - **Salter III:** An intra-articular fracture that extends through the growth plate and the epiphysis
   - **Salter IV**: An intra-articular fracture that involves the metaphysis, growth plate, and epiphysis
   - **Salter V:** A compression fracture of the growth plate. This injury is also unlikely to be detected initially by radiographs and often becomes evident only as the result of eventual growth arrest in the affected limb.

   Salter RB, Harris WR: Injuries involving the epiphyseal growth plate. J Bone Joint Surg 45A:587–622, 1963.

4. **Why is the Salter-Harris classification important?**
   The Salter-Harris classification of fractures categorizes fractures that involve the growth plate. The classification has implications for both prognosis and treatment. Fractures categorized within the higher numbers of the classification are more likely to affect joint congruity and disrupt blood supply to the growth centers of the bone, leading to greater potential for future growth disturbance.

5. **What is the Thurston-Holland sign?**
   This is the triangular fracture segment of the metaphysis found in Salter-Harris type II fractures.

6. **What are the four zones in the physis? Through which zone do fractures commonly occur?**
   There are four zones in the physis, which are found in the following order from the epiphysis to the metaphysis:
   1. The zone of resting cells
   2. The zone of proliferating cells
   3. The zone of hypertrophic/maturing cells
   4. The zone of provisional calcification
   Fractures typically occur through the zone of hypertrophic/maturing cells. The blood supply enters the bone through the epiphysis and is most crucial to the resting and proliferating cell layers.

7. **At what age are physeal injuries most likely to occur?**
   Eighty percent occur between 10 and 16 years of age, with a median age of 13 years. Hypertrophy of the physis during the growth spurt and increased participation in physical activity and sports at this age are responsible for the increased incidence.

   Peterson CA, Peterson HA: Analysis of the incidence of injuries to the epiphyseal growth plate. J Trauma 12:275–281, 1972.

8. **How does a mallet finger deformity differ in children and adults?**
   The adult mallet finger is the result of disruption of the extensor tendon. In young children, the underlying injury involves a fracture through the growth plate—a Salter I fracture with displacement of the epiphysis. In older children or teenagers, the injury is an avulsion or Salter III fracture through the epiphysis. Such injuries may cause difficulty in reducing the finger and may require open reduction.

9. **In what order do the growth centers in the elbow ossify? Why is this clinically important?**

The mnemonic **CRITOE** is a useful reminder of the order in which these ossified growth centers appear:

- **C** = **C**apitellum
- **R** = **R**adial head
- **I** = **I**nternal (medial) epicondyle
- **T** = **T**rochlea
- **O** = **O**lecranon
- **E** = **E**xternal (lateral) epicondyle

An ossified fragment that is present out of its expected order suggests a fracture rather than a normal ossification center.

Radiology cases in pediatric medicine: elbow ossification centers in a child: www.hawaii.edu/medicine/pediatrics/pemxray/v1c11.html

10. **What are plastic fractures?**

Plastic fractures result from the pliability of the bones in childhood. Pediatric bones respond to compressive and transverse forces through plastic deformation. With a small amount of force, the bone is capable of bending slightly and then returning to its natural state. If excessive force is applied, the bone eventually exceeds its capacity for full elastic recoil and deforms. Depending on the degree of force and how it is applied, one of the three plastic fractures of childhood may result.

11. **Name the three types of plastic fractures of childhood.**
    1. Buckle or torus fracture
    2. Greenstick fracture
    3. Bowing or bending fracture

12. **Why is it important to reduce a forearm bowing fracture?**

These fractures do not include injury to the periosteum and therefore do not undergo as vigorous stimulation to remodel. This may result in permanent angulation of the bone, which can have deleterious effects on the normal range of motion and function of the involved forearm.

Vorlat P, De Boeck H: Bowing fractures of the forearm in children. Clin Orthop Relat Res 413:233–237, 2003.

KEY POINTS: PEDIATRIC FRACTURES ✓

1. Any fracture can be the result of abuse, although certain extremity fractures are specific for abuse.

2. Because of its increased pliability, the pediatric bone can go through several stages of deformity prior to fracture.

3. Salter-Harris fractures are those involving the growth plate.

DIAGNOSIS

13. **In what situations are comparison films most useful?**
    - Suspicion of a bowing fracture
    - Suspicion of a nondisplaced Salter I fracture

- Discriminating a secondary or accessory site of ossification from a fracture
- Discriminating a possible anatomic variant from a fracture

14. **How do you evaluate distal nerve function in an uncooperative or preverbal child following extremity or digit injury?**
Placing the fingers in a bowl of warm water for several minutes results in wrinkling of the skin on the finger pads if distal nerve function is intact.

Eberlein R: Hand and finger injuries. In King C, Henretig FM (eds): Textbook of Pediatric Emergency Procedures. Baltimore, Williams & Wilkins, 2007.

15. **What is a FOOSH? What is its significance to pediatric extremity injuries?**
A **FOOSH** is a fall on an outstretched hand. This is the most common mechanism of forearm, elbow, and wrist injuries in children.

Perron AD, Miller MD, Brady WJ: Orthopedic pitfalls in the ED: Pediatric growth plate injuries. Am J Emerg Med 20:50–54, 2002.

16. **What name is associated with a Salter III fracture of the distal tibia? How is this fracture related to the age and growth of a child?**
A Salter III fracture of the distal tibia is called a Tillaux fracture (Fig. 54-1). It classically occurs in teenagers shortly before growth plate closure. The medial segment of the distal tibial physis fuses last, and the medial aspect of the distal epiphysis remains anchored to the fibula by the anterior tibiofibular ligament. External rotation of the foot with sufficient force produces an avulsion fracture through the unfused medial segment of growth plate and down through the epiphysis.

Koury SI, Stone CK, Harell G, et al: Recognition and management of Tillaux fractures in adolescents. Pediatr Emerg Care 15:37–39, 1999.

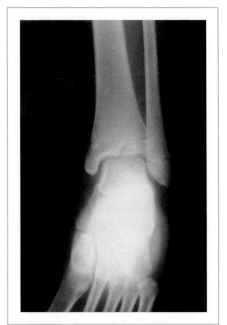

Figure 54-1. Salter III fracture of the distal tibia, commonly called a Tillaux fracture.

17. **What is a "wagon wheel injury"?**
Fracture of the distal femoral epiphysis. In the 19th century, such fractures resulted when the child's leg became entrapped between the wagon and the spokes of a wagon wheel. The femoral physis is at particular risk of injury. The medial and lateral collateral ligaments of the knee insert on the femoral epiphysis and provide no support for the growth plate.

18. **What is the difference between Galeazzi and Monteggia fractures?**
Both injuries involve a combination forearm fracture and dislocation. The Galeazzi fracture is a fracture of the radius with dislocation of the radioulnar joint. The Monteggia fracture is an ulnar fracture with radial head dislocation. The dislocations associated with these fractures are at risk of being overlooked once the fracture has been identified.

19. **What is a toddler's fracture?**

A toddler's fracture is described most commonly as a hairline, nondisplaced spiral or oblique fracture of the distal third of the tibia. It occurs, as its name suggests, in ambulatory children up to approximately 4 years of age. It often results from relatively minor force, such as a fall from a step or the end of a sliding board.

   Tenenbein M, Reed MH, Black GB: The toddler's fracture revisited. Am J Emerg Med 8:208–211, 1990.

20. **What is the apprehension test? When is it useful?**

The apprehension test is a provocative test consisting of lateral force applied to the patella with the leg in full extension. It is useful when a recent patella dislocation with spontaneous reduction is suspected. In a positive test result, the child resists the examiner for fear of recurrence of the dislocation.

21. **How do you differentiate an avulsion fracture at the proximal fifth metatarsal from the normal secondary site of ossification?**

Avulsion injuries of the proximal fifth metatarsal occur during inversion of the ankle. Stress is transmitted through the peroneus brevis ligament, which inserts on the proximal fifth metatarsal. The resulting fracture line is transverse to the foot, whereas the secondary site of ossification (os vesalianum) occurs in a longitudinal orientation. A comparison view of the normal foot may be helpful. Palpating for tenderness over the area is a simpler means of making the distinction.

22. **What is the mechanism of injury in a "boxer's fracture"?**

Fractures of the fourth or fifth metacarpal ("boxer's fractures") are sustained when a person strikes an object with a closed fist. Destructive infections of the hand and metacarpophalangeal joint can occur when one person strikes another in the teeth and mouth flora are introduced into the resulting lacerations.

MANAGEMENT

23. **Describe the initial approach to the trauma victim with a significantly deformed extremity fracture.**

The initial approach to any trauma patient should focus on potential life-threatening injuries. The primary survey consists of evaluation and stabilization of the airway, breathing, and circulation. The physician should not be distracted by the more obvious extremity injuries, which are rarely life-threatening. Extremity fractures are more appropriately addressed as part of the secondary survey.

24. **What factors determine the need for fracture reduction?**

Pediatric bones have a high capacity to remodel. As a general rule, remodeling should not be relied upon to correct all deformities. Fractures should be immobilized as close to anatomic position as possible. No degree of deformation is considered acceptable in all cases. The decision to actively reduce a particular fracture or to rely on remodeling depends on several factors:

- **Patient's age:** The older the child, the less time for growth and remodeling.
- **Location of the fracture:** Fractures farther from the physis have less capacity to remodel.
- **Bone involved:** Different bones are subjected to different muscular stresses that in part determine their growth and healing capacity.
- **Type of fracture:** In general, the greater the disruption of periosteum, the greater the stimulation for repair and remodeling.
- **Degree and direction of disruption:** Rotational deformities are particularly poor at remodeling.

25. **What pediatric extremity injuries require emergent orthopedic consultation?**
  - Femur fracture
  - Complete fractures of the tibia or fibula
  - Open fracture
  - Fractures associated with neurovascular compromise
  - Dislocation of a large joint, with the possible exception of the shoulder
  - Fractures with significant displacement
  - Fractures involving a large joint
  - Displaced supracondylar fractures

    Bachman D, Santora S: Orthopedic trauma. In Fleisher G, Ludwig S, Henretig FM (eds): Textbook of Pediatric Emergency Medicine, 5th ed. Philadelphia, Lippincott Williams & Wilkins 2006, pp 1525–1569.

26. **List the key factors that should be communicated when an orthopedic consultation is requested.**
  - Age and sex of the patient
  - Mechanism of injury
  - Bone or bones involved in the injury
  - Type of fracture
  - Neurovascular status of the extremity
  - Presence and amount of displacement
  - Presence and degree of angulation
  - Presence or absence of an open fracture

27. **Describe the appropriate acute management for the vast majority of extremity injuries.**
  The mnemonic **PRICE** summarizes the key elements:
  - **P** = **P**ain control
  - **R** = **R**est
  - **I** = **I**ce
  - **C** = **C**ompression
  - **E** = **E**levation

    The various components of this therapy help to reduce hemorrhage, posttraumatic edema, and pain. Immobilization prevents extension of soft tissue and neurovascular injury. The lack of consistent attention to pain management is a major problem in the care of injured children.

    Cimpello LB, Khine H, Avner JR: Practice patterns of pediatric versus general emergency physicians for pain management of fractures in pediatric patients. Pediatr Emerg Care 20:228–232, 2004.

28. **How do you reduce a dislocated patella?**
  A dislocated patella almost always reduces spontaneously when the leg is placed in extension; it remains dislocated only when the patient maintains the leg in flexion. Flexion of the hips to relax the quadriceps muscles may aid in the reduction. Occasionally a small amount of pressure applied on the medial side of the patella is necessary. After reduction the joint should be immobilized and radiographs obtained to rule out associated fractures. Whether prereduction radiographs are useful or simply prolong the patient's discomfort remains controversial.

    Young G: Reduction of common joint dislocations and subluxations. In King C, Henretig FM (eds): Textbook of Pediatric Emergency Procedures. Baltimore, Williams & Wilkins, 2007.

COMPLICATIONS

29. **What clinical findings suggest a compartment syndrome?**
  In addition to a tense, swollen area at the injury site, clinical findings may include the 5 Ps:
  - Pain
  - Paresthesia

- Paresis
- Pallor
- Pulselessness

Pain out of proportion or distal to the injury is the earliest and most sensitive sign of compartment syndrome and frequently the only one present. One study found pain and an increasing requirement for pain medications in 90% of children with compartment syndrome. Of the other Ps, only paresthesia was present in greater than 50% of patients. Pain is increased with passive extension of involved muscles. Notably, the absence of a distal pulse is not necessary for the diagnosis.

Bae DS, Kadiyala RK, Waters PM: Acute compartment syndrome in children: Contemporary diagnosis, treatment and outcome. J Pediatr Orthop 21:680–688, 2001.

30. **What extremity injuries are at the highest risk for compartment syndrome?**
Compartment syndrome can occur in the hand, foot, forearm, thigh, or leg, but most frequently involves the anterior tibial and peroneal compartments of the leg and the deep flexor compartment of the arm. Most compartment syndromes in children involve fractures (75–85%). Open fractures are at twice the risk of compartment syndrome as closed fractures. Specific injuries associated with compartment syndrome include:
- Displaced supracondylar fractures
- Forearm crush injuries or midshaft radius and ulna fractures
- Proximal tibia fractures
- Elbow dislocations
- Distal femoral physeal fractures with anterior displacement

Grottkau BE, Epps HR, Discala CD: Compartment syndrome in children and adolescents. J Pediatr Surg 40:678–682, 2005.

31. **What is Volkmann's contracture?**
Volkmann's contracture is the deformation that results from ischemia of the muscles and other soft tissues. It occurs most commonly in the forearm as the result of a compartment syndrome. The predisposing injury in children is frequently a supracondylar fracture.

32. **What is a gunstock deformity?**
A gunstock deformity or cubitus varus deformity occurs when a supracondylar fracture heals with poor alignment. This results in medial displacement of the distal humerus. It is the most common complication of supracondylar fractures. Cubitus varus is most often a cosmetic rather than a functional deformity.

Labelle H, Bunnell WP, Duhaime M, et al: Cubitus varus deformity following supracondylar fractures of the humerus in children. J Pediatr Orthop 1:539–546, 1982.

ABUSE INJURIES

33. **Describe the diagnosis and management of metaphyseal chip fractures.**
The radiograph in Fig. 54-2 depicts metaphyseal chip or "corner" fractures. The finding is highly suggestive of child abuse. The likely mechanism is vigorous pulling or shaking of the limbs. Corner fractures are most common in the distal femur and proximal tibia. Treatment should consist of splinting and pain management as well as a search for other evidence of abuse, including a skeletal survey. Social work services and child welfare should be involved.

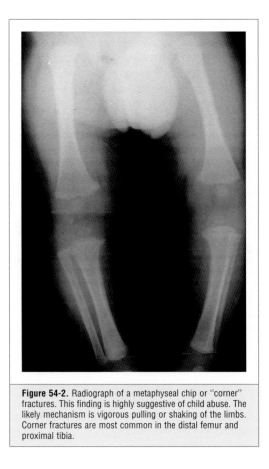

Figure 54-2. Radiograph of a metaphyseal chip or "corner" fractures. This finding is highly suggestive of child abuse. The likely mechanism is vigorous pulling or shaking of the limbs. Corner fractures are most common in the distal femur and proximal tibia.

34. **What extremity fractures are associated with abuse?**
    Up to 10% of all extremity injuries in children are inflicted. Almost any extremity injury may be the result of abuse. Classic extremity fractures that are more specific for abuse include:
    - Metaphyseal chip fractures
    - Multiple fractures in different stages of healing
    - Fractures inconsistent with the history or developmental abilities of the child
    - Bucket handle fractures
    - Femur fractures in children under a year of age or in preambulatory children
    - Spiral long bone fractures in preambulatory children
    - Fractures in association with injuries suggestive of abuse

ELBOW INJURIES

35. **Explain the term *nursemaid's elbow*.**
    The term refers to the most common mechanism for obtaining a radial head subluxation injury. A nursemaid may abruptly lift a young child by the wrist while crossing a street or attempting to prevent a stumbling child from falling. Traction is applied to the forearm with

the elbow extended and the forearm in pronation. A nursemaid's elbow can occur without a history of this classic mechanism.

36. **What is the typical clinical presentation for a nursemaid's elbow?**
Children typically do not appear to be in pain, but refuse to use the affected arm. The arm is held in pronation and slight flexion at the side of the body. The examiner detects no swelling, point tenderness, bruising, or warmth over the joint. The child may hold the wrist on the affected side to support the extremity, often leading the parents to believe that the wrist is involved. Mild dependent edema of the hand may appear as swelling and further confuse the picture. There is no point tenderness over the elbow, but resistance to supination, flexion, and pronation is noticeable.

37. **Name the classic radiographic findings for a radial head subluxation (nursemaid's elbow).**
There are no diagnostic radiographic findings for a radial head subluxation. Radiographs appear normal. They should be obtained only when the diagnosis is in question after the history and physical examination. In this setting, radiography is performed to rule out alternative causes of elbow pain.

Swischuk LE: Emergency Imaging of the Acutely Ill or Injured Child, 4th ed. Philadelphia, Lippincott Williams & Wilkins, 2000.

38. **Describe two accepted maneuvers for reducing a radial head subluxation.**
In both procedures, the child is seated in the parent's lap, facing the examiner. The examiner grasps the elbow and provides stabilization with the nondominant hand. With the dominant hand, the examiner holds the wrist or hand of the child's affected side and either (1) hyperpronates or (2) supinates the forearm and then flexes the elbow in one smooth motion so that the child's hand comes up to the ipsilateral shoulder. A palpable "pop" may be appreciated at the elbow as the reduction occurs. Over 90% of patients begin using the elbow normally within 15 minutes of successful reduction.

Supination or pronation with the elbow in extension also has been described as a successful means of reducing radial head subluxations.

Macias CG, Bothner J, Wiebe R: A comparison of supination/flexion to hyperpronation in the reduction of radial head subluxations. Pediatrics 102:e10, 1998.

KEY POINTS: FINDINGS IN RADIAL HEAD SUBLUXATION ✓

1. History of forearm traction in pronation

2. Refusal to use arm

3. Lack of swelling or bruising

4. Negative radiographs

39. **What radiologic findings on a lateral elbow film suggest the presence of an occult fracture?**
A visible posterior fat pad or outward displacement of the anterior fat pad away from the humerus is evidence of an elbow effusion. A fracture should be assumed to be present when an elbow effusion is seen in the setting of elbow trauma.

A malaligned anterior humeral line (one that does not pass through the middle or posterior third of the capitellum) suggests the presence of a supracondylar fracture with dorsal displacement of the capitellum and distal humerus.

Malalignment of the radiocapitellar line, as determined by a line through the center of the radius that does not pass through center of the capitellum on either the anteroposterior or lateral radiograph, is evidence of a dislocated radius.

Swischuk LE: Emergency Imaging of the Acutely Ill or Injured Child, 4th ed. Philadelphia, Lippincott Williams & Wilkins, 2000.

40. **What is the most frequently fractured bone in a pediatric elbow injury?**
In one study of children with elbow fractures, 81% of elbow fractures involved the distal humerus. Radial head fractures accounted for 9% of elbow fractures, and proximal ulnar fractures for 10%. Supracondylar fractures were found in 60% of the total, with medial epicondylar fractures in 7% and lateral condyle fractures in 19%.

John SD, Wherry K, Swischuk LE, et al: Improving detection of elbow fractures by understanding their mechanics. Radiography 16:1443–1460, 1996.

41. **What are the three classifications of supracondylar fractures?**
The three Gartland classifications of supracondylar fractures are:
- **Type I:** Nondisplaced fracture
- **Type II:** Mild displacement with intact posterior cortex
- **Type III:** Displaced fracture with no anterior and posterior cortical contact

All type III fractures and most type II supracondylar fractures (Fig. 54-3) require percutaneous pinning to obtain appropriate reduction and to reduce complications.

Pediatric supracondylar fractures of the humerus. Wheeless' Online Textbook of Orthopedic Surgery: www.wheelessonline.com/ortho/pediatric_supracondylar_fractures_of_the_humerus

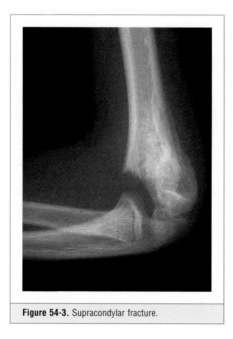

Figure 54-3. Supracondylar fracture.

KEY POINTS: ELBOW TRAUMA ✓

1. The most common mechanism of pediatric elbow injury is a fall on an outstretched hand.

2. The presence of a posterior fat pad or elevated anterior fat pad is evidence of a supracondylar fracture until proven otherwise.

3. Type II and type III Gartland fractures typically require surgical pinning for adequate reduction.

4. Secondary ossification centers in the elbow appear in a predictable order.

WEBSITES ⊕

1. Radiology cases in pediatric medicine
   www.hawaii.edu/medicine/pediatrics/pemxray/pemxray.html

2. Reviews and radiology cases in pediatric orthopedics
   www.pemdatabase.org/ortho.html

3. Wheeless' Online Textbook of Orthopedic Surgery
   www.wheelessonline.com

CHAPTER 55

EYE INJURIES

Martha W. Stevens, MD, MSCE

1. **Define an ophthalmologic "emergency" and give two common examples.**
   An ophthalmologic emergency is any injury that may lead to incremental vision loss without early recognition and prompt initiation of treatment. Two common examples are chemical burn and globe rupture. Both of these presentations warrant emergent (same-day) ophthalmologic consult after beginning initial treatment/stabilization.

2. **What is the initial treatment/stabilization for globe rupture?**
   Stop the examination, place a rigid eye shield, and keep the patient calm to avoid increased pressure to the globe, which may cause further extrusion of vitreous or aqueous humor. Administer pain medications, tetanus, and IV antibiotic prophylaxis, if possible. Order an imaging study if a retained foreign body is suspected.

3. **List the important aspects of the history in all patients with eye injuries.**
   - Change in visual acuity
   - Change in appearance of eyes
   - Discomfort or pain (including photophobia)
   - History of trauma, including details of the mechanism (blunt/sharp, significant impact, soil contamination, foreign-body risk) and tetanus immunization history
   - Corrective lenses (contacts currently in place?)
   - Medications
   - Eye surgeries
   - History of ocular problems
   - Systemic disease (sickle cell, connective tissue, or rheumatologic disease; hypertension; diabetes; HIV infection)

4. **What is included in the routine physical examination for all pediatric patients with eye injuries (except when temporarily deferred in absolute emergencies)?**
   - Visual acuity
   - Extraocular muscles
   - Pupillary reactions
   - External examination (including lids and conjunctivae)
   - Direct ophthalmoscopy/red reflex
   - Other tests as indicated: visual field testing (confrontational), slit-lamp examination, intraocular pressure (palpation or tonometer). The last two tests usually are performed by an ophthalmologist for pediatric patients.

5. **What are the common pitfalls in evaluating children with eye injuries?**
   - Failure to treat life-threatening injuries before the most obvious but less serious eye injury
   - Failure to examine both eyes
   - Failure to consider globe injury (after finding a more superficial injury)

   Levin AV: Eye trauma. In Fleisher GR, Ludwig S, Henretig FM (eds): Textbook of Pediatric Emergency Medicine, 5th ed. Baltimore, Lippincott Williams & Wilkins, 2006, pp 1485–1496.

6. **How do you test visual acuity in infants?**
   Check for pupillary reaction to light and fixation reflex. Infants should be able to fix on a high-contrast object held in their central vision, such as the caretaker's or examiner's face or a bright toy. By 2–3 months of age, they should be able to fix on and start to follow an object or light, and by about 6 months to fix and follow to all visual fields. Central, steady, maintained fixation is estimated to be equivalent to 20/40 vision, unsteady fixation equivalent to 20/100, and eccentric wandering gaze to < 20/400.

7. **How do you test visual acuity in preschool and school-aged children?**
   - 2½–3½ years old: Allen object recognition (picture) chart
   - 3½ and older: Picture chart, tumbling E chart, or Sheridan-Gardner visual acuity test
   - School age: Snellen chart (letters in rows of diminishing size)

8. **What pearls should be kept in mind for visual acuity testing in children?**
   - Have the child identify the objects on the chart up close before testing at a distance.
   - Test one eye at a time, "bad" eye first.
   - Use a card or the child's palm to cover the other eye; children "peek" between fingers.
   - Always test with corrective glasses if available.

9. **For patients without their glasses or contact lenses, how can you differentiate between decreased acuity and baseline refractive error?**
   Pinhole testing—with a premade device, a card with a hole punched with an 18-gauge needle, or multiple pinholes in a rigid eye shield—corrects refractive errors to about 20/30.

10. **How do you record decreased acuity in patients unable to visualize a chart?**
    - Ability to count fingers from a specified number of feet
    - Ability to perceive hand motion
    - Light perception (with or without directionality)

11. **What are the causes of an irregularly shaped pupil?**
    - Ocular rupture/corneal or other globe perforation
    - Prior ocular surgery
    - Scarring from previous iritis

12. **What are the causes and expected course of subconjunctival hemorrhage?**
    Subconjunctival hemorrhage, the localized rupture of small subconjunctival vessels, may be spontaneous or may be due to direct trauma or increased intrathoracic pressure (e.g., coughing, noseblowing, vomiting). It usually is benign and resolves in 2–3 weeks without treatment or sequelae. Very large hemorrhages or those that fully encircle the iris raise concern for an underlying injury, such as globe perforation, or a bleeding diathesis.

13. **What is the most common pediatric eye injury?**
    Corneal or conjunctival abrasion.

14. **Which eye injuries are possible when a child is a restrained passenger in the front seat and is involved in a car crash with air bag deployment?**
    Airbags have reportedly caused monocular and binocular injuries. Some injuries to the eyes are "mechanical," caused by the force of the airbag hitting the child's face. These injuries include eyelid trauma, corneal injury, orbital fracture, lens dislocation, corneoscleral laceration, and hyphema. Chemical injury to the eyes is also possible, and alkaline burns have been reported. An alkaline substance that triggers the airbag inflation has occasionally caused burns to the

eyes. Wearing glasses at the time of the crash protects against the chemical injury but may increase the risk of penetrating trauma to the eyes.

Lee WB, O'Halloran HS, Pearson A, et al: Airbags and bilateral eye injury: Five case reports and a review of the literature. J Emerg Med 20:129–134, 2001.

15. **How does a child with corneal abrasion typically present?**
The common presentation is a red eye with epiphora (tearing), intense pain, resistance to eye opening, and, less frequently, lid swelling or photophobia. The child often does not know what caused the injury.

16. **How is a corneal abrasion diagnosed?**
Larger abrasions often can be visualized with tangential light as an irregularity or dry-appearing area of the eye surface. Fluorescein staining and cobalt blue light (or Woods lamp) best delineate abrasions of any size. Use of a topical anesthetic facilitates the examination and aids in the diagnosis. If topical anesthesia fully alleviates the pain, an ocular surface problem, such as a superficial foreign body, abrasion, or superficial ulcer, is suggested. Persistent pain after use of a topical anesthetic suggests pathology of deeper structures. Be sure to check thoroughly for a retained foreign body when evaluating corneal or conjunctival abrasions. Any concern for a corneal or scleral laceration or an imbedded foreign body should prompt an ophthalmology consultation.

Pediatric pearl: Consider application of a topical anesthetic *before* your first examination attempt in suspected corneal or conjunctival abrasions. In young children, this is most easily accomplished by letting the child keep the eye shut, having the child lie in a supine position, and pooling several drops of the topical anesthetic medially at the corner of the eye. Gentle traction caudally on the cheek will crack apart the lids, and the drops will run onto the eye surface. Let the child sit up, and in a few seconds he or she will usually spontaneously open the eye and your examination can proceed without a fight!

17. **Describe the management of a corneal or conjunctival abrasion.**
Most abrasions heal quickly without sequelae. Antibiotic ophthalmic ointment or artificial tears provide lubrication and some pain relief. Small lesions do not need to be patched and, if asymptomatic in 24 hours, do not require follow-up. Large abrasions and those involving the visual axis are treated with antibiotic ointment, consider soft eye patching, and daily follow-up until they have healed. Patients should be instructed to return or see an ophthalmologist for pain or foreign-body sensation that persists for more than 2 or 3 days, or if pain and redness worsen at any time. Instruct those who wear contact lenses to discontinue their use until the patient is seen by an ophthalmologist.

LeSage N, Verreault R, Rochette L: Efficacy of eye patching for traumatic corneal abrasions: A controlled clinical trial. Ann Emerg Med 28:129–134, 2001.

18. **Describe the management of the child with "something in my eye."**
Most patients with an external foreign body (conjunctival or superficial corneal) report just that. If there is no suspicion of a perforated globe or deep corneal laceration, a topical anesthetic allows thorough examination of the bulbar conjunctival surface, cornea, palpebral conjunctivae, and superior and inferior fornices. Evert the upper lid to examine its inner aspect; outward traction on the lower lid with upward gaze provides good visualization of the lower bulbar and palpebral conjunctivae.

The foreign body usually can be loosened and removed with saline irrigation. A moistened sterile swab or gauze also can be used. If the foreign body is still adherent, consider removal under slit-lamp magnification or ophthalmologic referral. Be sure to complete a full eye examination after removal of the foreign body; look for and treat associated corneal abrasions if necessary.

19. **What is a hyphema?**
A hyphema is bleeding into the chamber between the cornea and iris or lens after blunt or sharp trauma. It may range from microscopic bleeding to a full-chamber or "eight-ball" hyphema.

20. **How are hyphemas diagnosed and treated?**
A hyphema (Fig. 55-1) should be suspected in any child with a tearing, painful eye and injected bulbar conjunctiva immediately after blunt eye trauma. It is often diagnosed by careful physical examination—many are visible without microscopic slit-lamp examination. Smaller hyphemas may require microscopic slit-lamp examination. All hyphemas require urgent ophthalmologic consultation for management, although in 66–97% of isolated hyphemas the hemorrhage resorbs without complication.
   Children with large hyphemas are sometimes managed as inpatients, particularly if they are young or if inadequate follow-up is a concern. Some ophthalmologists prefer home management. The patients are treated with cycloplegics, topical or systemic steroids, and bedrest (with sedation, if needed). Some ophthalmologists recommend the use of an antifibrinolytic agent, such as aminocaproic acid (Amicar). Children with hyphema should be cared for in consultation with an ophthalmologist.

Hertle RW, Bacal D: Traumatic hyphema: Evaluation and management. Contemp Pediatr 14:51–68, 1997.
Recchia FM, Saluja RK, Hammel K, et al: Outpatient management of traumatic microhyphema. Ophthalmology 109:1465–1470, 2002.

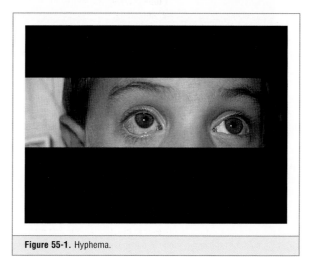

Figure 55-1. Hyphema.

21. **What is the major potential vision-threatening sequela of hyphemas? Who is at risk?**
Rebleeding with development of acute glaucoma or corneal staining. Rebleeding is most likely within 3–5 days of the initial injury. Patients with sickle cell disease are at particularly high risk of ocular complications; a screening test or hemoglobin electrophoresis is recommended for patients at risk for an undiagnosed hemoglobinopathy.

22. **When and how does traumatic iritis present?**
Traumatic iritis (Fig. 55-2), which may accompany other ocular injury or be the sole manifestation of blunt eye trauma, usually presents later than microscopic hyphema (24–72

hours after injury). Physical examination reveals a painful, red eye (typically perilimbal conjunctival injection), tearing, and pain with pupillary constriction (on accommodation or concentric constriction to light). The affected eye also may have slight miosis and a decreased or sluggish pupillary response. The pain is secondary to inflammation in the anterior chamber. Slit-lamp evaluation is diagnostic when it reveals white cells and a protein "flare" in the aqueous humor.

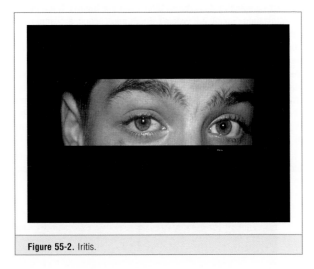

Figure 55-2. Iritis.

23. **How is traumatic iritis treated?**
    In children, an ophthalmology consultation should be requested for definitive diagnosis and initial management, which includes mydriatics for pain control, topical steroids, and close follow-up.

24. **What is an orbital "blow-out" fracture?**
    An orbital blow-out fracture involves one of the bony orbital walls and is usually caused by blunt trauma to the face. The presentation may include periorbital ecchymosis, facial asymmetry, lid swelling or ptosis, proptosis or enophthalmos, ophthalmoplegia, localized anesthesia of the face, and, in rare cases, orbital emphysema. The patient may have entrapment or restriction of the extraocular muscle adjacent to the fracture site and restriction of extraocular movement may be evident on examination. In particular, the patient may be unable to look up with the affected eye. The most common fracture sites are the inferior and medial walls (rarely lateral). Superior wall fractures have the potential to communicate with the intracranial space. Plain radiographs and computed tomography or magnetic resonance imaging may help delineate the fracture. A full ocular examination is needed to rule out other eye injuries, including retinal trauma.

25. **What is the major pitfall when diagnosing an orbital wall fracture?**
    Failure to consider and appropriately rule out other eye injuries. The incidence of concomitant globe injury with orbital fractures has been reported at 5–10%.

26. **What physical examination findings are consistent with a ruptured or perforated globe?**
   - Significantly decreased visual acuity and severe pain
   - Characteristic tear-drop pupil, pointing toward perforation
   - Plugging of perforation or rupture by choroid or iris, leading to fleshy or pigmented-appearing mass on ocular surface (do not mistake this for a foreign body!)
   - Large, overlying subconjunctival hemorrhage (often fully around iris) or hyphema
   - An unusually shallow anterior chamber

   Note: When a globe rupture or perforation is suspected, stop your examination, place a rigid eye shield, avoid patient agitation, keep the patient in bed with the head elevated, and request an emergent ophthalmologic consultation (see Question 2).

   Levin AV: Eye trauma. In Fleisher GR, Ludwig S, Henretig FM (eds): Textbook of Pediatric Emergency Medicine, 5th ed. Baltimore, Lippincott Williams & Wilkins, 2006, pp 1485–1496.

KEY POINTS: REASONS TO SUSPECT GLOBE PERFORATION OR RUPTURE ✔

1. History of hammering/grinding metal

2. Significant eye trauma causing decreased vision

3. Physical examination findings of a subconjunctival hemorrhage encircling the iris or cornea, large hyphema, posttraumatic corneal conjunctival edema, enophthalmos, extruded vitreous, iris, or choroid

4. The more difficult it is to examine the patient after trauma (because of pain, edema, hyphema, or vitreous hemorrhage), the greater the concern for globe rupture

27. **What aspects of the history or physical examination place patients at high risk for globe perforation or rupture?**
   - Hammering/grinding metal
   - Significant eye trauma causing decreased vision
   - Subconjunctival hemorrhage encircling the iris or cornea
   - Large hyphema
   - Posttraumatic corneal conjunctival edema
   - Enophthalmos
   - Extruded vitreous, iris, or choroid

   Note: It is sometimes difficult to see a globe rupture, especially if the etiology was a rapidly penetrating foreign body (from hammering). The more difficult it is to examine the patient after trauma (because of pain, edema, hyphema, or vitreous hemorrhage), the greater the likelihood of globe rupture.

   Handler JA, Ghezzi KT: General ophthalmologic examinations. Emerg Med Clin North Am 13:521–537, 1995.

KEY POINTS: MANAGEMENT OF GLOBE RUPTURE/ LACERATION ✔

1. Stop your examination.

2. Place shield over affected eye.

3. Keep patient at rest, with head elevated.

4. Avoid agitation of the child.

5. Ensure patient consumes nothing by mouth.

6. Consult ophthalmologist urgently.

7. Consider IV antibiotics.

28. **What are the important considerations for evaluating lacerations of the eyelids?**
It is important to consider the potential for a full-thickness laceration and underlying orbital injury. Even if the laceration is superficial in appearance, be sure to check the inner (conjunctival) surface. In upper lid lacerations, always assess the integrity of the levator muscle (both lids raise equally with upward gaze). Full-thickness lacerations, lacerations through the lid margin or tarsal plate, and lacerations potentially involving lacrimal canaliculi *(any laceration of the medial canthal angle)* require ophthalmologic consultation for multilayer repair. Consider consultation for lacerations with ptosis or significant avulsions or if you are unable to rule out other ocular injury. Adipose tissue exposed in an upper lid laceration indicates full-thickness lid laceration (this is exposed orbital fat).

29. **Describe the emergency initial management of chemical burns to the eye.**
    - Begin immediate lavage at the scene of injury with any bland fluid.
    - In the emergency department, irrigate immediately and copiously with normal saline or lactated Ringer's solution (at least 1–2 L via IV tubing set).
    - Use topical anesthetic every 20 minutes and lid retractors, if needed.
    - Evert the lids to ensure thorough irrigation.
    - Remove particulate matter.
    - Monitor pH of conjunctival fossa after irrigation, and recheck 10–20 minutes later. Continue irrigation until a pH of 7.4–7.6 is maintained on rechecks.
    - Arrange emergent (same day) ophthalmologic consultation for patients with evidence of a significant burn (such as persistent pain, corneal lesions, or decreased acuity).

    Blende MS: Irrigation of conjunctivae. In Henretig FM, King C (eds): Textbook of Pediatric Emergency Procedures. Baltimore, Williams & Wilkins, 1997, pp 605–608.

30. **Which are more severe—alkali or acid burns?**
Alkali burns are potentially more severe. Alkali substances penetrate more deeply than acids, which coagulate with surface proteins. Common alkaline agents include lye, lime, ammonia, and aluminum- or magnesium hydroxide–containing fireworks (flares and sparklers).

31. **An emergency physician attempts to repair a forehead laceration of a young child using cyanoacrylate glue. Some of the glue drips down the child's face and the child's eyelashes are noted to be stuck together. The child's parent is quite concerned. Which eye injuries are likely?**

    Usually none. The eyelashes may be stuck together by the glue, but the eye is very rarely injured in this scenario. Parents may be concerned, as the child cannot open his/her eye. Avoid forceful attempts to pry open the eye lids. Instead, place petroleum jelly on the eyelashes and wait patiently or massage with a cotton swab until the glue dissolves.

CHAPTER 56

HEAD TRAUMA

Sara A. Schutzman, MD

GENERAL

1. **How common and important is head trauma in children?**
   Head trauma accounts for approximately 650,000 emergency department (ED) visits and 50,000 hospitalizations per year. Traumatic brain injury is the most common cause of death and disability in childhood.

   > Palchak MJ, Holmes JF, Vance CW, et al: A decision rule for identifying children at low risk for brain injuries after blunt head trauma. Ann Emerg Med 42:492–506, 2003.

2. **What kinds of head injuries commonly present to the ED?**
   Head trauma includes injuries to the scalp, skull, and intracranial contents. Although most injuries are minor, there is a wide spectrum ranging from simple contusion to lethal brain injury. Lacerations and contusions are common scalp injuries. Injuries to the cranial vault result in skull fractures, and intracranial injuries include concussion, cerebral contusion, hematoma (epidural, subdural, subarachnoid, and intracerebral), and acute brain swelling. Most head injuries result from blunt head trauma, but penetrating injuries rarely occur and are caused by bullets, teeth (e.g., dog bites), or other sharp objects (e.g., dart, pellet, pencil).

3. **How is head trauma severity defined?**
   There is no standard definition for minor head trauma, which accounts for about 80% of injuries evaluated. Many definitions of minor head trauma have been based on the Glasgow Coma Scale (GCS) score; however, there has been no consistency, with various sources, including children with GCS scores of 13–15, 14–15, or 15. The American Academy of Pediatrics defined children with minor head injury as those who have normal mental status at the initial examination, normal neurologic examination, and no physical evidence of skull fracture. Moderate head trauma is typically defined as a GCS score of 9–12, and severe head trauma as a GCS score of 3–8.

   > Committee on Quality Improvement, American Academy of Pediatrics: The management of minor closed head injury in children. Pediatrics 104:1407–1415, 1999.
   > Schutzman S, Greenes D: State of the art: pediatric minor head trauma. Ann Emerg Med 37:65–74, 2001.

4. **How many children evaluated for minor head trauma have intracranial injuries?**
   Approximately 3–7% of children with minor head injury have an intracranial injury noted on computed tomography (CT). Approximately 0.5–1.5% require surgical intervention. Overall, about 50% of intracranial injuries occur in kids with a GCS score of 15.

   > Schutzman S, Greenes D: State of the art: Pediatric minor head trauma. Ann Emerg Med 37:65–74, 2001.

5. **Name the ways in which infants differ from older children with regard to head trauma.**
   Children younger than 1–2 years of age differ in several ways that make a low threshold for head imaging prudent:

- Clinical assessment is more difficult.
- Intracranial injury is frequently asymptomatic.
- Skull fractures and intracranial injuries may result from relatively minor trauma.
- Inflicted injury occurs more often.

Schutzman SA, Barnes P, Duhaime AC, et al: Evaluation and management of children younger than two years of age with apparently minor head trauma: Proposed guidelines. Pediatrics 107:983–993, 2001.

6. **How common is abuse in infants and young children with head trauma?**
   Although most head trauma is accidental, up to 10% of children brought to the ED with traumatic injury are victims of intentional injury, and abusive head trauma is the most common cause of traumatic death in children. Because these children are preverbal and abusive caretakers are rarely forthcoming, the clinician must have a heightened sense of awareness to diagnose nonaccidental trauma. This is important to guide appropriate therapy and to prevent further trauma.

Jenny C, Hymel KP, Ritzen A, et al: Analysis of missed cases of abusive head trauma. JAMA 281:621–626, 1999.
Ludwig S: Child abuse. In Fleisher G, Ludwig S, Henretig FM (eds). Textbook of Pediatric Emergency Medicine, 5th ed. Philadelphia, Lippincott Williams & Wilkins, 2006, pp 1761–1801.

SKULL FRACTURES

7. **Why are skull fractures important?**
   Skull fractures are important because they are predictors of intracranial injury (the presence of a skull fracture increases the likelihood of an intracranial injury by approximately twentyfold). In addition, fractures themselves occasionally lead to complications and may be important evidence of child abuse.

Quayle KS, Jaffe DM, Kuppermann N, et al: Diagnostic testing for acute head injury in children: When are head computed tomography and skull radiographs indicated? Pediatrics 99:E11, 1997.

8. **Describe the different types of skull fractures.**
   Skull fractures are described in terms of location and characteristics. They may occur in the frontal, parietal, occipital, and temporal bones of the skullcap (calvarium). The skull base consists of portions of the temporal and occipital bones, along with the maxillary, sphenoid, and palatine bones. Fractures in this area are referred to as basilar skull fractures.
   Fractures may be linear, depressed (if the inner table of the skull is displaced by more than the thickness of the entire bone), or diastatic (traumatic separation of the cranial bones at one or more suture sites). Compound fractures communicate with lacerations, and comminuted fractures are those with several fragments.

9. **Since CT is available, are skull films ever indicated?**
   CT is the imaging modality of choice to evaluate for acute injury since skull radiography gives no direct information about intracranial injuries (ICI). Rarely, skull radiography may be considered in:
   - Alert, asymptomatic infants with scalp hematomas: These infants are at risk for harboring occult ICIs, and skull fractures are one of the best predictors for ICI. Skull radiography offers the advantage of requiring no sedation and having significantly less radiation. The practitioner or radiologist should be proficient at reading skull radiographs (if ordered) since they may be challenging to interpret. CT should be performed if a fracture is identified.
   - Possible nonaccidental injury: Skull radiography sometimes detects fractures missed by CT, and are indicated (as part of a skeletal survey) for the evaluation of possible abuse.
   - Suspicion of possible depressed fracture, penetrating trauma, or foreign body.

Chung S, Schamban N, Wypij, et al: Skull radiograph interpretation of children less than age two: How good are pediatric emergency physicians? Ann Emerg Med 43:718–722, 2004.

10. **Name the most important complications of basilar skull fractures.**
    - **Intracranial injury:** 10–40% of patients with basilar skull fracture have an associated ICI, and about 20% of alert children with basilar skull fractures and a normal neurologic status have an ICI.
    - **Cerebrospinal fluid (CSF) leak:** An associated dural tear may lead to CSF leak through the nose or ear and occurs in approximately 15–30% of children with basilar skull fractures.
    - **Meningitis:** Meningitis occurs in 0.7–5% of children with BSF (due to CSF leak and exposure to microorganisms); the rate is < 1% for children with GCS score > 13 and no ICI.
    - **Cranial nerve impairment:** This occurs in 1–23% of cases, with cranial nerves VI, VII, and VIII most commonly injured. The impairment may be transient or permanent.
    - **Hearing loss:** This occurs in up to half of patients with basilar skull fracture; it can be conductive (from hemotympanum or otic canal disruption) or sensorineural.

    Kadish HA, Schunk JE: Pediatric basilar skull fracture: Do children with normal neurologic findings and no intracranial injury require hospitalization? Ann Emerg Med 26:37–41, 1995.

KEY POINTS: HEAD INJURIES IN CHILDREN YOUNGER THAN 2 YEARS OF AGE ✔

1. Children younger than age 2 differ from older children in significant ways that make a lower threshold for imaging prudent.

2. Up to 20–45% of infants with ICI have no signs or symptoms of brain injury (occult ICI).

3. Most infants with occult ICI have an associated skull fracture, which is usually associated with scalp hematoma (more concerning if larger, nonfrontal, and in younger child).

4. Clinicians should always be alert to the possibility of nonaccidental injury in this age group.

11. **How are CSF leaks treated?**
    Most CSF leaks through dural tears resolve spontaneously without complications within 1 week, and are thus managed conservatively. Operative intervention may be needed for persistent leaks. Given the potential for developing meningitis with CSF leaks, there has been significant controversy regarding the use of prophylactic antibiotics. Current data do not indicate that routine use of prophylactic antibiotics significantly reduces the incidence of meningitis.

INTRACRANIAL INJURY

12. **Define primary and secondary brain injury.**
    Primary brain injury is the neural damage sustained at the time of trauma. Secondary brain injury is neuronal damage sustained after the initial traumatic event to cells not initially injured, and results from numerous causes including hypoxia, hypoperfusion, and metabolic derangements. Because many causes of secondary brain injury are potentially preventable, the clinician's main goal is to monitor for and attempt to prevent these complications in order to limit further neuronal damage.

13. **What is a concussion? How are concussions graded?**
    A concussion is defined as head trauma–induced alteration in mental status that may or may not involve loss of consciousness. The American Academy of Neurology has defined three grades of concussion, summarized by the Centers for Disease Control and Prevention as follows:
    - **Grade 1 concussion:** Transient confusion, no loss of consciousness, and duration of mental status abnormalities < 15 minutes

- **Grade 2 concussion:** Transient confusion, no loss of consciousness, and a duration of mental status abnormalities > 15 minutes
- **Grade 3 concussion:** Concussion involving loss of consciousness, either brief (seconds) or prolonged (minutes or longer)

Centers for Disease Control and Prevention: Sports-related recurrent brain injuries—United States. MMWR Morb Mortal Wkly Rep 46:224–227, 1997.

14. **What is the second impact syndrome?**
The second impact syndrome, a very rare event, is acute, usually fatal, brain swelling that occurs when a second concussion is sustained before complete recovery from a previous concussion. The pathophysiology of the second impact syndrome is not well understood; the initial blow may be associated with alteration in cerebral blood flow and failure of normal autoregulation, making the second impact so much more devastating, with resulting brain swelling and increased intracranial pressure.

Evans R: Concussion and mild traumatic brain injury. In Rose BD (ed): Waltham, MA, UpToDate, 2006.

15. **What imaging modality is recommended for acute injuries?**
CT identifies essentially all significant ICI requiring intervention.

16. **If CT identifies major complications, why not image all children with head injuries?**
CT carries disadvantages, including exposure to ionizing radiation and the possible requirement for pharmacologic sedation, as well as additional health care costs. Therefore, CT ideally should be used selectively.

Brenner DJ, Elliston CD, Hall EJ, et al: Estimated risks of radiation-induced fatal cancer from pediatric CT. AJR 176: 289–296, 2001.

17. **Which children are at high risk for intracranial injuries and should undergo CT?**
Evidence indicates that children with a GCS score < 15, abnormal neurologic examination, evidence of skull fracture, or seizure should undergo CT. Additional criteria for infants include irritability, bulging fontanel, or suspected abuse.

Dunning J, Batchelor J, Stratford-Smith P, et al: A meta-analysis of variables that predict significant intracranial injury in minor head trauma. Arch Dis Child 89:653–659, 2004.
Palchak MJ, Holmes JF, Vance CW, et al: A decision rule for identifying children at low risk for brain injuries after blunt head trauma. Ann Emerg Med 42:492–506, 2003.
Quayle KS, Jaffe DM, Kuppermann N, et al: Diagnostic testing for acute head injury in children: When are head computed tomography and skull radiographs indicated? Pediatrics 99:E11, 1997.

18. **What are the indications for imaging in those who are alert with a nonfocal neurologic examination and no signs of skull fracture?**
To date, studies have not found consistent signs or symptoms that are completely sensitive for identifying ICI in this group. Headache, vomiting, and loss of consciousness have been variably significant as predictors. CT should be considered for children with these symptoms, and the longer the duration and the more intense the symptoms, the more strongly the clinician should consider imaging, especially if more than one symptom is present. For children with mild symptoms, careful observation in the ED or at home may be an alternative approach, with reevaluation and CT for persistent or worsening symptoms.

Dunning J, Batchelor J, Stratford-Smith P, et al: A meta-analysis of variables that predict significant intracranial injury in minor head trauma. Arch Dis Child 89:653–659, 2004.
Palchak MJ, Holmes JF, Vance CW, et al: A decision rule for identifying children at low risk for brain injuries after blunt head trauma. Ann Emerg Med 42:492–506, 2003.

19. **Are there additional factors to consider for alert, nonfocal children younger than 1–2 years old?**

    Symptoms in these children can be subtle, so in addition to vomiting, headache, and loss of consciousness, possible signs of ICI include a history of lethargy or irritability (now resolved), and caretakers' concern about the child's behavior. Additionally, these children may have "occult intracranial injuries" (i.e., injuries with no signs of brain injury). Since most occult injuries have an associated skull fracture, which is typically associated with scalp swelling, a scalp hematoma in these young patients is of concern. Hematomas of greatest concern are those that are larger in size, nonfrontal in location, and present in younger children. The youngest infants (particularly those younger than 2–3 months of age) may have no signs or symptoms with ICI; therefore, a very low threshold for imaging (unless very trivial trauma) is prudent.

    Greenes DS, Schutzman SA: Clinical indicators of intracranial injury in head-injured infants. Pediatrics 104:861–867, 1999.

    Greenes DS, Schutzman SA: Clinical significance of scalp abnormalities in head-injured infants. Pediatr Emerg Care 17:88–92, 2001.

    Palchak MJ, Holmes JF, Vance CW, et al: A decision rule for identifying children at low risk for brain injuries after blunt head trauma. Ann Emerg Med 42:492–506, 2003.

    Schutzman SA, Barnes P, Duhaime AC, et al: Evaluation and management of children younger than two years of age with apparently minor head trauma: Proposed guidelines. Pediatrics 107:983–993, 2001.

20. **What is the cerebral perfusion pressure (CPP)?**

    CPP is the difference between the mean arterial pressure (MAP) and the intracranial pressure (ICP) (CPP = MAP − ICP). Therefore, significant decreases in mean arterial pressure or significant increases in ICP can lead to inadequate CPP, with resultant cerebral ischemia and secondary brain injury.

21. **How does increased ICP occur?**

    After infancy (when the cranial sutures fuse), the cranial vault becomes stiff and poorly compliant. The normal intracranial contents include brain, blood, and CSF. Because intracranial volume is fixed, any increase in the volume of one of the components (e.g., cerebral edema, expanding epidural hematoma) must be accompanied by a proportional decrease of the others; otherwise, ICP will increase.

KEY POINTS: INTRACRANIAL INJURY ✔

1. Most head injury is minor; most children with minor head injury don't have ICI, but about 5% do; and about 50% of ICIs occur in children with minor head trauma.

2. The clinician's goal is to identify children with ICI in order to avoid further neuronal injury, while limiting unnecessary neuroimaging procedures.

3. No small group of signs or symptoms have been consistently sensitive for identifying all ICIs, but altered mental status, focal neurological examination, skull fracture, and seizure are predictors for increased risk of ICI.

4. Other signs and symptoms (including loss of consciousness, headache, vomiting) have been variably predictive for ICI.

5. All head-injured children who are discharged should be accompanied by a responsible adult who is given clear discharge instructions and able to return if concerning signs/symptoms of possible ICI develop.

22. **What is the cerebral herniation syndrome?**
The cranial cavity is separated by dural folds and bony prominences into the anterior, middle, and posterior fossa. Cerebral herniation occurs when increased ICP causes the brain parenchyma to shift into an anatomic area that it does not normally occupy.

   Uncal herniation is the most common form, in which the uncus (inferomedial-most structure of the temporal lobe) slides through the tentorial notch, passing from the middle to the posterior fossa. Initial symptoms include headache and decreased level of consciousness, followed by ipsilateral pupillary dilatation and contralateral hemiplegia. Altered respirations, bradycardia, and systemic hypertension may ensue with decerebrate posturing or flaccid paresis; if the process continues unchecked, ultimately brain stem failure with respiratory arrest, cardiovascular collapse, and death occur.

23. **Outline the ED treatment for increased ICP.**
   - Manage the ABCs. This is essential to avoid hypoxia and hypercarbia, and to maintain adequate cerebral perfusion pressure.
   - Avoid secondary brain injury from other metabolic causes, including hypoglycemia, hyperthermia, and seizures.
   - Ensure appropriate positioning with elevation of the head of the bed 30 degrees, and the neck midline. This promotes venous drainage and can lead to a significant decrease of ICP.
   - Perform emergent head CT to identify mass lesions that require surgical evacuation.
   - Consider osmotic agents: Mannitol (dose of 0.5–1 gm/kg)/kg can be used to lower the ICP.
   - Use sedation: Conscious patients who are paralyzed for intubation require sedation.

24. **Isn't hyperventilation used to treat elevated ICP?**
Although hyperventilation had been a mainstay of emergency treatment for increased ICP, its use has become controversial. Carbon dioxide is one of the main determinants of cerebrovascular tone, with low levels producing vasoconstriction and decreased blood flow, thus lowering ICP. However, if cerebral blood flow diminishes too much, substrate delivery of oxygen and glucose is impaired and cerebral perfusion pressure may be inadequate, resulting in ischemic injury. Mild hyperventilation (PCO_2 of 30–35) may be considered for periods of intercranial hypertension.

   Skippen P, Seear M, Poskitt K, et al: Effect of hyperventilation on regional cerebral blood flow in head-injured children. Crit Care Med 25:1402–1409, 1997.

25. **Are steroids indicated for treating increased ICP?**
Steroids have not been shown to improve outcome for patients with head trauma; therefore, their use is not recommended.

DISPOSITION

26. **Which children need to be admitted following acute head trauma?**
Children with intracranial injuries or depressed or basilar skull fractures will usually require hospital admission. A neurosurgeon should be consulted regarding their management and disposition. Hospital admission should also be considered for patients with persistent neurologic deficits (despite normal CT scan), significant extracranial injuries, unremitting vomiting, or caretakers who are unreliable or unable to return if necessary. Any child with suspected nonaccidental trauma should also be considered for admission.

27. **Why are discharge instructions important in patients with head trauma?**
Even well-appearing children with head trauma who have no evidence of complications (either clinically or radiographically) have a small chance of subsequent deterioration. Therefore, it is

mandatory that competent caretakers are available to observe the child at home. They should be educated about the signs and symptoms of complications of head trauma, and instructed to bring the child to medical care for reevaluation should concerning symptoms arise.

28. **When can a child return to sports after a concussion?**

Recommendations for the management of concussion in sports are designed to prevent second impact syndrome. They have been summarized as follows:

- **Grade I concussion:** No sports until the patient is asymptomatic. If a second grade I concussion occurs, no sports activity until the patient has been asymptomatic for 1 week.
- **Grade II concussion:** No sports until 1 week after symptoms resolve.
- **Grade III concussion:** No sports for 1–2 weeks after symptoms resolve, depending on the duration of loss of consciousness. For a second grade III concussion, no sports activity until the patient has been asymptomatic for 1 month. If intracranial pathology is detected on CT or magnetic resonance imaging, the athlete should not engage in any sports activity for remainder of the season and should be discouraged from future return to contact sports.

Centers for Disease Control and Prevention: Sports-related recurrent brain injuries—United States. MMWR Morb Mortal Wkly Rep 46:224–227, 1997.

CHAPTER 57

MINOR TRAUMA

Sabina B. Singh, MD, FAAP, and Magdy W. Attia, MD

1. **What are the major considerations in wound assessment?**
   - **Local factors** include location, mechanism of injury, wound age, possibility of foreign body, and degree of contamination. Soil contamination with organic matters has the highest rate of wound infection if not properly cleansed. The possibility of a retained foreign body should be entertained in wounds caused by broken glass or other debris. Imaging studies should be obtained if a foreign body is suspected.
   - **Host factors** include disease states, tetanus immunization, allergies, sedation, and pain control.

2. **How does location of injury affect assessment?**
   - **Injuries over a joint or adjacent to tendons** should be checked for crepitus, which may signify disruption of the joint capsule. Loss of function may indicate tendon injury.
   - **Lacerations close to the neurovascular bundle** are at risk for nerve damage. Assess capillary refill and pulses and conduct a careful neurologic examination of motor and sensory functions.
   - Wounds in proximity to **areas of high bacterial concentration,** such as the perineum, axilla (particularly in adolescents), and exposed parts (hands, feet) are at a higher risk for infection.

3. **Why are bites and crush injuries of special concern?**
   Bites and crush injuries are more difficult to repair. They are often associated with devitalized tissue and are more likely to become infected. Injury over a metacarpophalangeal joint from a fist punch should be managed as a human bite.

4. **How do disease states affect wound assessment?**
   Higher infection rates are seen in conditions such as diabetes, immunosuppressed states (e.g., AIDS, long-term steroid use), and chronic disease (e.g., renal insufficiency, cyanotic heart disease). Exposure to smoke delays proper healing.

5. **Which allergies are of particular relevance to wound assessment?**
   Allergy to latex, anesthetic agents, and antibiotics.

6. **What is the ideal time frame for repair of wounds?**
   Ideally wounds should be repaired within 6 hours of injury. Clean wounds can be closed within 12–24 hours after injury.

7. **When should delayed closure of a wound be considered?**
   Delayed closure is usually carried out 3–5 days after the original injury. Wounds that should be considered for delayed closure are those with high potential for infection (heavily contaminated wounds, bite wounds, puncture wounds) and wounds in immunocompromised patients in areas of low cosmetic concern. Facial and scalp wounds should be considered for primary closure for best results.

8. **Which wounds are allowed to heal by secondary intention?**
    Infected wounds and small puncture wounds in areas of low cosmetic concern may be allowed to close by secondary intention. A small wick of iodoform gauze may be placed in the wound to decrease chances of infection.

9. **How should the emergency physician approach sedation and pain control?**
    Options, risks, and benefits should be discussed with parents and older children. Parents often can predict the level of cooperation expected from the child.

10. **When should a consultation be obtained for wound care?**
    Consider consultation with a surgical or orthopedic specialist for wounds associated with:
    ■ Fracture or violation of a joint cavity
    ■ Injury to tendon, nerve, or large vessel
    ■ Difficult-to-repair wounds located in areas of high cosmetic concern

    Selbst SM, Attia M: Minor trauma—lacerations. In Fleisher GR, Ludwig S, Henretig FM (eds): Textbook of Pediatric Emergency Medicine, 5th ed. Philadelphia, Lippincott Williams & Wilkins, 2006, pp 1571–1586.

11. **When are radiographic studies indicated as a part of wound management?**
    Radiographs should be obtained for wounds associated with fractures or joint disruption or if a foreign body is suspected. Plain radiographs identify fragments of metal and glass if they are larger than 0.5 cm. Wood is identified in only 15% of cases because air trapped in the wood is resorbed within 48 hours. Ultrasonography has 90% sensitivity and specificity for nonopaque foreign bodies if the location is not near a bony or gaseous structure. Computed tomography or magnetic resonance imaging should be considered if a surgical approach is planned for the removal of a foreign body near vital structures.

12. **How can you decrease the chances of missing a retained foreign body in a wound?**
    A detailed history of the mechanism and circumstances surrounding the injury is important. Good exploration with visualization of the base of the wound significantly reduces the risk. In one study, wounds less than 0.5 cm deep had a low risk of an embedded foreign body.

13. **What are the signs of retained foreign body?**
    Extreme pain, pain on passive movement, or a mass with discoloration at the site of a wound is highly suggestive of a retained foreign body.

14. **When should a retained foreign body be removed?**
    The material, location, and tissue response to a foreign body determine the necessity of its removal. Attempts at removal in the emergency department (ED) should be limited to 30 minutes. The foreign bodies listed below should be removed.
    ■ **Location:** Intra-articular, intravascular, or in close proximity to vital structures or has the potential to migrate towards vital structures (e.g., lung, spleen)
    ■ **Material:** Risk of toxicity (e.g., lead, venom from spines)
    ■ **Tissue response:** Production of inflammatory response (e.g., organic matter, silica that causes large granuloma formation), persistent pain, infection, or cosmetic disfigurement

15. **What are the contraindications to the removal of a foreign body in the ED?**
    Foreign bodies associated with penetrating injuries to the abdomen, neck, or chest should be explored and removed in the operating room. Small, deeply embedded foreign bodies may be difficult to locate without ultrasound guidance. They can be left in place with close follow-up or removed electively.

16. **Should hair be removed from a wound site before repair?**
The presence of hair usually does not interfere with repair of the wound. Petroleum jelly can be used to keep hair away from the wound site during repair. If hair removal is needed, clippers should be used because they have a lower rate of infection than do razors. *Eyebrows should not be removed because regrowth can be slow or absent.*

17. **Outline the steps in preparing a wound for closure.**
   - Follow standard precautions.
   - Prepare the child and the family. An honest and caring explanation of the various steps is important to reduce anxiety.
   - Determine whether sedation is required.
   - Cleanse and irrigate the wound.
   - Use local anesthesia.
   - Always use sterile draping and technique.

18. **How is irrigation and cleansing of the wound best achieved?**
Irrigation is best achieved with normal saline or tap water under pressure using a 20- or 30-mL syringe on a 19- or 22-gauge plastic intravascular catheter. Splash shields (e.g., Zerowet) decrease splattering of irrigation fluid. A volume of 50–100 mL/cm of laceration should be used; for contaminated wounds, larger volumes may be needed. Avoid excessive pressure during irrigation because it can distort the anatomy and damage the tissues. Road rash (tar), dirt, and foreign material should be removed gently with irrigation and mild scrubbing to prevent tattooing. Scrubbing should be limited because it can damage tissues, leading to poor cosmetic outcome. The use of povidone-iodine is controversial. Several studies have shown that it affects fibroblasts and hence wound defenses. A study by Gravett et al showed that use of 1% of povidone-iodine for 1 minute reduces the risk of infection. If irrigation is not well tolerated, repeat it after giving a local anesthetic.

   Gravett A, Stener S, Clinton JE, et al: A trial of povidone-iodine in the prevention of infection in sutured lacerations. Ann Emerg Med 16:167, 1987.
   Valente JH, Forti RJ, Freundlich LF, et al: Wound irrigation in children: Saline solution or tap water? Ann Emerg Med 41:609–616, 2003.

19. **What agents are used for local anesthesia?**
Topical anesthetics such as LET (lidocaine 4%, epinephrine 1:1000, tetracaine 0.5%) are very useful. When applied to the wound locally in the form of a gel for 15–20 minutes, LET produces local anesthesia with 97% efficacy. It can be used for all superficial wounds as the sole local anesthetic agent. Topical agents should be avoided in areas of end-blood supply, such as the fingers, ears, nose, toes, and penis (do not use epinephrine for end-arterial structures). Occasionally, deeper wounds require infiltration with another agent, such as lidocaine 1% with or without epinephrine. Bupivacaine is an alternative in lidocaine-allergic patients. Bupivacaine has a longer duration of action.

20. **What is the maximum dose of epinephrine in local anesthetic medications?**
The does of lidocaine with epinephrine should not exceed 7 mg/kg body weight; the dose of lidocaine alone should not exceed 4 mg/kg.

21. **How can the pain of infiltration of a local anesthetic be decreased?**
The pain of infiltration can be decreased by:
   - Prior application of LET gel (time permitting)
   - Rubbing the skin near the site of injection (stimulates other nerve endings and thereby decreases the perception of pain)

- Buffering lidocaine with 8.4% sodium bicarbonate (ratio, 9:1)
- Warming the buffered lidocaine to 40°C
- Use of 27- or 30-gauge needle to slow the rate of injection
- Injecting from inside the wound through devitalized tissue

Ernst AA, Gershoff L, Miller P, et al: Warmed versus room temperature saline for laceration irrigation—a randomized clinical trial. South Med J 96:436–439, 2003.

22. **What is the best method of obtaining hemostasis during wound repair?**
A tourniquet, such as a rubber band or blood pressure cuff, and a local anesthetic with epinephrine can decrease the amount of bleeding during wound repair. The blood pressure cuff should be inflated to just above systolic blood pressure. A tourniquet should be used for only 20–30 minutes at a time. It should be released periodically for 2–3 minutes to allow reperfusion. Prolonged continuous use can lead to nerve and vascular damage, with subsequent thrombosis and gangrene.

KEY POINTS: TIPS TO REDUCE PAIN OF ANESTHETIC INFILTRATION ✓

1. Apply LET in advance.

2. Rub the skin near the site of injection.

3. Use buffered lidocaine.

4. Warm the buffered lidocaine.

5. Use a small needle (27- or 30-gauge) for infiltration.

6. Infiltrate slowly.

7. Inject from inside the wound through devitalized tissue.

23. **What are the key points for proper wound approximation?**
Some physicians find it helpful to place the first suture at midpoint for good alignment, but this technique is not necessary as long as the approximation is preplanned. Slight eversion of the wound edges throughout the procedure is important to avoid future tethering of the scar line. Removal of clot from gaping wounds also helps to avoid tethering and decrease tension. Keep the amount of tension on the wound to a minimum. In layered closure, close each layer individually.

24. **What are the appropriate types of sutures and techniques for closure of various wounds?**
For skin closure, synthetic nonabsorbable, monofilament nylon (Ethilon or Dermalon) should be used. Fine absorbable synthetic sutures (e.g., coated Vicryl or Dexon) are used for deeper layers or nail-bed repairs. Suture size depends on the site and size of the wound. Smaller needles (e.g., PS or P1) are used for wounds that require fine cosmetic outcome. Table 57-1 lists suggested suture types for various locations.

TABLE 57-1. SUGGESTED SUTURE TYPES FOR VARIOUS LOCATIONS

Wound Site	Suture Type	Recommended Technique	Removal (d)
Scalp	4.0 or 5.0 SNA	Simple, interrupted	7
Face	6.0 SNA for skin 5.0 AS for deeper layers	Simple interrupted or continuous for skin; interrupted for deeper layers	3–5
Extremity	3.0 or 4.0 SNA 4.0 or 5.0 AS	Simple interrupted mattress or continuous for skin; interrupted for deeper layers	7–10
Hands or feet	5.0 SNA 4.0 AS	Simple interrupted or continuous for skin; interrupted for deeper layers	7–10
Joints	3.0 or 4.0 SNA 4.0 AS	Simple interrupted mattress, or continuous for skin; interrupted for deeper layers	10–14

AS = absorbable synthetic, SNA = synthetic nonabsorbable.

KEY POINTS: ACHIEVING IDEAL WOUND APPROXIMATION ✓

1. Plan ahead.

2. Consider placing the first suture at the midpoint for good alignment.

3. Ensure slight eversion of the wound edges.

4. Remove clots from gaping wounds.

5. Keep wound tension to a minimum.

6. In layered closures, close each layer individually.

25. **How do alternative wound care techniques compare?**
    See Table 57-2.

26. **When can tissue adhesives be used?**
    Tissue adhesives are nearly painless, do not require local anesthesia or removal, and have cosmetic results similar to those of sutures in most instances. They should be used in wounds with straight edges that are less than 5–6 cm long. Wounds should be no wider than 2–4 mm, and should not be located over a joint or hair-bearing area. During application, good approximation of the wound must be ensured, and care must be taken to prevent the adhesive from dripping into the wound, eyes, or eyelashes. The presence of adhesive in the wound acts like a foreign body and can produce intense inflammation. Parents should be instructed to

TABLE 57-2.	COMPARISOIN OF ALTERNATIVE WOUND CARE TECHNIQUES					
Type of Closure	Wound Type	Ease of Application	Cosmetic Result	Pain	Cost	Need for Removal
Suture	Any	Poor	Excellent	High	High	Yes
Staple	Scalp*	Good	Poor	High	Medium	Yes[†]
Surgical glue	Small	Good	Good	None	Medium	None
Steri-Strips	Small[‡]	Good	Fair	None	Low	Yes

*Should be avoided in areas of cosmetic concern or in patients needing computed tomography or magnetic resonance imaging.
[†]Requires special removal forceps.
[‡]Small, straight lacerations or located over joints, hair-bearing areas, or moist areas.
Data from Farion K, Osmond MH, Harling L, et al: Tissue adhesives for traumatic lacerations in children and adults. Cochrane Database Syst Rev (3):CD003326, 2002; Karounis H, Gouin S, Eisman H, et al: A randomized, controlled trial comparing long-term cosmetic outcomes of traumatic pediatric lacerations repaired with absorbable plain gut versus nonabsorbable nylon sutures. Acad Emerg Med 11:730–735, 2004; and Bayat A, McGrouther DA, Ferguson, MWJ: Skin scarring. BMJ 326:88–92, 2003.

avoid the use of ointments or cream at the site of the wound because they lead to premature peeling of the adhesive. Tissue adhesive (cyanoacrylate) polymerize on the surface of the approximate wound edges, forming a strong bond to maintain the achieved approximation.

Mattick A, Clegg G, Beattie T, et al: A randomized controlled trial comparing a tissue adhesive (2-octylcyanoacrylate) with adhesive strips (Steristrips) for pediatric laceration repair. Emerg Med J 19:405–407, 2003.

27. **What are the complications of tissue adhesives?**
Occasionally, skin folds are inadvertently glued together, the glove of the operator may become glued to the patient's skin, or adhesive drips into the patient's eyelashes. If these complications occur, petroleum jelly or eye ointment should be massaged into the site to help dissolve the glue. Refrain from clipping the eyelashes because their regrowth is uncertain. The strength of the wound after repair with an adhesive is 10–15% less than that of wounds closed by sutures. Dehiscence occurs in 1–5% of all wounds, closed by adhesives. If the wound dehisces, it should be left to heal by secondary intention unless the result will be cosmetically unacceptable.

28. **What are some important considerations in the evaluation of puncture wounds?**
Puncture wounds account for 3–5% of all injuries. The most common site is the forefoot (50%). The rate of complications is directly proportional to the depth of penetration. Infection occurs in 6–10% of all puncture wounds, with staphylococci, streptococci, and anaerobes being the most common organisms. Injuries penetrating through a foam or rubber insole of a sneaker are often contaminated by *Pseudomonas aeruginosa*. The most common offending object in puncture wounds is a nail (> 90%). It is essential to examine the wound well for the possibility of damage to deeper structures and for retained foreign bodies. Puncture wounds have a greater incidence of infectious complications, such as cellulitis, soft tissue abscess, pyarthrosis, osteomyelitis (0.4–0.6% of wounds), and foreign-body granuloma.

29. **A 10-year-old boy presents with persistent pain in his right forefoot after sustaining a puncture wound from a nail 10 days ago. Some redness and swelling are seen at the site. What are your major concerns and management course?**

Osteomyelitis is a major concern with a puncture wound when persistent pain is accompanied by local signs of infection, even without systemic involvement. A complete blood count and erythrocyte sedimentation rate, along with imaging studies, should be obtained. Bone scanning or MRI is more sensitive in detecting periosteal reaction or bony destruction than radiography in the first week. Osteomyelitis should be treated with IV antistaphylococcal and antipseudomonal antibiotics. If no improvement is noted in 48 hours, surgical debridement may be necessary.

30. **What is coring of a puncture wound?**

Coring removes a 2-mm circular rim of the puncture track. The area should be prepared with povidone-iodine, local anesthetic, or regional nerve block, followed by irrigation and packing with iodoform gauze. The patient should be instructed to avoid weight-bearing for 5 days. Coring should be considered in wounds that are grossly contaminated or have a foreign body in an area of low cosmetic concern and high risk for infection, such as the foot.

31. **How are forehead lacerations repaired?**

Superficial transverse lacerations of the forehead are easy to repair with interrupted or continuous cuticular sutures using 6–0 nonabsorbable materials. Deeper transverse lacerations involving the deep fascia, frontalis muscle, or periosteum should be repaired in layers. If the deeper tissue planes are not closed, the function of the frontalis muscle (eyebrow elevation) may be compromised. Vertical forehead lacerations tend to have wider scars because they traverse the tension lines if proper tension and coaptation are not achieved. Forehead lacerations are rarely associated with skull fractures, but facial, neck, and intracranial injuries should be ruled out.

32. **Describe the appropriate technique for repair of eyebrow lacerations.**

The eyebrow should not be shaved for wound preparation because it serves as a landmark during repair. In addition, eyebrow regrowth is unpredictable; it may be slow or incomplete, leading to poor cosmetic outcome. Attention must be paid to avoid inverting the hair-bearing edges into the wound. It is also important to pay attention to proper alignment of both ends along the eyebrow wound.

33. **How are lacerations of the eyelid repaired?**

Lacerations of the eyelid are mostly simple transverse wounds of the upper eyelid just inferior to the eyebrow. Repair does not require special skills. Consider ophthalmology referral for complicated lacerations potentially involving the levator palpebrae muscle or medial canthal ligament or those close to the lacrimal duct. Evaluation for associated injuries to the globe is imperative.

34. **How are lacerations of the external ear treated?**

To avoid necrosis and auricular deformity, every attempt must be made to minimize debridement and to cover the perichondrium with the lacerated thin but vascular skin. Simple closure with the least possible tension is usually advised. The perichondrium should be included in the sutures to ensure that the suture material does not tear through the friable cartilage and to restore nutrient and oxygen supply. If ear trauma has led to auricular hematoma, it should be drained promptly to avoid necrosis of the cartilage, which leads to a deformed auricle or cauliflower ear. After repair of ear lacerations or evacuation of an auricular hematoma, a pressure dressing should be applied. Follow-up in 24 hours is recommended to evaluate vascular integrity.

35. **What is the recommended technique for repair of lip lacerations?**
Lip lacerations are important because of their highly visible nature. The vermilion border is
a relatively paler line that identifies the junction of the dry oral mucosa and facial skin. It is an
important landmark for proper repair. The use of epinephrine with local anesthesia should be
avoided because it causes local swelling that distorts the border. A mental nerve block provides
good anesthesia while preserving the landmarks. Lacerations involving the vermilion border
should be precisely aligned. Parents should be warned that, while the lip is still anesthetized,
the child might bite off the sutures. They should distract the child from doing so. After local
anesthesia has worn off, the site typically is sore enough that the child does not attempt to
manipulate the area.

36. **Describe the proper approach to lacerations of the tongue and buccal mucosa.**
   - Small isolated lacerations of the buccal mucosa, usually due to teeth impaction after falls,
     require no suturing. Lacerations > 2–3 cm in length or with flaps are best closed with simple
     interrupted stitches using absorbable material.
   - Tongue lacerations often bleed excessively at the time of injury, but the bleeding usually
     ceases quickly as the lingual muscle contracts. Most tongue lacerations can be left alone with
     good results. Large lacerations involving the free edge, large flaps, and bleeding lacerations
     should be repaired. Full-thickness repair with interrupted 4–0 absorbable sutures is
     recommended.
   - Local or regional anesthesia is often sufficient.
   - Attention must be paid to potential airway problems during repair.
   - The mouth should be held open with a padded tongue depressor. The tongue can be
     maintained in the protruded position by a gentle pull by using a towel clip or by placing
     a suture through the tip.
   - As in lip lacerations, children may chew off the stitches; parents must be warned of this
     possibility. They should attempt to distract the child, at least until the local anesthesia has
     worn off.

37. **How are fingertip avulsions repaired?**
Most fingertip avulsions are contused lacerations or partial avulsions. Sharp injuries are
more common in older children and less likely to be associated with fractures. Evaluate for
associated nail bed injury and obtain radiographs for possible fracture of the phalanx. In general,
this type of injury is managed by the emergency physician. The management is mostly
conservative, especially in preadolescent children, because tissue regeneration is remarkable.

38. **Describe the approach to nail bed injuries.**
Trauma to the distal fingers is often associated with nail and nail bed (matrix) injuries. Nail
avulsion may be partial or complete; it may or may not be associated with nail bed laceration.
An underlying fracture of the distal phalanx is not uncommon. Injury to the fingertip often is
associated with subungual hematoma. Unrepaired nailbed lacerations may permanently
disfigure new nail growth from the cicatrix nail bed. If the nail is partially avulsed but is firmly
attached to its bed, exploring the nail bed is difficult and probably not warranted. Good outcome
is expected because the nail holds the underlying lacerated nail bed tissues in place.
   When the nail is completely avulsed or attached loosely, the nail should be lifted and the nail
bed assessed for laceration. If the nail bed is lacerated, it should be repaired by using 6–0 or
smaller absorbable material. After its soft proximal portion is cleansed and trimmed, the nail
should be replaced between the nail bed and nail fold (eponychium) and then anchored in place
with a few stitches. This technique splints the nail fold away from the nail bed and prevents
obliteration of the space between the two. Preserving this space allows the new nail to grow
undisturbed. The preferred method of local anesthesia for nail bed repair is digital block, and use
of a finger tourniquet during repair allows a bloodless field. Application of a finger splint after
repair, especially in patients with an associated fracture, is recommended.

39. **How should a subungal hematoma be managed?**

Subungual hematoma (Fig. 57-1) is a collection of blood in the interface of the nail and nail bed. It is commonly seen with blunt fingertip injuries. The usual presentation is throbbing pain and discoloration of the nail. Subungual hematoma may be associated with nail bed injury or fracture of the distal phalanx. A subungual hematoma involving 50% or more of the nail should be drained. Drainage of the hematoma relieves symptoms. In general, no local anesthesia is required for a simple trephination by cauterization of the nail. Postdrainage care includes elevation of the hand and warm soaks for a few days. The possibility of nail deformity in the future should be discussed with the family.

When the injury is more involved, digital block is advised. If the hematoma is large and extends to the tip of the nail, separation of the nail from the nail bed allows drainage. In the presence of a distal phalangeal fracture, be careful not to transform a closed fracture into an open fracture by communicating a subungual hematoma to the exterior surface of the nail. If this possibility exists, antibiotic coverage and close follow-up are appropriate.

Roser SE, Gellman H: Comparison of nailbed repair versus nail trephination for subungual hematomas in children. J Hand Surg 24:1166–1170, 1999.

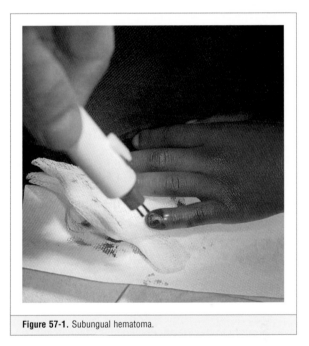

Figure 57-1. Subungual hematoma.

40. **What are the signs of wound infection?**

Signs of wound infection include marked or worsening pain or tenderness at the wound site beyond that expected from the initial trauma. Local erythema, warmth, swelling, and discharge, such as pus or serosanguineous fluid, also are signs of infection. In severe infections, fever, phlebitis (streaking), regional lymphadenopathy, and other systemic manifestations may be seen.

41. **For which wounds should prophylactic antibiotics be considered?**
    - Human bites
    - Cat bites
    - Crush injuries
    - Extensive wounds
    - Exposed cartilage
    - Open fractures
    - Joint cavity violated
    - Hand and foot wounds
    - Moist areas (axilla, perineum)
    - Contaminated wounds
    - Immunocompromised host

    Use a first-generation cephalosporin to cover staphylococci and streptococci or use clindamycin or trimethoprim-sulfamethoxazole if methicillin-resistant *Staphylococcus aureus* is a concern. Amoxicillin–clavulanic acid should be used for bites to provide additional coverage against anaerobes. Clindamycin is a suitable alternative.

42. **What are the key elements of postrepair wound care?**
    - Apply antibiotic cream to reduce infection by preventing scab formation.
    - Elevate the affected area to decrease edema.
    - Immobilize wounds over joints with a splint or apply a bulky dressing.
    - Provide discharge instructions regarding wound care, signs of infection, and follow-up.
    - Instruct patient to avoid bathing for 24–48 hours; after that time, the wound should be washed with mild soap and water and gently dried.
    - Recheck patient in 24–48 hours for healing and signs of infection.
    - Remove sutures in a timely manner to prevent scars from suture tracks.
    - Instruct patient to use sunscreen for 6–12 months after injury to prevent hyperpigmentation of the scar.

43. **When does a wound regain its strength?**
    A wound regains 5% of its strength in 2 weeks, 30% in 1–2 months, and full strength by 6–8 weeks. The scar achieves its final appearance in 6–12 months.

44. **What are the indications for tetanus prophylaxis?**
    Tetanus is a potential risk in all wounds. Wounds at a higher risk for tetanus are those contaminated by soil or feces and those with devitalized tissue (e.g., puncture, crush, missile, or avulsion wounds). Burns and frostbite are also prone to tetanus. Prophylaxis depends on the type of wound and the patient's immunization status (Table 57-3).

    Advisory Committee on Immunization Practices (ACIP): Preventing tetanus, diphtheria, and pertussis among adolescents: Use of tetanus toxoid, reduced diphtheria toxoid and acellular pertussis vaccines recommendations of the Advisory Committee on Immunization Practices (ACIP). MMWR Recomm Rep. 55:1–34, 2006.

45. **A young boy is brought to the ED after being stuck by a needle on the playground. The needle has crusted blood along the metallic edge. What are your concerns? What is the best course of management?**
    A needlestick injury raises concerns about exposure to tetanus and blood-borne pathogens, such as hepatitis B virus (HBV), hepatitis C virus (HCV) and human immunodeficiency virus (HIV). HBV can survive on fomites for several days. Table 57-4 summarizes the American Academy of Pediatrics *Red Book* recommendations for hepatitis prophylaxis after a needlestick exposure.

    For HCV exposure, the risk of transmission from a discarded needle is low and the need for testing is uncertain. If testing is done, antibodies for anti-HCV should be assessed by enzyme

TABLE 57-3. GUIDELINES FOR TETANUS PROPHYLAXIS

Dose of Tetanus Toxoid	Time Since Last Dose	Clean Wound		All Other Wounds	
		DPT/ Tdap/Td*	TIG	DPT/ Tdap/Td	TIG
>3	<5 y	No	No	No	No
	5–10 y	No	No	Yes	Yes
	>10 y	Yes	No	Yes	Yes
<3 or unknown		Yes	No	Yes	Yes

DPT = diphtheria, tetanus, pertussis toxoid for children <7 years of age; Td = tetanus toxoid, reduced diphtheria; Tdap = tetanus toxoid, reduced diphtheria toxoid, acellular pertussis vaccine; TIG = tetanus immunoglobulin.
*Tdap is preferred to Td for adolescents who have never received Tdap.

TABLE 57-4. HEPATITIS PROPHYLAXIS AFTER A NEEDLESTICK EXPOSURE

Number of Doses of HBV Vaccine Already Received	Immunoprophylaxis
>3	None
1–3	Additional dose of HBV vaccine; complete the rest of the schedule with or without HBIG
None	Begin vaccination series + HBIG

HBIG = hepatitis B immunoglobulin, HBV = hepatitis B.

immunoassay at the time of injury and 1 month later. The risk of infection with HIV is low but causes the greatest concern to the family and victim. No data evaluate the risk of acquiring HIV in this scenario. Baseline testing is controversial, and testing the syringe is neither practical nor reliable. Consult a specialist in HIV before using prophylaxis. Antiretroviral therapy should be started if the syringe had fresh blood. Testing the patient for HIV is controversial, but if testing is elected, it should be done at the time of injury, 6 weeks, 12 weeks, and 6 months after exposure.

American Academy of Pediatrics: Red Book Online: http://aapredbook.aappublications.org

46. **When is rabies prophylaxis indicated?**
    Various animals transmit rabies. The virus is shed in the saliva of infected animals for 10–14 days before they become symptomatic. Postexposure guidelines are summarized in Table 57-5.

TABLE 57-5. GUIDELINES FOR RABIES PROPHYLAXIS		
Type of Animal	Availability of Animal for Observation	Postexposure Prophylaxis
Dog or cat	Healthy or can be observed for 10 d Suspected to be rabid or unknown	Only if animal develops signs of rabies RIG + HDCV
Livestock, ferrets, rodents	Consider individually	As per advice of public health official
Skunks, raccoons, bats, fox, woodchuck, other carnivores	Consider rabid unless geographic area is known to be free of rabies	RIG + HDCV
HDCV = human diploid cell vaccine, RIG = rabies immunoglobulin.		

Bites from animals such as squirrels, hamsters, guinea pigs, gerbils, chipmunks, rats, mice, rabbits, hares, and other rodents rarely require rabies prophylaxis.

American Academy of Pediatrics: Red Book Online: http://aapredbook.aappublications.org

47. **What is the regimen for postexposure rabies prophylaxis?**
Active immunization with rabies human diploid cell (HDCV) vaccine is given on the day of injury and on days 3, 7, 14, and 28. The vaccines are administered as a 1.0-mL intramuscular injection in the deltoid. In small infants, the gluteal area is used. If the vaccine is not available, rabies immunoglobulin (RIG) should be given. The dose of RIG is 20 IU/kg body weight. It is given concomitantly with the first does of vaccine but at a different site. Infiltrate as much as possible of the total dose of RIG at the wound site and inject the remainder intramuscularly. RIG should be given as soon as possible, and within 7 days after exposure. Patients previously immunized with rabies vaccine should receive only two doses of HDCV on days 0 and 3.

48. **What is the best course of management for a fishhook embedded in soft tissue?**
Fishhooks have a straight shank and a curved belly that has an eyelet with a barb pointed away from the tip. Do not attempt removal in the ED if the fishhook is buried near vital structures. If the fishhook is not in a dangerous location, use a digital block or local infiltration. Wear protective eyewear to avoid injury during the removal. Remove lures and additional hooks first with a hemostat and wire cutter.

There are several methods of removal. The push-through method is most effective when the barb is close to the skin. The barb is pushed forward (antegrade) through the skin. It is then clipped with a wire cutter and the rest of the barb is pulled back through the original wound.

With the string technique, a long piece of string is looped around the hook at the point of entry and around the clinician's finger. While the clinician applies pressure downward over the straight part of the fishhook to disengage the barb, the hook is pulled away rapidly.

49. **What is the best way to remove a ring that is stuck on a child's finger?**

    If vascular compromise is present, the constricting ring should be removed as soon as possible. Risk of gangrene is present in any obstruction that persists beyond 10–12 hours. A ring cutter is useful. It is easiest to cut the thinnest portion of the ring or on the palmar surface of the hand. Once cut, the ends should be separated manually. The string-pull method is best used for broad or metallic bands. One end of a suture is slipped under the band. After application of lubricant, the string is grasped with a hemostat and pulled in a circular motion until it slides off.

CHAPTER 58

MULTIPLE TRAUMA

Laurie H. Johnson, MD, and Richard M. Ruddy, MD

1. **What is the importance of trauma to the health of children?**
   Injury is the leading cause of death in children older than 1 year (Fig. 58-1). Although injury death rates in the U.S. population have declined since 1991 (except for 2001 because of September 11), trauma is still the number one killer of children. Most injury is responsible for intermediate morbidity, with significant impact on the functioning of children and their progress to adulthood. Trauma is responsible for about 22,000 deaths per year in children age 19 years and younger. The number of permanently disabled may approach over 100,000 per year. Hospital admissions in the 0–14 age group for trauma is estimated to exceed 250,000 per year (> 51/100,000 population).

   Peclet MH, Newman KD, Eichelberger MR, et al: Patterns of injury in children. J Pediatr Surg 25:85–91, 1990.

   Centers for Disease Control and Prevention: National Vital Statistics Report. Deaths: Preliminary data for 2002: www.cdc.gov/nchs/data/nvsr/nvsr53/nvsr53_15.pdf

   Centers for Disease Control and Prevention, National Center for Health Statistics. National trends in injury hospitalizations: 1971–2001: www.cdc.gov/nchs/data/injury/InjuryChartbook79–01.pdf

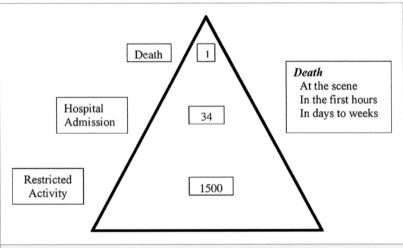

Figure 58-1. Iceberg of pediatric injuries—the American College of Surgeons Advanced Trauma Life Support guidelines, 1999.

2. **What specific mechanisms of injury are seen typically in children?**
   - Motor vehicle–related crashes are the leading cause of death from injuries in children, both as passengers and as pedestrians struck.
   - Drowning is the second leading cause of pediatric injury death in most areas.
   - Deaths from burns and smoke inhalation have declined but remain third.
   - Mortality rates (%) are highest for gunshot wounds, especially in teens, but also in the young.
   - Falls are the most common mechanism; severity of injury is minor except in falls greater than 10–20 feet.

   Centers for Disease Control and Prevention: Web-based Injury Statistics Query and Reporting System: www.cdc.gov/ncipc/wisqars/

KEY POINTS: THE CHALLENGE OF PEDIATRIC TRAUMA ✓

1. "Multiple trauma" is injury to two or more body areas.
2. Patients with severe head injuries are at high risk of poor outcome or death.
3. Lack of cooperation with examination due to age or fear, initially occult injuries, altered mental status due to alcohol or illicit substances, and nonaccidental trauma may interfere with rapid determination of isolated versus multiple trauma.

3. **Discuss the importance of sports-related injuries.**
   Sports-related injuries are common but do not often lead to death. Neck injury due to falls from equestrian sports or football spearing is an important cause of severe injury and death despite a fairly low incidence. Blunt trauma from sports can lead to serious head, intra-abdominal solid-organ, and eye injury. In terms of visits for emergency care, sports injuries are responsible for large numbers of musculoskeletal injuries, fractures, and joint injuries.

4. **Describe the prehospital care capability for children with potentially serious injuries.**
   Emergency medical technicians have a great deal of adult experience in advanced life support, which transfers to older children and adolescents. Important skills, such as endotracheal intubation and IV access, can be more of an issue in younger patients. Early studies reported successful field intubation rates of 50% in infants < 1 year of age and 64% in children < 18 years of age. Rates of success with IV access have been fair in infants, good in preschoolers, and excellent in adolescents. Even with programs conducted to improve these rates (such as procedures in the operating room and field courses), in settings with less experienced providers and short transit distances, the best procedure is safe extrication/preparation and immediate transfer to the hospital.

   Gausche M, Lewis RJ, Stratton SJ, et al: Effect of out of hospital endotracheal intubation on survival and neurological outcome. JAMA 283:783–790, 2000.
   Losek JD, Szewczuga D, Glauser PW: Improved prehospital pediatric ALS care after an EMT-paramedic clinical training course. Am J Emerg Med 12:429–432, 1994.

KEY POINTS: ABNORMAL VITAL SIGNS IN THE INJURED CHILD ✓

1. Tachycardia in an injured patient may be due to pain or loss of blood volume.

2. Carefully evaluate the tachycardic trauma patient for the possibility of compensated shock.

3. An older child in compensated shock may be deceivingly responsive and alert.

4. Shock in the trauma patient should be treated with a 20-mL/kg bolus of normal saline or lactated Ringer's solution, which should be repeated once if shock persists.

5. If the patient is refractory to treatment with crystalloid, rapidly infuse packed red cells and emergently seek operative intervention.

5. **Describe the initial approach to children with potentially serious injuries.**
   The ABCDEs are used during the primary assessment to define underlying injury and to reverse potential life-threatening problems:
   - **A**irway management with cervical spine control
   - **B**reathing: Maximize oxygen delivery
   - **C**irculation: Establish vascular access, control external hemorrhage, and restore circulatory volume
   - **D**isability: Assess potentially critical injury to the central nervous system
   - **E**xposure: Visualize every part of the patient to assess for injury and control body temperature (especially important in young infants and children)

   The team must assess and stabilize each step in order (i.e., control of airway always precedes control of circulation).

6. **How can one appropriately "clear the cervical spine" in a trauma patient?**
   In the alert patient with no distracting injury and no midline cervical pain with palpation, the patient can be cleared clinically by assessing active range of motion. Anteroposterior, lateral, and odontoid radiographs of the cervical spine should be obtained and proper immobilization should be continued if the cervical spine is tender to palpation, if the patient has altered mental status or neurologic deficits (even the presence or history of numbness, tingling sensation, decreased sensory, or motor function), or if a distracting injury exists (such as an extremity fracture or abdominal pain).

   Slack SE, Clancy MJ: Clearing the cervical spine of paediatric trauma patients. Emerg Med J 21:185–189, 2004.

7. **Is hypertonic saline beneficial in the fluid resuscitation of the multiply injured trauma patient with severe head injury?**
   Studies performed in pediatric and adult trauma patients in the intensive care unit setting have demonstrated the safety and efficacy of hypertonic saline for acutely decreasing intracranial pressure compared to traditional therapies. The proposed mechanism for use of hypertonic solutions is that increased serum osmolality decreases intracranial pressure via the osmotic pressure gradient. Initial fluid resuscitation with hypertonic saline may therefore be helpful in supporting blood pressure as well as decreasing intracranial pressure in this patient population.

   Simma B, Burger R, Falk M, et al: A prospective, randomized, and controlled study of fluid management in children with severe head injury: Lactated Ringers solution versus hypertonic saline. Crit Care Med 26:1265–1270, 1998.

KEY POINTS: INITIAL MANAGEMENT OF POTENTIALLY SERIOUS INJURIES ✓

1. Always assess the airway first.

2. Once airway is secure, stabilize breathing.

3. Confirm or establish stable circulation.

4. Always maintain cervical spine immobilization and control.

8. **Explain the secondary survey.**
It is the detailed head-to-toe physical examination that follows the initial ABCDE survey and resuscitation. The head, neck, and face are surveyed first for evidence of blood or occult injury with control of the cervical spine. Assessment of maxillary and mandibular stability, eyes, ears, and oropharynx follows. Careful assessment of the bony thorax, lungs, and cardiovascular system are next, followed by assessment of the abdomen, pelvis, and external genitourinary tract. The child should be logrolled in a neutral position to assess the back, posterior chest, and spine. Lastly, the extremities are assessed carefully for obvious and occult injury, along with neurovascular status. Observers may integrate evaluation of the central nervous system during each part of the examination or perform the entire central nervous system evaluation at the end.

9. **What components of the neurologic examination should be conducted during the primary and secondary surveys?**
A rapid neurologic evaluation is indicated rather than a detailed examination. It is not appropriate to assess the child's reflexes or fine-motor coordination during the primary survey. Instead, pupillary size, symmetry, and reactivity should be evaluated. The child's level of consciousness should be assessed by the **AVPU** mnemonic:
- **A** = **A**lert
- **V** = responds to **V**oice
- **P** = responds to **P**ain
- **U** = **U**nresponsive

The secondary survey should ascertain whether there is disability from a "quick" neurologic assessment based on the child's responsiveness.

10. **What initial radiographic and laboratory studies are important in trauma?**
In unstable or high-risk patients, the most important studies to be obtained in the first 5–10 minutes include a complete blood count with differential, type and cross-match for packed red blood cells, and coagulation studies (prothrombin time, partial thromboplastin time), the aminotransferases, and amylase. Initial radiographs should consist of lateral cervical spine, chest, and pelvis views. Urinalysis should be obtained to look for hematuria, evidence of a genitourinary injury.

In patients with mild to moderate trauma, screening blood studies and radiographs, although standard in the past, should not be routine and are usually of low utility. It is always appropriate to reassess the patient and obtain studies later if needed.

11. **Discuss the uses and complications of medical antishock trousers or pneumatic antishock garments in children.**
The only indicated use in children has been unstable pelvic fractures, but with the advent of pelvic wraps, they are rarely indicated. Medical antishock trousers are associated with problems such as:
- Lower-extremity compartment syndrome
- Ischemic events
- Increased rate of bleeding above the garment

12. **List the major signs of intra-abdominal bleeding caused by organ rupture.**
- Abdominal tenderness
- Abdominal distention that does not improve after nasogastric decompression
- Shock
- Bloody nasogastric aspirate

13. **Describe the presentation and treatment of tension pneumothorax. Define open pneumothorax. How is it managed?**
Tension pneumothorax results from penetrating chest trauma or acute barotrauma during blunt injury. Air is trapped behind a one-way flap-valve defect in the lung. The child presents with severe respiratory distress and contralateral tracheal deviation. Systemic perfusion is compromised significantly by obstructed venous return. Treatment requires needle decompression followed by chest tube placement.
Open pneumothorax, or "sucking chest wound," which may occur after a penetrating chest wound, allows free bidirectional flow of air between the affected hemithorax and surrounding atmosphere. Sucking chest wounds are extremely rare in children. Management centers on positive-pressure ventilation and covering the wound with an occlusive dressing.

14. **In a child who has suffered blunt abdominal trauma, what class of hemorrhage results in diminished pulse pressure, prolonged capillary refill, and normal systolic blood pressure?**
These findings are associated with a class II hemorrhage (15–30% blood loss). This level of blood loss is associated with tachycardia, tachypnea, minimal decrease in urine output, decreased pulse pressure, prolonged capillary refill, and normal blood pressure. Hypotension is a late finding, associated with ongoing hemorrhage, and indicates that the child is near decompensation.

15. **What is the "3-for-1" rule in trauma fluid resuscitation?**
The 3-for-1 rule is a rough guideline for the total amount of crystalloid required in the acute management of hypovolemia. Each milliliter of lost blood should be replaced with 3 mL of crystalloid fluid. This amount allows replacement of plasma volume lost into the interstitial space. The patient's response to fluid therapy remains the most important guideline for further fluid resuscitation (Fig. 58-2).

16. **Which visceral injuries are more common in children?**
Duodenal hematoma and blunt pancreatic injury may occur when a handle bar strikes the child in the right upper quadrant, due to undeveloped abdominal muscular tone. Small bowel perforations at or near the ligament of Treitz and mesenteric small bowel avulsion injuries are more common in children. The shallowness of the pelvis in a child leads to more frequent occurrences of bladder rupture. Because of the proximity of the peritoneum to the perineum, intraperitoneal injuries occur more commonly after straddle injuries in children.

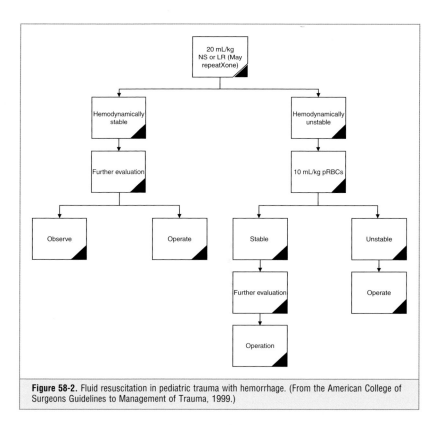

Figure 58-2. Fluid resuscitation in pediatric trauma with hemorrhage. (From the American College of Surgeons Guidelines to Management of Trauma, 1999.)

KEY POINTS: PITFALLS IN RESUSCITATION OF INJURED CHILDREN

1. Failure to recognize impending respiratory failure or potential airway obstruction

2. Failure to recognize early shock when the patient has a "normal" blood pressure with other signs of hemorrhage (e.g., tachycardia, delayed capillary refill, diaphoresis, altered mental status)

3. Failure to recognize impending neurologic deterioration from unsuspected head injury

17. **True or false: To open the airway in a pediatric trauma patient, the head-tilt chin-lift maneuver is the recommended procedure.**
    False. The cervical spine must be immobilized in a neutral position. This goal is best accomplished with the **jaw-thrust spinal-stabilization maneuver**. Place two fingers on each side of the lower jaw and lift the jaw upward and outward. This maneuver can be performed

without extension of the neck. The head-tilt chin-lift maneuver may cause manipulation of the neck, which can convert an incomplete to a complete spinal cord injury.

18. **What are the factors that may interfere in the detection of multiple injuries in the pediatric patient?**
    - Lack of cooperation of the child due to any of the following: preverbal or nonverbal, fearful, in pain, or with altered mental status due to injury or ingested substances
    - No trauma team activation
    - Occult injuries that are not initially apparent
    - Presentation without trauma as the history (physical abuse/nonaccidental trauma)

19. **What is the most appropriate way to intubate the trachea of a seriously injured child?**
    The orotracheal route is preferred. The nasotracheal route is contraindicated because it is very difficult without direct visualization. The patient's neck must remain in the neutral position and should not be hyperextended during the procedure. Always precede tracheal intubation with ventilation by a bag-valve-mask device. Ideally, one rescuer should stabilize the neck (bimanually) while another performs the endotracheal intubation. Perform the Sellick maneuver before the intubation if the child is unresponsive. Have a rigid suction device immediately available. If the child is conscious, especially if increased intracranial pressure is a concern, administer a short-acting neuromuscular blocking agent (succinylcholine) and a sedative or anesthetic (thiopental) before intubation. Sedatives are a risk if the patient is hypotensive or on the "edge."

20. **What can lead to gastric distention in an injured child? Why is gastric distention important?**
    Gastric distention can occur when the child swallows air at the time of injury. It also may be due to ventilation with a bag-valve-mask device or a leak around an endotracheal tube. Gastric distention can compromise ventilation. It limits diaphragmatic motion, reduces lung volume, and increases the risk of vomiting and aspiration.

21. **How should gastric distention in an injured child be managed?**
    A nasogastric tube should be placed as soon as the airway is controlled, and the stomach should be decompressed. An orogastric tube should be used instead of nasogastric decompression if the child has significant facial trauma or a maxillofacial or basal skull fracture. The orogastric route prevents possible intracranial placement of the tube.

22. **Which signs indicate shock in injured children?**
    Shock may be difficult to recognize because the signs are subtle and mimic those of fright or pain. Injured children with loss of about 15% of blood volume exhibit tachycardia, cool extremities, delayed capillary refill beyond 2 seconds, and possibly weak pulses. Confusion and clammy skin also may be present. Hypotension may not be evident until the child has lost 25–40% of blood volume and is thus a late finding.

23. **How might airbags and pediatric restraint devices in vehicles influence motor vehicle crash–related injuries?**
    Children younger than 10 years of age seated in the front seat of the car are at risk for minor injuries from airbag deployment, such as facial burns, lacerations, contusions, abrasions, and eye injuries. More devastating injuries of spinal cord transection and blunt head and neck trauma have also been reported, even in children who were restrained in the front seat. Unrestrained and improperly restrained children are at risk of being ejected during a motor vehicle collision.

Age-appropriate restraint devices have been shown to decrease mortality and significant injury in children 6 years old and younger.

American Academy of Pediatrics: Car safety seats: A guide for families 2007: www.aap.org/family/carseatguide.htm

National Highway Traffic Safety Administration: www.nhtsa.dot.gov

Scheidler MG, Shultz BL, Schall L, et al: Risk factors and predictors of mortality in children after ejection from motor vehicle crashes. J Trauma 49:864–868, 2000.

Tyroch AH, Kaups KL, Sue LP, et al: Pediatric restraint use in motor vehicle collisions. Arch Surg 135:1173–1176, 2000.

24. **Can the intraosseous route be used to establish vascular access in an injured child?**
Yes. The intraosseous route may be life-saving if an IV line cannot be established quickly. It is ideal for children younger than 6 years and can be used to deliver crystalloid fluids, blood, or medications. Avoid use through a fractured long bone to avoid extravasation.

25. **When is a blood transfusion indicated for an injured child?**
If signs of shock persist despite two or three boluses of crystalloid (20 mL/kg each) or if hypotension is present, a blood transfusion is warranted. Blood should be administered as a bolus of packed red blood cells in aliquots of 10 mL/kg. Warming the blood to body temperature is recommended to increase the speed of transfusion and prevent hypothermia. Boluses may be repeated until systemic perfusion improves. It is best to give type-specific, cross-matched blood, but O-negative blood may be imperative if shock is present and type-specific blood is not available.

26. **What is the most likely injury in a child with blunt head trauma and no evidence of external bleeding who presents with signs of shock?**
The child most likely has a serious injury of the chest, abdomen, or pelvis with internal bleeding. Isolated head trauma rarely results in shock, although a significant scalp laceration can produce excessive blood loss. Femur fractures from high impact injuries in adolescents may lead to shock.

27. **How does the anatomy of a child relate to the type of injury sustained?**
Because of their small size, children sustain more multiple organ system injuries than adults. Children have larger heads relative to their bodies and are more likely to land on their heads when they fall. The large head also contributes to a higher level of cervical spine injuries (C2–C3) in children than in adults. Because of their immature skeletons, children sustain less frequent bone injuries and more frequent soft tissue injuries and internal organ damage. Bone injury may be more subtle because of open growth plates at the epiphyses of children. These growth plates are not as strong as the connected tendons, and radiographs may not show the injury. The ribs are mainly cartilage and are softer than in adults. They do not fracture easily. The chest wall is flexible, and rib fractures and flail chest are uncommon in children. Because the chest wall is not muscular, forces are easily transmitted to internal organs. Likewise, the solid organs in the abdomen are disproportionately larger and more exposed than in adults. Because children have more skin surface area in relation to their overall size than adults, they can lose heat quickly after injury. Hypothermia is a potential problem.

28. **What are the important aspects of medical history in seriously injured children?**
In managing a critically injured child, it is not appropriate to divert attention to a long, detailed history. Instead, the American College of Surgeons recommends an **AMPLE** history:
- **A** = **A**llergies
- **M** = **M**edications
- **P** = **P**ast illnesses

- **L** = **L**ast meal
- **E** = **E**vents surrounding the injury

29. **What are the indications for endotracheal intubation of the injured child?**
    - Inability to ventilate with a bag-valve-mask device
    - Need for prolonged airway control
    - Prevention of aspiration in a comatose child
    - Serious head injury

30. **What are the criteria for admission to a pediatric trauma center?**
    - Glasgow Coma Scale score of 12
    - Decompensated shock (low systolic blood pressure for age)
    - Abnormal respiratory rate (adjusted for age)
    - Flail chest
    - Shock unresponsive to fluid resuscitation

31. **When a trauma patient requires transfer to a trauma center, what are the responsibilities of the transferring physician?**
    - Identification of the patient requiring transfer
    - Initiation of the transfer process via phone contact with the receiving doctor
    - Maximal stabilization using the capabilities of the local institution
    - Determination of the best mode of transport
    - Assurance that the level of care remains stable and does not deteriorate
    - Transfer of all relevant records, results, and radiographs to the receiving facility

    Waltzman ML, Mooney DP: Major trauma. In Fleisher GR, Ludwig S, Henretig F (eds): Textbook of Pediatric Emergency Medicine, 5th ed. Philadelphia, Lippincott, 2006.

BIBLIOGRAPHY

1. Advanced Trauma Life Support for Doctors: Student Manual. Chicago, American College of Surgeons, 1997, 2005.
2. Tepas III JJ, Fallat ME, Moriarty TM: Trauma. In Gausche-Hill M, Fuchs S, Yamamoto L (eds): APLS: The Pediatric Emergency Medicine Course, 4th ed. Dallas, American College of Emergency Physicians, American Academy of Pediatrics, 2004, pp 268–323.
3. Trauma. In Dieckman RA (ed): Pediatric Education for Prehospital Professionals (PEPP). Elk Grove Village, IL, American Academy of Pediatrics, 2000, pp 129–155.
4. Trauma resuscitation and spinal immobilization. In Zaritsky AL, Nadkarni VM, Hickey RW, Schexnayder SM, Berg RA (eds): Pediatric Advanced Life Support. Dallas, American Academy of Pediatrics, American Heart Association, 2002, pp 253–286.

CHAPTER 59

NECK AND CERVICAL SPINE TRAUMA

Howard Kadish, MD

1. **What are the differences in neck anatomy between children and adults?**
   Compared with adults, children have a larger head and mandible and a shorter neck in proportion to the rest of their body. These differences protect the child's anterior neck at the time of injury; the head, neck, and face absorb the major force of impact. In infants and young children, the larynx is not only smaller in overall size but also has smaller relative dimensions compared with adults. In children, the arytenoids are larger, the epiglottis has an omega shape, and the larynx has a funnel shape, which is narrowest in the subglottis. In adults, the narrowest point of the trachea is located at the level of C7, whereas in children it is at the cricoid cartilage (C3). These anatomic differences, along with the ringlike cricoid cartilage, result in a narrowed laryngeal inlet. Adolescents and adults can tolerate up to 50% narrowing of the airway without obvious respiratory distress. Infants and children experience significant respiratory embarrassment with this degree of restriction.

2. **Name the major signs and symptoms of a laryngotracheal injury.**
   - Neck pain/tenderness
   - Drooling
   - Stridor
   - Crepitus
   - Odynophagia
   - Pneumomediastinum
   - Retractions
   - Aphonia
   - Dysphagia
   - Airway obstruction
   - Subcutaneous emphysema
   - Hoarseness
   - Pneumothorax
   - Cough
   - Neck deformity
   - Dysphonia

3. **How should I manage a patient with a blunt or penetrating neck injury?**
   The goals of management should follow trauma guidelines, with strict adherence to airway, breathing, and circulation. After the airway is assessed and breathing stabilized, control any hemorrhage and maintain good cervical spine precautions rapidly. Stabilize all penetrating objects in the neck but keep them in place until they can be removed under surgical care in the operating room. Obtain routine trauma laboratory studies, including type and cross-match of blood for packed red blood cells. Minimal radiographic evaluation includes cervical spine films and chest radiograph.

4. **How should the airway and breathing be managed in a child with neck injury?**
   Give all patients supplemental oxygen and treat them as if they were considered to have cervical spine injury until proved otherwise. Therefore, any airway manipulation should include

cervical spine stabilization. Elective endotracheal intubation is not recommended unless back-up measures, such as a surgical airway or fiberoptic intubation equipment, are available. Attempted placement of an endotracheal tube through an already injured airway may cause a small mucosal laceration to progress to complete transection. In cases of laryngotracheal separation, the transected ends of the trachea may separate by as much as 8 cm. Successful passage of an endotracheal tube across this distance is difficult and may delay or preclude airway control. Trauma to the airway also may produce a blind path and inability to pass an endotracheal tube successfully. In the unstable airway, blind nasotracheal intubation is not recommended. If orotracheal intubation needs to be performed emergently, back-up measures, such as surgical and anesthesia consultation, fiberoptic bronchoscopy, cricothyrotomy, and tracheostomy, should be available in case complications occur.

5. **What are the major indications for surgical evaluation in patients with neck trauma?**
   - Unstable vital signs
   - Hematemesis
   - Exposed cartilage
   - Hemothorax
   - Cord paralysis
   - Neurologic deficits
   - Dysphagia
   - Foreign bodies
   - Airway obstruction
   - Hemoptysis
   - Displaced fracture
   - Pneumothorax
   - Active bleeding
   - Decreased level of consciousness
   - Dysphonia
   - Gun, rifle, or explosion wounds

6. **How common are cervical spine injuries in children?**
   Cervical spine injuries are rare, occurring in only 1–2% of pediatric patients with injuries due to blunt trauma. Unfortunately, a cervical spine injury can result in permanent disability or death. Therefore, patients with suspicious mechanisms of injury at least should be evaluated for cervical spine injury.

7. **Which methods are helpful to immobilize a patient with suspected cervical spine injury?**
   Soft cervical collars offer no stability to a potentially unstable cervical spine. Even hard collars (Philadelphia, Stifneck) allow a significant amount of motion. A Philadelphia collar allows approximately 60% of cervical flexion and rotation. Patients with a suspected cervical spine fracture should be placed in a hard cervical collar and immobilized on a hard spine board. Even with adequate immobilization on a spine board, the patient may be able to flex or extend the neck approximately 20%.

8. **What are the major differences between pediatric and adult cervical spines?**
   Upper cervical spine fractures are more common in younger pediatric patients because they have relatively large heads, weak neck muscles, and higher fulcrums. The large amount of cartilage in the pediatric cervical spine makes identification of radiographic injuries difficult, and the retropharyngeal space may change with crying or respiratory patterns. Pediatric patients also may present with pseudosubluxation rather than actual subluxation of C3 over C4 and C2 over C3.

9. **What is the NEXUS?**
   The National Emergency X-Radiography Utilization Study (NEXUS) is a multicenter, prospective, observational study of emergency department (ED) patients with blunt trauma for whom cervical spine imaging is ordered. The results of the study suggested that patients with an abnormal neurologic examination, depressed or altered level of consciousness, distracting or painful injury (femur fracture), intoxication, or midline cervical tenderness should be evaluated for a possible cervical spine injury. Patients without these findings have a low risk for cervical spine injury and may not need radiographic imaging.

   Hoffman JR, Mower WR, Wolfson AB, et al: Validity of a set of criteria to rule out injury to the cervical spine in patients with blunt trauma. National Emergency X-Radiography Study Group. N Engl J Med 343:94–99, 2000.

10. **What is the Canadian C-spine rule?**
    The Canadian C-spine rule was developed from a prospective cohort study in Canada evaluating patients with head or neck trauma. If there is a high-risk factor (dangerous mechanism, paresthesias) then radiography should be performed. A low-risk factor (simple rear-end motor vehicle collision, sitting position in ED, ambulatory at any time since injury, delayed onset of neck pain, or absence of midline C-spine tenderness) would allow for the clinician to assess the patient's range of motion. If the patient is able to actively rotate his or her neck 45° to the left and right, then cervical spine radiography may not be needed.

    Stiell IG, Wells GA, Vandemheen KL: The Canadian C-spine rule for radiography in alert and stable trauma patients. JAMA 286:1841–1848, 2001.

11. **What type of cervical spine radiographs should I order for a child with suspected neck injury?**
    A lateral cervical spine view misses approximately 20% of cervical spine injuries. At a minimum, three views—lateral, anteroposterior, and odontoid—should be ordered. The three views miss approximately 3–6% of cervical spine injuries. Therefore, if a patient is still symptomatic, further imaging tests, such as oblique views, flexion/extension, or cervical spine computed tomography, should be performed.

12. **When a cervical spine injury is suspected, when should computed tomography (CT) or magnetic resonance imaging of the cervical spine be ordered?**
    Magnetic resonance imaging is not ideal for identifying bony fractures and should be used when trying to evaluate a patient for an acute ligamentous or a spinal cord injury. CT identifies fractures, but is not ideal for evaluation of the spinal cord or ligaments. CT is useful in the secondary evaluation of a possible cervical spine fracture when plain radiographs are difficult to obtain or to interpret or are noted to be abnormal. Given the low incidence of pediatric cervical spine injuries and the increased radiation exposure with CT, it is not recommended to use CT as a primary radiographic evaluation in patients with a possible cervical spine fracture.

13. **What is the best way to read cervical spine radiographs?**
    A systematic approach using the ABCS method should be used:
    - **A** = **A**lignment (Four lines are assessed: the anterior vertebral bodies, posterior vertebral bodies, spinolaminal line, and spinous process tips.)
    - **B** = **B**ones (Evaluate for fractures.)
    - **C** = **C**artilage (Because cartilage is radiolucent on cervical spine radiographs, the intervertebral space, where cartilage is present, should be evaluated. Compression or widening of the intervertebral space may indicate a cartilage disruption.)
    - **S** = **S**oft tissues (Because a child's spinal column contains a significant amount of cartilage, prevertebral soft tissue swelling may be the only clue to cartilage or ligament injury. The prevertebral space at C2 or C3 should not be greater than half the width of the adjacent vertebral body. Abnormal swelling of the prevertebral space may be due to blood or edema.)

KEY POINTS: NECK AND CERVICAL SPINE TRAUMA ✓

1. Cervical spine injuries occur in only 1–2% of pediatric patients

2. Any pediatric trauma patient with an altered mental status, abnormal neurologic examination, point tenderness of the cervical spine, or pain with rotation should be evaluated radiographically.

3. One view is no view—at a minimum, patients with suspected cervical spine injury should undergo lateral, anteroposterior, and odontoid radiography.

4. The administration of high-dose steroids is controversial in spinal cord injury and should be preceded by consultation with a neurosurgeon.

5. When in doubt, immobilize, obtain imaging studies, and consult neurosurgery.

14. **What is a pseudosubluxation of C2 on C3? How do you differentiate it from an anterior subluxation of C2 on C3?**
Pseudosubluxation, which is a normal variant, is caused by ligamentous laxity and can be seen in patients up to 16 years of age, whereas anterior subluxation of C2 on C3 is usually caused by a hyperextension injury and possible spinal cord injury. Swischuk's "posterior cervical line" is helpful in distinguishing a pseudosubluxation from a more serious fracture. A line is drawn from the cortex of the spinous process of C1 to the cortex of the spinous process of C3. The line should not be greater than 2.0 mm anterior to the cortex of the spinous process of C2. If it is, then a fracture should be suspected and further imaging should be undertaken.

    Swischuk L: Emergency Radiology of the Acutely Ill or Injured Child, 3rd ed. Baltimore, Williams & Wilkins, 1994.

15. **What is a Jefferson fracture?**
A Jefferson fracture is a burst fracture of C1 secondary to an axial load, such as a diving injury. Patients may present with severe neck pain, especially with rotation. Although patients rarely have neurologic symptoms because the fracture burst outward, the Jefferson fracture is unstable and needs to be immobilized immediately. The odontoid view may show the lateral masses offset or overriding the vertebral body of C2. This fracture can be confused with a pseudo-Jefferson fracture. Children's lateral masses of C1 grow faster than the vertebral body of C2; often the lateral masses override C2 either unilaterally or bilaterally. If you are in doubt, CT of the cervical spine at C1 and C2 is helpful in making the diagnosis.

16. **Why should patients with Down syndrome receive cervical spine radiographs before participating in sports?**
Approximately 15% of patients with Down syndrome have atlantoaxial subluxation. Atlantoaxial subluxation occurs because ligament instability or a fractured dens allows movement between C1 and C2. It has been associated with minor trauma in patients with connective tissue disorders, arthritis, pharyngitis, and Down syndrome. The lateral cervical spine radiograph shows a widening of the preodontoid space. A normal preodontoid space should be < 3 mm in adults and < 5 mm in children. Neurologic symptoms may be seen if the preodontoid space is 7–10 mm.

    Elliot S, Morton R, Whitelaw R: Atlantoaxial instability and abnormalities of the odontoid in Down's syndrome. Arch Dis Child 63:1484–1489, 1988.

17. **What is SCIWORA?**

    SCIWORA is an abbreviation for **s**pinal **c**ord **i**njury **with**out **r**adiographic **a**bnormality. It usually is seen in children younger than 8 years because of the increased amount of cartilage and elastic nature of the younger child's spinal column. The child may present with an abnormal neurologic examination caused by vascular or ligamentous injury and no evidence of a fracture on radiography or CT.

18. **Describe the appropriate treatment of a child with a spinal cord injury.**

    Adherence to the ABCs of trauma management should be the first priority. Children may present with hypotension, bradycardia, and warm or flushed peripheral extremities (spinal shock) because of the loss of sympathetic input. They need fluid resuscitation and inotropic support (dopamine). A common mistake is to treat patients with spinal shock as if they have hypovolemic shock and to overload them with fluids. If the child is not improving after aggressive fluid resuscitation, spinal shock should be considered part of the differential diagnosis.

19. **Why is the administration of steroids in pediatric spinal cord injuries controversial?**

    Experts in emergency medicine and neurosurgery have recently questioned the potential benefit of steroids for a traumatic cervical spine injury. Children younger than 13 years of age were excluded in the studies, and some experts feel the potential risks of steroids are greater then the potential neurologic benefits. Consultation with neurosurgery and trauma surgery should occur prior to starting steroids.

    Qian T, Campagnolo D, Kirshblum S: High-dose methylprednisolone may do more harm for spinal cord injury. Med Hypotheses 55:452–453, 2000.

    Short DJ, El Masry WS, Jones PW: High dose methylprednisolone in the management of acute spinal cord injury: A systematic review from a clinical perspective. Spinal Cord 38:273–286, 2000.

CHAPTER 60

PELVIC TRAUMA AND GENITOURINARY INJURY

Javier A. Gonzalez del Rey, MD, MEd

1. **Why are children more likely to sustain renal injuries than adults?**

   A child's kidneys are disproportionately larger in relation to body size and have less perinephric fat, more lobulations, and a more intra-abdominal location. Because children have a weaker anterior abdominal wall and a less well-ossified thoracic cage with a more flexible thoracolumbar spine, the kidneys and other genitourinary structures are more susceptible to blunt trauma. Preexisting congenital renal abnormalities have been documented in 10–15% of patients evaluated for renal trauma. Approximately 10% of trauma patients have urogenital injuries. Common associated injuries include head injuries, fractures (extremities, pelvis, ribs, spine, and skull), spinal cord injuries, and liver or spleen injuries. Blunt trauma accounts for up to 90% of renal injuries.

   Abou-Jaoude WA, Sugarman JM, Fallat ME, et al: Indicators of genitourinary tract injury or anomaly in cases of pediatric blunt trauma. J Pediatr Surg 31:86–90, 1996.

2. **Describe the immediate and delayed complications of renal trauma.**

   Contusions and minor cortical lacerations usually heal without sequelae. More severe injuries may be associated with delayed bleeding, renal failure, abscess formation, urinary extravasation with sepsis, and ureteral obstruction secondary to clot formation. Late complications include hypertension, arteriovenous fistulas, hydronephrosis, pseudocyst formation, and renal calculi. Children with renal trauma (radiologically or operatively confirmed) should be followed closely with serial scans for at least 1 year after injury to evaluate renal anatomy and to ensure prompt diagnosis and treatment of possible complications.

   Gotschall CS, Eichelberger MR: Predictors of abdominal injury in children with pelvic fracture. J Trauma 31:1169–1173, 1991.

   McAleer IM, Kaplan GW: Pediatric genitourinary trauma. Urol Clin North Am 22:177–188, 1995.

3. **Which is the cardinal laboratory marker of renal injury?**

   Hematuria is the most important laboratory evidence of renal injury. Gross hematuria is the hallmark sign of severe injury. However, this finding may be absent in up to 50% of patients with vascular pedicle injuries and in 29% of patients with penetrating injuries. Radiographic evaluation is needed for children with gross hematuria, hematuria of more than 20 red blood cells/high-powered field, microscopic hematuria with shock, or clinical findings indicative of renal trauma.

   Garcia CT: Genitourinary trauma. In Fleisher GR, Ludwig S, Henretig FM (eds): Textbook of Pediatric Emergency Medicine, 5th ed. Philadelphia, Lippincott Williams & Wilkins, 2006.

4. **How are renal injuries classified?**

   The Organ Injury Scaling Committee of the American Association for Surgery of Trauma developed a new scaling system that unifies previous classifications for research purposes:
   - **Grade I:** Contusions or nonexpanding subcapsular hematomas with associated hematuria
   - **Grade II:** Hematomas confined to the retroperitoneum or laceration < 1 cm in depth without urinary extravasation

- **Grade III:** Lacerations extending into the perinephric fat > 1 cm in depth without involvement of the collecting system or extravasation
- **Grade IV:** Deep lacerations into the collecting system and vascular injuries with contained hemorrhage
- **Grade V:** Fractured or completely shattered kidneys and avulsion of the renal pedicle with organ devascularization

Moore EE, Shackford SR, Pachter HL, et al: Organ injury scaling: Spleen, liver, and kidney. J Trauma 29:1664–1666, 1989.

5. **Which imaging modality is considered the diagnostic test of choice for evaluation of renal injuries in stable pediatric patients?**
   Contrast-enhanced computed tomography (CT) is considered the diagnostic test of choice for detection of renal injury in stable pediatric patients with trauma. It not only delineates the degree of renal parenchymal injury with high accuracy (98%) but also assesses other intra-abdominal, retroperitoneal, and pelvic injuries simultaneously. However, this test is relatively expensive and requires a hemodynamically stable patient who can tolerate transport to the radiology suite. CT is useful for identifying genitourinary injury in children with penetrating trauma to the abdomen or other significant injuries.

   Stubbs DM: Emergency radiology of urinary tract injuries. Am J Emerg Med 10:242–250, 1992.

KEY POINTS: INDICATIONS FOR RADIOLOGIC EVALUATION OF THE GENITOURINARY TRACT IN PEDIATRIC TRAUMA ✓

1. Gross hematuria

2. Hematuria of more than 20 red blood cells/high-powered field

3. Microscopic hematuria with shock or clinical findings indicative of renal trauma

4. Penetrating trauma to the abdomen or other significant injuries

6. **Which diagnostic modality should be used in unstable patients?**
   Traditionally, IV pyelography has been used for the evaluation of renal trauma or isolated urogenital trauma in unstable patients. It is available in most institutions and is relatively inexpensive, and it provides evidence of renal function (including contralateral function in patients with penetrating injuries) and visualization of the calyceal system or extravasation. One-shot IV pyelography usually is indicated for unstable patients and can be performed in the emergency department or operating room. However, results of this study may be falsely negative in patients with pedicle injuries and, in general, correlates in only 50–75% of patients with injuries found at exploratory laparotomies.

   Stevenson J, Battistella FD: The "one-shot" intravenous pyelogram: Is it indicated in unstable trauma patients before celiotomy? J Trauma 36:828–833; discussion, 833–834, 1994.

7. **Which are the most commonly found symptoms in bladder injuries?**
   Hematuria and dysuria are usually present in patients with blunt or penetrating trauma to the pelvis. During childhood, the bladder has a higher abdominal location, which renders the organ more susceptible to injury. Radiologic evaluation is indicated in patients with pelvic or lower abdominal trauma who experience difficulty in voiding or gross hematuria. However,

catheterization must be avoided if physical examination reveals blood at the urethra or a high-riding prostate on rectal examination.

Corriere JN Jr, Sandler CM: Bladder rupture from external trauma: Diagnosis and management. World J Urol 17:84–89, 1999.

8. **What clinical findings should make you suspect ureteral injury?**
   Signs and symptoms of ureteral injuries are nonspecific and often overlooked. Fewer than 50% of patients are diagnosed within 24 hours because the presentation may develop gradually. An enlarging flank mass in the absence of retroperitoneal bleeding suggests the possibility of urinary extravasation. Hematuria is not a reliable sign because it may be absent in > 40% of patients with urethral injuries. Common symptoms in delayed presentation include fever, chills, ileus, lethargy, pyuria or bacteriuria, and flank pain. Ureteral injuries usually are discovered during evaluation of other traumatic injuries.

9. **Describe the most common mechanisms for ureteral injuries.**
   Ureteral injuries are uncommon in children, accounting for < 1–3% of patients with genitourinary tract injury. They may result from blunt trauma (involving the ureteropelvic junction) or penetrating trauma (gunshot wounds), but most ureteral injuries are iatrogenic (urologic, gynecologic, colonic, and vascular surgery procedures). Iatrogenic injury is less common in children than adults because of the nature of the procedures and easier identification of the ureters because of lack of retroperitoneal fat.

Tarman GJ, Kaplan GW, Lerman SL, et al: Lower genitourinary injury and pelvic fractures in pediatric patients. Urology 59:123–126, 2002.

10. **What clinical findings indicate urethral injuries?**
    The presence of blood at the meatus has been reported in more than 90% of patients with anterior urethral injury. Such injuries are commonly due to motor vehicle crashes, straddle injuries (bulbar urethra), or instrumentation. Patients may present with hematuria, difficulty or inability to void, swelling, and ecchymosis or hematoma of the perineum or penis. Anterior urethral injuries may produce extravasation of blood and urine into the abdominal wall, scrotum, or perineum.

11. **What are the indications for urethrography in pediatric trauma patients?**
    Retrograde urethrography is the radiologic method of choice for diagnosis. It should be performed in any child with penetrating trauma and suspected genitourinary injuries; perineal trauma with hematuria; inability to void or to advance a urinary catheter; vaginal laceration or bleeding; swelling, hematoma, or ecchymosis of the perineum; blood at the urethral meatus; and high-riding or boggy prostate.

Kotkin L, Brock JW: Isolated ureteral injury caused by blunt trauma. Urology 47:111–113, 1996.

12. **How does traumatic testicular dislocation present?**
    Forceful displacement of the testicle from its anatomic position is uncommon in children because of their brisk cremasteric reflex; however, a straddle-type injury may produce enough force to dislocate the testicle. Patients may present with nausea, vomiting, scrotal pain, and absence of the testicle in the involved hemiscrotum or a testis palpated in another location. Dislocation may be found in various ectopic locations: superior inguinal, pubic, abdominal, penile, acetabular, or perineal. Associated injuries, such as pelvic fractures, are common.

13. **How does testicular rupture present?**
    The tunica albuginea ruptures, and testicular contents extravasate into the scrotal sac. It is a surgical emergency because there is a higher chance of testicular salvage if exploration is done within 24 hours from the injury.

14. **Describe the management for zipper entrapment of the penis or foreskin.**
    Using a bone or wire cutter, split the median bar of the zipper. With the fastener intact, the zipper falls apart, freeing the foreskin or penis (Fig. 60-1). Warm soaks may be used after the procedure to control edema. Some children may require conscious sedation and, in severe cases, a penile block. Alternatively, mineral oil can be applied liberally to the entrapped tissue and allowed to soak for 15 minutes. The trapped skin may then be easily released.

    Fein J, Zderic SA: Management of zipper injuries. In Henretig FM, King C (eds): Textbook of Pediatric Emergency Procedures, Baltimore, Williams & Wilkins, 2007.

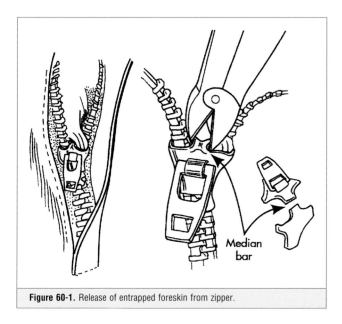

Figure 60-1. Release of entrapped foreskin from zipper.

15. **When should I consider the possibility of sexual abuse in a child with vaginal injury?**
    Young girls frequently suffer straddle injuries on a bicycle or a fall. However, injury to the perineum in which the history fails to explain the findings, a history of possible abuse from the child or another source, or presence of other suspicious injuries on physical examination obligates a report to appropriate agencies.

16. **What is the best predictor of abdominal injury in children with pelvic fractures?**
    Several classifications for pelvic fractures have been devised, but none has been used extensively in children. Several reviews of pelvic fractures in children have found that stable pelvic ring fractures and unstable fractures with anterior and posterior ring fractures were associated with urologic injury rates of 12–42%. However, the best predictor of abdominal injury in children with pelvic fractures is the presence of multiple fractures to the pelvic ring.

    Livne PM, Gonzales ET Jr: Genitourinary trauma in children. Urol Clin North Am 12:53–65, 1985.

17. **What are the most common diagnostic findings in children with pelvic fractures?**

Most patients have a history of a major mechanism of injury and associated multiple trauma. Some patients present with unstable vital signs due to internal hemorrhages and massive retroperitoneal hematomas. This presentation is most common in older children and adults. Pain and instability elicited by pelvic rocking (while holding the anterior iliac spines) suggest fractures in the pelvic ring. Pressure over the pubis also may produce pain and crepitus. Other findings, such as obturator, femoral, and sciatic nerve injuries, are infrequent in children because of the flexibility of the pelvic ring.

Straddle injury is the most common mechanism and it is usually the cause of vulvar hematomas and lacerations. Vaginal lacerations must always be suspected in patients with severe trauma to the external genitalia. Sedation or general anesthesia may be required for a complete evaluation that may include endoscopic evaluation.

Hendren WH, Peters CA: Lower urinary tract and perineal injuries. In Touloukian RJ (ed): Pediatric Trauma, 2nd ed. St. Louis, Mosby, 1990, pp 371–398.

CHAPTER 61

SPORTS INJURIES

Lauren P. Daly, MD, and Maria Carmen G. Diaz, MD

EPIDEMIOLOGY

1. **Which sports are associated with the highest injury rates in children? What are the most common types of injuries seen?**
    In boys, the most injuries are seen with football. In girls, soccer accounts for the highest injury rates. Other sport activities that commonly lead to the emergency department evaluation of pediatric injuries include basketball, baseball/softball, inline skating, and hockey.

    The most common types of ac ute injuries are soft tissue injuries, including sprains, strains, and contusions. Fractures and lacerations occur less frequently. However, in adolescents, overuse injuries are more common than acute injuries.

    Patel DR, Nelson TL: Sports injuries in adolescents. Med Clin North Am 84:983–1007, 2000.
    Taylor BL, Attia MW: Sports-related injuries in children. Acad Emerg Med 7:1376–1382, 2000.

OVERUSE INJURIES

2. **What are overuse injuries? How are they managed?**
    Overuse injuries are chronic injuries that are related to constant high levels of physiologic stress without sufficient recovery time. These injuries are characterized by repetitive microtrauma and the development of inflammation that lead to significant pain and loss or limitation of function.

    Overuse injuries are treated with rest and supportive bracing. Additionally the athlete should partake in proper training regimens that emphasize flexibility and stretching.

3. **What is "Little League shoulder"? How does it present?**
    "Little League shoulder," also known as proximal humeral epiphysitis, is most often seen in high-performance pitchers between 11 and 16 years of age. It may also be seen in tennis players, swimmers, and gymnasts. It is caused by overuse and subsequent inflammation of the proximal humeral physis. The chief complaint is gradual pain localized to the proximal humerus during the act of throwing or serving. The physical examination may be negative, or there may be tenderness to palpation of the proximal humerus. Radiographs may reveal a widening of the proximal humeral physis. Treatment is almost always nonsurgical and includes a rest period of 2 to 3 months, along with physical therapy.

    Walter KD, Congeni JA: Don't let little league shoulder or elbow sideline your patient permanently. Contemp Pediatr 21:69–92, 2004.

4. **What is "Little League elbow"?**
    "Little League elbow", or medial epicondylar apophysitis, results from stress to the medial epicondyle of the humerus. It is most commonly seen in children between the ages of 9 and 12 years who are baseball pitchers, infielders, or tennis players. An excessive number of pitches thrown and a sidearm pitching style have both been implicated as causes. The athlete presents

with gradual onset of pain in the medial elbow and proximal forearm while throwing. Radiographs may be normal or reveal medial epicondylar apophyseal widening. Treatment is complete rest from throwing activities, ice, nonsteroidal anti-inflammatory drugs (NSAIDs), and physical therapy.

Saperstein AL, Nicholas SJ: Pediatric and adolescent sports medicine. Pediatr Clin North Am 43:1013–1033, 1996.

5. **Why is the early identification of "gymnast's wrist" important?**
Left untreated, "gymnast's wrist," a stress injury to the distal radial physis, may lead to premature fusion of the physis, growth arrest, and radial shortening. These patients present with activity-related pain of the dorsal aspect of the wrist, especially with floor exercises and vaulting, where there is an excessive load on a dorsiflexed wrist. There is tenderness over the distal radius, and radiographic findings may be normal or exhibit widening, beaking, or an indistinct appearance of the physis. Treatment is rest for 2–4 weeks. If there are radiographic changes, immobilization may be necessary.

Patel DR, Nelson TL: Sports injuries in adolescents. Med Clin North Am 84:983–1007, 2000.

6. **Name the two types of apophysitis syndromes that occur surrounding the patellar tendon.**
   - **Osgood-Schlatter disease:** An apophysitis at the anterior tibial tubercle due to traction by the inferior aspect of the patellar tendon.
   - **Sinding-Larsen-Johansson syndrome:** An apophysitis of the inferior pole of the patella due to traction by the superior aspect of the patellar tendon. Treatment is analogous to that for Osgood-Schlatter disease. Sinding-Larsen-Johansson syndrome is differentiated from "jumper's knee" in that the latter is not an apophysitis but rather an inflammation within the proximal patellar tendon itself.

Ganley TJ, Lou JE, Pryor K, et al: Sports medicine. In Dormans JP, Bell LM (eds): Pediatric Orthopedics and Sports Medicine: The Requisites in Pediatrics. St. Louis, Mosby, 2004, pp 278–279.

7. **Which is the most common overuse injury in the young athlete?**
Osgood-Schlatter disease commonly affects adolescents during periods of rapid growth. Symptoms include tenderness and a prominence at the tibial tubercle, with pain worsened by high-impact sports, kneeling, or squatting. The diagnosis is usually made clinically. However, plain radiographs will demonstrate enlargement or fragmentation at the anterior tibial tubercle due to the traction force at the insertion of the patellar tendon. Management includes rest, ice, NSAIDs, and stretching regimens to increase flexibility of the quadriceps and hamstrings. The problem usually resolves with closure of the physis, but children rarely may develop ossicles within the patellar tendon that require surgical removal.

Adirim TA, Cheng TL: Overview of injuries in the young athlete. Sports Med 33:75–81, 2003.
Ganley TJ, et al: Sports medicine. In Dormans JP, Bell LM (eds): Pediatric Orthopedics and Sports Medicine: The Requisites in Pediatrics. St. Louis, Mosby, 2004, pp 278–279.

8. **What is the recommended management for Sever disease?**
Sever disease, an apophysitis resulting from repetitive stresses on the calcaneal ossification center by the Achilles tendon, is often seen in young runners. The athlete will report heel pain and often has had a recent growth spurt and increase in activity level. Management includes rest, NSAIDs, Achilles tendon stretching, and the use of heel cups in cleats or sneakers. It usually resolves in 2–4 months without the need for surgery.

Ganley TJ, et al: Sports medicine. In Dormans JP, Bell LM (eds): Pediatric Orthopedics and Sports Medicine: The Requisites in Pediatrics. St. Louis, Mosby, 2004, pp 273–298.
Simons SM, Sloan BK: Foot injuries. In Birrer RB, Griesemer BA, Cataletto MB (eds): Pediatric Sports Medicine for Primary Care. Philadelphia, Lippincott Williams & Wilkins, 2002, pp 443–444.

9. **List the most common locations for stress fractures in pediatric athletes.**
   - Tibia   51%
   - Fibula   20%
   - Pars interarticularis 15%
   - Femur   3%
   - Metatarsal   2%
   - Tarsal navicular   2%

   Coady CM, Micheli LJ: Stress fractures in the pediatric athlete. Clin Sports Med 16:225–238, 1997.

10. **In which sports are participants most likely to sustain stress fractures?**
    - Running
    - Basketball
    - Gymnastics
    - Football
    - Ice skating

    Saperstein AL, Nicholas SJ: Pediatric and adolescent sports medicine. Pediatr Clin North Am 43:1013–1033, 1996.

KEY POINTS: OVERUSE INJURIES ✓

1. They are the most common sports injuries seen in adolescents.

2. They are due to repetitive stress or trauma to an area that has had inadequate time for recovery between injuries.

3. Rest and proper conditioning regimens are crucial elements in management.

4. Osgood-Schlatter disease is the most common overuse injury in young athletes.

11. **Describe the most likely diagnosis in a gymnast who reports gradual-onset, recurrent, activity-associated, midline low back pain.**
    The most likely diagnosis is spondylolysis, a defect of the pars interarticularis that occurs with repetitive axial loading of the lumbar spine. The most common site is at L5. Radiographs may be normal or may show a pars defect in the oblique view, often described as a "Scotty dog with a collar" appearance. Treatment requires restriction of activity and an aggressive rehabilitation regimen that includes abdominal strengthening and flexion exercises. Bracing is reserved for athletes who are unresponsive to these measures.

    Herman MJ, Pizzutillo PD, Cavalier R: Spondylolysis and spondylolisthesis in the child and adolescent athlete. Orthop Clin North Am 34: 461–476, 2003.

ACUTE INJURIES

12. **What is the most dreaded complication of returning to sports too soon following a concussion?**
    Second impact syndrome. This results from acute brain swelling when a second head trauma is sustained prior to full recovery from an initial concussion. Second impact syndrome is thought to occur because the athlete reinjures the head during a period of disordered cerebral autoregulation following the initial head injury. The American Academy of Neurology guidelines on return to sports (Table 61-1) theoretically allow for this critical time period to

TABLE 61-1.   SUMMARY OF RECOMMENDATIONS FOR MANAGEMENT OF CONCUSSION IN SPORTS

A *concussion* is defined as head trauma–induced alteration in mental status that may or may not involve loss of consciousness. Concussions are graded in three categories. Definitions and treatment recommendations for each category are presented below.

Grade 1 Concussion

- **Definition:** Transient confusion, no loss of consciousness, and a duration of mental status abnormalities of > 15 minutes

- **Management:** The athlete should be removed from sports activity, examined immediately and at 5-minute intervals, and allowed to return that day to sports activity only if postconcussive symptoms resolve within 15 minutes. Any athlete who incurs a second grade 1 concussion on the same day should be removed from sports activity until asymptomatic for 1 week.

Grade 2 Concussion

- **Definition:** Transient confusion, no loss of consciousness, and a duration of mental status abnormalities of > 15 minutes

- **Management:** The athlete should be removed from sports activity, examined frequently to assess the evolution of symptoms, with more extensive diagnostic evaluation if the symptoms worsen or persist for > 1 week. The athlete should return to sports activity only after he or she has been asymptomatic for 1 full week. Any athlete who incurs a grade 2 concussion subsequent to a grade 1 concussion on the same day should be removed from sports activity until he or she has been asymptomatic for 2 weeks.

Grade 3 Concussion

- **Definition:** Loss of consciousness, either brief (seconds) or prolonged (minutes or longer)

- **Management:** The athlete should be removed from sports activity for 1 full week without symptoms if the loss of consciousness is brief or 2 full weeks without symptoms if the loss of consciousness is prolonged. If the athlete is still unconscious or if abnormal neurologic signs are present at the time of initial evaluation, the athlete should be transported by ambulance to the nearest hospital emergency department. An athlete who suffers a second grade 3 concussion should be removed from sports activity until he or she has been asymptomatic for 1 month. Any athlete with an abnormality on computed tomography or magnetic resonance imaging of the brain consistent with brain swelling, contusion, or other intracranial pathology should be removed from sports activities for the season and discouraged from future return to participation in contact sports.

From Quality Standards Subcommittee, American Academy of Neurology. www.aan.com/professionals/practice/guidelines/concussion_sports

pass and for the vascular autoregulatory mechanisms in the brain to heal and regain their normal function. Second impact syndrome, though quite rare, is not treatable and almost universally fatal.

Centers for Disease Control and Prevention: Sports-related recurrent brain injuries—US. MMWR Morb Mortal Wkly Rep 46:224–227, 1997.
Cantu RC: "Second impact syndrome." Clin Sports Med 17:37–44, 1998.

13. **Does posttraumatic seizure (the occurrence of a seizure directly after head trauma) increase the risk of intracranial injury?**
Posttraumatic seizure (PTS) can be divided into three categories based on when they occur in relation to the injury: Immediate (within seconds), early (within 1 week), and late (> 1 week). Most PTSs occur within 24 hours of injury, and they substantially increase the risk of intracranial injury. Computed tomography (CT) of the head is indicated in these patients to evaluate for traumatic brain injury. There is debate as to whether children with negative CT scans and normal neurologic examinations may safely be discharged to home. Immediate PTSs rarely recur, whereas early PTSs and late PTSs are more likely to recur.

Holmes JF, Palchak MS, Conklin MS, Kupperman N: Do children require hospitalization after immediate post-traumatic seizure? Ann Emerg Med 43:706–710, 2004.

Schutzman SA: Injury—head. In Fleisher GR, Ludwig S (eds): Textbook of Pediatric Emergency Medicine. Philadelphia, Lippincott Williams & Wilkins, 2000, pp 332–333.

14. **What is commotio cordis?**
Commotio cordis is a sudden cardiac arrest in a patient without preexisting heart disease following a relatively minor blow to the chest. The pathophysiology involves the mechanical force of the blow leading to a depolarization of the myocardium on the T-wave of the cardiac cycle, precipitating cardiac arrest. It is the second leading cause of sudden death in the young athlete and occurs most frequently in the sport of baseball. In animal models, commotio cordis is seen most often with balls thrown between 30 and 50 miles per hour, the speed of most Little League pitches. Chest protectors and softer-core balls have been marketed in an attempt at prevention, but most leagues do not mandate their use.

Maron BJ: Sudden death in young athletes. N Engl J Med 349:1064–1075, 2003.

15. **Why are children at greater risk for commotio cordis than adults?**
Children are more vulnerable than adults because of their thin and flexible chest walls and their lower agility.

16. **What is the most common cause of sudden death in the young athlete?**
Hypertrophic cardiomyopathy. This condition is a congenital heart deformity resulting in left ventricular outflow obstruction with asymmetric septal hypertrophy. It predisposes the athlete to arrhythmias that are likely to cause syncope or death. Unfortunately, most athletes are asymptomatic before the development of the lethal event, and preparticipation screening examinations (even with electrocardiography) may be normal.

Maron BJ, Epstein SE, Roberts WC: Causes of sudden death in competitive athletes. J Am Coll Cardiol 7:204–214, 1986.

17. **What are some clinical characteristics of burners/stingers?**
A stinger is a brachial plexus injury following a traumatic stretching or compression force on the neck. Symptoms include unilateral arm pain or burning especially in the C5–C6 nerve root distribution. There may be associated weakness. The symptoms often resolve within minutes but may persist. Of note, if the symptoms are persistent or bilateral, involve the lower extremities, or are accompanied by neck pain, more significant spinal cord injury may have occurred.

Vegso JJ, Lehman RC: Field evaluation and management of head and neck injuries. Clin Sports Med 6:1–15, 1987.

18. **What is the most commonly injured nerve in acute shoulder dislocation?**
The axillary nerve, which innervates the upper arm, must be carefully examined with acute shoulder dislocation. Shoulder dislocation is most likely to occur when the arm is abducted and externally rotated, is far more likely anterior than posterior, and is often recurrent.

Ganley TJ, et al: Sports medicine. In Dormans JP, Bell LM (eds): Pediatric Orthopedics and Sports Medicine: The Requisites in Pediatrics. St. Louis, Mosby, 2004, pp 283–284.

19. **Describe the mechanism of injury in gamekeeper's thumb.**
Gamekeeper's thumb, also known as skier's thumb, is a sprain of the ulnar collateral ligament of the metacarpophalangeal joint of the thumb. The injury is the result of a forced abduction and extension of the thumb that occurs when falling on an outstretched hand or colliding with an object. Patients with this injury exhibit point tenderness over the ulnar collateral ligament and may have no radiographic findings. Treatment includes immobilization and compression with a thumb spica splint. If the patient has an open physis, this mechanism of injury will produce a Salter-Harris III fracture of the proximal phalanx.

Garrick JG, Webb DR: Sports Injuries Diagnosis and Management, 2nd ed. Philadelphia, W.B. Saunders, 1999, pp 183–187.

20. **What is the difference between a mallet finger and a jersey finger?**
See Table 61-2.

TABLE 61-2.	MALLET FINGER VS. JERSEY FINGER	
Variable	Mallet Finger	Jersey Finger
Injury	Extensor digitorum tendon disruption	Flexor digitorum tendon disruption
Physical examination	Forced flexion of an extended distal interphalangeal joint	Forced extension of a flexed distal interphalangeal joint
Mechanisms	Finger struck on the tip by a ball	Football player grabs another player's jersey
	Forcefully tucking in a bedspread	Lifting a latch on a car door
	Pushing off a sock with an extended finger	

21. **How do pelvic avulsion fractures occur?**
Avulsion fractures (Fig. 61-1) result from sudden muscular contractions and are usually associated with vigorous running or jumping. These are seen in sports that require rapid acceleration or deceleration, or quick changes of direction.

Kim SS, Thomas M: A football player with thigh pain. Pediatr Emerg Care 17:267–268, 2001.

22. **What are the most common locations of pelvic avulsion fractures? What muscle attachment contributes to the fracture?**
See Table 61-3.

23. **A running football player was struck in the thigh by another player's helmet. Radiographs are negative, yet the patient has marked pain at the site of the injury and with ambulation. What is the likely diagnosis, and what treatment should be initiated?**
This patient probably sustained a quadriceps contusion. Initial treatment involves halting the hemorrhage and preventing spasm by rest, ice, compression, and elevation for 24–48 hours. Bracing with 90° of knee flexion may be needed in cases of severe swelling. The patient should then undergo progressive isometric strengthening and active range-of-motion exercises. Vigorous massage and passive stretching should be avoided because both have been

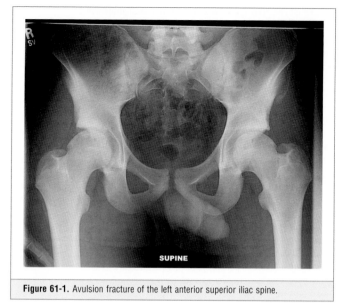

Figure 61-1. Avulsion fracture of the left anterior superior iliac spine.

TABLE 61-3. PELVIC AVULSION FRACTURES	
Location	Involved Muscle
Ischial tuberosity	Hamstrings and adductors
Anterior superior iliac spine	Sartorius
Anterior inferior iliac spine	Rectus femoris
Lesser trochanter of the femur	Iliopsoas

associated with myositis ossificans, a condition in which heterotopic bone growth occurs within the quadriceps muscle.

24. **What is the typical mechanism for an injury to the anterior cruciate ligament in children?**
As in adults, injury to the anterior cruciate ligament (ACL) results from a sudden deceleration accompanied by hyperextension and a rotatory force on a planted foot. This is often accompanied by a popping sensation and the acute onset of hemarthrosis. Whereas adults and older adolescents will probably tear the ligament itself, younger children may avulse a bony segment of tibia at the ACL insertion site. Plain radiography followed by magnetic resonance imaging is used to delineate the specifics of the injury. Management of the ACL injury is complicated by the open physes in skeletally immature children, requiring careful consideration of operative versus nonoperative treatment plans by the orthopedist.

Bernhardt DT: Knee and leg injuries. In Birrer RB, Griesemer BA, Cataletto MB (eds): Pediatric Sports Medicine for Primary Care. Philadelphia, Lippincott Williams & Wilkins, 2002, pp 409–410.

Ganley TJ, et al: Sports medicine. In Dormans JP, Bell LM (eds): Pediatric Orthopedics and Sports Medicine: The Requisites in Pediatrics. St. Louis, Mosby, 2004, pp. 288–290.

25. **What is the rate of recurrence of acute patellar dislocation?**

Approximately 1 in 6 pediatric patients with patellar dislocation will be affected by recurrent patellar instability. The patient most prone to recurrence will have an increased Q angle. The Q angle is created by two lines drawn from the anterior superior iliac spine to the center of the patella, and from the center of the patella to the center of the tibial tubercle. Q angles greater than 20° predispose to instability by increasing the lateral force of the patella during knee extension.

Ganley TJ, et al: Sports medicine. In Dormans JP, Bell LM (eds): Pediatric Orthopedics and Sports Medicine: The Requisites in Pediatrics. St. Louis, Mosby, 2004, pp 285–287.

26. **What are the limitations to the Ottawa Ankle Rules in children?**

The Ottawa Ankle Rules are criteria developed for predicting ankle fractures based on examination features in adults with the goal of reducing unnecessary radiographs. They allow, however, for "insignificant fractures" (such as small avulsion fractures) to be undiagnosed. They are not universally applicable to the pediatric population because of the questionable significance of Salter-Harris I and avulsion fractures on children's future growth and development. Though studies have attempted to validate them in children, they have been limited by small sample size and debate as to whether any fracture can be considered "insignificant" in a child.

Clark KD, Tanner S: Evaluation of the Ottawa Ankle Rules in children. Pediatr Emerg Care 19:73–78, 2003.

Plint AC, Bulloch B, Osmond MH, et al: Validation of the Ottawa Ankle Rules in children with ankle injuries. Acad Emerg Med 6:1005–1009, 1999.

27. **What are some unique characteristics of young athletes that make them more prone to heat-related illness than the adult?**

The larger body surface area of a child allows them to absorb more external heat, and they have a limited ability to produce sweat as compared to adults. They are also less able to cognitively appreciate the need to adequately hydrate and may not ask for hydration breaks often enough. Other risk factors for heat illness include obesity, dehydration, deliberate water restriction in order to "make weight," use of laxatives, practices early in the season without adequate acclimatization, and the use of dark clothing or heavy equipment (such as padding).

Gambrell RC: Environmental conditions and youth sports. In Birrer RB, Griesemer BA, Cataletto MB (eds): Pediatric Sports Medicine for Primary Care. Philadelphia, Lippincott Williams & Wilkins, 2002, pp 95–96.

28. **What measures can be used to prevent pediatric sports injuries?**

A thorough preparticipation sports evaluation by a physician should be conducted to detect potential risks and determine possible medical contraindications to participation in certain sports. A carefully planned conditioning regimen should start 6–8 weeks before the athletic season begins. This should emphasize overall fitness rather than focusing on skills specific to only one athletic activity. The athletes should slowly adapt to increases in intensity and frequency of exercise. Equipment and playing sites must be of appropriate size and satisfactory condition.

Christopher NC, Congeni J: Overuse injuries in the pediatric athlete; evaluation, initial management, and strategies for prevention. Clin Pediatr Emerg Med 3:118–128, 2002.

WEBSITE

National Center for Catastrophic Sport Injury Research
www.unc.edu/depts/nccsi

CHAPTER 62

THORACIC TRAUMA

Howard Kadish, MD

1. **What are the most common injuries in blunt and penetrating thoracic trauma?**
   - **Blunt thoracic trauma:** Lung contusions (58%), pneumothorax or hemothorax (38%), and rib fractures (38%)
   - **Penetrating thoracic trauma:** Pneumothorax or hemothorax (64%), diaphragmatic lacerations (15%), cardiac injuries (13%), and vascular injuries (10%)

2. **How does thoracic trauma differ in children and adults?**
   Pediatric thoracic trauma differs from adult thoracic trauma in mechanism of injury, type of injury, and other organ systems involved. Falls are the most common mechanism of injury in infants and children. Older children are often injured as pedestrians or unrestrained passengers in motor vehicle accidents. Adolescents are more likely to be occupants in motor vehicle–related accidents and to experience penetrating injuries secondary to violence.

   Lung contusion is the most common pediatric thoracic injury, with intrapleural injury second. Only 30% of children, compared with 50–75% of adults, sustain rib fractures because of increased compliance in the pediatric thoracic cage secondary to increased cartilage content and greater elasticity of the bones. Thus, a child may have an internal injury (lung contusion) without external evidence of trauma (rib fracture, laceration, bruising). The pediatric trachea has a smaller internal diameter than the adult trachea; therefore, a small amount of obstruction secondary to blood, secretions, or edema can cause significant respiratory distress and hypoxia. The younger pediatric patient is also more sensitive to hypoxia and may develop reflex bradycardia or asystole. In evaluating pediatric patients with thoracic trauma, the health care provider must consider head, neck, and intra-abdominal injuries because approximately 80% of cases of thoracic trauma in children are part of multisystem injury. Thoracic trauma is routinely associated with abdominal trauma in children because the chest and abdominal cavities lie in close proximity.

3. **How do I evaluate a patient with thoracic trauma?**
   The ABCs (airway, breathing, circulation) of trauma management apply regardless of the organ system injured. The injured child should be evaluated according to the primary survey of trauma management. Indications for endotracheal intubation in thoracic trauma patients include depressed neurologic status, inadequate oxygenation or ventilation, compromised circulatory status, or unstable airway (including burns). If a patient has an abnormal examination but appears to be oxygenating and ventilating well and is not in shock, chest radiography is indicated. If breathing is inadequate after endotracheal intubation, with asymmetry of breath sounds, intervention is required prior to chest radiography. Pericardial tamponade, tension pneumothorax, or hemothorax should be considered in poorly perfused patients with signs of shock in whom other sources of blood loss have been excluded and volume resuscitation has not improved clinical status. Once the patient is stabilized and immediate life-threatening injuries, such as airway obstruction, tension pneumothorax, hemothorax, and pericardial tamponade, are treated, chest radiography and thoracic computed tomography provide valuable information about other potentially life-threatening and operative injuries.

4. **What are the predictors of thoracic injury in children sustaining blunt trauma?**
   - Low systolic blood pressure
   - Elevated respiratory rate
   - Abnormal results of thoracic examination
   - Abnormal chest auscultation findings
   - Femur fracture
   - Glasgow Coma Scale score < 15

5. **Which thoracic injuries require operative intervention?**
   - Tracheal/bronchial rupture
   - Laceration of lung parenchyma, internal mammary artery, or intercostal artery
   - Esophageal disruption
   - Diaphragmatic hernia
   - Pericardial tamponade
   - Great vessel laceration

6. **Describe signs and symptoms related to each operative thoracic injury.**
   See Table 62-1.

TABLE 62-1. SIGNS AND SYMPTOMS OF THORACIC INJURIES	
Injury	Signs and Symptoms
Tracheal/bronchial rupture	Active chest tube air leak
Lung parenchyma	Chest tube bleeding > 2–3 mL/kg/hr
Internal mammary or intercostal artery laceration	Hypotension unresponsive to transfusions
Esophageal disruption	Abnormal esophagogram (leak) or esophagoscopic result Gastric contents in the chest tube
Diaphragmatic hernia	Abnormal gas pattern in hemithorax Displaced nasogastric tube in hemithorax
Pericardial tamponade	Positive pericardiocentesis
Great vessel laceration	Widened mediastinum Tracheal or nasogastric tube deviation Blurred aortic knob Abnormal aortogram (gold standard)

7. **What signs and symptoms are associated with pulmonary contusion?**
   Patients with moderate to severe pulmonary contusions may be tachypneic, with abnormal breath sounds and an oxygen requirement secondary to shunting within the lung. In one study of patients with mild pulmonary contusions, a finding of tachypnea, tenderness, or abnormal breath sounds was 100% sensitive for all positive radiographs in trauma.

Gittelman M, Gonzalez-del-Rey J, Brody A, et al: Clinical predictors for the selective use of chest radiographs in pediatric blunt trauma evaluations. J Trauma 55:670–676, 2003.
Ruddy R: Trauma and the paediatric lung. Paediatr Respir Rev 6:61–67, 2005.

8. **What signs and symptoms are associated with pneumothorax?**
   Patients may be asymptomatic, report pleuritic chest pain, have tachypnea, or be in severe respiratory distress. Physical examination may be normal or reveal diminished or absent breath sounds, crepitus, or hyperresonance to percussion on the side of the pneumothorax.

9. **How do I diagnose and treat patients with pneumothorax?**
   In asymptomatic or mildly symptomatic patients, a chest radiograph is helpful in diagnosing and determining type of treatment. If the pneumothorax is small and the patient asymptomatic, hospital observation and administration of 100% oxygen are all that is necessary. A small pneumothorax is classically described as < 15%, although it is common to underestimate the size of a pneumothorax on plain films and to find a much more extensive lesion on a CT scan. If the patient is in respiratory or cardiovascular distress, the diagnosis is made clinically. Tube thoracostomy should be performed. It is also indicated in patients undergoing positive-pressure ventilation or requiring air transport. An asymptomatic patient may rapidly become symptomatic if a small, simple pneumothorax progresses to a tension pneumothorax.

10. **Should thoracic helical CT replace chest radiography in the initial management of blunt trauma in the pediatric patient?**
    No, even though helical CT has been shown to be more sensitive than chest radiography in diagnosing thoracic injuries, thoracic trauma makes up less than 20% of all pediatric traumas. Performing thoracic CT on all pediatric trauma patients would increase costs and patient radiation dose, with little clinical improvement. Thoracic CT should be used only in patients with suspected thoracic injury (see question 4).

    Renton J, Kincaid S, Ehrlich P: Should helical CT scanning of the thoracic cavity replace the conventional chest x-ray as a primary assessment tool in pediatric trauma? An efficacy and cost analysis. J Pediatr Surg 38:793–797, 2003.

11. **What is the most common complication of an intrapleural injury?**
    Tension pneumothorax is the most common complication of an intrapleural injury, developing in up to 20% of children after simple pneumothorax. Tension pneumothorax occurs with progressive accumulation of air within the pleural cavity, which not only collapses the ipsilateral lung but also compresses the contralateral lung. Patients may present in severe respiratory distress, with decreased breath sounds on the side of the pneumothorax and a shift of mediastinal structures to the contralateral side. Because the inferior vena cava is relatively fixed in place and cannot shift as much as the superior vena cava, venous return to the heart is reduced. The patient may appear tachycardic, peripherally vasoconstricted, and in hypotensive shock. Whenever a trauma patient suddenly deteriorates, the treating physician must return to assessing the airway and breathing before focusing on circulation.

12. **How do I treat a patient with a tension pneumothorax?**
    Initial treatment consists of needle decompression performed in the midclavicular line, at the level of the second intercostal space of the ipsilateral side. With a tension pneumothorax, an immediate release of air should be noted. If this sign is positive, needle decompression is only a temporizing measure and must be followed by tube thoracotomy. Tube thoracotomy usually is done in the midaxillary line at the level of the fifth intercostal space (nipple level). Chest radiography is performed only after insertion of the chest tube and should not be used to diagnose tension pneumothorax in symptomatic patients. If significant air leak continues after chest tube placement, a tracheobronchial rupture must be considered.

13. **How can I tell if a patient has a tracheobronchial injury?**
    Injury to the tracheobronchial tree in children is rare (incidence < 1%). It is caused most commonly by acceleration or deceleration forces. Mechanism of injury (fall, crush, and direct

blow) provides an important clue. Clinical signs include cyanosis, hemoptysis, tachypnea, and subcutaneous emphysema (cervical, mediastinal, or both). A continued air leak after insertion of a thoracostomy tube should alert the physician to the possibility of a bronchial tear. In the absence of pneumothorax, suspect tracheal rupture if pneumomediastinum or cervical emphysema is present. Immediate surgical consultation is indicated.

14. **How is tracheobronchial injury treated?**
Treatment includes initial airway stabilization followed by bronchoscopic evaluation of the airway. According to numerous reports in the literature, a partial tracheal tear may become complete after endotracheal intubation. Therefore, if the airway is stable, perform oral tracheal intubation in the operating room under bronchoscopic guidance. If the airway is unstable and emergent endotracheal intubation is needed, prepare for backup measures, such as cricothyroidotomy, tracheostomy, or fiberoptic bronchoscopy.

15. **How can I tell if a patient has an esophageal injury?**
Esophageal injury is rare in children but presents a diagnostic challenge when it does occur. The most common cause for esophageal perforation in children is iatrogenic, followed by penetrating trauma (gunshot or stab wound). Patients with an esophageal rupture in the cervical region may report neck stiffness or neck pain. They may regurgitate bloody material and have cervical subcutaneous emphysema or odynophagia. A lateral neck radiograph may show retroesophageal emphysema. In the thoracic region, patients may present with abdominal spasms and guarding, chest pain, subcutaneous emphysema, tachycardia, or dyspnea. A chest radiograph may show pneumothorax, pneumomediastinum, or an air–fluid level in the mediastinum.

16. **How are esophageal injuries treated?**
Patients with suspected esophageal perforation should receive adequate volume resuscitation, placement of a nasogastric tube, and antibiotics covering gram-positive, gram-negative, and anaerobic organisms. Esophagography, esophagoscopy, or both can make the diagnosis of esophageal perforation. Once the diagnosis is made, prompt surgical correction is mandatory. If the diagnosis is made within 24 hours, the mortality rate is approximately 5%. Diagnosis delayed for more than 24 hours after injury is associated with a mortality rate of 70%.

17. **On which side is a diaphragmatic injury seen more commonly?**
Approximately 80% of diaphragmatic injuries occur on the left. The left diaphragm is relatively unprotected, whereas the liver protects the right side. Right-sided diaphragmatic injuries are associated with increased mortality; patients usually have a greater physiologic insult and more associated injuries.

18. **How is the diagnosis of a traumatic rupture of the aorta (TRA) made?**
The gold standard for diagnosing TRA is aortography. Thoracic CT is only 55–65% accurate but helps to diagnose associated injuries. In one study, transesophageal echocardiography was shown to be highly sensitive and specific for detecting injury to the thoracic aorta. If the patient is stable and TRA is a concern, aortography should be performed. Life-threatening intracranial, thoracic, or intra-abdominal injuries must be evaluated and stabilized before aortography is done. If the patient is unstable, transesophageal echocardiography can be performed in the operating room while other life-threatening injuries are treated. Early diagnosis is imperative in patients with TRA. Morbidity and mortality increase threefold if operative intervention is delayed more than 12 hours.

19. **How do patients with pericardial tamponade present?**

Pericardial tamponade initially may be difficult to diagnose because associated injuries obscure the clinical signs and symptoms. Patients may present with distant heart sounds, low blood pressure, poor perfusion, narrow pulse pressure, or electromechanical dissociation. Pulsus paradoxus, with blood pressure falling more than 10 mmHg during inspiration, occurs in less than half of patients with pericardial tamponade and should not be relied on to make the diagnosis. Chest radiography may show an enlarged heart, and an electrocardiogram may show low-voltage QRS waves. Neither of these tests is diagnostic for pericardial tamponade, and treatment (pericardiocentesis) should not be delayed in unstable patients. In stable patients, an echocardiogram can demonstrate fluid within the pericardial sac.@

20. **How concerned should I be about blunt cardiac injury in patients with thoracic trauma?**

Blunt cardiac injury should be considered in any patient with thoracic trauma (e.g., a child hit by a fast-pitched baseball) who develops cardiac arrhythmia, a new murmur, or congestive heart failure. Patients with suspected blunt cardiac injury can be monitored in the emergency department or hospital; if no arrhythmias develop on electrocardiography, they can safely be sent home. Creatine phosphokinase–MB ratios have a high false-positive rate and are not a helpful screening tool. Transesophageal echocardiography should be performed in patients with thoracic trauma who have an abnormal electrocardiogram, arrhythmia, or new heart murmur. It is more sensitive in detecting myocardial injury than transthoracic echocardiography. A child with suspected blunt cardiac injury who is hemodynamically stable and has no arrhythmias is unlikely to develop a serious life-threatening arrhythmia or pump failure. Any patient with suspected blunt cardiac injury who is hemodynamically unstable or has arrhythmias should undergo transesophageal echocardiography and be admitted to the intensive care unit.

KEY POINTS: THORACIC TRAUMA ✔

1. The most common injuries in blunt thoracic trauma are lung contusions (58%), pneumothorax or hemothorax (38%), and rib fractures (38%).

2. Thoracic CT should be part of the initial evaluation of pediatric trauma patients if a lung contusion, pneumothorax, or a hemothorax is suspected or if the cause of the patient's respiratory distress is unknown.

3. Myocardial contusion is the most common and ventricular rupture the most lethal of blunt cardiac injuries.

4. Patients with a traumatic rupture of the aorta may present with hypotension, paraplegia, anuria, or absent/diminished femoral pulses.

5. Radiographic findings of a traumatic rupture of the aorta may include a widened mediastinum, blurred aortic knob, pleural cap, or tracheal or nasogastric tube deviation.

6. Suspect commotio cordis and ventricular fibrillation in any patient who has become unconscious immediately after blow to the chest.

21. **What are the four conditions that must be present for sudden circulatory arrest to occur after a nonpenetrating blow to the chest (commotio cordis)?**
    1. The blow must strike the chest in the area of the heart with force.
    2. The object must have sufficient mass (baseball, hockey puck, knee).
    3. The blow must strike the chest during the ventricular vulnerable period (T wave).
    4. The ventricles must have a large enough mass (> 3.5 kg).

    Geddes L, Roeder R: Evolution of our knowledge of sudden death due to commotio cordis. Am J Emerg Med 23:67–75, 2005.

BITES AND STINGS

Kate M. Cronan, MD, FAAP

1. **True or false: Bites from imported fire ants** *(Solenopsis invicta)* **can cause severe systemic reactions.**
   True. Local reactions can consist of a wheal, a pustule, or a large local reaction. Systemic reactions may range from urticaria to life-threatening anaphylaxis.

   deShazo RD, Williams DF, Goddard J, et al: Medical consequences of stings of imported fire ants, 2006: www.uptodate.com

2. **Describe the bite of the imported fire ant. How is it treated?**
   Imported fire ants are nonwinged hymenoptera found in the Southeastern and South Central United States. They bite with their jaws, then pivot around and sting at multiple sites in a circular pattern. Within 24 hours a sterile pustule develops at the site of the stings. This lesion can be diagnostic of a fire ant sting. Stings often occur on the legs and feet of children. Treatment consists of local wound care, antihistamines, and steroids for severe cases.

   Hodge D, Tecklenburg F: Imported fire ants. In Fleisher G, Ludwig S, Henretig F (eds): The Textbook of Pediatric Emergency Medicine, 5th ed. Philadelphia, Lippincott Williams & Wilkins, 2006, p 1053.

3. **What are the common microbiological organisms of dog, cat, and human bites?**
   - **Dog bites**: *Staphylococcus aureus*, streptococci, *Pasteurella canis*
   - **Cat bites**: *Pasteurella multocida*, *Staphylococcus aureus*, streptococci
   - **Human bites**: *Streptococcus viridans*, *Staphylococcus aureus*, anaerobes, *Eikenella corrodens*

   Talan DA, Citron DM, Abrahamian FM, et al: Bacteriologic analysis of dog and cat bites. N Engl J Med 340:85, 1999.

4. **Which bites should be routinely treated with prophylactic antibiotics?**
   - All dog bites involving hands and feet
   - All human bites
   - All cat bites
   - Puncture wounds
   - Bites for which treatment has been delayed for more than 24 hours
   - Bites in immunosuppressed patients

KEY POINTS: BITES THAT SHOULD NOT BE SUTURED ✓

1. Puncture wounds

2. Bites on the hands

3. Cat bites

4. Human bites

5. Crush injuries

6. Dog bites with delayed presentation

5. **How can one tell if a human bite was inflicted by an adult or a child?**
   If the intercanine distance is greater than 3 cm, it is most likely caused by an adult. This should raise concerns about child abuse.

   American Academy of Pediatrics. Committee on Child Abuse and Neglect. American Academy of Pediatric Dentistry. Ad Hoc Work Group on Child Abuse and Neglect: Oral and dental aspects of child abuse and neglect. Pediatrics. 104:348–350, 1999.

6. **What is the preferred hand position for evaluation of a fist injury from a bite?**
   Evaluate the wounds when the hand is in a *clenched* position. This permits more accurate assessment of the injuries. Once the hand is relaxed, it is difficult to assess the extent of injury because the deeper tissues form a closed space permitting the growth of bacteria.

7. **What causes rat-bite fever?**
   Rat-bite fever is caused by one of two organisms: *Streptobacillus moniliformis* or *Spirillum minus*. Mice, squirrels, cats, and weasels can also carry these organisms. Transmission to humans occurs via bites, scratches, handling infected rats, or ingestion of food or water contaminated by rat excreta.

   American Academy of Pediatrics: Red Book 2006: Report of the Committee on Infectious Diseases; 27th ed. Elk Grove, IL, American Academy of Pediatrics, 2006, p 559.

8. **How does rat-bite fever present?**
   Exposure to either organism results in abrupt onset of fever, chills, myalgia, extremity rash, and headache. The rash usually begins as a maculopapular eruption and often involves the palms and soles. With *Streptobacillus moniliformis* infection, the rat bite heals quickly and is followed by migratory polyarthritis in approximately 50% of patients. Pneumonia, endocarditis, myocarditis, and meningitis may occur. With *Spirillum minus* infection, the bite heals and is followed by local ulceration, lymphangitis, and lymphadenopathy. Occasionally arthritis also develops.

   Fatal rat-bite fever—Florida and Washington, 2003. MMWR Morb Mortal Wkly Rep 53:1198–1202, 2005.

9. **What is the best multipurpose insect repellent?**
   DEET (*N,N*-diethyl-m-toluamide) is the best multipurpose insect repellent. DEET is the active ingredient in most commercial insect repellents. It is available in various forms, including sprays, gels, liquids, and sticks, and in concentrations of 4–100%. DEET can be applied to skin or clothes. It should not be applied under clothes. It does not work against stinging insects but is quite effective against mosquitoes, gnats, chiggers, ticks, and other insects. DEET washes off with water and perspiration. It is important to note that application of DEET may reduce the efficacy of sunscreen.

10. **What are the major disadvantages of DEET?**
    DEET can be toxic, and use of low concentrations (10%) is recommended in children. It should be applied to the clothes more than to the skin. Application to areas around the eyes, mouth, and open skin lesions should be avoided. For children, DEET should be applied once per day. It should be avoided completely for children younger than 2 months of age. Oral ingestion of large quantities of DEET may cause seizures, coma, or death. For those concerned about the possible toxicity of DEET, citronella, a plant-derived insect repellent, is a good alternative.

    Fradin MS, Day JF: Comparative efficacy of insect repellents against mosquito bites. N Engl J Med 347:13–18, 2002.

11. **What is papular urticaria?**
    Papular urticaria is a skin condition that consists of intensely pruritic wheals and papules. These lesions are attributable to arthropod bites in specifically sensitized children. Sensitization

may occur in infancy, but the lesions do not appear until the second year of life in many cases. Various arthropods have been identified as culprits: dog lice, mosquitoes, bedbugs, fleas, mites, and chiggers. The wheals represent an immediate hypersensitivity reaction to insect bites. Wheals then evolve into papules, which represent a delayed hypersensitivity reaction. New lesions form continually, and the eruption may persist for many months. The lesions usually appear on exposed areas, such as the extremities, head, neck, and shoulders. The differential diagnosis includes scabies, varicella, pediculosis, urticaria, and insect bites without papular urticaria.

12. **How is papular urticaria treated?**
Treatment should focus on an multipurpose insecticide for the entire home. Household pets should be included in the treatment. When the cause of the lesions is removed, clinical symptoms should improve greatly, but supportive treatment is necessary. Oral antihistamines and topical steroid creams help to control the itching.

13. **Name the tick-borne infectious diseases that occur in the United States.**
   - **Bacterial:** Lyme disease, tularemia, relapsing fever
   - **Rickettsial:** Rocky Mountain spotted fever, ehrlichiosis
   - **Viral:** Colorado tick fever
   - **Protozoal:** Babesiosis

   American Academy of Pediatrics: Red Book 2006: Report of the Committee on Infectious Diseases, 27th ed. Elk Grove, IL, American Academy of Pediatrics, 2006, p 195.

14. **In penicillin-allergic patients who present with a human bite or a high-risk animal bite, what antibiotic regimen is recommended?**
Prophylaxis and treatment for penicillin-allergic children are challenging problems. Erythromycin and tetracycline activity against *Staphylococcus aureus* and anaerobes is unreliable. Tetracycline is effective against *Pasteurella* sp., but the risk of dental staining in children younger than 8 years must be considered. Therefore, combination treatment with oral or parenteral trimethoprim-sulfamethoxazole (effective against *Staphylococcus aureus*, *Eikenella corrodens*, and *Pasteurella* sp.) and clindamycin (effective against anaerobes, streptococci, and *Staphylococcus aureus*) may be effective for preventing or treating bite wound infections. Ceftriaxone may be used if the patient can tolerate cephalosporins. Metronidazole provides excellent anaerobic coverage and may be used as an alternative to clindamycin.

   American Academy of Pediatrics: Red Book 2006: Report of the Committee on Infectious Diseases; 27th ed. Elk Grove, IL, American Academy of Pediatrics, 2006, p 195.

15. **Define *Hymenoptera* sting.**
A sting consists of an injection of venom via a tapered shaft that projects from the venom sac located in the abdomen of females of the *Hymenoptera* species. Stings usually occur in warm weather.

16. **Which group of the order *Hymenoptera* is considered aggressive—apids or vespids?**
Bees, wasps, and hornets are responsible for many of the anaphylactic reactions to venomous insects in the United States. Apids include honeybees and bumblebees; vespids include yellow jackets, hornets, and wasps. Apids tend to be docile and sting only when provoked. The bumblebee is large, slow-moving, and very noisy. Honeybees may cause problems among beekeepers. Vespids are aggressive; the yellow jacket is the most aggressive in this family. Yellow jackets are thought to be the principal cause of allergic reactions to insect stings in the United States.

17. **How are reactions to bee stings categorized?**
    - The most common reaction is a **small local reaction** that presents as a painful pruritic lesion < 5 cm at the site of the sting and lasts briefly (several hours).
    - A **large local reaction** occurs in approximately 10% of people after a sting and manifests with swelling and erythema in the area of the sting. It is usually > 5 cm in diameter, often very painful and itchy, and lasts for > 24 hours, sometimes up to 1 week. The features of this reaction may be confused with cellulitis, but cellulitis rarely develops after a bee sting.
    - **Systemic reactions**, which occur in approximately 0.5% of *Hymenoptera* stings, begin within minutes to hours after the sting and can be mild or severe.
    - **Mild systemic reactions** most commonly consist of dermal signs and symptoms: generalized urticaria, pruritus, flushing, and angioedema. Gastrointestinal symptoms, such as abdominal pain, nausea, and diarrhea, may also occur.
    - **Severe systemic reactions** include life-threatening signs, such as upper airway edema with hoarseness and stridor; shock, manifested by pallor and fainting; and bronchospasm, characterized by coughing, dyspnea, and wheezing.
    - **Unusual reactions** to bee stings include vasculitis, nephrosis, encephalitis, and serum sickness. Symptoms usually occur several days to several weeks after the sting and tend to last for a long time.

18. **What is the best way to remove a stinger from a bee sting?**
    If a stinger remains in the skin after a bee sting, it should be swiped sideways away from the direction in which it points. A credit card or other similar card works well to do the swiping. Grasping and pulling the stinger may squeeze the remaining venom from the venom sac into the sting site. The stinger should be removed as soon as possible to avoid further deposition of venom.

19. **What is the treatment for anaphylaxis due to an insect sting?**
    The treatment is the same as for anaphylaxis from other causes. Attention must be paid first to airway, breathing, and circulation. Intramuscular epinephrine in a 1:1000 dilution should be given immediately; the dose may be repeated every 30 minutes as needed. Intravenous epinephrine is rarely indicated except in the case of profound shock. Antihistamines, such as diphenhydramine or hydroxyzine, given parenterally, may reduce urticaria and pruritus. Steroids, such as methylprednisolone, should be administered early in the treatment plan. Depending on the severity of the reaction, other treatment modalities may be indicated (vasopressors, supplemental oxygen, IV fluids, bronchodilators).

    After recovery, emergency kits for self-administration of epinephrine should be prescribed. Detailed instructions about technique and appropriate use must be provided to the patient and family.

    Vankawala H, Park R: Bee and Hymenoptera stings: www.emedicine.com/emerg/topic55.htm

20. **What is the significance of the Southwestern desert scorpion, *Centruroides exilicaida*?**
    It is the only scorpion species of medical importance in the United States. Also called the Arizona bark scorpion, it is found mainly in Arizona, Texas, and California. Arizona bark scorpions are yellow or brown and are usually 5 cm in length. Their appearance resembles that of the shrimp. Their long, very mobile tails contain the stinger. They tend to reside in brush areas and trees and sting mostly at night. Children are usually stung on their extremities.

21. **How does the venom of the Arizona bark scorpion work?**
    The venom is mostly neurotoxic. It overstimulates the parasympathetic and sympathetic nervous systems and results in agitation, tachycardia or bradycardia, hypertension, dysrhythmias, and increased secretions. Cranial nerve dysfunction may cause rapid

dysconjugate eye movements and contractions of muscles of the face and tongue. Peripheral motor neuron involvement presents as muscle contractions and uncontrolled jerking movements of the extremities, which may be mistaken for seizures. Respiratory distress may result from decreased pharyngeal tone and uncoordinated contraction of respiratory muscles.

22. **How are scorpion envenomations treated?**
Treatment of scorpion envenomation is usually supportive; focus must be placed on airway control. Local wound care should be provided along with tetanus prophylaxis. Children with systemic signs and symptoms should be admitted to the hospital. Analgesics and benzodiazepines should be administered for pain and agitation. Many authorities prefer a continuous infusion of midazolam. A hyperimmune goat serum antivenin is known to be effective but has not been approved by the Food and Drug Administration. It is therefore available only in Arizona, where the Arizona State Board of Pharmacy has approved its use.

 Bush S, Gerardo C: Scorpion envenomations: www.emedicine.com/emerg/topic524.htm

23. **What are the four kinds of sharks in the United States that are responsible for most shark bites?**
Gray reef, great white, blue, and mako sharks. Bites from these sharks can cause extensive injury, including fractures, amputations, and penetration of internal organs.

 Hodge D, Tecklenburg FW: Bites and stings. In Fleisher GR, Ludwig S, Henretig FM (eds): Textbook of Pediatric Emergency Medicine, 5th ed. Philadelphia, Lippincott Williams & Wilkins, 2006, p 1045.

24. **Which two spiders in the United States cause significant envenomations?**
The black widow spider *(Latrodectus mactans)* and the brown recluse spider *(Loxosceles reclusa)* are the only two spiders known to cause significant envenomations. Brown recluse spider bites occur much more frequently than black widow spider bites. Brown recluse spiders are nonaggressive and usually bite only when threatened. They have a brown or yellow violin-shaped marking on the dorsal thorax and are found most commonly in the Southern and Midwestern states. They prefer dark, warm, protected areas, such as closets and garages. Black widow spiders inhabit all states except Alaska and are found most commonly in the South, Ohio Valley, Southwest, and West Coast. They are found in attics, barns, trash piles, and other dimly lit areas. Bites are more frequent in the warmer months. The black widow spider is jet black, with an hourglass-shaped red mark on the underside of the abdomen.

25. **What are the symptoms of the bite of a brown recluse spider?**
At the time of the bite, a stinging sensation may be felt. Increased pain and pruritus may develop within several hours. The clinical course ranges from mild local irritation to large necrotic skin lesions and systemic reactions. Most bites go unnoticed or result in only a mild red papule that heals quickly. A central vesicle with surrounding erythema is discovered at the site of the bite. In some scenarios, vasospasm and hemorrhage in the first few hours after the bite account for the red, white, and blue discoloration. Systemic signs and symptoms occur in approximately 40% of envenomations, including fever, nausea, vomiting, headache, and arthralgias. A scarlatiniform rash may occur simultaneously. Systemic loxoscelism is rare and seen almost exclusively in children. It is characterized by anemia, hemolysis and thrombocytopenia, shock, and renal failure.

26. **How is the bite of a brown recluse spider treated?**
Treatment consists of local wound care; extensive dermal injury may require skin grafting. Analgesics and tetanus immunization are mainstays of therapy. If extensive intravascular hemolysis occurs, it is crucial to maintain high urinary flow rates with alkalinization of the urine via sodium bicarbonate infusion.

 Stibich A, Schwartz R: www.emedicine.com/DERM/topic598.htm

27. **What is latrodectism?**
This term applies to systemic symptoms due to the spread of the neurotoxin from black widow spider bites. There are three phases of latrodectism:
   - The **exacerbation** phase, which occurs from < 6 up to 24 hours and is characterized by muscle spasms at the site of the bite or elsewhere
   - The **dissipation** phase, which occurs 1–3 days after the bite and is a time when symptoms subside
   - The **residual** phase, which occurs weeks to months after the bite and may consist of persistent tremors and weakness and fatigue
   Castells M: Spider bites: www.uptodate.com

28. **How is the bite of a black widow spider treated?**
Treatment consists of analgesia, including oral narcotics for milder cases and IV morphine for more severe cases. Benzodiazepines can relieve anxiety. An antivenin is available, but it is indicated only for the most severe cases unresponsive to the above measures. Life-threatening tachycardia and hypertension are indications for this antivenin. Death is extremely uncommon.

29. **What infectious agent should be considered when treating an iguana bite?**
Iguanas are becoming popular pets. They can inflict injury via scratching, biting, and tail whipping. They frequently carry unusual subtypes of fecal salmonella. The Centers for Disease Control and Prevention recommends that children under age 5 and those who are immunocompromised should not have iguanas and other salmonella-carrying pets, such as turtles, in the home.
   Reptile-associated salmonellosis—selected states, 1998–2002. MMWR Morb Mortal Wkly Rep 52:1206–1209, 2003.

30. **What are the poisonous snakes indigenous to the United States?**
Snakes in the Crotalidae family (pit viper) family and Elapidae family (coral snakes) are poisonous. Rattlesnakes, copperheads, and water moccasins are pit vipers and account for 99% of poisonous snakebites. The coral snake accounts for less than 1% of poisonous snakebites.

31. **How can pit vipers be distinguished from nonpoisonous snakes?**
Pit vipers have two pits, one on either side of their head, and their pupils are elliptical and vertically oriented. The head is triangular and they have two curved fangs that are widely spaced. The scales caudal to the anal plate continue in a single row. Nonpoisonous snakes have oval heads with round pupils. The anal plate has a double row of subcaudal plates.
   Hodge D, Tecklenberg F: Snake bites. In Fleisher G, Ludwig S, Henretig F (eds): The Textbook of Pediatric Emergency Medicine, 5th ed. Philadelphia, Lippincott, Williams & Wilkins, 2006, p 1054.

32. **What causes tularemia?**
Francisella tularensis, a gram-negative pleomorphic coccobacillus, is the causative agent. Sources of this organism include many species of wild mammals, some domestic animals (e.g., sheep, cattle, cats), and the blood-sucking arthropods that bite these animals (e.g., ticks and mosquitoes). In the United States, rabbits and ticks are major sources of infection.
   American Academy of Pediatrics: Red Book 2006: Report of the Committee on Infectious Diseases, 27th ed. Elk Grove, IL, American Academy of Pediatrics, 2006, p 705.

33. **How does tularemia present? How is it treated?**
Most patients present with an abrupt onset of fever, chills, myalgia, and headache. There are several tularemic syndromes. The most common is the ulceroglandular syndrome, which presents with a painful maculopapular lesion at the bite site and painful, acutely inflamed lymph

nodes. Other less common syndromes are the glandular, oropharyngeal, oculoglandular typhoidal, intestinal, and pneumonic presentations.

The treatment is streptomycin. Gentamycin is an effective alternative.

American Academy of Pediatrics: Red Book 2006: Report of the Committee on Infectious Diseases, 27th ed. Elk Grove, IL, American Academy of Pediatrics, 2006, p 706.

34. How soon after an exposure should immunoprophylaxis for rabies begin?

After thorough wound care is completed, passive and active immunoprophylaxis is required for optimal therapy. Begin prophylaxis as soon as possible after exposure, ideally within 24 hours. However, a delay of several days or more may not compromise effectiveness; begin prophylaxis, if indicated, regardless of the time of exposure.

American Academy of Pediatrics: Red Book 2006: Report of the Committee on Infectious Diseases, 27th ed. Elk Grove, IL, American Academy of Pediatrics, 2006, p 556.

35. Which type of jellyfish sting is highly toxic?

Stings from the common purple jellyfish *(Pelagia noctiluca)* and the sea nettle jellyfish *(Chrysaora quinquecirrha)* are only mildly toxic. Local skin irritation is the usual clinical manifestation. However, stings from **lion's mane** *(Cyanea capillata)* are highly toxic. This jellyfish is found along both coasts of the United States. Contact with the tentacles of lion's mane causes severe burning; prolonged exposure results in muscle cramps, and respiratory failure may ensue.

36. How are toxic jellyfish stings treated?

Treatment of toxic jellyfish stings focuses on relieving pain, alleviating effects of the venom, and supportive therapy. The first goal is to remove the tentacles to avoid further nematocyst discharging. It is possible to inactivate the remaining nematocysts by topical application of vinegar (acetic acid) for 30 minutes. Alternative solutions include baking soda slurry or meat tenderizer. The sting area should be washed with normal saline or sea water. The residual tentacles should be removed with instruments or gloved hands. No antivenin is available. Antihistamines, steroids, and analgesics may be indicated. Cardiac and respiratory support may be required.

37. How should one remove a tick embedded in the skin?

Grasp the tick by the head or the mouth with blunt angled forceps as close to the skin as possible. This action should be perpendicular to the patient's skin. With steady traction, pull the tick and do not twist as you pull back. It is best not to squeeze, puncture, or crush the tick as it could regurgitate material into the wound during removal. If any residual parts or cement is noted on the skin, remove it with forceps. Alternatively, use a large-gauge needle to swipe residual parts away. Cleanse the bite wound after removal. Do *not* apply petroleum jelly, a hot match, alcohol, or other irritants.

Howard J, Loiselle J: A clinician's guide to safe and effective tick removal. Contemp Pediatr 23:36–42, 2006.

38. How important is the duration of attachment of ticks to the skin?

Duration of attachment to the host plays a major role in the transmission of pathogens. *Borrelia burgdorferi* from an infected tick has a higher likelihood of transmission after 24 hours, and this likelihood increases after 72 hours. On the other hand, *Ehrlichia chaffeensis* requires a shorter period for transmission.

Howard J, Loiselle J: A clinician's guide to safe and effective tick removal. Contemp Pediatr 23:36–42, 2006.

39. **What are the most effective precautions to avoid Lyme disease?**
    - **Personal protection consists of wearing appropriate clothes:** Wear long sleeves and long pants in at-risk areas.
    - **Use of repellants:** DEET applied to the skin and clothes. Consider the use of Permethrin applied to the clothes in conjunction with DEET.
    - **Inspection:** Parents should inspect their children after times spent in risky areas. If a tick is found on the skin, washing can be effective before attachment occurs.
    - **Modification of outdoor environment:** Replace brush with wood chips.

CHAPTER 64

DROWNING

Linda Quan, MD, and Brian Coleman, MD, MS

1. **How should the terms *near drowning* and *drowning* be applied to submersion victims? What is a drowning?**

   In 2002, the World Congress on Drowning developed universal terminology to improve interpretation and comparison of reported data. Previously used terminology, such as *near-drowning*, *secondary*, *wet*, *dry*, and *silent* drowning have been abandoned. Drowning is immersion in a liquid medium that results in some degree of primary respiratory impairment and may result in survival or death. The term *drowning* should not reflect clinical course or final outcome.

   > Bierens J: Handbook on Drowning. Springer, Netherlands, 2004.
   > Idris AH: Recommended guidelines for uniform reporting of data from drowning: The "Utstein style." Resuscitation 59:45–57, 2003.
   > Zuckerbraun NS: Pediatric drowning: Current management strategies for immediate care. Clin Pediatr Emerg Med 6 49–56, 2005.

2. **Is cardiopulmonary resuscitation indicated for every patient in cardiac arrest following a drowning?**

   Survival rates from cardiac arrest following drowning are among the highest, 20–31%, reported in pediatric cardiac arrest, although it is unclear why. To be effective, resuscitation should begin as soon as possible after retrieval from the water, at the scene. However, survival from prolonged (> 25 minutes) non–icy water drownings is essentially zero, as is survival following cardiopulmonary resuscitation for > 25 minutes without return of spontaneous circulation (a perfusing blood pressure). There are clearly some patients who are dead at the scene for whom efforts are futile.

   > Orlowski JP: Prognostic factors in pediatric cases of drowning and near-drowning. JACEP 8:176–179, 1979.

3. **What is a cold water drowning?**

   The term *cold water* should be abandoned for the evidence-based predictor *icy water*. While there are rare, isolated cases of successful resuscitation and intact survival after long drowning in cold waters, these dramatic cases usually occurred in waters colder than 10° C. Nonicy cold water, unfortunately, is still too warmly defined by some enthusiastic resuscitators and is assigned greater powers than are supported by well-done studies.

   > Wollenek G: Cold water submersion and cardiac arrest in treatment of severe hypothermia with cardiopulmonary bypass. Resuscitation 52:255–263, 2002.

4. **Is hypothermia protective?**

   Hypothermia can dramatically decrease the cerebral metabolic rate, with a resultant decrease in the oxygen requirements of the brain and greater tolerance of hypoxia. However, for hypothermia to be protective, it must precede the onset of hypoxic injury. The very rapid cooling required to produce protective hypothermia is usually not accomplished in the usual nonicy water drowning; in these patients, hypothermia upon arrival to the emergency department (ED) predicts a bad, not a good, outcome.

Biggart MJ: Effect of hypothermia and cardiac arrest on outcome of near-drowning accidents in children. J Pediatr 117:179–183, 1990.

5. **How should an icy cold water drowning be managed differently from a warm water drowning?**

A patient who has had a truly icy water drowning should be managed aggressively because of the possibility of intact survival. Prolonged and maximal resuscitative efforts, including cardiopulmonary bypass or extracorporeal membrane oxygenation, may be indicated for the icy water submersion but have not been effective for warm water submersion patients. Because icy water drownings are anecdotal reports, predictors and likelihood ratios for survival from icy water submersions are not available. Most would agree, however, that for nonicy water drownings, failure to restore a circulating cardiac rhythm within about 30 minutes after rewarming to 32–35°C suggests that further efforts are unlikely to be successful.

Wollenek G, Honarwar N, Golej J, Marx M: Cold water submersion and cardiac arrest in treatment of severe hypothermia with cardiopulmonary bypass. Resuscitation 52:255–263, 2002.

6. **Is there a clinical difference between a salt water AND fresh water drowning?**

There is none. A large clinical study showed no real difference in the clinical presentation of adults who drowned in salt or fresh waters, thus invalidating the mythic physiologic changes reported in one animal study. Clinical experience dictates that both salt water– and fresh water–drowned patients may develop pulmonary edema, anemia is rare, and electrolytes are usually normal. The explanation may lie in the fact that most humans do not aspirate large volumes of water. Furthermore, the pulmonary response to drowning, especially the development of pulmonary edema, relates to other factors besides the salinity of the aspirated fluid.

Modell JH: Drowning. N Engl J Med 328:253–256, 1993.

7. **What are the tenets of management in resuscitation of the unresponsive drowning patient?**

The injury of drowning is hypoxia, and the goal of resuscitation should be directed toward the ABCs. Those who are unconscious or who have respiratory compromise should undergo rapid sequence intubation and endotracheal intubation to protect their airway from vomiting and aspiration. Positive-pressure ventilation is the single most effective method for reversing hypoxemia. Poor perfusion is usually the result of significant myocardial hypoxia. It should first be treated with one to two boluses of normal saline (20 mL/kg body weight) for the possibility of hypovolemia; if this fails to restore adequate perfusion, cardiac dysfunction should be treated with inotropic agents. Additionally, regardless of the water temperature in which the drowning occurred, all drowning patients should be assumed to be at risk for hypothermia. Management includes continuous monitoring of core body temperature and careful rewarming to achieve and maintain a core temperature between 32–34°C as part of present mild hypothermia cerebral resuscitation protocols.

After successful resuscitation, attention must be directed toward preventing secondary brain injury. This can be achieved by monitoring for hypoxia, hypercapnia, and hypothermia.

Zuckerbraun NS: Pediatric drowning: Current management strategies for immediate care. Clin Pediatr Emerg Med 6:49–56, 2005.

KEY POINTS: DROWNING ✓

1. Failure to restore a perfusing rhythm within about 30 minutes of resuscitation in a patient with a core temperature of 32–35° C, following a nonicy water drowning, suggests that further efforts are unlikely to be successful.

2. Patients who had a drowning but are asymptomatic after 6–8 hours of observation can be safely sent home if the social situation permits.

3. Social work involvement is important in the evaluation of any drowning patient for possible abuse, homicide, suicide, or risk-taking behaviors, especially alcohol use.

8. **Should prophylactic antibiotics be given to the drowning patient?**
No. The only indication for the prophylactic use of antibiotics is drowning in grossly contaminated water (e.g., sewage, retention pond). Instead, antibiotics should be initiated once signs of sepsis or pneumonia become apparent.

Orlowski JP: Drowning. Rescue, resuscitation, and reanimation. Pediatr Clin North Am 48:627–646, 2001.

9. **Which tests are helpful in managing the drowning patient?**
The patient's clinical examination should guide what tests are needed. The full work-up panel of blood gas, chest radiography, complete blood count, and electrolytes can be reserved for the unresponsive patient; full evaluation is needed if this patient incurred a more serious hypoxic injury and is at great risk for complications and bad outcome. Additionally, a glucose level should be included because it is a useful prognostic factor. Hyperglycemia (glucose level > 250 mg/dL) portends a poor outcome. It is unclear if hyperglycemia should be treated. On the other hand, hypoglycemia must be treated. For the alert patient with no or mild respiratory distress, oximetry monitoring may be all that is needed and is a more reliable treatment guide than chest radiography. Several studies have recommended against using an abnormal radiograph as the sole criterion for hospital admission. Electrolytes are usually normal.

Noonan L: Freshwater submersion injuries in children: A retrospective review of seventy-five hospitalized patients. Pediatrics 98:368–371, 1996.

10. **What is the most common cause of death and disability in hospitalized drowning victims?**
Cerebral edema secondary to hypoxic ischemia is the usual cause of death and becomes a clinical challenge at 6–18 hours after the drowning event. Hypoxic encephalopathy in survivors of severe drownings usually results in severe neurologic sequelae, including loss of self-help skills.

Orlowski JP, Szpilman D: Drowning: Rescue, resuscitation, and reanimation. Pediatr Clin North Am 48:627–646, 2001.

11. **Can some drowning patients be sent home from the ED?**
Some postsubmersion patients arrive looking cheery but wet. They have usually had a short submersion interval, have minimal signs (mild metabolic acidosis) of a hypoxic insult, and are asymptomatic. These patients should be observed in the ED for a minimum of 6–8 hours with evaluation of neurologic and pulmonary status, including cardiorespiratory monitoring. Some initially asymptomatic, alert patients can develop mild respiratory distress (tachypnea, mild hypoxia) and cough at the scene or within a few hours of the submersion. In many cases,

their symptoms respond to a brief period of low-flow oxygen and do not mandate hospital admission if they are asymptomatic at 8 hours.

Causey AL: Predicting discharge in uncomplicated near-drowning. Am J Emerg Med 18:9–11, 2000.

Noonan L, Howrey R, Ginsburg CM: Freshwater submersion injuries in children: A retrospective review of seventy-five hospitalized patients. Pediatrics 98:368–371, 1996.

Quan L: Near-drowning. Pediatr Rev 20:255–259, quiz 260, 1999.

12. **Does every drowning patient need evaluation for cervical spine injury?**
    No. Routine cervical spine imaging is not indicated for the overwhelming majority of patients. Cervical spine injury is very rare (< 1%) in drowning patients, and is almost never seen in preadolescent children. It occurs when there has been a high-velocity injury and when concern for multiple major trauma coexists, such as drowning associated with motor vehicle, boating, or personal watercraft accidents; diving; or surfing. In two large retrospective studies of over 2000 patients, all cases of cervical spine injury had a history consistent with high-speed mechanism, or clinical signs of serious injury on physical examination. A careful history and examination of the neck are sufficient screening for cervical spine injury for most patients.

Hwang V: Prevalence of traumatic injuries in drowning and near drowning in children and adolescents. Arch Pediatr Adolesc Med 157:50–53, 2003.

Watson RS: Cervical spine injuries among submersion victims. J Trauma 51:658–662, 2001.

13. **Who will survive a drowning?**
    The victim whose drowning interval is less than 5 minutes will most likely (90%) survive. Following longer drowning intervals, survival drops precipitously. Young children are more likely to survive than adolescents, who are more likely to be declared dead at the scene. The marked difference in survival between young children and adolescents or adults is explained by their different submersion scenarios. Young children tend to drown where supervision is nearby but has lapsed; they also tend to drown in bodies of water, such as bathtubs or swimming pools, where rescue is easy. On the other hand, adolescents and adults get to larger, deeper, murkier bodies of water, such as lakes and rivers, where rescue is more difficult and the drowning interval is lengthy. When these factors are controlled for, age is not a predictor of outcome.

Quan L: Characteristics of drowning by different age groups. Inj Prev 9:163–168, 2003.

14. **What are predictors of outcome in drowning?**
    The key predictor is the patient's mental status after the drowning. Patients who are alert on arrival to the ED or at hospital admission will survive with normal neurologic status. In patients arriving unresponsive to the ED, ultimate neurologic outcome is more difficult to predict. Factors upon presentation that will identify patients who will remain in a persistent vegetative state or die include duration of submersion > 10 min., absent pupillary reflexes, Glasgow Coma Scale score ≤ 5, hyperglycemia after resuscitation (glucose level > 250 mg/dL), acidosis (pH < 7.10), and duration of cardiopulmonary resuscitation greater than 25 minutes until return of spontaneous circulation. A poor prognosis is most likely when all of these bad prognostic factors are present. However, no single factor or combination of factors at the time the patient arrives in the ED has achieved greater than 96% accuracy in predicting poor outcome (persistent vegetative state or death), so some recommend resuscitation attempts for all drowning victims on arrival in the ED. As the time interval from the drowning event increases, predicting outcome becomes more reliable; most of those who remain comatose at 24 hours will die or survive with severe neurologic sequelae.

Ashwal S: Prognostic implications of hyperglycemia and reduced cerebral blood flow in childhood near-drowning. Neurology 40:820–823, 1990.

Causey AL, Tilelli JA, Swanson ME: Predicting discharge in uncomplicated near-drowning. Am J Emerg Med 18:9–11, 2000.

Graf WD: Predicting outcome in pediatric submersion victims. Ann Emerg Med 26:312–319, 1995.

Jacinto SJ: Predicting outcome in hypoxic-ischemic brain injury. Pediatr Clin North Am 48:647–660, 2001.

Lavelle JM: Near drowning: Is emergency department cardiopulmonary resuscitation or intensive care unit cerebral resuscitation indicated? Crit Care Med 21:368–373, 1993.

Quan L: Outcome and predictors of outcome in pediatric submersion victims receiving prehospital care in King County, Washington. Pediatrics 86:586–593, 1990.

Suominen PK: Does water temperature affect outcome of nearly drowned children? Resuscitation 35:111–115, 1997.

KEY POINTS: POOR PROGNOSTIC SIGNS ✓

1. Duration of submersion > 10 minutes

2. Absent pupillary reflexes

3. Glasgow Coma Scale score ≤ 5

4. Hyperglycemia (glucose level > 250 mg/dL)

5. Acidosis (pH < 7.1)

6. No spontaneous circulation after 25 minutes of cardiopulmonary resuscitation

15. **How does one recognize child abuse as the etiology for drowning?**
Drowning as child abuse or homicide is most often recognized in the young child whose submersion occurred in the bathtub. Drowning may be the primary injury as well as a secondary injury when the abuser attempts to revive the child or to conceal other physical injury by placing the child in the tub. The physical examination must include a careful search for signs of physical abuse and signs of multiple traumas. However, radiographs for fractures are usually not helpful. The key to recognition of intentional trauma is usually in the history. A caregiver's explanation for the injury that is not compatible with the child's developmental status or a changing or vague history should prompt consideration of child abuse. A critical part of any childhood drowning, regardless of the concern for abuse, is evaluation by social services.

Gillenwater JM: Inflicted submersion in childhood. Arch Pediatr Adolesc Med 150:298–303, 1996.

Kemp AM: Accidents and child abuse in bathtub submersions. Arch Dis Child 70:435–438, 1994.

16. **How can pediatric drowning be prevented?**
Drownings are preventable with active and passive interventions. For children younger than 5 years of age, falling into swimming pools is the most common cause of drowning. Four-sided, isolation fencing with self-closing, self-latching gates around residential pools is effective in preventing more than 50% of these drownings. Adult supervision of young children around any water is essential and can prevent all bath tub–related drownings. Infant bath seats, supporting rings, or the care provided by another young child are not suitable substitutes for adult supervision. Adequate supervision entails that the adult be constantly present, focused on the child, and within an arm's length. The American Academy of Pediatrics also recommends swimming lessons as soon as the child is developmentally ready, after the age of 4 years, and caregiver training in cardiopulmonary resuscitation. For adolescents, drownings occur while swimming with friends or while boating. Many of these deaths could be prevented by wearing life vests and avoiding alcohol.

Prevention of drowning in infants, children, and adolescents. Pediatrics 112:437–439, 2003.

Quan L, Liller K, Bennett E. Water-related injuries of children and adolescents. In: Liller K. Injury Prevention for Children and Adolescents: Research, Practice and Advocacy. Washington DC, American Public Health Association, 2006.

17. **Should patients with seizures be allowed to participate in water-related activities?**

    Seizures are the most common predisposing event for drowning in all age groups, and drowning is the major cause of death in patients with epilepsy. This group of patients has 10 times the risk for drowning and death from drowning of those without seizures. In these children, the bath tub actually is the highest risk site. Health care providers should advise patients with seizures to take showers, not baths. Involvement in water sports should include wearing of life jackets when by and in the water and swimming in pools where lifeguards supervise and are notified of the patient's increased risk.

    Diekema DS: Epilepsy as a risk factor for submersion injury in children. Pediatrics 91:612– 616, 1993.

ELECTRICAL AND LIGHTNING INJURIES

Amanda Pratt, MD

1. **What characteristics of electrical energy predispose to severe injury?**
   - In general, the higher the voltage and current, the worse the injury.
   - Alternating current (AC) causes intense muscle contractions, thus prolonging the exposure.
   - Direct current (DC) can cause significant trauma by throwing the victim from the source.
   - AC is three times more dangerous than DC of the same voltage.

2. **Which body tissues offer the highest resistance?**
   From greatest to least resistance: bone > fat > tendon > skin > muscle > nerve. The most important resistor of current flow is skin, because it is typically the site of first contact. Dry skin over palms and soles can have a resistance of 100,000 ohms. When skin is wet, the resistance drops to 2500 ohms; when skin is immersed in water, resistance can be as low as 1500 ohms. Lowered resistance allows more current to penetrate deeper tissue.

   Jain S, Bandi V: Electrical and lightning injuries. Crit Care Clin 5:319–331, 1999.

3. **How does the pathway of the current through the body affect the degree of injury?**
   The path that a current takes determines the number of organs affected and thus the severity of injury. A vertical path parallel to the body involves almost all vital organs and is thus the most dangerous. A horizontal path from hand to hand spares the brain but can still be fatal because it can involve the heart, spinal cord, or respiratory muscles. A horizontal path through the lower body may cause severe local damage but is not typically fatal.

   Koumbourlis AC: Electrical injuries. Crit Care Med 30:S424–S430, 2002.

4. **Do electrical injuries cause significant external signs that provide a clue to the severity of injury?**
   No. Injury potential ranges from a superficial wound to multisystem failure. Deep injury may not be immediately apparent, particularly if the resistance of the skin has been lowered by moisture. Low-resistance structures sustain significant injury and necrosis that may not be apparent on initial physical examination.

   Martinez JA, Nguyen T: Electrical injuries. South Med J 93:1165–1168, 2000.

5. **What are the cardiac manifestations of electrical injuries?**
   - Sinus tachycardia, premature ventricular contractions, reversible QT prolongation, and other arrhythmias have been reported.
   - Low-voltage AC may cause ventricular fibrillation.
   - High-voltage AC or DC is likely to cause ventricular asystole.

6. **How may electrical injuries affect the respiratory system?**
   - Primary central nervous system dysfunction at the respiratory center of the brain can induce apnea.
   - Paralysis or tetany of the respiratory muscles and diaphragm may occur.

7. **How are the kidneys affected in electrical injuries?**
Myoglobinuria with subsequent renal failure is possible; direct renal injury is rare.

8. **Describe the neurologic effects of electrical injuries.**
Acute findings may include altered mental status, loss of consciousness, seizures, and paralysis.
    Delayed findings (days to years) may include depression, memory loss, motor neuropathy, and transverse myelitis.

9. **What are the dermatologic manifestations of electrical injuries?**
    - Entrance and exit burns may be seen and should be evaluated to determine the path of current.
    - Burns across joints at the flexor creases on both flexor surfaces may be seen, known as "kissing burns."
    - Mouth commissure burns are a unique problem in children; other issues are associated with their management (see Question 14).

10. **How do I manage patients with significant electrical exposure?**
    1. Most patients with significant electrical exposure (i.e., high-voltage, DC, or AC injury with respiratory, hemodynamic, or neurologic sequelae) should undergo rapid trauma assessment and resuscitation.
    2. Provide the ABCs of trauma care (airway, breathing, and circulation).
    3. In patients with DC exposure, immobilize the cervical spine until further clinical and radiographic evaluations are done.
    4. Aggressive fluid resuscitation should be initiated to treat presumed myonecrosis and prevent renal failure.
    5. Assess for compartment syndrome due to myonecrosis.
    6. Provide local burn care and tetanus prophylaxis.
    7. Obtain laboratory data: complete blood count, seven-panel chemistry study, creatine phosphokinase, urinalysis, urine for myoglobin, electrocardiography (12 lead), and appropriate radiography. If severe injury or suspected abdominal trauma, add liver function tests, amylase, prothrombin time, partial thromboplastin time, and type and crossmatch.

KEY POINTS: INITIAL MANAGEMENT OF VICTIMS OF SIGNIFICANT ELECTRICAL INJURY ✔

1. Treat the victim as a trauma patient.
2. Initiate the ABCs.
3. Provide cervical spine immobilization.
4. Aggressive fluid resuscitation.

11. **How should fluid resuscitation be approached in victims of electrical injury?**
Fluid resuscitation should not be based on the rule of nines as in thermal burns because there is typically more extensive internal injury than manifested by the skin findings. Patients with rhabdomyolysis should be given fluids to maintain urine output of 1–1.5 mL/kg/hr. If there is no evidence of blood in the urine, the goal is 0.5–1 mL/kg/hr.

12. **For the typical child with short-sustained exposure to household current, how do I approach evaluation and management?**
Most pediatric electrical exposures are minor. A tailored evaluation with specific attention to cardiac and neurologic issues, as well as local wound care, is warranted. For household, low-voltage exposures (120–240 volt), any patient with loss of consciousness, history of tetany, wet skin, or current path across heart (hand-to-hand contact) should be monitored for 4 hours for delayed cardiac rhythm disturbances before a disposition is made. If injury is regarded as minor, risk factors are absent, and the general physical examination is normal, brief observation, local wound care, and discharge with appropriate follow-up are sufficient.

13. **What are the admission criteria for cardiac monitoring in children who sustain electrical injuries?**
An electrocardiogram should be obtained if there is a history of tetany or decreased skin resistance by water or burns, or if it is an unwitnessed event. Patients should be admitted to the hospital for 24 hours of cardiac monitoring if there is an abnormal electrocardiogram, past cardiac history, loss of consciousness, or voltage greater than 240 volts.

Bailey B, Gaudreault P, Thivierge RL: Experience with guidelines for cardiac monitoring after electrical injury in children. Am J Emerg Med 18:671–675, 2000.

14. **What are the special concerns in children with mouth commissure burns sustained from biting an electric cord?**
Such burns occur most frequently from 6–36 months of age. The burn is caused by direct contact with the electrical source as well as an arc burn in contact with the wet mouth surface. Patients are often stable on initial presentation, but as the eschar begins to loosen (after approximately 7–14 days), labial artery bleeding may occur. Local care, along with use of an acrylic oral splint, is the mainstay of treatment. Discharge instructions should include an understanding of the risk of rebleeding during the following 1–2 weeks. For the best cosmetic results, surgical reconstruction should be delayed until the burn has fully healed (at least 6–9 months).

15. **List the common pitfalls in evaluation and treatment of electrical injuries.**
- Rescuer injuries at the scene due to inappropriately secured, active electrical lines
- Failure to immobilize the cervical spine and perform the ABCs of trauma assessment
- Failure to consider occult blunt trauma injuries in children with DC exposure
- Underestimating fluid requirements for the severity of the burn, specifically depth of thermal injury

16. **What are the four mechanisms of a lightning strike?**
Direct strike (to either the victim or an object held by the victim) has the highest mortality rate.
Side flash, the most common form, involves a lightning strike that jumps from a primary strike area through the surrounding air to the nearby victim.
Ground strike impacts the ground near the victim. The current enters the victim usually from one foot and exits the other.
Blast phenomenon can occur when rapid cooling of air superheated from lightning causes an explosion with enough force to create blunt trauma, including concussive symptoms.

17. **What is the voltage potential in a lightning strike?**
A typical lightning strike usually exceeds 1 million volts, but its duration is short (on the order of 1/1000 to 1/10,000 of a second). Because of the extreme voltage potential, the mortality rate is approximately 30% and the morbidity rate approximately 70% for all lightning injuries.

Whitcomb D, Martinez JA, Daberkow D: Lightning injuries. South Med J 95:1331–1334, 2002.

18. **How successful is cardiopulmonary resuscitation in victims of a lightning strike?**
If resuscitation is initiated promptly, the survival rate is significantly higher than in other causes of cardiopulmonary arrest. Because of the high voltage and DC, asystole is the usual initial rhythm, whereas ventricular fibrillation results from AC. Aggressive and persistent efforts should be provided.

19. **Discuss the rules of triage for lightning victims.**
Lightning injuries frequently involve more than one victim because people tend to seek shelter in groups. The rules of triage are reversed for lightning injuries, and attention should first be given to those not breathing. Victims with signs of life at the scene are highly likely to survive and should not be treated first. Victims with cardiac or respiratory arrest should receive the greatest efforts because they have a high likelihood of survival with aggressive cardiopulmonary resuscitation.

   Stewart CE: When lightning strikes. Emerg Med Serv 29:57–67, 2000.

20. **Explain feathering burns.**
Feathering burns are microburns due to the electron shower that results in the lightning exposure. They are seen within several hours of injury and resolve within 24 hours. These are called Lichtenberg figures and are pathognomonic for lightning injuries.

21. **How are hearing and vision affected by a lightning strike?**
Perforated tympanic membranes and sensorineural hearing loss have been reported in up to 50% of victims. Fixed, dilated pupils can result from autonomic effects of the lightning strike and are not a reason to terminate resuscitative efforts. Retinal detachment and optic nerve injury also have been reported.

KEY POINTS: APPROACH TO VICTIMS OF A LIGHTNING STRIKE ✔

1. Reverse the rules of triage. Treat those who are not breathing.
2. Pursue aggressive cardiopulmonary resuscitation.
3. Remember that a blown pupil is not an ominous sign and continue resuscitation.

22. **Define keraunoparalysis.**
Keraunoparalysis is the vasospastic paralysis of limbs unique to lightning strikes. It may last several hours before resolution. *Keraunos* is Greek for "thunderbolt" and is used as a prefix to describe lightning-related phenomena.

23. **What are the risks of sustaining a lightning injury indoors?**
The dangers of lightning injury to persons who are indoors are not well known. The two potential risks are telephone and plumbing lines. A current surge on a telephone line, due to a direct lightning strike or, more commonly, to current traveling along the ground, may result in a large voltage difference between telephone apparatus and user. Deaths are rare. Acoustic trauma is the most common form of injury. Current also may travel in grounded pipes to bathtubs and showers. Such injuries have high morbidity and mortality rates because the ground current is highly conductive by the water in the bathtub or shower.

24. **What is the "30–30 Rule"?**

    This is an easy way to remember how to avoid lightning injury. If the time between seeing lightning and hearing thunder is less than 30 seconds, an individual should be seeking shelter. Outdoor activities should not resume until 30 minutes after the last sound of thunder or sighting of lightning. Another easy reminder that can be taught to children is, "If you can see it, flee it; if you can hear it, clear it."

    Zimmermann C, Cooper MA, Holle RL: Lightning safety guidelines. Ann Emerg Med 39:660–664, 2002. National Lightning Safety Institute: www.lightningsafety.com

CHAPTER 66

HEAT-RELATED ILLNESSES

Kathy Palmer, MD

1. **Explain the four methods of heat loss from the body.**
   - Conduction by direct contact of the body with objects and surrounding air
   - Convection to air or liquid that surrounds body tissues
   - Evaporation through perspiration
   - Radiation of infrared energy directly into the environment

   Ewald MB, Baum CR: Environmental emergencies. In Fleisher GR, Ludwig S, Henretig FM (eds): Textbook of Pediatric Emergency Medicine, 5th edition, Philadelphia, Lippincott Williams & Wilkins, 2006, pp 1017–1021.

2. **What environmental conditions predispose to heat-related illnesses?**
   High ambient temperature and humidity. Once ambient temperature equals or exceeds skin temperature, conduction, convection, and radiation cease to be effective methods of heat dissipation. The only remaining method of heat loss is evaporation (perspiration). Evaporative heat loss begins to decrease once ambient humidity reaches 75% and is minimal once it reaches 90–95%. In the presence of high ambient temperature and humidity, the body can no longer dissipate heat by any mechanism and the core temperature inevitably rises, causing heat-related illnesses.

   Ewald MB, Baum CR: Environmental emergencies. In Fleisher GR, Ludwig S, Henretig FM (eds): Textbook of Pediatric Emergency Medicine, 5th edition. Philadelphia, Lippincott Williams & Wilkins, 2006, pp 1017–1021.

3. **What is the best type of clothing to prevent heat-related illness?**
   Light-colored clothing permeable to moisture but impervious to radiant heat from the environment allows heat loss by evaporation but prevents heat gain by radiation from the environment. During longer periods of activity, dry clothes should replace sweat-saturated garments.

4. **Why are children at a greater risk for heat-related illnesses than adults?**
   - Larger ratio of body surface area to mass (greater heat exchange with the environment)
   - Higher set point (change in rectal temperature at which sweating starts)
   - Greater endogenous heat production
   - Lower output of sweat
   - Greater thermoregulatory impairment by dehydration
   - Blunted thirst response in comparison with adults

   Neonates are at greatest risk because they have poorly developed thermoregulatory mechanisms and depend on others to remove them from a hot environment and provide adequate hydration.

   Bytonski JB: Heat illness in children. Curr Sports Med Rep 2:320–324, 2003.

5. **What situations or activities are associated with a high risk for heat-related illnesses in children?**
   - **Saunas, steam rooms, whirlpools, and hot tubs:** Severe hyperthermia secondary to rapid conduction of heat from the water
   - **Unventilated automobiles in the hot sun:** Temperatures can reach 60° C within 15 minutes when a car is left in the sun at 30–40° C.

6. **What patient factors predispose to heat-related illnesses?**
   1. Conditions associated with excessive fluid loss (fever, gastrointestinal infection, diabetes insipidus, and diabetes mellitus)
   2. Suboptimal sweating (spina bifida)
   3. Excessive sweating (some cyanotic heart disease)
   4. Diminished thirst (cystic fibrosis)
   5. Inadequate drinking (mental retardation, young children who rely on others for liquid intake)
   6. Abnormal hypothalamic thermoregulatory function (anorexia nervosa, prior heat-related illness)
   7. Obesity

   American Academy of Pediatrics Committee on Sports Medicine and Fitness: Climactic heat stress and the exercising child and adolescent. Pediatrics 106:158–159, 2000.

7. **What is the most important risk factor for heat-related illnesses?**
   Dehydration. Participants in sports associated with intentional weight loss immediately before competition (wrestlers, jockeys, and boxers) are at increased risk for heat-related illnesses. Attempts at rapid oral rehydration after weighing in are not successful at preventing heat-related illness because plasma volumes remain decreased despite return to normal body weight.

8. **What problems are considered minor heat emergencies?**
   Heat edema, heat cramps, and heat syncope.

   Pratt A: Putting the chill on heat-related illness Contemp Pediatr June:23–28, 2005.

9. **What is heat edema? How is it treated?**
   Heat edema is mild swelling of the feet and ankles during the summer months, usually worse in the first few days of exposure. No treatment is necessary except reassurance.

10. **What are heat cramps? How are they treated?**
    Heat cramps are painful involuntary spasms of major muscle groups during or immediately after exercise in a hot environment. Symptoms may be exacerbated by excessive intake of hypotonic fluids during exercise. Heat cramps are treated by placing the victim in a cool environment and replacing fluid and salt losses. Oral electrolyte solutions (or 1 tsp of table salt in 500 mL of water) are appropriate for milder cases; IV fluids (20 mL/kg of 0.9 normal saline solution) are used in more severe cases. Appropriate conditioning, acclimation, and adequate hydration can prevent heat cramps.

    Bytonski JB: Heat illness in children. Curr Sports Med Rep 2:320–324, 2003.

11. **What is heat syncope? How is it treated?**
    A syncopal event caused by prolonged standing in hot weather is seen most often in military recruits and marching band members. High temperatures, vasodilatation, and relative dehydration are the precursors. Heat syncope is treated by placing the victim in a recumbent position in a cool environment and administering oral fluids. Minimal knee bending can prevent future syncopal events while standing at attention for prolonged periods.

    Lugo-Amador NM: Heat-related illness. Emerg Med Clin North Am 22:315–327, 2004.

12. **What is the difference between heat exhaustion and heat stroke?**
Heat exhaustion and heat stroke are a continuum of heat-related illnesses that occur when the body's heat loss mechanisms are overwhelmed or insufficient to respond to environmental demands. Heat exhaustion is the less severe of the two and is believed to represent reversible heat overload, whereas heat stroke is characteristically associated with irreversible tissue damage.

13. **What are the clinical characteristics of heat exhaustion? How is it treated?**
Heat exhaustion is a precursor to heat stroke and therefore warrants vigorous treatment. Symptoms include temperature elevation, nausea, vomiting, headache, excessive sweating, hyperventilation, and intense fatigue. Victims have a relatively normal mental status except for mild confusion, clumsiness, unsteadiness, dizziness, or weakness. Tachycardia, tachypnea, and orthostatic hypotension are often present. Hemoconcentration, hypernatremia, hyperchloremia, and urinary concentration are common. Treatment includes allowing the victim to rest in a cool environment, administering oral fluids (IV fluids in more severe cases), external cooling (e.g., fans, ice, sponge baths), and monitoring for signs of heat stroke. An adolescent or adult should consume 1–2 L of cold water over 2–4 hours. Cooling to the point of shivering should be avoided because shivering increases the body's endogenous heat load.

   Glazer JL: Management of heatstroke and heat exhaustion. Am Fam Phys 71:2133–2142, 2005.

14. **What are the two variants of heat stroke?**
Classical and exertional.
   Classical heat stroke presents with coma, elevated temperature, and hot, dry skin. Heat stroke is often seen in epidemic proportions during heat waves when victims are constantly exposed to elevated temperature and humidity for several days without relief. The typical pediatric victim initially becomes dehydrated; if left untreated over a period of days, symptoms progress to lethargy, coma, and ultimately death. The disease process may advance more rapidly if the child is exposed to extremely high temperatures (e.g., if left in an unventilated car in the summer).
   Exertional heat stroke most often is associated with strenuous physical activity in hot weather; poorly conditioned and poorly acclimated patients are at the highest risk. Exertional heat stroke most often presents with an acute deterioration of mental status.

   Ewald MB, Baum CR: Environmental emergencies. In Fleisher GR, Ludwig, S, Henretig FM (eds): Textbook of Pediatric Emergency Medicine, 5th edition, Philadelphia, Lippincott Williams & Wilkins, 2006, pp 1017–1021.

15. **What are the central nervous system manifestations of heat stroke?**
Central nervous system dysfunction can be manifested in many ways, including a sense of impending doom, headache, dizziness, weakness, confusion, euphoria, gait disturbance, combativeness, seizures, posturing, and coma. The early clinical symptoms are sometimes overlooked because they often are perceived to be the normal result of exertion. Often the severity of the problem is realized only when the victim collapses suddenly.

   Glazer JL: Management of heatstroke and heat exhaustion. Am Fam Phys 71:2133–2142, 2005.

16. **Describe the clinical characteristics of heat stroke.**
Shock (hypovolemic), altered mental status, and rectal temperature > 40° C are suggestive but not diagnostic for heat stroke. Sweating may or may not be present. Dehydration, tachycardia, tachypnea, and postural or frank hypotension may be seen. In more severe cases, seizures, posturing, or coma is present.

   Ewald MB, Baum CR: Environmental emergencies. In Fleisher GR, Ludwig S, Henretig FM (eds): Textbook of Pediatric Emergency Medicine, 5th edition, Philadelphia, Lippincott Williams & Wilkins, 2006, pp 1017–1021.

17. **How is heat stroke treated?**
The goals of therapy are to restore intravascular volume and to lower core body temperature. Treat the victim as you would any other patient with shock:
1. Address airway, breathing, and circulation while moving the victim to a cool, shaded environment.
2. Obtain large-bore IV access, and place a Foley catheter to monitor urine output.
3. Attach the patient to a cardiac monitor and supply supplemental oxygen.
4. Administer crystalloid solutions (normal saline or lactated Ringer's) to address hypovolemia or hypotension.
5. Begin external cooling as soon as possible.
6. Order initial laboratory studies: blood gas, complete blood count, clotting studies, electrolytes, glucose, renal and liver function tests, and electrocardiography. Be prepared to treat arrhythmias and seizure activity and to correct electrolyte imbalances.
7. Cooling should be continued until the core temperature reaches 38.5° C.
8. More severe cases may require central venous pressure monitoring and inotropic support. α-Adrenergic drugs should be avoided because they decrease skin perfusion and limit heat dissipation.
9. All victims of heat stroke require hospitalization, the majority in an intensive care setting.
Lugo-Amador NM: Heat-related illness. Emerg Med Clin North Am 22:315–327, 2004.

18. **List the possible complications of heat stroke.**
Acidosis, electrolyte imbalance, adynamic ileus, dysrhythmias, shivering, seizures, rhabdomyolysis, disseminated intravascular coagulation, renal failure, hepatic damage, permanent neurologic sequelae, and death.
Glazer JL: Management of heatstroke and heat exhaustion. Am Fam Phys 71:2133–2142, 2005.

19. **Explain heat acclimatization.**
Acclimatization describes the body's physiologic adaptation to tolerate activity in a hot, humid environment. Acclimatized people demonstrate increased ability to sweat and improved conservation of total body sodium. Well-conditioned athletes acclimate to hot weather more efficiently than their poorly conditioned peers. People who are not acclimatized are at greater risk for heat-related illnesses.
American Academy of Pediatrics Committee on Sports Medicine and Fitness: Climactic heat stress and the exercising child and adolescent. Pediatrics 106:158–159, 2000.

20. **How long does it take to acclimate to a hot, humid environment?**
Eight to 12 days in adults. Children require a gradual increase in duration and intensity of activity over 10–14 days. The American Academy of Pediatrics recommends "as many as 8 to 10 exposures (30–45 minutes each) to the new climate to acclimatize sufficiently. Such exposures can be taken at a rate of one per day or one every other day." Athletes who plan to compete during the midday should include periods of training during the warmer midday hours.
American Academy of Pediatrics Committee on Sports Medicine and Fitness: Climactic heat stress and the exercising child and adolescent. Pediatrics 106:158–159, 2000.

21. **What is the best way to provide external cooling for victims of heat-related illnesses?**
The victim's clothing should be removed to allow maximal skin exposure and heat dissipation. The most traditional method of cooling involves covering the patient with sheets or towels that have been immersed in ice water and then allowing a fan to blow across them; sheets and towels should be changed frequently to keep them cool. Ice baths or ice water baths have been advocated by some authors, but they are impractical in more severe cases of heat stroke requiring cardiopulmonary resuscitation or defibrillation.

Evaporative cooling can be accomplished by spraying the skin with cool water and allowing a fan to blow across the moistened skin. Cooling by evaporation is more efficient than ice water baths in reducing core body temperature.

Alternative methods of cooling that require special training or equipment include peritoneal lavage with cold fluids, cardiopulmonary bypass, ice water enemas, and bladder and gastric lavage.

Stewart C, Ruddy R: The spectrum of heat illness in children. Pediatr Emerg Med Rep 4:41–52, 1999.

22. **What methods of cooling are ineffective or harmful?**
    - **Alcohol baths:** Children are susceptible to toxic absorption of alcohol through the skin
    - **Antipyretics:** Not successful in decreasing temperatures secondary to heat-related illnesses

    Stewart C, Ruddy R: The spectrum of heat illness in children. Pediatr Emerg Med Rep 4:41–52, 1999.

23. **How can heat-related illnesses be prevented?**
    Physical activity should be modified in the face of high ambient temperature and humidity. Athletes should be well hydrated before initiating physical activity and should continue to consume cold water throughout the exercise period and after exercise has been completed to avoid dehydration. Clothing should be lightweight and light-colored, with as much skin exposed as possible to allow evaporative dissipation of heat. Athletes should participate in a preseason conditioning program and allow a period of acclimation when exercising in the hot summer months.

    Glazer JL: Management of heatstroke and heat exhaustion. Am Fam Phys 71:2133–2142, 2005.

KEY POINTS FOR HEAT-RELATED ILLNESS ✓

1. Heat-related illness can be fatal but is most importantly PREVENTABLE.

2. Heatstroke is the third most common cause of exercise-related deaths in U.S. high schools (following head injuries and cardiac disorders).

3. Adequate hydration before, during, and after exercising is one of the key elements in prevention of heat-related illness.

4. Children may require as long as 2 weeks to acclimate safely to exercising in a hot climate.

24. **What is the Wet Bulb Globe Temperature (WBGT) Index?**
    The WBGT index is an attempt to standardize the effects of heat, humidity, and solar radiation on the body. It reflects the influence of ambient temperature, humidity, and solar radiation. Recommendations for modification of physical activity in hot weather are based on the WBGT index.

    The U.S. Armed Forces WBGT index can be found on the following website: www.usariem.army.mil/heatinjury.htm.

25. **What are the current recommendations for modification of activity in hot, humid weather?**
    See Table 66-1.

    American Academy of Pediatrics Committee on Sports Medicine and Fitness. Climactic heat stress and the exercising child and adolescent. Pediatrics 106:158–159, 2000.

TABLE 66-1. RESTRAINTS ON ACTIVITIES AT DIFFERENT LEVELS OF HEAT STRESS*

WBGT		
°C	°F	Restraints on Activities
<24	<75	All activities allowed, but be alert for prodromes of heat-related illness in prolonged events
24.0–25.9	75.0–78.6	Longer rest periods in the shade; enforce drinking every 15 min
26–29	79–84	Stop activity of unacclimatized persons and other persons with high risk; limit activities of all others (disallow long-distance races, cut down further duration of other activities)
>29	>85	Cancel all athletic activities

*WBGT is *not* air temperature. It indicates *wet bulb globe temperature*, an index of climatic heat stress that can be measured on the field by the use of a psychrometer. This apparatus, available commercially, is composed of three thermometers. One (wet bulb [WB]) has a wet wick around it to monitor humidity. Another is inside a hollow black ball (globe [G]) to monitor radiation. The third is a simple thermometer (temperature [T]) to measure air temperature. The heat stress index is calculated as WBGT = 0.7 WB temp + 0.2G temp + 0.1 T temp. It is noteworthy that 70% of the stress is due to humidity, 20% to radiation, and only 10% to air temperature.
From American Academy of Pediatrics Committee on Sports Medicine and Fitness: Climactic heat stress and the exercising child and adolescent. Pediatrics 106:158–159, 2000; with permission.

26. **How much fluid is required to maintain hydration during exercise?**
Exercising athletes may lose 2–3% of body weight before they become thirsty. Athletes should drink 8 ounces of cold water 10–15 minutes before exercising and consume an additional 8–12 ounces every 20–30 minutes during exercise. Heavier athletes require more fluid; smaller athletes may require less. When beginning training in the heat, athletes should weigh themselves before and after a workout to ensure adequate postexercise rehydration—a pint of water for every pound lost. Maintenance of clear, unconcentrated urine output indicates adequate hydration.

27. **Why is even mild dehydration and heat exposure a dangerous combination in children?**
Children who are dehydrated experience an excessive increase in core body temperature when exposed to a hot environment compared to their well-hydrated peers and similarly hydrated adults.

American Academy of Pediatrics Committee on Sports Medicine and Fitness. Climactic heat stress and the exercising child and adolescent. Pediatrics 106:158–159, 2000.

28. **How much fluid should a child drink while exercising in a hot climate?**
They should begin the exercise period well hydrated, and periodic drinking should be enforced during the exercise period. For every 20 minutes of exercise, 150 mL of cold tap water or a flavored salted beverage should be consumed for a 40-kg child (250 mL for a 60-kg adolescent). The child should be encouraged to drink even if he or she is not thirsty.

American Academy of Pediatrics Committee on Sports Medicine and Fitness. Climactic heat stress and the exercising child and adolescent. Pediatrics 106:158–159, 2000.

29.   **What are the benefits of flavored sports drinks?**
Flavored sports drinks were shown to increase voluntary drinking by 90% over plain water. Adding salt to sports drinks also enhances thirst. The recommended concentration is 15–20 mmol NaCl/L or 1 gm of NaCl in 2 pints of water.

American Academy of Pediatrics Committee on Sports Medicine and Fitness. Climactic heat stress and the exercising child and adolescent. Pediatrics 106:158–159, 2000.

WEBSITES

1. The American Red Cross: Heat-related illness
   www.redcross.org/services/hss/tips/heat.html

2. Centers for Disease Control and Prevention: Tips for preventing heat-related illness
   http://www.bt.cdc.gov/disasters/extremeheat/heattips.asp

CHAPTER 67

HYPOTHERMIA

Howard M. Corneli, MD

1. **Why are children more prone to hypothermia than adults?**
   - Children have larger body surface–to–mass ratios.
   - They may have less insulation, faster metabolism, and smaller energy reserves.
   - They may be more at risk for medical illness, trauma, or environmental exposure.

2. **Does hypothermia require severe cold exposure?**
   No. Unfortunately, clinicians may suspect hypothermia only when severe environmental exposure is evident. Any immersion in warm or cold water, or any major illness or trauma, may precipitate hypothermia. It is also seen in conditions as diverse as sepsis, hypoglycemia, drug ingestion, and child abuse, any of which may be occult.
   Children are more at risk than adults for iatrogenic hypothermia due to rescue, transport, and resuscitation.

3. **Why is hypothermia overlooked in pediatric patients in the emergency department (ED)?**
   Hypothermia victims only appear cold in the mild range of hypothermia. In deeper hypothermia, signs such as shivering, pallor, cyanosis, and agitation are replaced by flushing, edema, muscular rigidity, and decreased mental status. Standard clinical thermometers only measure down to 94° F (34° C).

4. **What are some risk factors for hypothermia?**

Trauma	Rescue
Severe illness	Transport
Immersion or submersion	Resuscitation
Exposure to wind or cold air	Intoxication, especially with:
Central nervous system illness or injury	Alcohol
Hypothalamic dysfunction	Barbiturates
Endocrine impairment	Phenothiazines
Metabolic impairment	Burns and weeping dermatoses
Iatrogenic causes	Child abuse (e.g., cold water baths)

5. **What clinical clues should prompt measurement of core temperature?**
   - Any of the above risk factors (including, but not limited to, any critical care patient)
   - Decreased mental status, respiration, or circulation without other obvious cause
   - A J (Osborne) wave on electrocardiogram (Fig. 67-1) is diagnostic when present, but is seen in only about 10–80% of cases in various series.

   Nolan J, Soar J: Images in resuscitation: The ECG in hypothermia. Resuscitation 64:133, 2005.

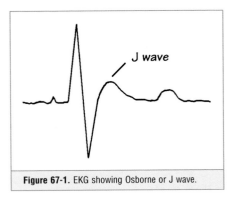

Figure 67-1. EKG showing Osborne or J wave.

6. **How should temperatures be taken to detect hypothermia?**
   A low-reading thermometer must be used. Oral and axillary temperatures are unreliable.
   Rectal temperatures are subject to damping, artifact, and time lags up to 1 hour. If used,
   rectal temperatures must be taken deep in the rectum for at least several minutes. The reliability
   of tympanic temperatures in the setting of significant hypothermia has not been established.
   Temperature probes in the bladder, esophagus, or nasopharynx are typically used to provide
   core temperatures of the trunk.

   Danzl DF, Pozos RS: Accidental hypothermia. N Engl J Med 331:1756, 1994.

7. **Define mild, moderate, and severe hypothermia.**
   - **Mild hypothermia:** Temperature ranges from approximately 32° to 35° C. In this range,
     the body attempts to combat heat loss by shivering, increasing metabolism and
     vasoconstriction.
   - **Moderate hypothermia:** Temperature spans the range from 28° to 32° C. In this range,
     compensatory mechanisms begin to fail, and mental status may be altered.
   - **Severe hypothermia:** Temperature ($<$ 28° C) leads to failed thermoregulation, metabolic
     shutdown, and paradoxical vasodilatation accompanied by hypovolemia, decreased
     perfusion, and stupor or coma.

   Corneli HM: Hot topics in cold medicine: Controversies in accidental hypothermia. Clin Pediatr Emerg
   Med 2:179–191, 2001.

8. **Describe some landmarks for converting between Celsius and Fahrenheit.**
   At the upper end of the hypothermic range, 35° C equals 95° F. The threshold of severe
   hypothermia, 28° C, can be inverted to yield 82° F. Starting with these landmarks, an
   approximate 2:1 ratio between degrees Fahrenheit and degrees Celsius gives workable
   conversions. For example, 30° C, an increase of 2° from 28° C, is equivalent to 86° F, an
   increase of 4° from 82° F.

9. **Describe the major causes of hypothermic death during rescue and
   resuscitation.**
   Afterdrop is the continued cooling of a body after removal from cold. Due in part to conduction,
   it can be increased markedly with peripheral rewarming or muscular exertion, which rapidly
   return cold acidotic blood from the periphery to the core circulation.
   Rewarming shock is almost universal in severe or prolonged hypothermia. Hypovolemia is
   caused by profound diuresis and fluid shifts out of the vasculature, worsened by sludging
   of cold thick blood, and augmented by cardiac collapse, vascular dilation, and loss of

autoregulation. Afterdrop, peripheral rewarming, and exertion all challenge the collapsed circulation. Shock and death often result unless copious warmed IV fluids can be provided. **Asystole** and **ventricular fibrillation** are common endpoints in severe hypothermia. Profound bradycardia and hypotension, often present initially, may be adequate to maintain the minimal metabolic needs of patients with core temperature below 28° C. Further cooling, rough handling, mechanical stress, and exertion have all been linked to deterioration from a perfusing to a nonperfusing rhythm.

10. **What rules of advanced life support may be altered in hypothermia?**
If the core temperature is known to be below 28° C, cardiopulmonary resuscitation (CPR) may be withheld in the presence of a pulse, no matter how slow or weak, and no matter the blood pressure. Some experts would withhold CPR in pulseless patients this cold if a narrow-complex QRS were seen on electrocardiography. In this temperature range, only minimal circulation is required, and CPR is relatively ineffective and may provoke ventricular fibrillation.

If, however, the temperature cannot be taken accurately, or if no pulse or narrow QRS can be established, CPR is indicated at standard rates. Earlier concerns about intubation have been put to rest by further study. Interventions should be made gently because cardiac arrest has been associated with rough handling, patient exertion, and iatrogenic cooling.

KEY POINTS: HYPOTHERMIA IN CHILDREN ✓

1. Children are particularly prone to hypothermia, especially with serious illness or injury.

2. Serious hypothermia often goes undetected by clinicians without a high degree of suspicion.

3. Although it may provide for an occasional remarkable recovery after prolonged resuscitation, hypothermia is generally harmful.

4. Moderate and severe hypothermia alter standard resuscitation measures.

11. **Should blood gases be corrected for patient temperature?**
The long-standing belief that blood gases are best corrected for patient temperature has been overturned by evidence that uncorrected gases better reflect the true physiology of the hypothermic state, lead to more appropriate therapy, and are associated with improved outcomes.

12. **What standard treatments are usually safe and effective in hypothermia?**
Almost all hypothermic patients are volume depleted, and volume replacement with warmed isotonic IV fluid is essential. Administration of oxygen and maintenance of the airway is indicated. Although some patients will be hyperglycemic, hypoglycemia is common, and infusion of dextrose in 5–10% solutions is indicated if the blood glucose is unknown. Lidocaine and vasopressors may be helpful at times if indicated. Cardioversion of ventricular fibrillation may not be effective until after rewarming, but case reports of success at low temperatures probably warrant at least one or two attempts with standard energy settings before further rewarming.

American Heart Association: 2005 guidelines for cardiopulmonary resuscitation and emergency cardiovascular care. Part 10.4. Hypothermia. Circulation 112:136–138, 2005.

13. **What commonly used treatments are *not* routinely recommended for hypothermia?**
The routine administration of antibiotics or corticosteroids is not beneficial in hypothermia. Sodium bicarbonate is probably contraindicated, as acidosis is relatively physiologic in the hypothermic state, and the use of bicarbonate has provoked dangerous alkalosis after rewarming. Insulin for hyperglycemia is contraindicated, since this condition will usually resolve with rewarming, and the insulin will become effective only at that time. The same caution applies to many other medications.

14. **Is room-temperature IV fluid thermally neutral?**
At approximately 70° F (21° C), room temperature fluid is colder than all but the coldest hypothermia patients. The infusion of room-temperature fluid has been associated with further cooling of patients and with shock, ventricular fibrillation, arrest, and death.

15. **What is the best way to deliver warm IV fluids in the ED?**
Immersion-bath and coil-sleeve warmers do not effectively warm IV fluids, and they markedly slow flow. Microwave ovens can be used in a pinch to warm IV fluids in plastic bags. This requires prior experimentation to see how long a particular oven requires to warm a standard IV bag to a temperature of 40–44° C. Unless these fluids are given very rapidly through specifically designed short, large-bore IV tubing, however, they cool before reaching the patient. The preferred method is to use countercurrent blood warmers designed for rapid warming and rapid infusion. These come with large-bore plumbed tubing to ensure the delivery of warm fluid to the patient.

16. **Describe three rewarming strategies.**
Passive rewarming involves placing the patient in a warm room, covering with dry (not warm) blankets, and allowing spontaneous gradual rewarming. This method has no demonstrated advantage in pediatrics, and is associated with increased morbidity and mortality.
Active external rewarming involves measures such as warm baths or blankets, plumbed pads, chemical heat packs, heat lamps, and forced-air warming. Although available in many settings, these techniques often promote the dumping of cold, acidotic blood from the periphery onto the core, and increase metabolic demand and circulatory work prior to volume expansion or cardiac rewarming. Thus, they are associated with afterdrop and rewarming shock, and may potentiate ventricular fibrillation. These methods should be reserved for stable patients with mild hypothermia. They are also useful to prevent cooling during the resuscitation of normothermic children.
Core rewarming methods range from the simplest, such as warmed IV fluids and heated, humidified oxygen; through warmed irrigation of the bladder, stomach, colon, peritoneum, or left pleural cavity; to extracorporeal circulation (i.e., the heart–lung pump). These methods are more effective and support the patient. They decrease the risk of afterdrop and rewarming shock. They are indicated in moderate to severe hypothermia; the more aggressive methods are preferred in the setting of hypothermia with circulatory compromise or cardiac arrest.

Walpoth BH, Walpoth-Aslan BN, Mattle HP, et al: Outcome of survivors of accidental deep hypothermia and circulatory arrest treated with extracorporeal rewarming. N Engl J Med 337:1500–1505, 1997.

17. **If active external rewarming is sought, what is the best method?**
Current evidence suggests that forced-air warming using devices such as the Bair Hugger (Arizant Healthcare, Eden Prairie, MN) may be most effective and associated with less afterdrop in patients with intact circulation. Such devices limit patient access to some degree. There is little evidence or logic to suggest that any external rewarming method would work well in patients with absent or severely depressed circulation.

18. **What is the ideal rewarming rate?**

There is no single ideal rate. Even if there were, achievable rewarming rates vary among patients with different degrees of metabolic and circulatory impairment. Rather, the method chosen should be matched to the patient's needs and the severity of hypothermia. Rapid or profound cooling warrants rapid rewarming. Most children suffer from acute hypothermia and will tolerate rapid rewarming if given aggressive volume expansion and other support. The core methods above are listed in approximate order of increasing effectiveness. If the method chosen does not produce rapid rewarming, a more effective method should be employed.

19. **Discuss the treatment of frostbite.**

After core rewarming to at least 35° C and after any risk of further chilling is past, frostbitten body parts should be rapidly rewarmed. This is done in a bath carefully maintained at 40° C to 42° C for 15–30 minutes, until flushing indicates reperfusion. Narcotic analgesia is indicated. Tetanus immunization should be updated, and the affected part should be elevated. Blisters that appear blue or black are left intact. Pink or white blisters should be opened because they contain thromboxane, which increases inflammation and promotes thrombosis. Either type of blister can be covered with aloe ointments. Prostaglandin inhibitors, such as ibuprofen, are administered orally to counteract the effects of thromboxane. Immediate amputation is never indicated. Admission and ongoing care are usually best directed by specialists in burn, plastic, or trauma surgery.

Koljonen V, Andersson, K, Mikkonen K, Vuola J: Frostbite injuries treated in the Helsinki area from 1995 to 2002. J Trauma 57:1315–1320, 2004.

Murphy JV, Banwell PE, Roberts AH, et al: Frostbite: Pathogenesis and treatment. J Trauma 48:171–178, 2000.

KEY POINTS: TREATMENT OF FROSTBITE ✓

1. Rapidly rewarm frostbitten parts in a bath of water at 40–42° C.

2. Give narcotic analgesics.

3. Leave blue or black blisters intact.

4. Open pink or white blisters.

5. Give oral ibuprofen to counteract effects of thromboxane.

6. Admit the patient and involve surgical colleagues.

20. **Does hypothermia alter usual prognostic indicators?**

Yes. Intact survival has been reported after submersion for up to 79 minutes, immersion for hours, exposure for days, core temperatures as low as 14° C, and CPR for up to 9 hours.

Gilbert M, Busund R, Skagseth A, et al: Resuscitation from accidental hypothermia of 13.7 degrees C with circulatory arrest. Lancet 355:375–376, 2000.

21. **Cite exceptions to the rule, "no one is dead until they're warm and dead."**

    This rule does not apply in the face of injuries incompatible with survival. It cannot be applied if the patient cannot be rescued from a cold environment in the first place, or if maximal available rewarming methods are ineffective and transport is not an option. Finally, failure to restore a circulating cardiac rhythm after 30 minutes of resuscitation above a core temperature of 32° C is usually a sign of irreversible death.

    Auerbach PS: Some people are dead when they're cold and dead. JAMA 264:1856–1857, 1990.

CHAPTER 68

CHEMICAL AND BIOLOGICAL TERRORISM

Fred M. Henretig, MD

1. **What happened in Tokyo on March 20, 1995?**
   On March 20, 1995, at the height of morning rush hour, members of the Japanese Aum Shinrikyo religious cult placed containers of the deadly nerve agent sarin in various downtown locations of the Tokyo subway system and unleashed a new era in terrorism. This same group attempted unsuccessfully to deploy anthrax and botulinum toxin weapons on several occasions. The chemical warfare attack on Tokyo affected more than 5000 victims and caused 12 deaths.

   Henretig FM, Cieslak TJ, Madsen JM, et al: Emergency department awareness and response to incidents of biological and chemical terrorism. In Fleisher GF, Ludwig S, Henretig FM (eds): Textbook of Pediatric Emergency Medicine, 5th ed. Philadelphia, Lippincott Williams & Wilkins, 2006, pp 135–162.
   Rotenberg JS, Newmark J: Nerve agent attacks on children: Diagnosis and management. Pediatrics 112:648–658, 2003.

2. **How is the Tokyo incident typical of recent terrorism?**
   Prior decades had witnessed numerous attacks targeted at military installations, government officials or representatives, or, on occasion, relatively small groups of ordinary civilians in highly visible circumstances. In the 1990s a new threshold was crossed, however, with the rise of religious terrorism that allows violence as a seemingly justifiable means to accomplish a sacred theological imperative. Several terrorist incidents over the past decade, such as the Oklahoma City bombing and, of course, the attacks of September 11, 2001, on the World Trade Center and the Pentagon have highlighted this new willingness to kill large numbers of innocent people indiscriminately. An especially disturbing scenario in terms of the medical management challenges posed is that of the use of biologic and chemical weapons as a means of terrorism. In 1984, the Rajneeshee cult sickened 750 citizens of The Dalles, a town in Oregon, by intentionally contaminating restaurant salad bars with *Salmonella typhimurium*. More recently, persons linked to white-supremacist militias have obtained anthrax, stockpiled the highly toxic substance ricin (a biotoxin extracted from castor beans), and have been arrested for transporting the bacterium *Yersinia pestis*, the etiologic agent of bubonic plague. In 1995, the FBI thwarted an attempt to release a chlorine gas bomb in Disneyland, an attack obviously targeted particularly at children. And then came the mysterious epidemic of illness that began in October 2001.

3. **What did we learn from the anthrax outbreak of 2001?**
   This outbreak was characterized by 22 confirmed or suspected cases (11 inhalational, 11 cutaneous), with five deaths, resulting from presumed or known exposure to anthrax-contaminated mail. At least five letters containing highly weaponized anthrax spores were sent to government and business offices in Florida, Washington, DC, and New York City from Trenton, New Jersey. This means of dispersal represents one mode of attack, but many bioterrorism defense experts fear even more a widespread aerosol release (e.g., from a small crop duster–type airplane) that could potentially sicken hundreds of thousands. As it was, even the 2001 attack resulted in enormous public anxiety and major demands for medical care and public health resources. Antibiotic prophylaxis was prescribed for over 30,000 persons, and decontamination of just the Hart Senate Office Building alone took months and cost more than $20 million.

   Centers for Disease Control and Prevention: Update: investigation of bioterrorism-related anthrax and interim guidelines for exposure management and antimicrobial therapy, October 2001. MMWR Morb Mortal Wkly Rep 50:909–919, 2001.

4. **Why are such incidents of particular importance to emergency department (ED) personnel?**

Such incidents illustrate the potential for biologic or chemical terrorist attacks, thus the imperative that health care workers, particularly first-responders and ED personnel, be familiar with the expedient diagnosis and management of chemical and biologic terrorist events.

5. **What are the four basic phases of disaster response?**
   1. Preparedness
   2. Actual response
   3. Mitigation
   4. Recovery, both short and long term

   Agency for Healthcare Research and Quality: Pediatric Terrorism and Disaster Preparedness: A Resource for Pediatricians: www.ahrq.gov./research/pedprep/resource.htm

6. **Why do terrorists use biologic and chemical weapons?**

The term *weapons of mass destruction* (WMD) has been used to denote weapons using nuclear, biologic, or chemical agents in devices intended to kill and injure large numbers of victims. Biologic and chemical weapons are believed by U.S. military and counterterrorism experts to constitute a likely mode of WMD attack on civilian populations by terrorist groups. These agents are relatively inexpensive and technically less difficult to produce and deploy than nuclear weapons, the raw materials for their production are less regulated, and there is wide access to biologic and chemical agent information via the Internet.

Chemical and biologic weapons can be deployed easily, using relatively simple devices, such as garden sprayers, aerial crop dusting equipment, or insect control vehicles. In addition, a conventional attack on factories, chemical production facilities, or tank cars may result in the release of toxic industrial chemicals, with effects similar to those of an attack by military chemical warfare agents. Biologic agents may involve aerosol dispersal or possible contamination of food or water supplies.

7. **What are the potential medical consequences of a chemical attack?**

Chemical attacks probably would combine elements of traditional mass disasters (e.g., earthquakes), in which large numbers of casualties occur almost immediately, and traditional hazardous materials (HAZMAT) incidents. However, they may be more catastrophic for several reasons:
- Intent to inflict mass casualties
- Hazardous materials of extreme lethality
- HAZMAT site that is extremely toxic to rescue workers
- Less information about agent(s) involved
- Potentially overwhelming numbers of patients requiring emergency medical services (EMS)
- Even larger number of mildly affected or "worried-well" patients self-transporting to EDs and placing additional demands on the health care system
- Mass hysteria and panic

   Henretig FM, Cieslak TJ, Eitzen EM Jr: Biological and chemical terrorism. J Pediatr 141:311–326, 2002.

8. **Which of these features were observed in the 1995 Tokyo sarin attack?**

One ED close to the scene received more than 500 patients, including three in cardiopulmonary arrest. Citywide, over 5000 persons sought emergency medical treatment at more than 200 facilities within a few hours, and about 25% required hospitalization. Of note, 90% of victims went to hospitals by taxi, private vehicles, or on foot rather than by formal EMS transport, further compounding the initial chaos. Until the identity of the agent was known, significant efforts at patient decontamination were lacking, resulting in many symptomatic exposures to hospital staff, although most were mild.

   Okumura T, Suzuki K, Fukuda A, et al: The Tokyo subway sarin attack: Disaster management Part 2: Hospital response. Acad Emerg Med 5:618–624, 1998.

9. **How would a biologic attack differ from a chemical attack?**
   Because of incubation periods, attacks with biologic agents must be viewed differently than conventional and chemical terrorist attacks. The scenario is more like that of a public health crisis than an EMS or HAZMAT emergency. Exposed persons may well be unaware of the attack, and disperse from the site of initial exposure. Many diseases caused by high-threat agents begin with nonspecific febrile syndromes. The first indication of a biologic attack is likely to be an epidemic of an unusually large number of persons presenting to diverse locations, possibly several days after exposure, with either early nonspecific clinical findings or later findings of severe disease. Thus, patients may present to various medical offices and EDs in piecemeal fashion, reporting, for example, flulike symptoms. This was clearly illustrated by the mail-borne anthrax outbreak in the fall of 2001.

10. **What clues suggest a biologic attack?**
    Pediatricians and emergency physicians must maintain an index of suspicion if a biologic attack is to be diagnosed in time for useful measures to be undertaken. Several epidemiologic features may suggest a bioagent attack:
    - Epidemic presentation in a relatively compressed time frame (because most persons would be exposed at the same time)
    - Diseases that are rare or not endemic in the area of exposure
    - Especially high infection rate among exposed persons
    - More respiratory forms of disease than usual
    - Particularly high morbidity or mortality
    - Several epidemics at once
    - Attack rates lower in persons sheltered from the suspected route of exposure
    - Infected or dying animals
    - Discovery of suspicious actions or potential delivery systems

    The earliest suspicion of such an attack should be reported at once to appropriate public health authorities.

    Henretig FM, Cieslak TJ, Madsen JM, et al: Emergency department awareness and response to incidents of biological and chemical terrorism. In Fleisher GF, Ludwig S, Henretig FM (eds): Textbook of Pediatric Emergency Medicine 5th, ed. Philadelphia, Lippincott Williams & Wilkins, 2006, pp 135–162.

11. **Why may children be disproportionately affected by both chemical and biologic agents?**
    - Many agents are aerosolized as the intended route of exposure. Children have higher minute ventilation rates and live closer to the ground, which enhances respiratory exposure, especially for agents denser than air.
    - Children have thinner and more permeable skin, allowing greater injury from vesicant or corrosive chemicals and in some cases faster systemic absorption (e.g., nerve agents).
    - Children have age-related developmental vulnerabilities that may hamper their ability to escape exposure from a contaminated site.
    - Children may suffer unique psychological trauma in the context of separation from parents or witnessing the death of family members.
    - Pediatric experience with several of the relevant antibiotics, antidotes, and vaccines is limited; in several cases, thoughtful use of treatments usually considered contraindicated in children may be necessary.
    - The health care response to children would be hampered by the usual decrements in ability of EMS systems to handle pediatric patients.
    - All procedures are more difficult if providers are garbed in protective gear; this phenomenon would be exaggerated with small children.

- Massive numbers of pediatric casualties would require the definitive treatment of numerous children in centers that normally rely on expeditious interhospital transport to relieve them of the long-term responsibility for critical pediatric patients.
- Pediatric centers probably would be overwhelmed with both indigenous patients and those transferred.

Henretig FM, Cieslak TJ, Eitzen EM Jr: Biological and chemical terrorism. J Pediatr 141:311–326, 2002.

Henretig FM, Cieslak TJ, Madsen JM, et al: Emergency department awareness and response to incidents of biological and chemical terrorism. In Fleisher GF, Ludwig S, Henretig FM (eds): Textbook of Pediatric Emergency Medicine 5th, ed. Philadelphia, Lippincott Williams & Wilkins, 2006, pp 135–162.

Rotenberg JS, Newmark J: Nerve agent attacks on children: Diagnosis and management. Pediatrics 112:648–658, 2003.

KEY POINTS: REASONS THAT CHEMICAL AND BIOLOGIC ✔ AGENTS DISPROPORTIONATELY AFFECT CHILDREN

1. They have higher minute ventilation and live closer to the ground, enhancing respiratory exposure of aerosolized agents.

2. They have thinner and more permeable skin, allowing greater injury from vesicant or corrosive chemicals and possibly faster systemic absorption of nerve agents.

3. They have age-related developmental vulnerabilities that may hamper their ability to escape exposure.

4. They may suffer unique psychological trauma after separation from parents or witnessing death of family members.

5. There is limited study of relevant antibiotics, antidotes, and vaccines.

6. EMS systems may be unable to handle pediatric patients.

7. Procedures may be more difficult if providers are garbed in protective gear.

8. Massive numbers of pediatric casualties would overwhelm interhospital transport teams and pediatric treatment centers.

12. **What are the principal biologic agent threats?**
See Table 68-1. In most circumstances patients will present after a significant time interval from their exposure. In the event of an announced attack, some consideration to decontamination issues is appropriate. In most cases, simple disrobement of outer garments and soap and water washing is sufficient for biologic agents.

KEY POINTS: CATEGORY A BIOLOGIC AGENTS ✔

1. Variola virus

2. *Bacillus anthracis*

3. *Yersinia pestis*

4. *Francisella tularensis*

5. Botulinum toxin

6. Filoviruses and arena viruses (viral hemorrhagic fevers)

TABLE 68-1. PRIMARY BIOLOGICAL AGENTS OF TERRORISM

Disease	Etiology	Clinical Findings*	Incubation Period	Diagnostic Samples	Diagnostic Assay	Isolation Precautions	Initial Treatment†	Prophylaxis
Anthrax	*Bacillus anthracis*	*Inhalational:* febrile prodrome with rapid progression to mediastinal lymphadenitis, mediastinitis (chest radiograph findings: presence or absence of infiltrates, widened mediastinum, pleural effusions); sepsis; shock; meningitis. *Cutaneous:* papule progressing to vesicle, to ulcer, then to depressed black eschar, with marked edema	1–5 d (up to 6 wk?)	Blood CSF Pleural fluid Skin biopsy	Culture Gram stain ELISA PCR Immunohisto-chemical assay	Standard	Ciprofloxacin: 10–15 mg/kg (maximum, 400 mg) IV every 12 hr or doxycycline: 2.2 mg/kg (maximum, 100 mg) IV every 12 hr†	Ciprofloxacin: 10–15 mg/kg (maximum, 500 mg) orally Every 12 hr × 60 d, or Doxycycline: 2.5 mg/kg (maximum, 100 mg) orally every 12 hr × 60 days‡

Continued

TABLE 68-1.	PRIMARY BIOLOGICAL AGENTS OF TERRORISM—CONT'D							
Disease	Etiology	Clinical Findings*	Incubation Period	Diagnostic Samples	Diagnostic Assay	Isolation Precautions	Initial Treatment†	Prophylaxis
Plague	*Yersinia pestis*	Febrile prodrome with rapid progression to fulminant pneumonia with bloody sputum, sepsis, DIC	2–3 d	Blood Sputum Lymph node aspirate	Culture Gram or Wright-Giemsa stains ELISA, IFA Ag-ELISA	Pneumonic: droplet until patient treated for 3 d	Gentamycin: 2.5 mg/ kg IV every 8 hr§ or Doxycycline: 2.2 mg/ kg IV (maximum, 100 mg) IV every 12 hr, or Ciprofloxacin, 15 mg/kg (maximum, 500 mg) IV every 12 hr, or Chloramphenicol, 25 mg/kg (maximum, 1 gm) IV every 6 hr	Doxycycline, 2.2 mg/kg (maximum, 100 mg) orally every 12 hr × 7 d, or Ciprofloxacin, 20 mg/kg (maximum, 500 mg) orally every 12 hr × 7 d, or Chloramphenicol, 25 mg/kg (maximum, 1 gm) orally every 6 hr × 7 d
Smallpox	Variola virus	Febrile prodrome Synchronous vesicopustular eruption, predominately on face and extremities	7–17 d	Pharyngeal swab Scab material	ELISA, PCR Virus isolation	Airborne, droplet, contact	Supportive care	Vaccination within 4 d (consider vaccinia immunoglobulin: 0.6mL/kg IM within 3 d of exposure for vaccine complications, immunocompromised persons)

Disease	Organism	Clinical Features	Incubation	Specimens	Diagnostics		Treatment	Prophylaxis
Tularemia	*Francisella tularensis*	*Pneumonic:* abrupt-onset fever, fulminant pneumonia (chest radiograph findings: prominent hilar adenopathy) *Typhoidal:* fever, malaise, abdominal pain	2–10 d	Blood, sputum, Serum Tissue	Culture¶ Serology: agglutination EM	Standard	Gentamicin, 2.5 mg/kg IV every 8 hours¶, or Doxycycline, 2.2 mg/kg (maximum, 100 mg) IV every 12 hr, or Ciprofloxacin, 15 mg/kg (maximum, 500 mg) IV every 12 hr, or Chloramphenicol, 15 mg/kg (maximum, 1 gm) IV every 6 hr	Doxycycline, 2.2 mg/kg (maximum, 100 mg) orally every 12 hr, or Ciprofloxacin, 15 mg/kg (maximum, 500 mg) orally every 12 hr
Botulism	*Clostridium botulinum* toxin	Afebrile Descending flaccid paralysis Cranial nerve palsies Sensation and mentation intact	1–5 d	Nasal swab?	Mouse bioassay, Ag-ELISA	Standard	CDC trivalent antitoxin (serotypes A, B, E), 1 vial (10 mL) IV DOD heptavalent antitoxin (serotypes A–G) (IND) California Department of Health immunoglobulin (IND)	None

Continued

TABLE 68-1. PRIMARY BIOLOGICAL AGENTS OF TERRORISM—CONT'D

Disease	Etiology	Clinical Findings*	Incubation Period	Diagnostic Samples	Diagnostic Assay	Isolation Precautions	Initial Treatment[†]	Prophylaxis
Viral hemorrhagic fevers	Arenaviridae (e.g., Lassa fever) Filoviridae (Ebola, Marburg viruses)	Febrile prodrome; rapid progression to shock, purpura, bleeding diathesis	4–21 d	Serum, blood	Viral isolation Ag-ELISA RT-PCR Serology: Ab-ELISA	Contact, droplet; consider airborne if massive hemorrhage	Supportive care Ribavirin (arenaviruses) 30 mg/kg IV initially 15 mg/kg IV every 6 hr × 4 d 7.5 mg/kg IV every 8 hr × 6 d	None

Adapted from Henretig FM, Cieslak TJ, Eitzen EM Jr: Biological and chemical terrorism. J Pediatr 141:311-326, 2002.
Ab-ELISA = antibody detection enzyme-linked immunosorbent assay, Ag-ELISA = antigen detection enzyme-linked immunosorbent assay, CDC = Centers for Disease Control and Prevention, CSF = cerebrospinal fluid, DIC = disseminated intravascular coagulation, DOD = Department of Defense, ELISA = enzyme-linked immunosorbent assay, EM = electron microscopy, IFA = immunofluorescence antibody, IM = intramuscular, IND = investigational new drug, PCR = polymerase chain reaction, RT-PCR = reverse transcriptase polymerase chain reaction.
*Syndrome expected after aerosol exposure.
[†]Centers for Disease Control and Prevention (CDC) recommended one or two additional antibiotics for inhalational anthrax in fall 2001 outbreak: rifampin, vancomycin, penicillin or ampicillin, clindamycin, imipenem, or clarithromycin. Recommendations for future outbreaks may evolve rapidly, and urgent consultation with local health departments and CDC (1-770-488-7100; www.bt.cdc.gov) is encouraged.
‡Amoxicillin, 80 mg/kg/d divided every 8 hr, can be substituted if strain proves susceptible.
§Streptomycin, 15 mg/kg IM every 12 hr, may be substituted if available.
•Laboratory must be notified that tularemia is suspected.

13. **What is the most important biologic threat?**
The most important biologic threat is believed to be *inhalational anthrax*. This disease is caused by aerosol exposure to anthrax spores, which were weaponized by the United States (before 1969, when the United States renounced the use of biologic weapons and destroyed all existing stockpiles) and more recently by Russia and Iraq. The causative bacterium is *Bacillus anthracis*, a sporulating gram-positive rod. Endemic anthrax occurs in cutaneous and gastrointestinal as well as inhalational forms; generally it is contracted by close contact with hides, wool, or meat of infected herbivores (especially sheep, cattle, and goats).

14. **What are the signs and symptoms of inhalational anthrax exposure?**
After inhalation of anthrax spores, infection begins with pulmonary macrophage uptake and subsequent carriage to mediastinal lymph nodes, where necrotizing lymphadenitis and sepsis ensue. *Inhalational anthrax* has an incubation period of 1–6 days, and then begins with a flulike illness characterized by fever, myalgia, headache, cough, and chest "tightness." A brief period of improvement sometimes is seen 1–2 days later, but it is followed by rapid deterioration with high fever, dyspnea, cyanosis, and shock. Hemorrhagic meningitis is present in up to 50% of cases. Chest radiographs obtained late in the course of illness may demonstrate a widened mediastinum or prominent mediastinal lymphadenopathy; infiltrates or pleural effusions may also be present. Death is universal in untreated cases and may occur in as many as 95% of treated cases if therapy is begun more than 48 hours after symptom onset (even with modern intensive care). The diagnosis should be considered with this clinical picture and a chest radiograph demonstrating widened mediastinum and may be confirmed with positive blood cultures.

15. **What are the signs and symptoms of cutaneous anthrax exposure?**
Cutaneous anthrax occurs when organisms gain entry into skin, particularly through abrasions or cuts. It is characterized by the development of a papule at the inoculum site, which then progresses over days to a vesicle, then an ulcer, and finally to a depressed, black eschar. The surrounding tissue becomes markedly edematous, but not particularly tender, distinguishing this infection from more typical staphylococcal or streptococcal cellulitis. It is quite amenable to therapy with a variety of antibiotics; with timely institution of treatment, it is rarely fatal. In the fall 2001 outbreak, all 11 patients with cutaneous anthrax survived. The only pediatric victim of that attack was a 7-month-old boy with cutaneous anthrax on his arm, presumably contracted after a brief visit to a New York City television news studio that had received contaminated mail. He was initially suspected of having a brown recluse spider bite, and the correct diagnosis was confirmed only after the discovery of anthrax contamination at another television studio. Of note, he also developed hemolysis, thrombocytopenia, and renal insufficiency, features not usually observed in otherwise uncomplicated cases of cutaneous disease, thus raising the possibility of a particular vulnerability in infancy.

16. **What problems are associated with management of children exposed to anthrax?**
First, the anthrax vaccine is approved only for adults. Second, both quinolones and tetracyclines have relative contraindications in children, although dental staining seen with tetracyclines usually requires multiple courses, and the risk of cartilage problems associated with quinolones is theoretical. Current experience with the use of both classes of antibiotics in children suggests that short-term use is safe. It seems reasonable that the extreme danger posed by anthrax

exposure warrants use of any or all of these modalities in exposed children. Anthrax has little potential for person-to-person transmission; thus, standard precautions are adequate for health care workers.

17. **Why is smallpox of special concern?**
Because smallpox is highly contagious, protection of health care workers and prevention of secondary transmission are important factors. Smallpox was globally eradicated in 1980, and children are no longer vaccinated. Most American adults and all children are susceptible. Smallpox produces a febrile prodrome followed by a characteristic centrifugal vesicular rash; fatality rates approach 30% in unimmunized patients. Smallpox mandates the use of airborne isolation technique. Treatment is primarily symptomatic.

18. **What are the concerning features of plague?**
Like smallpox, plague is highly contagious. Inhalational exposure causes a severe, hemorrhagic pneumonia (pneumonic plague) characterized by respiratory distress and hemoptysis. Plague is highly lethal in untreated patients. Antibiotics, including aminoglycosides and doxycycline, are effective if begun within 24 hours of onset of illness. Droplet precautions are necessary in managing patients with plague.

19. **What are the primary chemical threats? Describe the general approach to their management.**
See Table 68-2.

20. **Which chemical weapons are most feared?**
Nerve agents are the most feared chemical weapons. These potent organophosphate compounds, similar to many pesticides, are toxic by inhalation, ingestion, and topical absorption and can result in profound muscarinic (cholinergic syndrome), nicotinic (initial muscle fasciculations, then paralysis), and central nervous system effects (seizures, coma, apnea). The clinical picture varies slightly by route of exposure, as noted in Table 68-2. Severe cases require antidotal therapy with atropine (adults, 2–5 mg; children, 0.02–0.05 mg/kg), pralidoxime (adults, 1–2 gm; children, 25–50 mg/kg), and usually diazepam for seizure control (adults, 5–10 mg; children, 0.1–0.3 mg/kg).

Rotenberg JS, Newmark J: Nerve agent attacks on children: Diagnosis and management. Pediatrics 112:648–658, 2003.

21. **What are the principal components of the federal response plan?**
The 1996 Defense Against Weapons of Mass Destruction Act lays out the federal response plan for management of chemical or biologic attacks. The lead federal agencies are the FBI and the Federal Emergency Management Administration. The Public Health Service may activate the National Disaster Medical System, which can deploy disaster medical assistance teams from military bases or coordination centers, such as the Centers for Disease Control and Prevention. Regionally, local EMS systems and hospitals need to coordinate planning and provide adequate training, protective gear, antidote and antibiotic availability, triage systems, protocols for isolation or quarantine, and potential utilization of alternative secondary care sites (e.g., schools, nursing homes as communal infectious disease wards).

TABLE 68-2. PRIMARY CHEMICAL AGENTS OF TERRORISM

Agent	Toxicity	Clinical Findings	Onset	Decontamination*	Management
Nerve agents: Tabun, sarin, soman, VX	Anticholinesterase: muscarinic, nicotinic and CNS effects	*Vapor:* miosis, rhinorrhea, dyspnea *Liquid:* diaphoresis, vomiting *Both:* coma, paralysis, seizures, apnea	*Seconds:* Vapor *Minutes to hours:* liquid	*Vapor:* breathe fresh air, remove clothes, wash hair *Liquid:* remove clothes, thoroughly wash skin and hair with soap and water, irrigate eyes	ABCs Atropine: 0.05 mg/kg IV†, IM‡ (minimum, 0.1 mg; maximum, 5 mg), repeat every 2–5 min as needed for marked secretions, bronchospasm Pralidoxime: 25 mg/kg IV, IM§ (maximum, 1 gm IV; 2 gm IM), may repeat within 30–60 min as needed, then again every hr for 1 or 2 doses as needed for persistent weakness, high atropine requirement Diazepam: 0.3 mg/kg (maximum, 10 mg) IV Lorazepam: 0.1 mg/kg IV, IM (maximum, 4 mg) Midazolam: 0.2 mg/kg (maximum, 10 mg) IM as needed for seizures or severe exposure
Vesicants: Mustard Lewisite	Alkylation Arsenical	*Skin:* erythema, vesicles *Eye:* inflammation *Respiratory tract:* inflammation	Hours (immediate pain with lewisite)	*Skin:* soap and water *Eyes:* water *Both:* major impact only if done within minutes of exposure	Symptomatic care (possibly BAL, 3 mg/kg IM every 4–6 hr for systemic effects of lewisite in severe cases)
Pulmonary agents: Chlorine phosgene	Liberate HCl, alkylation	Eyes, nose, throat irritation (especially chlorine) *Respiratory:* bronchospasm, pulmonary edema (especially phosgene)	*Minutes:* eyes, nose, throat irritation, bronchospasm *Hours:* pulmonary edema	Fresh air *Skin:* water	Symptomatic care

Continued

TABLE 60-2. PRIMARY CHEMICAL AGENTS OF TERRORISM—CONT'D

Agent	Toxicity	Clinical Findings	Onset	Decontamination*	Management
Cyanide	Cytochrome oxidase inhibition: cellular anoxia, lactic acidosis	Tachypnea, coma, seizures, apnea	Seconds	Fresh air *Skin:* soap and water	ABCs, 100% oxygen Sodium bicarbonate as needed for metabolic acidosis Sodium nitrite (3%): <u>Dose (mL/kg) Estimated Hgb (g/dL)</u> 0.27 10 0.33 12 (estimated for average child) 0.39 14 (maximum, 10 mL) Sodium thiosulfate (25%): 1.65 mL/kg (maximum, 50 mL)
Riot control agents: CS CN (Mace) Capsaicin (pepper spray)	Neuropeptide substance P release; alkylation	*Eye:* tearing, pain, blepharospasm Nose and throat irritation Pulmonary failure (rare)	Seconds	Fresh air *Eyes:* lavage	Ophthalmics topically, symptomatic care

ABCs = airway, breathing, and circulatory support, BAL = British antilewisite, CN = chloroacetophenone, CNS = central nervous system, CS = 2-chlorobenzalmalononitrile, HCl = hydrogen chloride, Hgb = hemoglobin concentration, IM = intramuscular, VX = O-ethyl-S-[2(diisopropylamino)ethyl] methylphosphonothiolate.
*Health care providers garbed in adequate personal protective equipment should perform decontamination, particularly for patients with significant nerve agent or vesicant exposure. For emergency department staff, this consists of nonencapsulated, chemically resistant body suit, boots, and gloves with a full-face air purifier mask/hood.
†Intraosseous route is probably equivalent to the IV route.
‡Atropine might have some benefit via endotracheal tube or inhalation, as might aerosolized ipratropium. As of July 2004, the Food and Drug Administration has approved pediatric autoinjectors of atropine in 0.25-, 0.5-, and 1-mg sizes. Recommendations are:

Approximate Age	Approximate Weight (lb)	Autoinjector Size (mg)
<6 mo	<15	0.25
6 mo–4 yr	15–40	0.5
5–10 yr	41–90	1
>10 yr	>90	2 (adult-sized)

§Pralidoxime is reconstituted to 50 mg/mL (1 gm in 20 mL water) for IV administration, and the total dose infused over 30 min, or may be given by continuous infusion (loading dose, 25 mg/kg over 30 min, then 10 mg/kg/hr). For intramuscular use, it might be diluted to a concentration of 300 mg/mL (1 gm added to 3 mL water; by analogy to the U.S. Army's Mark 1 autoinjector concentration) to effect a reasonable volume for injection. Pediatric autoinjectors of pralidoxime are not Food and Drug Administration approved or available at this time. The Mark 1 autoinjector kits contain 2 mg (0.7mL) atropine, and 600 mg (2 mL) pralidoxime, delivered into two separate intramuscular sites; while not approved for pediatric use, the pralidoxime autoinjector might be considered as initial treatment in dire (especially prehospital) circumstances; for children with severe, life-threatening nerve agent toxicity who lack IV access; and children for whom more precise, mg/kg intramuscular dosing would be logistically impossible. Suggested dosing guidelines are offered; note potential excess of initial pralidoxime dose for age/weight, although within general guidelines for recommended total over first 60–90 min of therapy of severe exposures:

Approximate Age (yr)	Approximate Weight (kg)	Number of Autoinjectors	Pralidoxime Dose Range (mg/kg)
3–7	13–25	1	24–46
8–14	26–50	2	24–46
>14	>51	3	≤35

Adapted from Henretig FM, Cieslak TJ, Eitzen EM Jr: Biological and chemical terrorism. J Pediatr 141:311–326, 2002.

22. **How does the federal plan apply to children?**

As noted earlier, many exposure and treatment issues are not settled in regard to children, and many EMS concerns would specifically relate to the provision of adequate care to pediatric mass casualties. Recently, the American Academy of Pediatrics has turned attention to many of these logistical and research issues as they pertain to children and has recommended extensive involvement of the pediatric emergency medicine community in this effort.

American Academy of Pediatrics: Chemical-biological terrorism and its impact on children: A subject review. Pediatrics 105:662–670, 2000.

EMERGENCY MEDICAL SERVICES AND PREHOSPITAL CARE

Hazel Guinto-Ocampo, MD

1. **Describe the American Heart Association's pediatric chain of survival link.**
   Prevention of injury or arrest → Early and effective cardiopulmonary resuscitation → Early emergency medical services (EMS) activation → Early advanced life support, including stabilization, transport, and rehabilitation.

   The chain of survival and emergency medical services for children. In Hazinski MF (ed): PALS Provider Manual. Dallas, TX, American Heart Association, 2002, pp 1–16.

2. **What is enhanced 911?**
   Enhanced 911 automatically provides computerized identification of the telephone number and location of the caller, regardless of the quality of information provided.

3. **What is the role of an EMS dispatcher?**
   An EMS dispatcher is a specialized operator who gathers essential information regarding the nature and location of the emergency, and relays this information to the EMS system for dispatch of a first responder. The dispatcher's responsibilities include calming the caller, learning the complaint, making a triage decision, and obtaining the location of the emergency.

4. **What are dispatcher protocols?**
   These are written guidelines, often computerized, that are developed and utilized so that dispatchers can accurately instruct callers in pediatric cardiopulmonary resuscitation, relief of foreign-body airway obstruction, and essential first aid maneuvers, until EMS personnel arrive. Their use reduces the variability of the information provided by the dispatchers, and ensures that accurate emergency information is provided to every caller.

5. **Name the three general categories of prehospital personnel.**
   1. First responders
   2. Basic life support (BLS) providers
   3. Advanced life support (ALS) providers
      The categories vary in levels of training and degrees of capabilities. At the federal level, the National Highway Traffic Safety Association (NHTSA) has developed the National Standard Curricula for certification for each category, but state or local requirements supersede these standards. Intermediate levels of providers with varied capabilities have evolved as many jurisdictions offer supplemental training modules.

   Blackwell T: principles of emergency medical services systems. In Marx JA, Hockberger RS, Walls RM (eds): Rosen's Emergency Medicine Concepts and Clinical Practice Vol. III, 5th ed. St. Louis, Mosby, 2002, pp 2616–2625.

6. **What is a first responder?**
   First responders have limited but significant life-saving capabilities. By definition, first responders are typically the first to arrive at the scene of an incident. The Department of Transportation (DOT) recommends a 40-hour didactic curriculum for certification, and 16–36 hours for refresher training. Most are trained to administer BLS, help clear an obstructed airway, control hemorrhage, and splint an injured extremity. The use of an automated external

defibrillator (AED) should be a mandatory procedure for first responders. Spinal immobilization is usually beyond the first responder's capabilities. Except in some rural EMS systems, first responders usually do not provide ambulance transport.

Woodward GA, King BR, Garrett AL, Baker MD. Prehospital care and transport medicine. In Fleisher GR, Ludwig S, Henretig FM (eds). Textbook of Pediatric Emergency Medicine, 5th ed. Philadelphia, Lippincott, Williams & Wilkins, 2006, pp 93–134.

7. What are BLS providers?

BLS providers are usually called emergency medical technician–basic, or simply emergency medical technicians (EMTs). They have capabilities that exceed those of the first responders. In 1995, NHTSA developed a revised BLS provider curriculum, which requires 110 hours of didactic and clinical instruction. The DOT recommends a 24-hour refresher course, 48 hours of continuing education, and a BLS course every 2 years, for recertification. BLS providers are capable of patient assessment, spinal immobilization, noninvasive ventilatory assistance, and application of pneumatic antishock garment. They are trained to recognize respiratory distress, shock, altered mental status, mechanisms of injury, and death. As ambulance transport personnel, they perform initial triage and route patients to receiving medical facilities.

Woodward GA, King BR, Garrett AL, Baker MD. Prehospital care and transport medicine. In Fleisher GR, Ludwig S, Henretig FM (eds). Textbook of Pediatric Emergency Medicine, 5th ed. Philadelphia, Lippincott, Williams & Wilkins, 2006, pp 93–134.

8. What are ALS providers?

ALS providers are usually referred to as emergency medical technician–paramedic, or simply paramedics/medics. They are more extensively trained and more capable than BLS providers. A recently revised National Standard Curriculum for ALS providers requires approximately 1000 to 1200 hours of didactic, clinical, and field instruction on advanced resuscitation techniques, such as ventilatory support, vascular access, and drug administration. They are capable of general diagnostic skills, rhythm disturbance recognition and treatment, and advanced, including invasive, airway management. Many ALS provider educational programs have advanced to a 2-year associate or a 4-year baccalaureate degree. A 48-hour refresher course, 24 hours of yearly continuing education, BLS, and adult and pediatric ALS courses are required for recertification.

Woodward GA, King BR, Garrett AL, Baker MD. Prehospital care and transport medicine. In Fleisher GR, Ludwig S, Henretig FM (eds). Textbook of Pediatric Emergency Medicine, 5th ed. Philadelphia, Lippincott, Williams & Wilkins, 2006, pp 93–134.

9. How can one become an intermediate provider?

Intermediate providers have met EMT-basic certification and undergo supplemental training. For example, some EMTs acquire additional training in defibrillation and are designated EMT-D.

KEY POINTS: CATEGORIES OF PREHOSPITAL PERSONNEL ✔

1. First responders

2. BLS providers or EMT–B (basic)

3. ALS providers or EMT–P (paramedic)

10. **Where can I find the list of minimum pediatric equipment and supplies for BLS and ALS units?**

    The most recent lists of recommended pediatric BLS and ALS ambulance equipment were published simultaneously in the following journals:

    - Committee on Ambulance Equipment and Supplies, National EMSC Resource Alliance. Guidelines for pediatric equipment and supplies for basic and advanced life support ambulances. Ann Emerg Med 28:699–701, 1996.
    - Committee on Ambulance Equipment and Supplies, National EMSC Resource Alliance. Guidelines for pediatric equipment and supplies for basic and advanced life support ambulances. Pediatr Emerg Care 12:452–453, 1996.

11. **What is medical command?**

    Medical command is the entity responsible for the supervision of the emergency medical services of the community. In general, paramedics are assigned to a specific operational base or base station, and these base stations are responsible to medical command. **Medical control** provides medical direction to prehospital personnel. Medical control can be off-line/indirect, or on-line/direct.

12. **Differentiate off-line and on-line medical control.**

    - **Off-line medical control** consists of patient care protocol development, personnel education and training, prospective and retrospective patient care review, and other process improvement activities.
    - **On-line medical control** involves real-time interaction between a physician or designee, and a field provider. On-line medical control can be centralized or decentralized. In a *centralized* system, a designated hospital is responsible for all direct medical control orders and notification, regardless of the receiving facility. In a *decentralized* system, each receiving hospital provides direction to EMTs transporting patients to their facility.

13. **Where can I find examples of pediatric EMS protocols?**

    National Association of EMS Physicians: Model Pediatric Protocols, 2003:www.naemsp.org/protocols.asp

14. **Describe the difference between single-tiered and multitiered EMS systems.**

    - In a **single-tiered** system, every response, regardless of the call type, receives the same level of personnel expertise and equipment (all BLS or ALS). The advantage of this design is the provision of advanced level of care to all calls, and overcomes under- or overtriaging by EMS dispatchers.
    - **Multitiered** systems respond with an ALS- or BLS-level unit depending on the nature of the call. This design reserves ALS units for higher-priority calls, and aims to ensure that an ALS unit is always available for potential critical responses.

    The ideal EMS system design provides quality patient care in the briefest possible period of time. Therefore, the efficiency of adopting a single-tiered versus multitiered response is affected by the availability of BLS and ALS providers in the community, and the distance from the scene of the incident to the nearest receiving hospital. Regardless of the response design, EMS systems usually include first responder services, often provided by the police or fire department, as part of the response.

15. **What is EMS-C?**

    Emergency Medical Services for Children (EMS-C) is a federally funded program administered by the Health Resources and Services Administration's Maternal and Child Health Bureau and NHTSA, which provides grant funding to states or medical schools in all 50 states, the District of Columbia, and five territories, to support pediatric emergency care initiatives at the state and local level. Funding supports all the components of the program, namely, education and training, systems development, data analysis and research, and public policy and future planning. EMS-C partners with numerous national organizations involved in the care of acutely ill or injured children.

Emergency Medical Services for Children: www.ems-c.org

16. **What resources are available through EMS-C?**

Numerous education and training resources regarding emergency care are available through EMS-C. These resources are geared toward various users, such as children, parents and families, school and child care professionals, prehospital care providers, and physicians and nurses. These resources are available, mostly for free, through the EMS-C website, which won the 1999 Gold Award for best government health care website.

Emergency Medical Services for Children: www.ems-c.org

17. **What is family-centered prehospital care?**

Family-centered prehospital care is a systematic approach to building collaborative relationships between prehospital personnel and the patients' families during on-site treatment, transport, and transition of care. The goal is to provide the best outcome for the patient through collaboration with his or her family members.

Emergency Medical Services for Children. Available at www.ems-c.org

18. **What is an AED?**

An AED is a device that recognizes rhythms amenable to shock, and directs the user to deliver the shock.

19. **In which pediatric age groups is it appropriate to use an AED?**

AEDs may be used for children 1 year of age or older. Ideally, the device should be equipped with pediatric pad/cable systems that reduce the energy delivered for patients younger than 8 years of age.

Samson RA, Berg RA, Bingham R: Use of automated external defibrillators for children: An update—an advisory statement from the Pediatric Advanced Life Support Task Force, International Liaison Committee on Resuscitation. Pediatrics 112:163–168, 2003.

20. **What is the doctrine of implied consent?**

This doctrine permits the treatment of minors without parental consent when an emergency exists. A minor with a condition that threatens either life or limb is viewed as an emergency and must be treated and transported.

CHAPTER 70

PATIENT SAFETY IN THE EMERGENCY DEPARTMENT

Melanie Pitone, MD, FAAP, and Steven M. Selbst, MD, FAAP, FACEP

1. **How extensive is the problem of medical errors in the emergency department (ED)?**
   The Institute of Medicine (IOM) estimated in 1998 that 44,000 to 98,000 deaths per year are due to medical errors. These data make medical errors the eighth leading cause of death. Medical errors in the United States cost $2 billion each year. The number of deaths noted above has been disputed, and some of the adverse events included in the above report may not have been due to medical error. However, the problem is significant. It is not known how many errors in the IOM report involved delivery of care to children in the ED. Many of these errors are preventable.

   Bates DW, Spell N, Cullen DJ, et al: The costs of adverse drug events in hospitalized patients. Adverse Drug Events Prevention Group. JAMA 277:307–311, 1997.
   Kohn LT, Corrigan JM, Donaldson MS (eds): To Err Is Human: Building a Safer Health System. Washington, DC, Institute of Medicine, National Academy Press, 1998.

2. **Which factors inherent to the ED contribute to medical errors?**
   1. Time pressures
   2. Incomplete medical and drug histories available
   3. Unscheduled care
   4. Inconsistency of patient arrival
   5. High-risk patients (high acuity)
   6. Environment in flux—patients have varied locations (rooms, x-ray, hallway)
      - 24-hour activity
      - No time to restore order and "reset" the environment
      - Circadian rhythm of staff is challenged
      - Transition of patient care among staff (consultants and change-of-shift)

   Schenkel S: Promoting patient safety and preventing medical error in emergency departments. Acad Emerg Med 7:1204–1219, 2000.

3. **What is a latent error?**
   Latent errors are design flaws or failures in the tools or systems and work environment that produces circumstances in which a worker (nurse, physician) is likely to err. Latent errors may persist for long periods of time before they are discovered and corrected.

4. **Why are children in the ED at particular risk for error?**
   - Variety of patient size and age
   - Need to calculate most medication doses
   - Limited time for pharmacist review of medication orders
   - Stressful/demanding environment
   - ED overcrowding
   - Fatigue (nurses and physicians)
   - Miscommunication (with patients or among staff)
   Seriously ill pediatric patients are at greatest risk for error in the ED.

   Chamberlain, JM, Slonim A, Joseph JG. Reducing errors and promoting safety in pediatric emergency care. Ambul Pediatr 4:55–63, 2004.

Selbst S, Levine S, Mull C, et al: Preventing medical errors in pediatric emergency medicine. Pediatr Emerg Care 20:702–709, 2004.

5. **How common are medication errors in the United States?**
The IOM report found that 20% of errors involved medications and the majority (75%) of these occurred at the physician ordering stage. Medication errors are the second most frequent and second most expensive precipitant of medical malpractice claims. About 42% of claims involving medication errors result in significant permanent injury, and 21% result in death. It is estimated that preventable adverse drug events cost U.S. hospitals $2 billion annually, not including malpractice costs. In a study by Kozer et al, 10% of all patients seen in a pediatric ED had a prescribing error. In a study by Taylor et al, almost 60% of prescriptions written in a pediatric ED contained an error.

Kohn LT, Corrigan JM, Donaldson MS (eds): To Err Is Human: Building a Safer Health System. Washington, DC, Institute of Medicine, National Academy Press, 1998.
Kozer E, Scolnick D, Macpherson A, et al: Variables associated with medication errors in pediatric emergency medicine. Pediatrics 110:737–742, 2002.
Physicians Insurers Association of America. Medication Errors Study. Philadelphia, Physicians Insurers, 1993, pp 1–44.
Taylor BL, Selbst SM, Shah AEC: Prescription writing errors in the pediatric emergency department. Pediatr Emerg Care 21:822–827, 2005.

6. **What are the most common types of medication errors in a pediatric ED?**
Medication dosing errors are the most common type. Pediatric medicines, for the most part, have weight-based dosing. Incorrect recording of weight or incorrect calculation of dose results in the largest amount of error. This can lead to severe morbidity because often the mistake is a "tenfold error" because of a misplaced decimal point. Giving an incorrect drug is the next most common type of medication error. This is usually due to similar packaging of drugs or medication names that sound alike. Administration of a medication to a child with a known allergy to the medication is another common type of medication error.

Kozer E, Scolnick D, Macpherson A, et al: Variables associated with medication errors in pediatric emergency medicine. Pediatrics 110:737–742, 2002.
Selbst S, Fein JA, Osterhoudt K, et al: Medication errors in a pediatric emergency department. Pediatr Emerg Care 15:1–4, 1999.

7. **What is the most common outcome of medication errors in the pediatric ED?**
Most commonly, no harm is done. There is, however, potential risk of prolonged hospital stay, additional care required, and death.

Selbst S, Fein JA, Osterhoudt K, et al: Medication errors in a pediatric emergency department. Pediatr Emerg Care 15:1–4, 1999.

KEY POINTS: MEDICATION ERRORS IN THE PEDIATRIC ED ✓

1. The largest threat to children in the ED is medication errors, most of which are dosing errors.

2. The ED environment is a challenge, largely because of its unstructured and hurried environment, with patients presenting with unpredictable issues, with varied patient size and levels of urgency, and at unscheduled times.

3. Better ED systems, communication, and teamwork can reduce errors. Knowing the risk of errors is a big first step.

8. **When are errors most likely to occur in a pediatric ED?**
Evening shift and overnight—specifically 4 AM to 8 AM. Fatigue, severity of patient illness, and less supervision of trainees are theoretical reasons for this trend.

   Kozer E, Scolnick D, Macpherson A, et al: Variables associated with medication errors in pediatric emergency medicine. Pediatrics 110:737–742, 2002.

   Selbst S, Fein JA, Osterhoudt K, et al: Medication errors in a pediatric emergency department. Pediatr Emerg Care 15:1–4, 1999.

9. **What is a transition? What makes it a risk in emergency medicine?**
Transition is the transfer of care between care providers. It is also known as "change of shift." Transitions in the ED interrupt continuity of care and are a source of potential error. Few studies have described transitions or promoted safe transition practices. Communication errors can result from the poor transfer of information and also from the transfer of poor information. Staff should be educated on the risks created by the transfer of a patient's care, and best practices for safe transitions should be promoted.

   Beach C, Croskerry P, Shapiro M: Profiles in patient safety: Emergency care transitions: Acad Emerg Med 10:364–367, 2003.

10. **Why are children with special health care needs vulnerable to error in emergency care?**
Children with special health care needs are a growing population representing 16–18% of children in the United States. They are at risk for medical error in the ED for several reasons:
   - Some of their problems are occult and difficult to recognize, thus delaying care.
   - Some conditions are recognizable but refractory to standard therapy, thus delaying receipt of the *best* care for that particular patient.
   - Their baseline condition (e.g., vital signs, mental status) may not be known to the ED provider. Thus, severity of illness can be underestimated or overestimated.
   - They often have rare conditions that are unfamiliar to the emergency care provider.
   - Many require technologic devices that are not available to the ED providers.

   Sacchetti A, Sacchetti C, Carraccio C, et al: The potential for errors in children with special health care needs. Acad Emerg Med 7:1330–1333, 2000.

11. **What can be done to make children with special health care needs safer when receiving emergency care?**
An emergency information form, promoted and conceptualized in part by the American College of Emergency Physicians and the American Academy of Pediatrics, can help ED physicians provide more efficient and appropriate care to children with special health care needs. The form may contain contact information, past medical history and procedures, common presenting problems, and suggestions for management strategies. Coupled with medical identification jewelry and electronic information transfer, the emergency information form has the potential to improve safety for this at-risk group.

   Sacchetti A, Sacchetti C, Carraccio C, et al: The potential for errors in children with special health care needs. Acad Emerg Med 7:1330–1333, 2000.

12. **When caring for a patient with limited English proficiency in the ED, would a family member interpreter be sufficient?**
No, it would not be ideal. In one pediatric study, one clinical encounter generated 31 errors in medical interpretation. Most errors were of omission and had potential for clinical consequences. Errors committed by ad hoc interpreters (hospital staff, family members, other patients in the ED) as opposed to hospital interpreters were more likely to have clinical consequence. The legal liability of not ensuring appropriate interpretation is large. A $71 million lawsuit was generated by one misinterpreted word in the ED. One family was

separated by social services for misinterpretation in a child abuse case. Efforts should be made to provide reliable, professional interpretation for ED patients and families.

Flores G, Laws MB, Mayo SJ, et al: Errors in medical interpretation and their potential clinical consequences in pediatric encounters. Pediatrics 111:6–14, 2003.

13. **Why would physicians conceal a medical error?**
   - The medical profession values perfection.
   - The doctor may feel shame or guilt.
   - The doctor may fear damage to reputation and decreased income.
   - There is a need to maintain trust with the patient/family.
   - There may be pressure from administration or other parties.
   - There is often fear of punishment.
   - There is often fear of a malpractice lawsuit.

Finkelstein D, Wu AW, Holtzman NA, et al: When a physician harms a patient by a medical error: Ethical, legal and risk management considerations. J Clin Ethics 8:330, 1997.
Selbst SM: The difficult duty of disclosing medical errors. Contemp Pediatr 20:51–63, 2003.

14. **Are physicians obligated to disclose medical errors to patients?**
   The American Medical Association Code of Ethics guidelines for professional conduct states: "The physician is ethically obligated to inform the patient of all the facts necessary to ensure understanding of what has occurred when a patient experiences a significant medical complication from a mistake." Disclosure regarding minor errors with little consequence is not specifically addressed. Several studies have found that patients and parents want the physician to disclose a medical error. Patients want the physician to apologize for an error. Families should be assured that everything is being done to discover how the error occurred and to prevent it from happening again.

American Medical Association, Council on Ethical and Judicial Affairs: Code of medical ethics: Current opinions with annotations. Chicago, Ill. American Medical Association 1997; Sect. 8. 12:125.
Gallagher TH, Waterman AD, Ebers AG, et al: Patients' and physicians' attitudes regarding the disclosure of medical errors. JAMA 289:1001–1007, 2003.

15. **Is disclosure of a medical error likely to lead to a malpractice lawsuit?**
   Most patients, when asked, would be more likely to distrust a doctor, take their care elsewhere, or bring a lawsuit against a physician who conceals an error as opposed to one who is truthful and forthcoming with information. In Hobgood's survey of parents who presented to an ED with a child, 99% wanted disclosure of hypothetical errors presented to them in scripted scenarios. Only 39% said they wanted the doctor to be reported to a disciplinary board because of the hypothetical error. Thirty-six percent said they were less likely to sue if the physician informed them of the error. However, if parents thought the error was severe, their desire for legal action was less amenable to reduction by disclosure.

Hobgood C, Tamayo Aarver JH, Elms A, et al: Parental preferences for error disclosure, reporting, and legal action after medical error in the care of their children. Pediatrics 116:1276–1286, 2005.
Whitman AB, Park DM, Hardin SB: How do patients want physicians to handle mistakes? Arch Intern Med 156:2565–2569, 1996.

16. **How should an ED physician approach a family after an error is discovered?**
   - Investigate the problem first: Make sure there was an error.
   - *Follow hospital policy.* Discuss the case with risk management according to policy.
   - Find an appropriate time (when the family might be less stressed) and place (quiet area) to talk with the family.
   - Sit with the family and speak at eye level.
   - If an error is uncertain, advise the family that the event will be investigated.
   - If a mistake is certain, apologize. *Say you are sorry.*

- Be plausible; do not mislead the parents or patient.
- Avoid placing blame on others.
- *Reassure the family* that any effects of the error will be managed to mitigate harm to the child.

17. What can be done to prevent errors in a pediatric ED?

Errors and error prevention must be addressed instead of hidden. An environment that encourages staff to detect and report errors is crucial. An environment that blames individuals hinders the reporting process. Physicians and administrators must focus on systems that lead to error. Medical errors are rarely the result of one individual and are most commonly due to the ED process. The system must be designed to decrease the likelihood of an error reaching the patient.

Address workforce fatigue issues. Ensure quiet areas for calculation and drawing-up of medications, and develop a system to allow for independent double-checking of medications. Use only approved abbreviations. Write the patient's weight and allergies in a clearly visible location, perhaps near the medication orders and on prescriptions for verification. Encourage staff to be less defensive and more receptive to helpful feedback. Carefully mentor and monitor trainees. Emphasize good communication skills to staff. Analyze "near-misses" (Table 70-1).

Selbst S, Levine S, Mull C, et al: Preventing medical errors in pediatric emergency medicine: Pediatr Emerg Care 20:702–709, 2004.

Wears RL, Leape LL: Human error in emergency medicine. Ann Emerg Med 34:370–372, 1999.

TABLE 70-1. PREVENTING MEDICATION ERRORS IN THE EMERGENCY DEPARTMENT

1. Educate physicians, nurses, pharmacists, and manufacturers about potential errors.
2. Create systems in the emergency department to make errors less likely.
   - Remove dangerous medications that are rarely used from emergency department shelves. For example, since tetanus immunoglobulin is rarely needed and sometimes confused with tetanus toxoid, do not keep this drug in the emergency department. When needed, order it from the hospital pharmacy.
   - Reduce the noise level in the area where medications are drawn.
   - Reduce calculations for drug ordering as much as possible. Use length-based tapes or books with precalculated doses based on the patient's weight.
3. Avoid abbreviations (such as q.d.) in drug ordering as much as possible.
4. Always place a zero before a decimal point (such as 0.5 mg), and avoid use of a terminal zero (such as 5.0 mg). Misinterpretation could result in a tenfold error.
5. Highlight patient drug allergies in the record.
6. Record weights of pediatric patients clearly and only in kilograms.
7. Note the child's weight in an easily located area of the medical record, perhaps near where orders are written.
8. Consider computerized order entry to help reduce computational errors and errors related to patient allergies.
9. Welcome a nurse or pharmacist who questions an order. Do not act defensively or refuse to investigate a possible error.
10. Consider bar coding of medications.
11. Consider using an automated drug dispensing system.

18. **How does Computer Physician Order Entry (CPOE) affect patient safety?**
CPOE, the process by which orders for patient care are directly entered into the computer by the treating physician, can improve patient safety by making medication ordering safer. The software can provide physician decision support, check allergies and weights, and eliminate transcription errors. CPOE avoids omitted information on generated prescriptions, and the prescriptions can be sent electronically to a given pharmacy, enhancing efficiency. Implementation of CPOE in one intensive care unit setting decreased medication errors by 99% and adverse drug events by 40%. Unfortunately, there can be new types of errors inherent in the system. Drug alerts may be overridden because of the frequency of inexact allergy matches conveyed. There can also be adverse events if allergy information is not updated, or if the patients' weight is entered incorrectly. CPOE has not been well studied in the ED setting.

Hsieh T, Kupperman G, Jaggi T, et al: Characteristics and consequences of drug allergy alert overrides in a computerized physician order entry system. J Am Med Inform Assoc 11:482–491, 2004.

Potts A, Barr F, Gregory D, et al: Computerized physician order entry and medication errors in a pediatric critical care unit. Pediatrics 113:59–63, 2004.

19. **What are potential causes for patient misidentification?**
- Similar or same patient names
- Language barriers
- Patient answers to wrong name
- ID bands removed
- ID bands illegible or incorrect
- Lack of patient ID process or failure to comply

O'Neill K, Shinn D, Starr K: Patient misidentification in a pediatric emergency department: Patient safety and legal perspectives. Pediatr Emerg Care 20:487–492, 2004.

20. **How is patient safety taught to physicians in training?**
Professional societies have been challenged by the Committee on Quality of Health Care in America to develop curricula to teach patient safety routinely, and include such knowledge in certification requirements. The Patient Safety Task Force of the Society for Academic Emergency Medicine has developed a suggested curriculum for this mission. Guidelines and case-based examples are available on their website (www.saem.org).

Cosby K, Croskerry P: Patient safety: A curriculum for teaching patient safety in emergency medicine. Acad Emerg Med 10:69–78, 2004.

21. **What resources are available?**
- Agency for Healthcare Research and Quality (AHRQ) (www.ahrq.gov/qual): A division of the U.S. Department of Health and Human Services with a mission to improve the quality, safety, efficiency, and effectiveness of health care for all Americans.
- National Guideline Clearinghouse (www.guideline.gov): A public resource for evidence-based clinical practice guidelines and an initiative of the AHRQ. Search terms can be entered.
- National Patient Safety Foundation (www.npsf.org): Nonprofit organization devoted to understanding patient safety issues and how to improve them, as well as promoting public awareness and fostering communication.
- Institute for Safe Medication Practices (www.ismp.org): Nonprofit organization devoted entirely to medication error prevention.
- The Leapfrog Group (www.leapfroggroup.org)

CHAPTER 71

RISK MANAGEMENT AND ADMINISTRATIVE ISSUES

Steven M. Selbst, MD, FAAP, FACEP

1. **Which diagnoses involving pediatric patients in an emergency department (ED) are most likely to result in malpractice suits?**

   Most malpractice suits involving children in an ED result from failure to diagnose meningitis, appendicitis, fractures, and testicular torsion. In addition, failure to diagnose sepsis (especially meningococcemia), medication errors, errors in wound management, failure to diagnose slipped capital femoral epiphysis, myocarditis, dehydration, and child abuse are among the common sources of lawsuits in pediatric emergency medicine.

   > Reynolds SL: Missed appendicitis and medical liability. Clin Pediatr Emerg Med 4:231–234, 2003.
   >
   > Rothschild JM, Federico FA, Gandhi, TK et al: Analysis of medication-related malpractice claims. Arch Intern Med 162:2414–2420, 2002.
   >
   > Selbst SM, Friedman MJ, Singh SB: Epidemiology and etiology of malpractice lawsuits involving children in US emergency departments and urgent care centers. Ped Emerg Care 21:165–169, 2005.

2. **Why are emergency physicians at high risk for involvement in a malpractice suit?**

   Whenever the outcome is poor, an emergency physician is likely to be the subject of a malpractice suit, especially if the family is angry during their visit to the ED. Anger is a major force in initiating a lawsuit. Families in the ED may be dissatisfied before they even interact with the physician. They may be angry because of a long waiting time to see the physician. Sometimes they are angry with a discourteous staff member. The impersonal setting in the ED may be another contributing factor. It is often difficult to establish rapport with a family during a brief visit to the ED, which also puts the physician at a disadvantage if the outcome is poor.

   > Selbst SM, Koren JB: Preventing Malpractice Lawsuits in Pediatric Emergency Medicine. Dallas, American College of Emergency Physicians, 1999, pp 1–196.

3. **Which physicians have the highest average settlement per case? Why?**

   Pediatricians have the fourth highest indemnity per case compared with physicians of all other fields of medicine. Only those cases from neurology, neurosurgery, and obstetrics/gynecology are higher. The average settlement for pediatricians is about $254,000 per case. Pediatricians face high payments because an injured child generally has the potential for a longer period of suffering than an adult patient.

   > Physician Insurers Association of America: www.thepiaa.org

4. **How is the "standard of care" defined?**

   The standard of care is defined as care that a reasonable physician in a particular specialty would give to a similar patient under similar circumstances. Physicians generally are held to the same standard of care across the country—a national level of competence. It is assumed that all physicians have the same knowledge of current procedures, treatments, and practices. Although not every doctor has the same access to specialists and technology, it is usually expected that an emergency physician will recognize a medical condition and attempt to get the proper care for the child as soon as reasonably possible.

5. **In addition to civil charges, can criminal charges be brought against an emergency physician in a malpractice setting?**
   Rarely. In some cases, such as failure to report a case of drug abuse, child abuse, or injury by a weapon, an emergency physician may be charged with a misdemeanor. Such charges usually are not made unless it is believed that the doctor was deliberately uncooperative. If the patient has died, the doctor can be charged with manslaughter if it is believed that an extreme or unusual breach of the physician's duty took place. The court may determine that the physician's actions were reckless or disregarded the rights and safety of others. Again, this event is very rare.

6. **What is the statute of limitations?**
   The statute of limitations sets the length of time in which a person may bring a lawsuit for an alleged injury. Each state sets its own statute of limitations, but most states set a limit for adult patients of 2–3 years from the time that an injury due to alleged negligence is discovered or should have been discovered. After that time has passed, a malpractice suit cannot be initiated, regardless of the merits of the case. In a malpractice case involving a child, the time period does not begin until the child has reached the age of majority (18–21 years of age) in many states, because the child is unable to initiate legal action on his or her own behalf. Thus, it is possible for a lawsuit to be filed 18–20 years after the alleged injury occurred.

   Selbst SM, Korin JB: Malpractice and emergency care—doing right by the patient and yourself. Contemp Pediatr 17:88–106, 2000.

7. **What percentage of malpractice lawsuits is brought to a jury for a verdict?**
   Only about 10% of malpractice cases reach a jury verdict. Most are settled out of court, and some are dropped altogether. Nonetheless, a malpractice lawsuit, once initiated, is a long and stressful event for most physicians.

8. **How are plaintiffs rewarded in malpractice lawsuits involving children in the ED?**
   Although millions of dollars are paid out in malpractice lawsuits each year, money is actually paid to plaintiffs in about one third of closed claims. The overwhelming majority of payments occur in pretrial settlements. If a case proceeds to trial, the plaintiff is rarely rewarded. Less than 2% of cases result in judgment for the plaintiff.

   Selbst SM, Friedman MJ, Singh SB: Epidemiology and etiology of malpractice lawsuits involving children in US emergency departments and urgent care centers. Pediatr Emerg Care 21:165–169, 2005.

9. **What role does good communication play in reducing malpractice suits?**
   Good communication with patients and families is crucial. A lawsuit is more likely when there is poor communication between family members and the medical staff. One study showed a direct correlation between good communication skills of physicians and fewer malpractice suits. A patient or family must perceive that the physician has a caring attitude, professional integrity, openness, and high standards of excellence. Another study of families who had sued physicians found that most mothers were dissatisfied with the doctor–patient communication. About 13% reported that the doctor would not listen to them, 32% noted that the doctor would not talk openly, 48% believed that the doctor attempted to mislead them, and 70% believed that the doctor did not warn them about long-term neurodevelopmental problems.

   Hickson GB, Clayton EW, Githens PB et al: Factors that prompted families to file medical malpractice claims following perinatal injuries. JAMA 267:1359–1363, 1992.
   Hickson GB, Federspiel, Pichert JW, et al: Patient complaints and malpractice risk. JAMA 287:2951–2957, 2002.

10. **How important is it to arrange for a follow-up examination of a child seen in the ED?**

Physicians have been found liable when they failed to instruct parents, instructed them inadequately, or could not prove that they gave instructions to return to the ED or to seek care elsewhere. In one case, a patient successfully sued because a doctor did not document that an incidental finding of hypertension had been addressed and follow-up arranged. The child eventually developed end-stage renal disease. Discharge instructions for patients or parents should include specific information about when to seek follow-up care with the child's primary care physician or specialist or when to return to the ED.

Selbst SM: The febrile child—missed meningitis and bacteremia. Clin Pediatr Emerg Med 1:164–171, 2000.

11. **What is the physician's obligation to inform parents about a procedure or treatment?**

Physicians are obligated to obtain informed consent from parents. Most states follow a "patient-focused" concept of informed consent. That is, the doctor must give the consenting person (guardian) a description of the procedure and the risks and alternatives so that a reasonably prudent person would be able to make an informed decision about the procedure. A physician must speak in "lay language" so that the guardian understands the information. A guardian or patient is entitled to know the diagnosis, nature of the proposed treatment or procedure, risks and side effects of the procedure, available alternatives, and risks involved with alternatives. Guardians or patients also are entitled to know the prognosis with and without treatment. A physician should disclose all but the most remote risks if the outcome may be serious, but only common risks if they are likely to result in only minor harm to the child.

Kassutto Z, Vaught W: Informed decision making and refusal of treatment. Clin Pediatr Emerg Med 4:124, 2003.

12. **How important is it to get parents to sign a consent form for a procedure?**

A signed consent form has some value. It provides documentation that an attempt was made to educate the guardian about a procedure. However, signing a form does not always equate with informed consent. A parent may still claim that risks and benefits were not adequately explained. The consent form must be clearly written in language that most parents would understand. If a signed consent form is not used, the medical record should contain documentation that specific risks and benefits were explained to the guardian before the procedure was performed.

13. **When is it permitted to treat a minor in the ED without consent from a parent or guardian?**

Any minor can and should receive medical care in the event of a true emergency. Most states define an emergency in vague terms such as one that "threatens life and limb" or "life and health" of a child. Such vague definitions are meant to protect a well-meaning physician. In reality, because an emergency is often difficult to define, every patient who presents to the ED should receive a medical screening examination, even if parents or guardians are not available to give consent. Generally, parental consent for treatment is not needed if a child presents to the ED with a chief complaint related to venereal disease, pregnancy, testing for HIV, or drug and alcohol abuse. However, many states require that the child be over the age of 14 before treatment can be rendered for these conditions.

14. **What is an emancipated minor?**

An emancipated minor is one who can seek and receive medical care without the consent of parents. In almost all 50 states, an emancipated minor is defined as one who is:
- Over the age of 18 years
- Has been married or self-employed

- Has graduated from high school
- Has served in the armed forces
- Is otherwise independent of parental care or control

Many states consider a pregnant minor to be emancipated and allow her to give consent for care for herself and her unborn baby.

Anderson SL, Shaechter J, Brosco JP: Adolescent patients and their confidentiality: Staying within legal bounds. Contemp Pediatr 22:54–64, 2005.

15. What is the "mature minor doctrine"?

This law, recognized by about 22 states, allows a minor over the age of 14 years (not necessarily emancipated) to consent to medical or surgical treatment even if it is not a true emergency. In the judgment of the treating physician, the minor must be "sufficiently mature to understand the nature of the procedure and its consequences." The treatment must be intended to benefit the minor rather than someone else and must not involve serious risks. For example, the mature minor doctrine was applied to the case of a 17-year-old girl who consented to receive treatment for a minor finger laceration without parental consent.

American Academy of Pediatrics Committee on Pediatric Emergency Medicine: Consent for emergency medical services for children and adolescents. Pediatrics 111:703–706, 2003.

Kassutto Z, Vaught W: Informed decision making and refusal of treatment. Clin Pediatr Emerg Med 4:124, 2003.

16. In which situations do parents *not* have the right to refuse treatment for their child?

If a life-threatening situation exists and the emergency physician believes that it is unsafe for a patient to leave the ED to seek care elsewhere, a family cannot sign out against medical advice or refuse care for their child. Likewise, if the patient or parent is under the influence of drugs or alcohol and cannot understand the risks and benefits of receiving or refusing care, the patient cannot be permitted to leave the ED. Finally, if child abuse is suspected, a guardian may not refuse care for the child.

17. What is the appropriate way to correct a written error in the medical record?

An error should be corrected with a single line drawn through the incorrect statement. The correction should be initialed and dated by the clinician. The emergency physician should not attempt to hide an error written on a patient's chart.

18. List guidelines for documentation in the medical record of a child who presents to the ED.

- Always document the child's chief complaint, even if it seems trivial.
- Be sure to record the child's medical history, allergies, immunization status, and current medications.
- Carefully describe the child's general appearance and state of hydration.
- Include important positive and negative findings, rather than just noting that the examination was "normal."
- Avoid derogatory or self-serving statements in the record.
- Make sure that the chart looks neat and professional.
- When appropriate, record a "progress note" to indicate a child has improved prior to discharge.
- *Never enhance or alter the record* after the child leaves the ED. Additions should be made cautiously and must be timed and dated so as not to appear misleading.

19. How should an ED physician proceed if the referring primary care doctor disagrees with the ED physician's assessment and plan for the child?

It is not uncommon for a referring physician to have a specific plan in mind for a pediatric patient. However, once the child arrives in the ED, the emergency physician probably will have some liability if the outcome is poor. The ED physician may be considered in a better position to determine the child's need for treatment and hospital admission, especially if the referring doctor has not actually examined the patient. Thus, the emergency physician should not automatically defer to the referring doctor on the telephone. The emergency physician should try to reach an agreement about the child's care without compromising what he or she believes is the best plan for the child. If the referring doctor does not agree with the decision to admit a child, it is best for that doctor to come to the ED (if he or she has staff privileges) to examine the child and assume responsibility for the disposition. Emergency care should not be delayed while waiting for a primary care physician or specialist requested by the primary care physician to arrive in the ED. Hospital policies should be in place to guide the staff in such situations.

20. **What is EMTALA?**

The Emergency Medical Treatment and Active Labor Act (EMTALA) states that all hospitals that receive Medicare funds and have an ED must provide an "appropriate medical screening examination" to all patients who present to the ED to determine whether a medical emergency exists. EMTALA was developed to protect patients without medical insurance from being "dumped" by some hospitals, but the law applies to patients with insurance as well as to those who belong to a managed care plan. Many experts recommend that an emergency physician perform the medical screening examination rather than a nurse. However, EMTALA has been updated, and hospitals may allow nonphysicians to perform the screenings as long as hospital policies define in writing that such individuals are authorized to perform the screenings. The acuity of the patient's illness may indicate whether a physician should perform the screening. A medical screening examination may range from a brief history and physical examination to a complex process involving ancillary studies and procedures. The screening examination must include all appropriate ancillary tests and services normally available to any patient. The tests must be ordered regardless of the patient's insurance if they are needed to determine whether an emergency exists.

Bittinger AM: Changes to EMTALA rules affect pediatric emergency departments. Pediatr Emerg Care 20:347–353, 2004.

Linzer JF, EMTALA: A clearer road in the future? Clin Pediatr Emerg Med 4:249–255, 2003.

KEY POINTS: TIPS TO PREVENT MALPRACTICE LAWSUITS IN PEDIATRIC EMERGENCY MEDICINE ✔

1. Use caution in treating children with fever and abdominal pain.

2. Use caution if the patient is unable to ambulate upon discharge without a good explanation.

3. Use caution in performing a lumbar puncture in a small infant, especially if the baby is in respiratory distress (risk of apnea).

4. Remember that care given by others in the hospital (and prehospital) will affect the liability of the ED staff.

5. Communicate carefully with colleagues, especially around change of shift.

6. Consider pathology beyond the gastrointestinal tract if a child has vomiting.

7. Do not allow consultants to avoid cases when their help is needed.

8. Ask for help when managing complex wounds.

9. Read the notes of others involved in the child's care.

10. Document patient improvement in a discharge note.

21. **When is transfer of a child from the ED in compliance with EMTALA?**

    A patient may be transferred from the ED if the transfer is medically indicated and the patient needs a level of care that is not available at the transferring hospital. An unstable child may be transferred if the patient or parents make the request. Informed consent should be obtained if the patient or parent requests the transfer. If the transfer is medically indicated, the emergency physician must document that the benefits of transfer outweigh the risks and must arrange for an "appropriate" or safe transfer.

    Woodward GA: Legal issues in pediatric interfacility transport. Clin Pediatr Emerg Med 4:256–264, 2003.

22. **Is a pediatric ED responsible for an adult with an emergency according to EMTALA?**

    If a patient is within 250 yards of the hospital, EMTALA rules apply. Thus, if a person (child or adult) collapses on the parking lot or sidewalk outside the ED, or in the hospital gift shop, the hospital is obligated to screen and appropriately stabilize the individual, regardless of the person's ability to pay. Pediatric ED staff should screen and attempt to stabilize the adult patient within their capabilities. Staff should not just call emergency medical services without first starting to treat the adult. The hospital should generate a medical record for the adult patient, and the physician may wish to certify that benefits of transfer to a hospital for adults outweighs the risks of continuing treatment in the pediatric hospital, which has limited capabilities.

23. **What is the policy of the American College of Emergency Physicians (ACEP) about providing telephone advice from the ED?**

    The ACEP policy (2000) states that most medical conditions cannot be accurately diagnosed by telephone. Each ED should have a procedure to identify the nature of all incoming calls. Persons making calls about life- or limb-threatening medical emergencies should be given information about how to access the emergency medical services system. Calls from patients recently discharged from the ED should be managed by prearranged protocols. In the interest of good patient care, the ACEP recommends that EDs do not attempt medical assessment or management by telephone. Callers should be advised that EDs are available at all times to assess their condition.

    American College of Emergency Physicians: www.acep.org

24. **What are the most important factors in patient satisfaction in the ED?**

    Patient satisfaction depends primarily on prompt treatment, the caring nature of the emergency nurses and physicians, and the degree of organization of the medical staff.

25. **What are the most common sources of complaints resulting from pediatric visits to the ED?**

    Most patient or parent complaints concern waiting time, quality of medical care (including an incomplete medical examination or failure to order enough tests), attitude of the ED staff, and misdiagnosis. In a general ED, complaints about billing are frequent, but billing accounts for only about 20% of complaints from a pediatric ED. Other complaints from families involve an unclean appearance and lack of privacy in the ED.

26. **What are "good Samaritan statutes"?**

    Good Samaritan statutes exist in almost every state and provide immunity to physicians and others who err while administering emergency medical care to ill or injured people. The laws were passed to encourage physicians and others to stop at the scene of an emergency and offer assistance without fear of a malpractice suit. The Good Samaritan statutes require that aid be given without compensation. They generally apply to care at the scene of an accident rather than in the ED or elsewhere in the hospital. Physicians are obligated to act in good faith but are not expected to put their own lives or their families in danger. Many statutes exclude "gross negligence" or "willful misconduct," but a physician who makes an honest mistake is likely to be protected. A lawsuit still may be initiated if the patient suffers a poor outcome after treatment at the scene of an accident, but the suit is likely to be unsuccessful if the physician acted in good faith.

27. **What should you do if named in a malpractice lawsuit?**
Contact your insurance carrier as soon as possible about any potential lawsuit, even a threatening letter from an attorney. Early notification allows the insurance carrier to investigate the claim and prepare a defense. It is possible that a "default judgment" against the physician may result if the doctor fails to notify his or her carrier and the defense team is not given adequate time to answer a claim.

28. **Which actions are reported to the National Practitioner Data Bank (NPDB)?**
   - Any adverse licensure action, whereby a physician is denied a medical license because of professional incompetence or misconduct.
   - Any action by a professional society, hospital, or other health care facility that adversely affects a physician's clinical privileges for more than 30 days. This includes voluntary surrender of clinical privileges while under investigation or in return for not conducting an investigation.
   - All medical malpractice payments. Payors must submit reports to the NPDB about payments to settle a claim within 30 days of payment.

29. **Who is permitted to access information from the NPDB?**
Hospitals *must* request information when screening an applicant for medical staff appointment or granting new clinical privileges and every 2 years for medical staff reappointment. State licensing boards and other health care entities *may* request information when screening applicants for licenses or privileges. Professional societies also *may* request information when a physician applies for membership. In some cases, a plaintiff's attorney *may* request information from the NPDB if there is evidence that a hospital failed to check on the status of a staff physician involved in a malpractice case. Currently, the lay public *may not* access information from the NPDB.

30. **What are some tips to prevent complaints in the pediatric ED?**
See Table 71-1. Complaints from parents in the ED are inevitable, but many are preventable. It generally requires less work to prevent a complaint than to manage a family after they have formally complained about their ED visit. Developing rapport with families is essential. Good communication skills are extremely important. Sitting at the bedside with a patient and family can improve patient satisfaction. When the physician takes time to sit in the examining room, patients perceive that they spent more time with the physician.

Cronan K: Pediatric complaints in a pediatric emergency department: Averting lawsuits. Clin Pediatr Emerg Med 4:235–242, 2005.

31. **What is the recommendation of ACEP to manage telephone orders called to the ED by outside physicians?**
ACEP believes that telephone orders for ED patients that are dictated by a physician from outside the ED can adversely affect the quality of medical care that patients receive and create legal liability for physicians. ACEP endorses the following principles:
   - Hospital policy should specify the criteria for accepting telephone orders in the ED.
   - Hospital policy should specify that all patients who come to the hospital for emergency care should be provided with an appropriate medical screening examination.
   - Telephone orders directed to ED personnel should be subject to the review and approval of the emergency physician on duty.

TABLE 71-1. TIPS TO PREVENT COMPLAINTS IN THE PEDIATRIC EMERGENCY DEPARTMENT

1. Meet or exceed the expectations of the patient and family.
2. Introduce yourself to the family.
3. Pay attention to the patient and family.
4. Tell them why they are waiting.
5. Make the patient and family comfortable while they wait.
6. Defuse potential complaints during the visit.

From Cronan K: Pediatric complaints in a pediatric emergency department: Averting lawsuits. Clin Ped Emerg Med 4:235–242, 2003.

It should also be noted that the Drug Enforcement Administration regulations prohibit dispensing controlled substances from ED stocks for treatment of patients by telephone order.

American College of Emergency Physicians: www.acep.org

32. **Does the presence of family members at the resuscitation of a relative increase the risk of litigation for emergency physicians?**
No data exist on family member presence and litigation. However, most families who witness a resuscitation report favorable opinions of the medical personnel involved. This is true even though the actual survival rate from resuscitation is far lower than the perception of the public. Family satisfaction after witnessing cardiopulmonary resuscitation may actually lower the risk of a malpractice lawsuit, even in the event of a poor outcome. Also, health care providers are more likely to consider the privacy of a patient and pain management when family members are present. Attention to these details may also reduce the risk of malpractice lawsuits.

Sacchetti AD, Guzzetta CE, Harris RH: Family presence during resuscitation attempts and invasive procedures: Is there science behind the emotion? Clin Pediatr Emerg Med 4:292–296, 2003.

CHAPTER 72

SEDATION AND ANALGESIA

Richard J. Scarfone, MD, FAAP

1. **Why is the term *conscious sedation* considered obsolete?**
   In the past, conscious sedation has been defined as a medically controlled state of depressed consciousness in which:
   - Protective reflexes are maintained
   - The airway remains patent
   - The patient responds purposefully to physical or verbal stimuli

   This term is now considered obsolete and has been replaced with the phrase *moderate sedation and analgesia*. For most clinical indications, emergency department (ED) physicians are attempting to achieve a deeper level of altered consciousness for their patients, referred to as *deep sedation and analgesia*. This state is characterized by:
   - Partial or complete loss of protective reflexes
   - An inability to independently maintain a patent airway
   - No purposeful response to stimulation

   American Society of Anesthesiologists: Continuum of depth of sedation: Definition of general anesthesia and levels of sedation/analgesia: www.asahq.org/publicationsAndServices/standards/20.pdf
   EMSC Grant Panel on Pharmacologic Agents Used in Pediatric Sedation and Analgesia in the Emergency Department: Clinical policy: Evidence-based approach to pharmacologic agents used in pediatric sedation and analgesia in the emergency department. Ann Emerg Med 44:342–377, 2004.

2. **What are some reasons for the mismanagement of pain in children?**
   - Lack of available data in children. The Food and Drug Administration studies and approves medications for use in adults. Physicians must extrapolate this information for pediatric patients. Until the past decade, few clinical trials assessed the safety and efficacy of sedatives or analgesics in children.
   - Fear of addiction from opioids. In both adult and pediatric patients, physicians have been overly concerned about inducing addiction with the use of opioid analgesics. In fact, addiction is a rare consequence of the legitimate use of opioids for medical purposes in children.
   - Belief that neonates and young children do not experience pain to the same degree as adults because of their immature nervous systems. Any physician who has attempted to intubate the trachea of an awake neonate or to perform a lumbar puncture in a struggling toddler can testify to the contrary. Young children cannot understand the purpose of a painful procedure or comprehend its time-limited nature. Therefore, they are likely to experience a greater degree of pain and anxiety compared to older children or adults and are more likely to benefit from the liberal use of procedural sedation and analgesia (PSA).

   Berde CB, Sethna NF: Analgesics for the treatment of pain in children. N Engl J Med 347:1094–1101, 2004.
   Lampell MS, Leder MS: Pediatric pain control. Pediatr Emerg Med Rep 4:73–84, 1999.
   Zempsky WT, Cravero JP, Committee on Pediatric Emergency Medicine and Section on Anesthesiology and Pain Medicine: Relief of pain and anxiety in pediatric patients in emergency medical systems. Pediatrics 114:1348–1356, 2004.

3. **What are tolerance, physical dependence, and addiction?**
   A child with sickle cell anemia who has been treated at home with acetaminophen and codeine for 2 weeks will probably require higher than usual doses of parenteral narcotics for

management of a vaso-occlusive crisis. Such a child may have developed *tolerance*, diminished effectiveness of the drug with repeated administration. A child with leukemia and bony pain who abruptly discontinues daily oral morphine after 10 days may experience headaches, sweating, tachycardia, and tachypnea. Such a child may have developed *physical dependence*. In contrast, *addiction* is a psychological syndrome marked by compulsive drug-seeking behavior and associated with desire for euphoric effects.

4. **Describe methods to reduce the pain of administration of local anesthetics.**
   Local anesthetics administered through intact skin or into an open wound can cause considerable pain. Techniques that may be employed to reduce the pain of injection include using a needle of small caliber, buffering the lidocaine with bicarbonate, warming the drug, injecting slowly, and providing counterstimulation to the adjacent skin. Many physicians employ topical formulations, such as lidocaine, epinephrine, and tetracaine, either in a liquid or a gel form. This may be administered, without using a needle, to exposed mucosa. These drugs should not be used in any regions of the body in which epinephrine is contraindicated, such as fingertips or ears.

   In addition, liposomal lidocaine (LMX) and a mixture of lidocaine and prilocaine (EMLA) may each be applied to intact skin to reduce the pain of venipuncture. Physicians have also found these topical mixtures to alleviate the pain associated with lumbar punctures incision of abscesses, and insertion of intravenous lines.

   > Berde CB, Sethna NF: Analgesics for the treatment of pain in children. N Engl J Med 347:1094–1101, 2002.
   > Eichenfield LF, Funk A, Fallon-Friedlander S, Cunningham BB: A clinical study to evaluate the efficacy of ELA-Max (4% liposomal lidocaine) as compared with eutectic mixture of local anesthetics cream for pain reduction of venipucture in children. Pediatrics 109:1093–1099, 2002.
   > Scarfone RJ, Jasani M, Gracey EJ: Pain of local anesthetics: Rate of administration and buffering. Ann Emerg Med 36:36–40, 1998.
   > Zempsky WT, Cravero JP, Committee on Pediatric Emergency Medicine and Section on Anesthesiology and Pain Medicine: Relief of pain and anxiety in pediatric patients in emergency medical systems. Pediatrics 114:1348–1356, 2004.

5. **Describe the key elements of the medical history for a child about to receive PSA.**
   Aspects of the history that should be known before drug administration include time since last meal, current medications, allergies, pregnancy status, significant medical history, history of complications with sedation or general anesthesia, and a complete review of systems.
   If the child was transported from another institution, the clinician must know whether he or she received sedation or analgesia at the referring hospital and, if so, what was given and when. In addition, physicians should ask questions pertinent to the specific medication that one is about to give. For example, active laryngotracheobronchitis should be considered a contraindication to the use of ketamine.

6. **Describe the key elements of the physical examination for a child about to receive PSA.**
   Clinicians must monitor the patient's vital signs (especially blood pressure), cardiac and pulmonary examinations, and mental status. Many agents cause hypotension and should be used cautiously or not at all for children with impending shock. Similarly, agents that may cause hypoventilation and hypoxemia are poor choices for any child with respiratory distress.

7. **How much time should elapse between the last oral intake of food or liquid and PSA?**
   This is perhaps the area of greatest controversy in the administration of PSA to children. These are the published fasting guidelines for elective procedures developed by the American Society of Anesthesiologists (ASA):

Ingested Material	Minimum Fasting Period
Clear liquids	2 hr
Breast milk	4 hr
Infant formula, nonhuman milk, light meal	6 hr

8. **What are the concerns about fasting guidelines for PSA?**
   Problems with these guidelines include:
   - They are arbitrary: For example, what evidence exists to support a longer fasting time after formula intake compared to breast milk? How does the age of the patient or the volume ingested influence these recommendations? In fact, the ASA states that "the literature does not provide sufficient evidence to test the hypothesis that preprocedural fasting results in a decreased incidence of adverse outcomes."
   - They were written for fasting prior to general anesthesia.
   - Physicians working in busy EDs with time and space constraints find these guidelines prohibitively conservative and difficult to adhere to.
   - Aspiration following moderate or deep sedation is extremely rare.

   Newer evidence suggests that prolonged fasting may not lead to fewer adverse events. In a recent report of over 1000 children receiving PSA, about half were not fasted as per the ASA guidelines. These children did not experience a greater incidence of aspiration or other adverse outcomes compared to the fasted group. A second study of over 2000 children and young adults found no correlation between preprocedural fasting time and adverse outcomes.

   A recently published clinical practice advisory recommends weighing several factors when deciding what is the appropriate fasting for elective procedures. These factors include the overall health of the patient, the desired length and depth of sedation and analgesia, and the urgency of the procedure.

   Agrawal D, Manzi SF, Gupta R, Krauss B: Preprocedural fasting state and adverse events in children undergoing procedural sedation and analgesia in a pediatric emergency department. Ann Emerg Med 42:636–646, 2003.

   American Society of Anesthesiologists: Practice guidelines for sedation and analgesia by non-anesthesiologists. American Society of Anesthesiologists task force on sedation and analgesia by non-anesthesiologists. Anesthesiology 96:1004–1017, 2002.

   Green SM.: Fasting is a consideration—not a necessity—for emergency department procedural sedation and analgesia. Ann Emerg Med 42:647–650, 2003.

   Green SM, et al. Fasting and emergency department procedural sedation and analgesia: a consensus-based clinical practice advisory. Ann Emerg Med 49:454–461, 2007.

   Roback, MG, Bajaj L, Wathen JE, Bothner J: Preprocedural fasting and adverse events in procedural sedation and analgesia in a pediatric emergency department: Are they related? Ann Emerg Med 44:454–459, 2004.

9. **What is the ASA physical status classification?**
   This is a physical status classification based on the ASA recommendations. This status should be assigned before the initiation of sedation. There are five classes.
   - **Class I:** Normally healthy patient
   - **Class II:** Patient with mild systemic disease (e.g., mild asthma)
   - **Class III:** Patient with severe systemic disease (e.g., poorly controlled diabetes mellitus)
   - **Class IV:** Patient with severe systemic disease that is a constant threat to life
   - **Class V:** Moribund patient who is unlikely to survive without the operation

10. **During PSA, which equipment is needed to monitor the patient and to be immediately available at the bedside?**
    The risks of sedating children are significant and include hypoventilation, apnea, airway obstruction hypotension, and aspiration. Equipment that should be immediately available at the bedside includes:

- Cardiorespiratory monitor
- Pulse oximeter
- Blood pressure cuff
- Suction catheters
- Oxygen source
- Airway equipment, such as self-inflating breathing bags with masks, and oropharyngeal and nasopharyngeal airways
  In addition, advanced airway equipment, such as laryngoscopes and endotracheal tubes, should be available in the ED.

American Academy of Pediatrics and American Academy of Dentistry: Guidelines for monitoring and management of pediatric patients during and after sedation for diagnostic and therapeutic procedures: an update. Pediatrics 118:2587–2602, 2006.

American Society of Anesthesiologists: Practice guidelines for sedation and analgesia by non-anesthesiologists. American Society of Anesthesiologists task force on sedation and analgesia by non-anesthesiologists. Anesthesiology 96:1004–1017, 2002.

11. **What is the optimal staffing for PSA?**
Ideally, a physician experienced in pediatric advanced life support should administer the medications and closely observe the child's response. The risk of respiratory depression is minimized by administering agents slowly, over about 60 seconds. The physician should remain at the bedside at least until the period of peak sedation and cardiorespiratory side effects has passed (typically about 20 minutes). A second physician should perform the procedure. In this way, a single physician is not dividing attention between two important tasks. A nurse should document the patient's response to medications and be available to assist in suctioning or administering oxygen or reversal agents.

12. **How frequently should the child be monitored? How should this be documented?**
A sedation and analgesia flow chart should supplement the patient's medical record, with a complete and accurate account of the encounter. Medications, times administered, doses, routes, and name of the person who gave the drugs should be recorded. The patient's vital signs, oxygen saturation, and mental status should be monitored continuously, with recordings documented every 5 minutes for the first 30 minutes after drug administration. One-on-one clinical monitoring should continue until the child is well into the recovery phase. The frequency of monitoring beyond the initial half-hour and the duration of observation depend on which agents were given and depth of sedation.

13. **Describe the characteristics of the ideal agent for sedation and analgesia.**
- Painless administration
- Onset of action within minutes
- Adequate and predictable sedation, analgesia, anxiolysis, and amnesia
- Excellent safety profile
- Duration of action longer than procedure time
- Rapid recovery
- Ready reversibility
  In fact, no agent has all of these desirable characteristics. Clinicians must decide what agent or agents can safely and efficiently achieve the goals for a particular clinical situation.

14. **What are the expected rates of success and complications for PSA in children?**
Recent data has demonstrated that when PSA is provided to children by pediatric emergency medicine physicians in a tertiary care children's hospital, success rates are very high and serious adverse outcomes are rare. In one report, over 1200 children received PSA in such a setting, with a variety of different medications being employed. For more than 98% of the children, the procedure was successfully completed while the patient remained minimally responsive. The rate of complications was 18%, with the most common complication being hypoxia.

In a study assessing more than 30,000 pediatric sedation/anesthesia events, there were no deaths, cardiopulmonary resuscitation was required once, and oxygen desaturation was uncommon.

Cravero JP, et al. Incidence and nature of adverse events during pediatric sedation/anesthesia for procedures outside the operating room: report from the Pediatric Sedation Research Consortium. Pediatrics 118:1087–1096, 2006.

Newman DH, Azer MM, Pitetti RD, Singh S: When is a patient safe for discharge after procedural sedation? The timing of adverse effect events in 1,367 pediatric procedural sedations. Ann Emerg Med 42:627–645, 2003.

Pitetti RD, Singh S, Pierce MC: Safe and efficacious use of procedural sedation and analgesia by nonanesthesiologists in a pediatric emergency department. Arch Pediatr Adolesc Med 157:1090–1096, 2003.

15. **What are the advantages and disadvantages of transmucosal drug administration?**

The main advantage of transmucosal (oral, intranasal, rectal) compared to parenteral (IV, intramuscular) drug administration is its painless nature. It seems counterintuitive to cause pain with a needle puncture in an attempt to ultimately relieve pain. However, important disadvantages of transmucosal administration include delayed onset of action, less predictable results, and difficulties in titrating the dose to the desired effect. It can be frustrating to the child, parents, and doctor if the child is fully alert 40 minutes after an oral sedative has been administered. Thus, for most ED indications, the parenteral route of administration is preferred because it allows finer minute-to-minute control of depth of sedation and analgesia.

16. **What are the advantages and disadvantages of chloral hydrate?**

The main advantages of chloral hydrate are that it may be given orally and it has a relatively good safety profile. Its use in the ED is limited by a prolonged time to onset of sedation (30–60 minutes for peak plasma concentrations), prolonged recovery time (several hours), frequent gastric irritation and emesis, and inability to titrate the dose effectively.

17. **Discuss the role of propofol for PSA.**

Propofol is a nonbarbiturate ultra–short-acting hypnotic agent. It has an extremely short onset (within 1 minute) of effect and duration of action, necessitating delivery by continuous IV infusion or frequent readministration for most procedures. Respiratory depression, hypoxemia, hypotension, and injection pain are common side effects. Its use requires vigilance on the part of physicians because of the likelihood of adverse effects. Its extremely rapid onset of action and potency make it difficult to titrate without inducing serious adverse effects. Unless physicians are experienced with its use, propofol would not be a good choice for sedating a child who will be leaving the ED, such as for a radiologic study. Even in the hands of practitioners experienced with its use, two thirds of children experienced decreases in systolic blood pressure below the fifth percentile and 12% had partial airway obstruction.

Bassett KE, Anderson JL, Pribble CG, et al: Propofol for procedural sedation in children in the emergency department. Ann Emerg Med 42:773–782, 2003.

Green SM, Krauss B: Propofol in emergency medicine: Pushing the sedation frontier. Ann Emerg Med 42:792–797, 2003.

Guenther E, Pribble CG, Junkins EP Jr, et al: Propofol sedation by emergency physicians for elective pediatric outpatient procedures. Ann Emerg Med 42:783–791, 2003.

Hertzog JH, Dalton HJ, Anderson BD, et al: Prospective evaluation of propofol anesthesia in the pediatric intensive care unit for elective oncology procedures in ambulatory and hospitalized children. Pediatrics 106:742–747, 2000.

18. **Discuss the role of etomidate for PSA.**

Etomidate is a nonbarbituate hypnotic without analgesic properties that has been used extensively as an anesthetic induction agent. It has a very rapid onset of action, short duration of action, and minimal effects on cardiovascular status. Myoclonus and injection pain are common side effects. There is a growing experience with its use for PSA in children. In a recent study, it compared favorably to pentobarbital for sedating children for CT scans. Similarly, it has been shown to be superior to midazolam for fracture reductions.

Baxter AL, et al. Etomidate versus pentobarbital for computed tomography sedations: Report from the Pediatric Sedation Research Consortium. Pediatr Emerg Care 23:690–695, 2007.

Liddo LD, et al. Etomidate versus midazolam for procedural sedation in pediatric outpatients: A randomized controlled trial. Ann Emerg Med 48:433–440, 2006.

Miner JR, et al. Randomized clinical trial of etomidate versus propofol for procedural sedation in the emergency department. Ann Emerg Med 49:15–22, 2007.

KEY POINTS: SEDATIVE/HYPNOTIC AGENTS USED IN SEDATION ✔

1. Midalozam

2. Propofol

3. Chloral hydrate

4. Barbiturates

5. Etomidate

19. **Can opioids be used safely in neonates?**

The greatest experience with the use of opioids in neonates is with the use of morphine. Morphine may be indicated to reduce the pain associated with a strangulated inguinal hernia or resulting from an inflicted injury, such as a fracture. Because a smaller proportion of an administered dose of morphine is protein-bound in young infants compared to older children, the proportion of drug reaching the brain is increased and the elimination half-life is prolonged. Thus, very young infants are particularly susceptible to apnea and respiratory depression with morphine. For those <6 months of age, a starting dose that is one-quarter to one-third the dose recommended for older infants and children should be used. Age from birth, rather than duration of gestation, determines how premature and full-term infants metabolize narcotics. Thus, a 4-month-old who was born at term metabolizes narcotics at the same rate as a 4-month-old who was born prematurely. The clinician must judge the infant's facial expressions, heart rate, and blood pressure to determine whether to administer additional morphine for the desired effect.

Berde CB, Sethna NF: Analgesics for the treatment of pain in children. N Engl J Med 347:1094–1101, 2002.

20. **A bead is located in the ear canal of an 8-year-old boy. Initial attempts to remove it cause considerable anxiety and discomfort, preventing successful removal. What are some sedation options for this patient?**

Because the boy does not have an inherently painful condition and because he does not require an IV line for any other reason, a pure sedative hypnotic such as midazolam given orally may be a reasonable option. However, it will take about 30 minutes for the full effects to be realized, the depth of sedation after oral administration is not predictable, and midazolam alone does not offer him analgesia. Intranasal midazolam administered with an atomizer is likely to result in more rapid and more reliable sedation than that given orally. Another option would be nitrous oxide, an odorless gas that patients inhale. Nitrous oxide causes mild analgesia, anxiolysis, sedation, and amnesia. Its ease of delivery and rapid onset of action makes it ideal for sedation before foreign-body removal. However, at a ratio of 50% nitrous oxide to 50% oxygen, it is not likely to be effective for more painful procedures, such as incision and drainage of an abscess.

21. **A 3-year-old girl fell down five cement steps and struck her head on the pavement. She has vomited repeatedly since the injury but is fully alert and awake in the ED. You want to perform computed tomography of the head to rule out an intracranial injury. What are some sedation options for this patient?**

Because the desired goal is to prevent the child from struggling and moving during the study, you wish to achieve sedation rather than analgesia. Pure sedative-hypnotics in common use in EDs include chloral hydrate, propofol, benzodiazepines, barbiturates, and etomidate. In addition to providing sedation before imaging studies, these drugs may also be useful as adjuncts to narcotics prior to painful procedures.

For this patient, midazolam or pentobarbital may be the best choices. The ability to titrate each drug offers an advantage over chloral hydrate. Their safety profiles and longer durations of action offer advantages over propofol and etomidate.

Midazolam may be administered by the IV, intramuscular, oral, nasal, or rectal routes. Its onset is within minutes after IV administration, and clinical effectiveness usually lasts about 30 minutes. One may expect mild reductions in blood pressure and dose-related respiratory depression. Significant hypoventilation is rare unless the drug is given concurrently with a narcotic or pushed too rapidly. Its effects may be reversed with the competitive antagonist flumazenil.

Pentobarbital is a short-acting barbiturate that produces sedation within 5 minutes, lasting 30–60 minutes. As with midazolam, hypoventilation may occur but responds readily to gentle stimulation. Hypotension is a common side effect, and the drug should not be used in children with possible cardiovascular compromise.

22. **An adolescent girl needs a lumbar puncture to rule out aseptic meningitis. What agent(s) should be used for PSA?**

For this procedure, an IV sedative alone does not provide analgesia for the painful local anesthetic that should be administered in the lumbar region. Topical anesthetics alone don't provide a great enough depth of analgesia for this indication. In response to the injection of the local anesthetic, an anxious patient may arch her back and move enough that it will be nearly impossible to perform the lumbar puncture.

Some physicians have had success combining midazolam with fentanyl, which is 100 times more potent than morphine. Fentanyl's onset and duration of action closely parallel that of midazolam, making this combination particularly potent. Fentanyl provides analgesia and potentiates the sedative effect of midazolam. Respiratory depression is common with this combination but may be minimized by administering each agent over 60 seconds with a 60-second interval in between and by titrating doses carefully. Gentle stimulation of the patient and supplemental oxygen almost always prevent hypoxemia.

Fentanyl has a more rapid onset and shorter duration of action than morphine, making it a better choice for most procedural analgesia. When more prolonged analgesia is desired (e.g., for vaso-occlusive crisis), morphine is the better choice. The combination of midazolam and fentanyl is also useful in the settings of laceration repair, burn care, and reduction of minimally displaced or angulated fractures.

23. **A 10-year-old boy has displaced and angulated fractures to his ulna and radius that require closed reduction. What agent(s) should be used for PSA?**

Clearly, the primary goal in this case is to achieve potent analgesia for what is anticipated to be a very painful procedure. With the midazolam/fentanyl combination it will be difficult to achieve the depth of analgesia required without producing significant hypoventilation. In this case, ketamine is a good choice. It causes dissociation between the cortical and limbic systems, resulting in potent sedation, analgesia, and amnesia. Unlike most other agents, it does not cause cardiovascular depression. In fact, patients typically experience an increased heart rate and blood pressure with its use. Onset of action after IV administration is 3–5 minutes, with return of coherence in 30–45 minutes. Because ketamine causes hypersalivation, concurrent administration of atropine or glycopyrolate is indicated. Two uncommon but potentially serious side effects are hallucinatory emergence reactions and laryngospasm. Many clinicians believe that the incidence of emergent reactions can be minimized with the concurrent administration of midazolam, but the results of recent studies have failed to prove this. In a study assessing the ED use of intramuscular ketamine among more than 1000 children, over 90% achieved acceptable sedation within 10 minutes and four young children experienced transient laryngospasm. The expected rate of laryngospasm with the use of ketamine is 1 in 250.

Green SM, Krauss B: Clinical practice guideline for emergency department ketamine dissociative sedation in children. Ann Emerg Med 44:1–21, 2004.

Green SM, Rothrock SG, Lynch EL, et al: Intramuscular ketamine for pediatric sedation in the emergency department: Safety profile in 1,022 cases. Ann Emerg Med 31:688–697, 1998.

Heinz P, et al. Is atropine needed with ketamine sedation? A prospective, randomized, double-blind study. Emerg Med J 23:206–209, 2006.

Roback MG, et al. A randomized, controlled trial of IV versus IM ketamine for sedation of pediatric patients receiving emergency department orthopedic procedures. Ann Emerg Med 48:605–612, 2006.

Sherwin TS, Green SM, Khan A: Does adjunctive midazolam reduce recovery agitation after ketamine sedation for pediatric procedures? A randomized, double-blind, placebo-controlled trial. Ann Emerg Med 35:239–244, 2000.

Wathen JE, Roback MG, Mackenzie T, Bothner JP: Does midazolam alter the clinical effects of intravenous ketamine sedation in children? A double-blind, randomized, controlled, emergency department trial. Ann Emerg Med 36:579–588, 2003.

24. **What are the contraindications to the use of ketamine?**
Absolute contraindications to the use of ketamine are age younger than 3 months (because of increased risk of laryngospasm) or psychosis. Other factors are considered to be relative contraindications because of the concern for laryngospasm, and physicians must weigh the risk/benefit ratio for individual patients. These factors include age younger than 12 months, intraoral procedures, upper airway problems (such as moderate upper respiratory tract infection, croup, tracheomalacia, active asthma, or anatomic abnormalities). Other relative contraindications include coronary artery disease, increased intracranial pressure, and glaucoma.

Green SM, Krauss B: Clinical practice guideline for emergency department ketamine dissociative sedation in children. Ann Emerg Med 44:1–21, 2004.

Lampell MS, Leder MS: Pediatric pain control. Pediatr Emerg Med Rep 4:73–84, 1999.

25. **For what period of time should a child be observed in the ED after PSA before being discharged home?**
A recent report of over 1300 sedation events in children found that 92% of adverse events occurred during the procedure and serious adverse events rarely occurred after 25 minutes from the final medication administration. In another study of over 1000 children who had received intramuscular ketamine, four experienced laryngospasm. Onset of this complication ranged from 15–25 minutes after ketamine administration.

Ideally, a child should return to his or her baseline verbal and motor skills and mental status before ED discharge. However, if the drugs are administered to a young child in the late evening or beyond, this state may not be achieved until the following morning. More practical endpoints are the ability to maintain normal spontaneous respirations and oxygen saturation for a period beyond the peak effect of the drugs and easy arousability. For most agents discussed above, the child will be ready for discharge 45–90 minutes after drug administration.

Green SM, Rothrock SG, Lynch EL, et al: Intramuscular ketamine for pediatric sedation in the emergency department: Safety profile in 1,022 cases. Ann Emerg Med 31:688–697, 1998.

Newman DH, Azer MM, Pitetti RD, Singh S: When is a patient safe for discharge after procedural sedation? The timing of adverse effect events in 1,367 pediatric procedural sedations. Ann Emerg Med 42:627–645, 2003.

26. **What are the top 10 pitfalls in administering sedation and analgesia to children in the ED?**
    1. Undersedation
    2. Oversedation
    3. Using reversal agents to speed recovery

4. Choosing a short-acting narcotic when prolonged pain relief is required
5. Combining two opioids or two sedative agents
6. Choosing a sedative when analgesia is required or vice versa
7. Choosing an improper route of administration
8. Failure to document appropriately
9. Failure to have proper equipment immediately available
10. Not including parents in the discussion about the need for sedation and analgesia

KEY POINTS: REQUIREMENTS FOR SAFE USE OF PSA ✓

1. Focused patient history

2. Careful physical examination

3. Available emergency equipment

4. Knowledge of sedative agents to be used

5. Appropriate staff

6. Careful monitoring

27. **What are the recommended starting doses for sedatives and analgesics commonly used in children?**
See Table 72-1.

TABLE 72-1. RECOMMENDED STARTING DOSE*		
Drug	**Route**	**Dose (mg/kg)**
Midazolam	IV	0.1
Midazolam	IM	0.2
Midazolam	IN	0.4
Midazolam	PO, PR	0.5
Pentobarbital	IM	4
Pentobarbital	IV	2
Chloral hydrate	PO	50–100
Propofol	IV	1–3 load, 25–100 µg/kg/min
Etomidate	IV	0.1–0.2
Ketamine	IV	1–2[†]
Ketamine	IM	4[†]
Morphine	IV	0.1[‡]
Fentanyl	IV	1 µg

IM = intramuscular, IN = intranasal, IV = intravenous, PO = oral, PR = rectal.
*All drugs should be titrated to desired effect.
[†]Premix with atropine or glycopyrolate.
[‡]Lower in neonates.

CHAPTER 73

TRANSPORT MEDICINE

George A. Woodward, MD, MBA

1. **List the goals of interfacility transport.**

   To meet the unique needs of ill and injured infants and children, to meet the needs of the medical community, to allow for regionalization, to provide high-quality care, and to deliver the patient to the receiving center in stable or improved condition.

   Woodward GA, Insoft RM, Pearson-Shaver AL, et al: The state of pediatric interfacility transport: Consensus of the second national pediatric and neonatal interfacility transport medicine leadership conference. Pediatr Emerg Care 18:38–43, 2002.

   Woodward GA, King BR, Garrett AL, Baker MD: Prehospital care and transport medicine. In Fleisher G, Ludwig S, Henretig F (eds): Textbook of Pediatric Emergency Medicine, 5th ed. Phildelphia, Lippincott Williams & Wilkins, 2006, pp 93–134.

2. **What issues should be considered at the time of transport?**
   - Current level of care
   - Stability of the patient
   - Options available to provider and patient
   - Type of care that the patient requires and urgency of need for advanced medical care

3. **List the advantages and disadvantages of the seven methods of ground transport.**

   See Table 73-1.

4. **True or false: When choosing an ambulance service or interfacility transport provider, the receiving hospital is legally responsible for ensuring the adequacy of transport service.**

   False. Under Emergency Medical Treatment and Active Labor Act (EMTALA) regulations, the *referring hospital* and clinicians are responsible for ensuring that the quality of care during transport does not diminish and that an unstable patient is not placed in a less sophisticated environment. The transporting system is responsible for ensuring that the medical care it delivers meets the defined standard of care.

   Woodward GA: Legal issues in pediatric interfacility transport. Clin Pediatr Emerg Med 4:256–264, 2003.

5. **What are the advantages and disadvantages of ambulance transport?**

   The ambulance leaves from a referring facility and travels directly to the receiving facility. It has the ability to stop if problems arise during transport. Team composition changes and additions are easy and safe. Ambulance transport is relatively inexpensive, family member(s) can accompany the patient, backup vehicles are often available, and there are few weather restrictions. Disadvantages include noise, vibration, motion sickness, road conditions, traffic, detours, delays, and accident risk.

6. **Describe the advantages and disadvantages of transport by helicopter.**

   Helicopters offer the advantage of rapid transport (often one-third to one-half of ground transport time to the same location). They have the ability to access difficult locations and avoid traffic. A major disadvantage is the need for a local landing zone or helipad, without which the

TABLE 73-1.	SEVEN METHODS OF GROUND TRANSPORT	
Method	Advantages	Disadvantages
Private vehicle	Immediate	Potential for nondirect transport
		No medical care available
Taxi	Direct transport to hospital	No medical care
Volunteer ambulance	Direct transport to hospital	Minimal medical care
Basic life support (BLS)	Direct transport to hospital	Limited medical care
Advanced life support (ALS)	Direct transport to hospital	Variable pediatric experience
	Emergency resuscitative care	Limited diagnostic and interventional capabilities
	Some interventions available	
Critical care ambulance	Direct transport to hospital	May have limited or no pediatric expertise
	Sophisticated medical care	
Pediatric specialty interfacility transport	Direct transport to hospital Pediatric expertise	Limited resource; may not be immediately available

speed advantage is diminished. Size and space limitations may limit patient assessment or intervention. Altitude physiology, including pressure changes and hypoxia, is important, but may not be a major issue for low-altitude helicopter transport. Other flight issues include stress on equipment, humidity, fatigue, gravitational forces, weight restriction, and emergency survival, as well as increased noise and vibration. Helicopter travel may be limited by weather; many systems are regulated by visual flight rules rather than instrument flight rules. (The capability for instrument flight rules enables safe flight in weather with diminished visibility.) Helicopter transport is expensive.

7. What are the advantages and disadvantages of transport with fixed-wing aircraft?

Fixed-wing (jet, airplane) transport offers the advantage of speed and is appropriate for transports over 100–150 miles. An airplane often can fly over or circumvent bad weather. The cabin can be pressurized to diminish problems with altitude physiology and often offers more room than a helicopter for patient assessment and intervention. A disadvantage is that the airport location may not be convenient to the hospital. Required additional ground or helicopter transport increases the time as well as the risk to the patient.

8. Without parental consent, can a minor be transported?

If a parent or legal guardian is not available for consent, the treating physician may decide and document that the benefits of transport exceed the risks of waiting for parents and may provide emergency consent. Consent would be provided for the treatment and transport for that emergent issue only. Consent from the legal guardians should be sought and obtained as soon as possible.

Woodward GA: Legal issues in pediatric interfacility transport. Clin Pediatr Emerg Med 4:256–264, 2003.

9. **Is it necessary for children to consent for transport?**
The parent/legal guardian is responsible for consent for treatment. Ideally, assent (or agreement) of the process is also obtained from the child but is not mandatory, unless the child is emancipated. Rules for emancipation and age of majority vary by state and should be understood prior to transport.

10. **What are the key elements of a pediatric transport system?**
Adequate preparation for transport involves designing and developing a transport process before it is needed. Educating all levels of providers, appropriate patient care during transport, and reviewing and addressing systems and quality issues during and after transport are imperative. Other key elements include medical supervision and involvement during transport, experienced on-site personnel, cooperation between referring and receiving hospitals and personnel, and adequate quality assurance and improvement.

   American Academy of Pediatrics, Section on Transport Medicine Editor in Chief: George A. Woodward, MD, MBA, FAAP. Guidelines for Air and Ground Transport of Neonatal and Pediatric Patients. 3rd ed. Elk Grove Village, IL: American Academy of Pediatrics; 2006.

11. **In what areas is medical oversight important?**
Medical oversight may be the most important element of the transport system. Knowledgeable physicians must be involved at all levels:
   - **Organizational physicians** design the transport system and evaluate operations.
   - **Referring physicians** should be experts in initial care and stabilization. They should know how and when to refer patients to an appropriate transport service.
   - **Command or supervising physicians** must be immediately available to the transport system for questions or issues that arise during transport.
   - **Receiving physicians** must be aware of the patient's arrival and capable of streamlining the transition to care at the receiving hospital.

12. **What degree or level of education should pediatric transport personnel possess?**
No singular optimal degree or level has been established. The most important qualifications are experience in pediatric critical care or neonatal care and an appropriate skill level, as determined by routine assessment. Personnel must have specific training and experience in the care of critically ill children. They may include physicians, registered nurses, nurse practitioners, paramedics, and respiratory therapists. All who are involved must be familiar with the transport environment and capable of recognizing and stabilizing any problems that arise in that transport population.

13. **What type of skills should be considered imperative for transport personnel?**
The level of skill required for transport personnel depends on the patient population. For a pediatric/neonatal critical care transport service, the personnel must be skilled in managing all routine and emergent pediatric and neonatal issues. Examples include airway stabilization and management with bag/mask ventilation, intubation, rescue airways, surgical airway placement, and ventilatory support. Ability to understand and use critical adjuncts, such as rapid-sequence intubation; expertise in establishing vascular access, including IV and intraosseous routes; understanding of fluid resuscitation; and ability to use pharmacologic adjuncts for cardiovascular support are imperative. Knowledge of infection control and ability to assess patients adequately and effectively at a referral center are also important.

   King BR, Foster RL, Woodward GA, McCans K: Procedures performed by pediatric transport nurses: How "advanced" is the practice? Pediatr Emerg Care 17:410–413, 2001.
   King BR, Woodward GA: Procedural training for pediatric and neonatal transport nurses. Part I: Training methods and airway training. Pediatr Emerg Care 17:461–464, 2001.
   King BR, Woodward GA: Procedural training for pediatric and neonatal transport nurses. Part II: Procedures, skills assessment and retention. Pediatr Emerg Care 18:438–441, 2002.

14. **What factor most increases the risk for transported patients?**

   Whenever the patient is moved from one location to another (e.g., bed to stretcher, incubator), the opportunity for line or tube displacement increases. Movement can cause appropriately immobilized patients to become malpositioned, perhaps decreasing desired protection, impeding respiratory efforts, or even worsening an existing injury. Multiple modes of transport increase movement needs and potentially increase risk to the patient. If a patient deteriorates during or shortly after movement, consider sequelae of the move as a potential cause.

15. **What equipment is important in a critical care ambulance environment?**

   The answer depends on the patient population. Minimal required equipment should include appropriate pediatric interventional supplies, medication, monitors, radios, and phones. Monitoring capability should include pulse oximetry, respiratory rate, blood pressure, temperature, end-tidal carbon dioxide monitors, and electrocardiography. One should strive for point-of-care laboratory testing, which allows rapid analysis of blood gases, chemistries, hemoglobin, and glucose.

   Woodward GA, King BR, Garrett AL, Baker MD: Prehospital care and transport medicine. In Fleisher G, Ludwig S, Henretig F (eds): Textbook of Pediatric Emergency Medicine, 5th ed. Philadelphia, Lippincott Williams & Wilkins, 2006, pp 93–134.

16. **How can referral for transport be streamlined?**

   Development of a specialized communication center with a centralized number is important. The ability to triage incoming calls efficiently to appropriate command physicians or transport personnel is vital. Transfer agreements and up-to-date knowledge of bed availability can markedly decrease time necessary for patient acceptance.

17. **What information should be gathered and documented at the time of patient referral?**

   - Referring physician's name, location (hospital and unit) and phone number
   - Patient data, including name, age, weight, acute medical history, working diagnosis, pertinent past medical history, current vital signs, clinical parameters, and laboratory and radiographic results
   - Brief summary of interventions performed and patient's response
   - Any confounders or projected issues with expected care

KEY POINTS: METHODS OF INCREASING EFFICIENCY OF TRANSPORT ✔

1. Central communication center
2. Centralized phone number
3. Personnel capable of triaging incoming calls
4. Predetermined transfer agreements
5. Current awareness of bed availability

18. **What are the responsibilities of the referring physician during the transport process?**

The referring physician must assess the patient to the best of his or her ability. He or she must ensure that the chosen transport service allows no decrease in the level of care. Plans for stabilization and intervention should be discussed with the receiving hospital or transport service, and, if at all possible, recommendations should be followed. Disagreements about patient stability or inability to perform a task for other reasons should be discussed with the command physician. If the patient's condition changes, the transport service should be notified immediately. The family must consent to the particular type of transport (air, ground) and to the receiving hospital. The agreement should be documented in writing. There should be a written order for transport services. The referring physician and care team should be available for discussion in person or by telephone when the transport service arrives.

In addition, the referring physician must ensure that:

- IV access has been secured.
- All tubes and lines are taped securely to help avoid dislodgment during transport.
- A copy of medical records, radiographs, and laboratory results accompany the patient.
- A medical summary is completed and included with transfer materials.
- Blood products or medications are ordered and available, if their use is considered for the transport.
- The referring physician and care team are available for discussion in person or by telephone when the transport service arrives.

Bolte RG: Responsibilities of the referring physician and referring hospital. In McCloskey K, Orr R (eds): Pediatric Transport Medicine. St. Louis, Mosby, 1995, pp 33–40.

19. **Can a general rather than a pediatric transport service adequately transport children?**

The optimal transport of patients depends on resource availability. If a pediatric critical transport service is available, it potentially offers the highest level of care for pediatric patients. If a pediatric transport service is not available, a general transport service may adequately transport the child. What one gains in availability and efficiency of response, however, may be minimized by an inability to optimally diagnose and intervene for the pediatric patient. General services often do not transport a significant number of critically ill pediatric patients; therefore, their pediatric expertise may be diminished by lack of experience. Referring and receiving physicians should take the opportunity to increase the pediatric expertise of general transport services to ensure adequate care.

20. **How can a transport service develop pediatric expertise?**

Many options are available. One is to visit and emulate the best practices of other services. The American Academy of Pediatrics publishes "Guidelines for Air and Ground Transports of Neonatal and Pediatric Patients" and also provides a course in pediatric education for prehospital professionals. Introduction to pediatric advanced life support is provided by the American Heart Association. The Committee on Accreditation of Medical Transport Systems offers standards and an accreditation process for transport systems. The Internet offers many opportunities for discussion of pediatric transport, including the pediatric interfacility transport e-mail list at PEDTPT-L@Listserv.brown.edu.

American Academy of Pediatrics, Section on Transport Medicine Editor in Chief: George A. Woodward, MD, MBA, FAAP. Guidelines for Air and Ground Transport of Neonatal and Pediatric Patients. 3rd ed. Elk Grove Village, IL: American Academy of Pediatrics; 2006.

21. **What is the appropriate response to inadequate care during transport?**

A review of patient care with care providers and involved facilities is important. This review must be done in a constructive fashion with a plan to increase the level of care for the next patient. Do not be view this as an opportunity to dictate standards of care or to take a position on one side of an issue.

22. **What time factors are involved in patient transport?**
    - Time from presentation of illness or injury to initial care
    - Initial assessment, stabilization, and management
    - Decision to transport
    - Acceptance of patient by the receiving center or transport service
    - Arrival of the transport team
    - Further stabilization at the scene or referring hospital
    - Arrival at the receiving hospital
    - Transition to in-hospital services

23. **What major issue should be considered in selecting a transport service?**
    Determine whether the immediate goal is to transport the patient to an intensive care setting or to bring intensive care capabilities to the patient. The answer may help to determine the type of transport and level of sophistication necessary for the transport personnel and service.

24. **How does EMTALA affect the transport of pediatric patients?**
    EMTALA places clear duties on both referring and receiving hospitals. The referring clinicians must do everything possible to stabilize the patient's medical condition before transport unless the facility cannot provide an adequate level of care. Patient or parent consent for transport must be obtained. EMTALA requires receiving hospitals to accept a patient for transport if space and appropriate level of care are, or can be, available. The patient's ability to pay should not be considered by the referring or receiving hospital. When considering critical care transport for an acute medical or surgical need, discussion with the patient or family about transport should not include financial ramifications of the decision.

    Woodward GA: Legal issues in pediatric interfacility transport. Clin Pediatr Emerg Med 4:256–264, 2003.

25. **What are two major concerns about altitude physiology?**
    - According to **Boyle's law**, an increase in altitude brings a decrease in barometric pressure. Decreased barometric pressure (P) results in an increase in volume (V) of gas (Boyle's law: $P_1V_1 = P_2V_2$). Boyle's law has ramifications for air in enclosed spaces, such as ear canals, endotracheal tube and blood pressure cuffs, mast trousers, intestinal gas, pneumothorax, and pneumocranium. There is approximately a 20% increase in gas volume between sea level and 5000 feet and a 100% increase between sea level and 18,000 feet.
    - **Dalton's law,** or the law of partial pressure ($P_T = P_1 + P_2 + P_3...$), states that the total pressure of a gas is a sum of its components. Although the concentration of oxygen in air is always 21%, air is less dense at higher altitudes; therefore, an increase in altitude results in a decrease in ambient oxygen available to the patient.

    Woodward GA, Vernon DD: Aviation physiology in pediatric transport. In Jaimovich DG, Vidyasagar D (eds): Handbook of Pediatric and Neonatal Transport Medicine, 2nd ed. Philadelphia, Hanley & Belfus, 2002, pp 43–54.

26. **How serious is the concern about problems related to altitude?**
    Most patients do not have problems with air physiology at the relatively low altitudes at which helicopters usually fly or with pressurized fixed-wing transport. However, if the patient has a small, unrecognized air collection, decompression sickness, or diving illness, or if the air transport must traverse significant altitude, associated problems may develop. The decrease in ambient oxygen is usually not a factor because of the availability of supplemental oxygen and positive-pressure delivery. For patients at maximal oxygen and pressure support at sea level, however, an increase in altitude may be of significant concern.

    Woodward GA, Vernon DD: Aviation physiology in pediatric transport. In Jaimovich DG, Vidyasagar D (eds): Handbook of Pediatric and Neonatal Transport Medicine, 2nd ed. Philadelphia, Hanley & Belfus, 2002, pp 43–54.

27. **What is on-line medical command?**

With on-line medical command, an off-site physician or other advanced provider offers medical advice to the on-site team in real time during the transport. Off-line medical support involves the development of protocols or guidelines, without interaction at the immediate time of transport.

28. **What is the value of exposing the pediatric resident to interfacility transport?**

The transport environment provides an opportunity for senior pediatric residents to apply skills developed during the first part of a residency program. Although the patient population and disease processes are similar to those in the hospital, the environment in which care is given is markedly different. Significant preparation is required for optimal participation in the transport process, including development of skills for communicating with transport team personnel and receiving and referring physicians and intimate knowledge of transport vehicles (ambulance or aircraft) and equipment (medications, monitors, interventional equipment). One also must be able to anticipate and respond to issues that do not occur within the hospital, including delays in transport, traffic, mechanical factors, and differences in skill levels and personalities at referring and receiving hospitals.

29. **What training and capabilities are required of a resident physician participant involved in transport?**

Any resident involved in the transport of critically ill children should have the experience of critical care rotations, including pediatric intensive care, emergency and neonatal care, and general pediatric experience. Capabilities for airway, breathing, and circulatory intervention and ability to access more sophisticated knowledge and expertise are imperative. Transport-specific training is also essential for all who care for patients during the process.

Aoki BY, McCloskey K: Evaluation, Stabilization, and Transport of the Critically Ill Child. St. Louis, Mosby, 1992.

30. **What makes transport medicine a high-quality educational experience?**

Pediatric transport medicine allows one to experience the delivery of pediatric care in facilities other than the home institution. Evaluating and participating in care at the referring hospital, as well as communicating directly with referring physicians, other clinicians, and parents of critically ill children, are often enlightening and rewarding growth experiences.

KEY POINTS: CRITICAL CARE TRANSPORT ✓

1. Critical care transport is an integral component of the care continuum for ill and injured pediatric and neonatal patients.

2. It requires specific equipment and training and expertise with pediatric critical care skills.

3. It demands understanding of transport personnel and modes of transport for all who participate in transport, whether as a referring, receiving or on-site care provider.

4. It offers significant educational opportunities for medical trainees.

31. **Should parents accompany a pediatric transport?**

Whenever possible, allow parents to be part of the transport process. Their presence can be invaluable for information and for patient comfort. It is also important to maintain the family support unit as much as possible during these transfers. If, however, parental involvement puts the patient at risk (weight or space limitations of the vehicle; a parent who abusive, is inebriated or belligerent; or a parent who may distract medical attention from the patient during the transport), reconsider their accompaniment.

Woodward GA, Fleegler EW: Should parents accompany pediatric interfacility ground ambulance transports? The parents' perspective. Pediatr Emerg Care 16:383–390, 2000.

Woodward GA, Fleegler EW: Should parents accompany pediatric interfacility ground ambulance transports? Results of a national survey of pediatric transport team managers. Pediatr Emerg Care 17:22–27, 2001.

32. **Identify potential personnel participants for pediatric transport.**
The transport personnel can include physicians, nurses, nurse practitioners, respiratory therapists, and emergency medical services personnel (emergency medical technician–paramedic [EMT-P] or emergency medical technician [EMT])

33. **True or false: Seat belts and restraint devices should be used during transport.**
True. Safety of the transport patient and personnel are paramount. *Unless the patient status dictates that personnel be temporarily mobile,* personnel must be restrained at all times when in a moving transport vehicle. In addition, any objects that might move during a rapid acceleration or deceleration must be secured to help ensure a safe environment. Objects that are in an area where one's head might strike them during an accident must be moved.

King BR, Woodward GA: Pediatric critical care transport—the safety of the journey: A five-year review of vehicular collisions involving pediatric and neonatal transport teams. PreHosp Emerg Care 6:449–454, 2002.

Woodward GA: Legal issues in pediatric interfacility transport. Clin Pediatr Emerg Med 4:256–264, 2003.

34. **List strategies for follow-up to a stressful transport or patient care experience.**
Critical incident stress management helps personnel to understand and cope with stressful events. These preparations and interventions include understanding stressful issues in the transport environment and education regarding coping skills prior to involvement, as well as defusing (discussing) and debriefing (formal incident review) processes after an incident has occurred.

American Academy of Pediatrics, Section on Transport Medicine Editor in Chief: George A. Woodward, MD, MBA, FAAP. Guidelines for Air and Ground Transport of Neonatal and Pediatric Patients. 3rd ed. Elk Grove Village, IL: American Academy of Pediatrics; 2006.

INDEX

Page numbers followed by *t* indicate tables; *f*, figures.

Colorimetric device, 14*f*
Commotio cordis, 533, 542
Compartment syndrome, 476–477
Compensation, 36
Complaints, 605–606, 606*t*
Computed tomography (CT), 47, 52
  abdomen, 383
  in abdominal trauma, 439–440
  in appendicitis, 382–383
  in child abuse, 453
  intracranial injury and, 485
  of retropharyngeal space, 420
  after seizures, 230
  skull fractures and, 483
  in thoracic trauma, 539
Computer Physician Order Entry (CPOE), 598
Concussions, 484, 531–532
  management of, 532*t*
  sports and, 496
Confusional migraine, 55
Congenital adrenal hyperplasia (CAH), 241, 242
Congestive heart failure, 223, 224
Conjugated hyperbilirubinemia, 129–131
  causes of, 131
  diagnostic approach to, 131–132
Conjunctival abrasion, 484
Conjunctivitis. *See also specific types*
  allergic, 161–162
  causes of, 158, 161
  neonatal, 159
Consent, 601
  transport and, 618
Constant infusions, calculating, 18
Contraception, emergency, 265
Corneal abrasion, 77, 405, 484
  management of, 484
  treatment of, 405
Corticosteroids, 315, 337, 361, 364
  delivery methods, 367
  for meningitis, 302
Cough
  antibiotic treatment of, 73
  asthma and, 71–72
  bronchitis and, 72–73
  choking and, 73
  differential diagnosis of, 71*t*
  habitual, 73–74
  medications, 73
  normal, 70
  persistent, 71, 72, 74
  reflex, 70
  strange causes of, 74
  suppression of, 70
CPOE. *See* Computer Physician Order Entry
CPP. *See* Cerebral perfusion pressure
C-reactive protein (CRP), 134, 277, 382
Criminal charges, 600
Crohn's disease, 255

Crotaline, 345
Croup, 180, 365, 366–367
  diagnosis of, 365, 366
  differential diagnosis of, 365
  radiographic findings in, 180–181
  spasmodic, 180
  steroids, 366–367
CRP. *See* C-reactive protein
Crush injuries, 497
Crying, 75
  cardiac etiologies, 78
  conditions associated with, 76*t*
  intractable, 77
  normal amounts of, 75
  screening tests and, 79
Crystalloids, 26
CSF. *See* Cerebrospinal fluid
CT. *See* Computed tomography
Cyanide toxicity, 324, 450
  treatments for, 450
Cyanosis, 341
Cyclic antidepressants, 330
Cystic hygromas, 143
Cystitis, 291, 429
Cytokines, 38

D
Dacryocystitis, 159
Dactylitis, 266–267
Dalton's law, 621
DEET, 544
Defense Against Weapons of Mass Destruction Act, 584–588
Defibrillation, 18
  in resuscitation, 18
Dehydration, 241
  bolus in, 244
  clinical examination in, 243–244
  clinical findings of, 243*t*
  extent of, 243, 244
  fluid rate in, 245
Delivery
  preterm, 20
  unexpected, 20
Dental caries, 377
Dental injuries
  alveolar ridge fracture, 465
  antibiotics in, 468
  avulsion, 467, 468
  chest radiographs in, 468
  consultation and, 468
  describing, 463
  fractures, 464
  frequency of, 462
  intrusion, 466–467
  luxation, 466
  root fractures, 464–465
  tooth concussion, 465

Kernicterus, 128
Kernig's sign, 173
Ketamine, 614
Kidney stone, 118*f*
Kingella kingae, 410
   isolation of, 411
Klippel-Feil syndrome, 175

L
Labial adhesions, 259
Lacerations
   external ear, 503
   eyebrow, 503
   eyelid, 503
   forehead, 503
   lip, 504
   tongue, 504
Lactic acidosis, 335
Language proficiency, 595–596
Laparotomy, 440*t*
Lap-belt complex, 437
Laryngeal mask airway, 11
Laryngomalacia, 181
   diagnosing, 181–182
Laryngotracheal injury, 519
Latent error, 593
Latrodectism, 548
Lead encephalopathy, 339
Lead point, 384
Legg-Calvé-Perthes disease, 135, 136
Lemierre syndrome, 380, 425
Lens dislocation, 405
Leukocyte esterase test, 430
Levalbuterol, 360
Lightning strikes, 559
   30-30 rule in, 561
   cardiopulmonary resuscitation in, 560
   hearing and vision in, 560
   risks of, 560
   rules of triage for, 560
   voltage potential in, 559
Limp
   causes of, 134
   etiology of, 140
   imaging tests in, 136–137
   pain location and, 139–140
   rashes and, 137
Lip lacerations, 504
Little League elbow, 529–530
Little League shoulder, 529
Long QT syndrome, 187, 221
   familial, 221
Lower airway disease, 30
   signs of, 30
Ludwig's angina, 380
Lumbar puncture, 98, 173, 613
   complications of, 173
   contraindications, 173

Lumbar puncture *(Continued)*
   in febrile seizures, 231
   in meningitis, 231
Lund and Browder chart, 445*f*
Luxation injuries, 466
Lyme disease, 155, 305, 306*t*, 550
Lymph nodes, 295, 296
Lymphadenitis, 277, 296
Lymphadenopathy, 295
   regional, 295*t*
Lymphoma, 272

M
Magnesium sulfate, 361
Magnetic resonance imaging (MRI), 53, 409–410
   after seizures, 230
Malaria, 319
Malignancy
   common, 270
   sepsis, 270
Mallet finger deformity, 472, 534*t*
Malpractice suits, 599, 605
   plaintiff rewards in, 600
   reducing, 600
   settlements, 599
Malrotation, 252, 253
Manual detorsion, 163–164
Marfan's syndrome, chest pain and, 67
MAST. *See* Military antishock garment
Mastoiditis, 88–89, 285, 421–422, 423
   coalescent, 422
   complications of, 89, 422
   defining, 421
   pathogens in, 422
   presentation of, 421–422
   treatment of, 89
Mature minor doctrine, 602
MDI. *See* Metered dose inhaler
Measles, 149
Mechanical bowel obstruction, 384
Mechanical ventilation, 362
Meckel's diverticulum, 254, 389
Meconium, 25
Medical antishock trousers, 514
Medical command, 591
   on-line, 622
Medical control
   off-line, 591
   on-line, 591
Medical errors, 593
   common, 595
   concealment of, 596
   disclosure of, 596
   family and, 596–597
   frequency of, 594
   outcomes of, 594–595
   prevention of, 597, 597*t*
   types of, 594